Edited by
László Urbán, Vinod F. Patel, and Roy J. Vaz

Antitargets and Drug Safety

Related Titles

Methods and Principles in Medicinal Chemistry

Edited by R. Mannhold, H. Kubinyi, G. Folkers
Editorial Board
H. Buschmann, H. Timmerman, H. van de Waterbeemd

Previous Volumes of this Series:

Keserü, György M./Swinney, David C. (Eds.)

Kinetics and Thermodynamics of Drug Binding

2015
ISBN: 978-3-527-33582-4
Vol. 65

Pfannkuch, Friedlieb/Suter-Dick, Laura (Eds.)

Predictive Toxicology

From Vision to Reality

2014
ISBN: 978-3-527-33608-1
Vol. 64

Kirchmair, Johannes (Ed.)

Drug Metabolism Prediction

2014
ISBN: 978-3-527-33566-4
Vol. 63

Vela, José Miguel/Maldonado, Rafael/Hamon, Michel (Eds.)

In vivo Models for Drug Discovery

2014
ISBN: 978-3-527-33328-8
Vol. 62

Liras, Spiros/Bell, Andrew S. (Eds.)

Phosphodiesterases and Their Inhibitors

2014
ISBN: 978-3-527-33219-9
Vol. 61

Hanessian, Stephen (Ed.)

Natural Products in Medicinal Chemistry

2014
ISBN: 978-3-527-33218-2
Vol. 60

Lackey, Karen/Roth, Bruce (Eds.)

Medicinal Chemistry Approaches to Personalized Medicine

2013
ISBN: 978-3-527-33394-3
Vol. 59

Brown, Nathan (Ed.)

Scaffold Hopping in Medicinal Chemistry

2013
ISBN: 978-3-527-33364-6
Vol. 58

Hoffmann, Rémy/Gohier, Arnaud/Pospisil, Pavel (Eds.)

Data Mining in Drug Discovery

2013
ISBN: 978-3-527-32984-7
Vol. 57

Dömling, Alexander (Ed.)

Protein-Protein Interactions in Drug Discovery

2013
ISBN: 978-3-527-33107-9
Vol. 56

Kalgutkar, Amit S./Dalvie, Deepak/Obach, R. Scott/Smith, Dennis A.

Reactive Drug Metabolites

2012
ISBN: 978-3-527-33085-0
Vol. 55

Edited by László Urbán, Vinod F. Patel, and Roy J. Vaz

Antitargets and Drug Safety

WILEY-VCH
Verlag GmbH & Co. KGaA

Series Editors

Prof. Dr. Raimund Mannhold
Rosenweg 7
40489 Düsseldorf
Germany
mannhold@uni-duesseldorf.de

Prof. Dr. Hugo Kubinyi
Donnersbergstrasse 9
67256 Weisenheim am Sand
Germany
kubinyi@t-online.de

Prof. Dr. Gerd Folkers
Collegium Helveticum
STW/ETH Zurich
8092 Zurich
Switzerland
gerd.folkers@collegium.ethz.ch

Volume Editors

László Urbán
Novartis Institutes for BioMedical Research Inc.
250 Massachusetts Ave.
Cambridge, MA 02139
USA

Vinod F. Patel
Sanofi US
LGCR-Boston Hub
153 2nd Ave.
Waltham, MA 02451
USA

Roy J. Vaz
Sanofi US
LGCR-Boston Hub
153 2nd Ave.
Waltham, MA 02451
USA

Library of Congress Card No.: applied for

British Library Cataloguing-in-Publication Data
A catalogue record for this book is available from the British Library.

Bibliographic information published by the Deutsche Nationalbibliothek
The Deutsche Nationalbibliothek lists this publication in the Deutsche Nationalbibliografie; detailed bibliographic data are available on the Internet at <http://dnb.d-nb.de>.

Print ISBN: 978-3-527-33511-4
ePDF ISBN: 978-3-527-67367-4
ePub ISBN: 978-3-527-67366-7
Mobi ISBN: 978-3-527-67365-0
oBook ISBN: 978-3-527-67364-3

Cover Design Grafik-Design Schulz, Fußgönheim, Germany
Typesetting Thomson Digital, Noida, India
Printing and Binding Markono Print Media Pte Ltd, Singapore

Printed on acid-free paper

Contents

List of Contributors

Daniel J. Antoine
University of Liverpool
Institute of Translational Medicine
Department of Molecular and
Clinical Pharmacology
MRC Centre for Drug Safety
Science
Liverpool L69 3GE
UK

Richard J. Brennan
Sanofi US
Preclinical Safety
DSAR
153 2nd Ave.
Waltham, MA 02451
USA

Kim L.R. Brouwer
The University of North Carolina
at Chapel Hill
UNC Eshelman School of Pharmacy
Division of Pharmacotherapy and
Experimental Therapeutics
Chapel Hill, NC 27599
USA

José S. Duca
Novartis Institutes for BioMedical
Research
Computer Assisted Drug Discovery
100 Technology Square
Cambridge, MA 02139
USA

Berengere Dumotier
Novartis Institutes for BioMedical
Research
Preclinical Safety/Cardiac
Electrophysiology
Klybeckstrasse 141, WKL.136.178
4057 Basel
Switzerland

Gül Erdemli
Novartis Institutes for BioMedical
Research
Center for Proteomic Chemistry
Ion Channel Group
250 Massachusetts Ave.
Cambridge, MA 02139
USA

Ramy Farid
Schrödinger, Inc.
120 West Forty-Fifth Street, 17th
Floor
New York, NY 10036
USA

Alexander Fekete
Novartis Institutes for BioMedical Research
Preclinical Safety
Preclinical Secondary Pharmacology
250 Massachusetts Avenue
Cambridge, MA 02139
USA

Oliver Flint
Bristol-Myers Squibb
Pharmaceutical Candidate Optimization
Discovery Toxicology
Liberty Drive
Newtown, PA 18940
USA

Gary Gintant
AbbVie
Integrated Science and Technology
Department of Integrative Pharmacology
Abbott Park Road
Abbott Park, IL 60064
USA

Andrea Greiter-Wilke
F. Hoffmann-La Roche Ltd.
Pharmaceuticals/Metabolic DTA
Grenzacherstrasse 124
4070 Basel
Switzerland

Brian Guth
Boehringer Ingelheim Pharma GmbH & Co. KG
General Pharmacology, Drug Discovery Support
Biberach an der Riss
Germany

Robert L. Hamlin
QTest Labs LLC and The Ohio State University
1900 Coffey Road
Columbus, OH 43210
USA

Jacques Hamon
Novartis Institutes for BioMedical Research
Preclinical Safety Profiling
Klybeckstrasse 141
4057 Basel
Switzerland

Andreas Hartmann
Novartis Institutes for BioMedical Research
Preclinical Safety
Klybeckstrasse
4057 Basel
Switzerland

Brett A. Howell
The Hamner Institutes for Health Sciences
The Hamner–UNC Institute for Drug Safety Sciences
Research Triangle Park, NC 27709
USA

Daniel Hoyer
The University of Melbourne
Faculty of Medicine, Dentistry and Health Sciences
School of Medicine
Department of Pharmacology and Therapeutics
Parkville, Victoria 3010
Australia

and

The University of Melbourne
The Florey Institute of
Neuroscience and Mental Health
30 Royal Parade
Parkville, Victoria 3052
Australia

and

The Scripps Research Institute
Department of Chemical Physiology
10550 North Torrey Pines Road
La Jolla, CA 92037
USA

Qi-Ying Hu
Novartis Institutes for BioMedical
Research
Global Discovery Chemistry
100 Technology Square
Cambridge, MA 02139
USA

Haisong Ju
Novartis Institutes for BioMedical
Research Head
Safety Pharmacology-US/Preclinical
Safety
Novartis Pharmaceuticals
Corporation
One Health Plaza
East Hanover, NJ 07936-1080
USA

Michael J. Keiser
University of California, San
Francisco
Department of Pharmaceutical
Chemistry
1700 4th Street
San Francisco, CA 94158
USA

and

University of California, San
Francisco
Department of Bioengineering and
Therapeutic Sciences
1700 4th Street
San Francisco, CA 94158
USA

and

University of California, San
Francisco
Institute for Neurodegenerative
Diseases
675 Nelson Rising Lane
San Francisco, CA 94158
USA

Douglas A. Keller
Sanofi US
Preclinical Safety
DSAR
55 Corporate Dr.
Bridgewater, NJ 08807
USA

Gerd A. Kullak-Ublick
University Hospital Zurich
Department of Clinical
Pharmacology and Toxicology
Raemistrasse 100
8091 Zurich
Switzerland

Pierre Lainée
Sanofi
DSAR
371, RUE DU PROF JOSEPH
BLAYAC
Montpellier 34184
France

Ellen R. Laird
Array BioPharma Inc.
Computational Chemistry
3200 Walnut Street
Boulder, CO 80301
USA

Karen L. Leach
Pfizer
Centers for Therapeutic Innovation
3 Blackfan Circle
Boston, MA 02115
USA

Eugen Lounkine
Novartis Institutes for BioMedical Research
Center for Proteomic Chemistry
In Silico Lead Discovery
250 Massachusetts Avenue
Cambridge, MA 02139
USA

K. Andrew MacCannell
Novartis Institutes for BioMedical Research
100 Technology Square
Cambridge, MA 02139
USA

Mateusz Maciejewski
Novartis Institutes for BioMedical Research
Center for Proteomic Chemistry
Preclinical Safety Profiling
250 Massachusetts Avenue
Cambridge, MA 02139
USA

Frederic Moulin
Bristol-Myers Squibb
Pharmaceutical Candidate Optimization
Discovery Toxicology
Clover Lane
Madison, CT 06443
USA

Lutz Müller
F. Hoffmann-La Roche Ltd.
Pharmaceuticals/Metabolic DTA
Grenzacherstrasse 124
4070 Basel
Switzerland

Patrick Y. Müller
Novartis Pharma
Global Pharma Development Strategy
Fabrikstrasse
4057 Basel
Switzerland

Mark C. Munson
Sanofi US
LGCR-Boston Hub
153 2nd Ave
Waltham, MA, 02451
USA

Eric J. Niesor
F. Hoffmann-La Roche Ltd.
Pharmaceuticals/Metabolic DTA
Grenzacherstrasse 124
4070 Basel
Switzerland

Vinod F. Patel
Sanofi US
LGCR – Boston Hub
153 Second Avenue
Waltham, MA 02451
USA

Robert A. Pearlstein
Novartis Institutes for BioMedical Research
Computer Assisted Drug Discovery
100 Technology Square
Cambridge, MA 02139
USA

Sarita Pereira[†]
Novartis Institutes for BioMedical Research
250 Massachusetts Avenue
Cambridge, MA 02139
USA

Dusty Sarazan
Data Sciences International
119 14th Street NW, Suite 100
St. Paul, MN 55112
USA

John R. Senior
Food and Drug Administration
Center for Drug Evaluation and Research
Office of Surveillance and Epidemiology
Office of Pharmacovigilance and Epidemiology
10903 New Hampshire Avenue
Silver Spring, MD 20993-0002
USA

Lisl K. Shoda
The Hamner Institutes for Health Sciences
The Hamner–UNC Institute for Drug Safety Sciences
Research Triangle Park, NC 27709
USA

Scott Q. Siler
The Hamner Institutes for Health Sciences
The Hamner–UNC Institute for Drug Safety Sciences
Research Triangle Park, NC 27709
USA

Matt Skinner
AstraZeneca R&D
Drug Safety and Metabolism
Alderley Park
Macclesfield SK10 4TG
UK

Bruno Stieger
University Hospital Zurich
Department of Clinical Pharmacology and Toxicology
Raemistrasse 100
8091 Zurich
Switzerland

Martin Traebert
Novartis Institutes for BioMedical Research
Preclinical Safety/Cardiac Electrophysiology
Klybeckstrasse 141, WKL.136.178
4057 Basel
Switzerland

Christian Trendelenburg
Novartis Institutes for BioMedical Research
Preclinical Safety
Klybeckstrasse 141,
4057 Basel
Switzerland

[†]Deceased

László Urbán
Novartis Institutes for BioMedical Research
Preclinical Safety
Preclinical Secondary Pharmacology
250 Massachusetts Avenue
Cambridge, MA 02139
USA

Jean-Pierre Valentin
UCB Biopharma
Investigative Toxicology, Non-Clinical Development
1420 Braine-l'Alleud
Belgium

Roy J. Vaz
Sanofi US
LGCR – Boston Hub
153 Second Avenue
Waltham, MA 02451
USA

Paul B. Watkins
The Hamner Institutes for Health Sciences
The Hamner–UNC Institute for Drug Safety Sciences
Research Triangle Park, NC 27709
USA

and

The University of North Carolina at Chapel Hill
UNC Eshelman School of Pharmacy
Division of Pharmacotherapy and Experimental Therapeutics
Chapel Hill, NC 27599
USA

Steven Whitebread
Novartis Institutes for BioMedical Research
Preclinical Safety
Preclinical secondary Pharmacology
250 Massachusetts Avenue
Cambridge, MA 02139
USA

Jeffrey L. Woodhead
The Hamner Institutes for Health Sciences
The Hamner–UNC Institute for Drug Safety Sciences
Research Triangle Park, NC 27709
USA

Kyunghee Yang
The Hamner Institutes for Health Sciences
The Hamner–UNC Institute for Drug Safety Sciences
Research Triangle Park, NC 27709
USA

Yuching Yang
The Hamner Institutes for Health Sciences
The Hamner–UNC Institute for Drug Safety Sciences
Research Triangle Park, NC 27709
USA

Preface

In drug discovery, target definition and validation are the first steps, followed by the search for biologically active hits. This can be performed by "wet" screening, optimally by high-throughput techniques, or by virtual screening of large compound libraries or even much larger virtual libraries of chemical structures. Nowadays, one- or two-digit micromolar hits result in most cases and in very short time. After a search for similar compounds that might also be active, medicinal chemists start to optimize their activities against the target under consideration. Nowadays chemists are aware of the problems of "fatty" and large compounds, resulting in poor bioavailability. But a mostly unsolved problem is the optimization with respect to undesired side effects. To understand and tackle these problems, Roy Vaz and Thomas Klabunde edited 7 years ago the book "Antitargets: Prediction and Prevention of Drug Side Effects," volume 38 of our series "Methods and Principles in Medicinal Chemistry," in which they discussed the most important targets that might generate undesired or even fatal side effects. Now it is time to discuss some more relevant antitargets and to add recently accumulated knowledge on such targets that were already presented in the earlier volume.

We are very grateful to the editors László Urbán, Vinod F. Patel, and Roy J. Vaz, and all chapter authors for their effort to review all relevant aspects and latest developments in the field of antitarget research. Last but not least, we thank the publisher Wiley-VCH, especially Heike Nöthe, Waltraud Wüst, and Frank Weinreich, for their ongoing support of our series "Methods and Principles in Medicinal Chemistry."

Düsseldorf — *Raimund Mannhold*
Weisenheim am Sand — *Hugo Kubinyi*
Zürich — *Gerd Folkers*
February 2015

A Personal Foreword

The concept represented by the book *Antitargets* [1] was revolutionary when it was published in 2008 with the clear intention to alert the pharmaceutical industry and the medical community to the fact that some therapeutic or unintended off-target activities could translate into serious side effects also known as adverse drug reactions (ADRs). The important message was that one needs to consider all biological effects of a drug or drug candidate, link the adverse drug reactions to molecular targets, and then devise a plan to de-risk these properties in the drug optimization phase. To a great extent, knowledge concerning ADRs has emerged from clinical side effects that were not intended when drugs were initially marketed. One of the first drugs was terfenadine (Seldane) that was withdrawn from use due to sudden deaths caused by torsades de pointes [2]. This drug in the presence of other drugs, such as ketoconazole, prolonged the cardiac QT interval due to unintended modulation of (anti-)targets, including hERG, CYP3A4/5, and P-glycoprotein, among others. The development of *in vitro* assays for these antitargets rapidly followed, and these assays were introduced into the process of drug discovery. The first book, *Antitargets*, tried to provide information on the regulatory and human clinical viewpoints, preclinical biology, pharmacology, and medicinal chemistry (structure–activity relationships (SARs)) of these antitargets. In addition, examples were included to demonstrate derisking of these antitarget activities resulting in a cleaner antitarget profile of new clinical candidates. During the writing of the first book, other antitargets emerged and were included, for example, the unexpected cardiac toxicity with 5-HT_{2B} agonism on the use of the anorexigen, fenfluramine.

Black box warnings, failures in drug trials, and drug withdrawals have always been, and continue to be, part of the drug discovery and development and marketed use of drugs. Thus, a new book on antitargets has warranted to continue to capture antitarget information and knowledge not discussed previously and capture broader coverage of related, emerging topics. It is on this basis that sections in this book were assembled. Systems pharmacology, a newer field, has gained prominence and chapters dedicated to the utility in deciphering and modeling antitargets have been included in this book (see Chapters 2 and Chapter 9).

The first section deals with novel technologies and includes description of the utility of adverse event reports to drug discovery, the translational aspects of preclinical safety findings, broader computational prediction of drug side effects, and a description of the serotonergic system – GPCRs, enzymes, and a transporter.

The importance of hepatotoxicity in drug safety warranted several chapters solely on this subject matter. Chapter 5 starts with a view of hepatotoxicity from a clinician's perspective. Chapter 6 includes a review of the most promising predictive biomarkers for hepatotoxicity. A description of the *in vitro* systems – both assays and their readouts utilized in the early phases of drug discovery – follows in Chapter 7. The role of transporters in the liver, from a pragmatic perspective, provides a deeper understanding of how drugs and their metabolites are distributed throughout the liver. As a case example (http://www.medicinenet.com/bosentan-oral/article.htm), the recent drug labeling of bosentan, resulting from the inhibition of the bile secretion export pump (BSEP) and its consequent drug-induced liver injury (DILI), is described. Finally, description of DILIsym®, an *in silico* approach combining known mechanisms in a mathematical framework and its application to two drugs, troglitazone and bosentan, is included.

Then follows a collection of chapters on cardiac safety and ion channels, an ever-interesting topic in toxicology. It begins with a review of inotropy and functional safety of the heart followed by updated understandings of three well-known antitarget cardiac ion channels that are important in the action potential generation in a cardiomyocyte, namely, $Na_v1.5$, $Ca_v1.2$, and hERG. There is an analysis of a systems pharmacology model and the latest update on hERG channel mechanisms. Also included is a chapter describing common circulating biomarkers for human subjects and preclinical species as a more sensitive method for early safety signals.

The kinase class of antitargets was not discussed in the first book and due to the numerous entries of kinase inhibitors into clinical trials a wealth of human safety data has accumulated on clinical adverse events (AEs) associated [3] with kinase inhibition. This, together with a lack of previous efforts to discuss important side effect profiles of this class of drugs, leads us to dedicate a section to kinase antitargets and their inhibitors. Chapter 15 reviews the known side effects of approved kinase inhibitors, including preclinical and clinical observations. The pharmacological and systems biology approach to understanding and predicting adverse on-mechanism effects is now being systematically applied to each of the targets, which is described in the second chapter. A chapter on cardiotoxicity and protection, specifically related to kinases and their inhibitors, is included. Application of drug discovery tools (structural biology, medicinal chemistry, and *in vitro* biological assays) to design safer kinase therapeutics is exemplified in the case study.

Some time ago [4], work on the anti-atherosclerotic compound torcetrapib by Pfizer was terminated, due to an increase in blood pressure. This event caused many other research efforts to pause and re-evaluate the development of drugs toward the target, cholesterylester transfer protein (CETP). As in all these types of cases, the question of on-mechanism versus off-mechanism arises. An example of Roche's efforts and how the question was addressed and the outcome are included in this section.

The final chapter of the book is dedicated to those compounds that inadvertently elicit CNS-mediated adverse events and lead to relabeling or withdrawal from the market. A pragmatic description of ways to mitigate these types of safety risks is provided in the last chapter.

Our deep thanks go to our contributing authors for making this book possible through their hard work, dedication, and enthusiasm.

Cambridge, MA
Acton, MA
Bridgewater, NJ
February 2015

László Urbán
Vinod F. Patel
Roy J. Vaz

References

1 Vaz, R.J. and Klabunde, R. (eds) (2008) *Antitargets*, Wiley-VCH Verlag GmbH, Weinheim.

2 Estelle, F. and Simons, R. (1999) H1-receptor antagonists: safety issues. *Annals of Allergy, Asthma, and Immunology*, **83** (5), 481–488.

3 Yang, X., Huang, Y., Crowson, M., Li, J., Maitland, M.L., and Lussier, Y.A. (2010) Kinase inhibition-related adverse events predicted from *in vitro* kinome and clinical trial data. *Journal of Biomedical Informatics*, **43** (3), 376–384.

4 Barter, P.J., Caulfield, M., Erikson, M., Grundy, S.M., Kastelein, J.J.P., Komajda, M., Lopez-Sendon, J., Mosca, L., Tardif, J.C., Waters, D.D., Shear, C.L., Revkin, J.H., Buhr, K.A., Fisher, M.R., Tall, A.R., and Brewer, B. (2007) Effects of torcetrapib in patients at high risk for coronary events. *The New England Journal of Medicine*, **357** (11), 2109–2122.

Section 1
General Concept for Target-based Safety Assessment

Antitargets and Drug Safety, First Edition. Edited by László Urbán, Vinod F. Patel, and Roy J. Vaz.

1
Side Effects of Marketed Drugs: The Utility and Pitfalls of Pharmacovigilance

Steven Whitebread, Mateusz Maciejewski, Alexander Fekete, Eugen Lounkine, and László Urbán

1.1
Introduction

Drug discovery projects can learn a lot from existing drugs, for instance, how well they perform in a particular indication and patient population, but also which side effects they cause. While efficacies for a particular indication may be quite similar between compounds, their side effect profiles may vary considerably. Many diseases are managed by drugs acting at various targets and diverse chemical structures might be available for the same target. Incidence of adverse drug reactions (ADRs) could vary for drugs acting at the same target due to different off-target profiles and different levels of required exposure of parent and metabolites. These are strongly dependent on the pharmacological interaction with the target (e.g., potency and binding kinetics [1]) and availability in different organs (e.g., blood–brain barrier penetration and high concentrations in the gastrointestinal system or liver).

One can differentiate between ADRs associated with on- and off-targets and we recognize that on-target-related side effects could also vary by exposure in a particular organ (e.g., presence or absence of brain access of H1 antihistamines [2]) or the mode of interaction with the therapeutic target (e.g., inhibition, full or partial agonism, and allosteric modulation [3]). One can learn a considerable lesson from on-target-related side effects and apply this knowledge when the same target emerges as an off-target with a different drug in a different indication [4]. In this respect, monoclonal antibodies (mAbs) can provide excellent opportunities for the study of on-target ADRs due to their high target specificity. mAbs for various kinase targets in oncology indications highlighted pathways that were involved in various physiological functions in addition to pathways associated with cancer [5].

To unequivocally identify off-targets for clinical ADRs is not an easy matter. Common symptoms such as headache, chest pain, or cough could

Antitargets and Drug Safety, First Edition. Edited by László Urbán, Vinod F. Patel, and Roy J. Vaz.

be associated with several targets or not associated with any, just developing as concomitant symptoms during treatment with a drug. However, when the same side effect is observed with drugs for different indications or with diverse structural features, a common off-target can be suspected. These clinical observations do not always manifest during clinical trials, either because their incidence is low and linked to a particular patient subpopulation [6] or because the development of the side effect takes a long period of time [7]. Until recently, there was little knowledge of the underlying mechanisms of most ADRs, and they were often denoted as "idiosyncratic" adverse reactions. The vast majority of hepatic and cardiac side effects fall into this nebulous category. Recent increase in off-target and pathway profiling has opened the door to the understanding of many side effects [8–10]. The concept is very simple: drugs or any new molecular entity (NME) can be tested in assays representing targets that are closely associated with clinical side effects [8]. This method was applied to marketed drugs and environmental chemicals/toxins in various formats and recently applied to over 8000 compounds in the frame of a federal collaboration called "Toxicity Testing in the 21st Century" (Tox21), comprised of EPA, the National Institute of Environmental Health Sciences/National Toxicology Program, National Center for Advancing Translational Sciences, and the Food and Drug Administration. Data from this orchestrated effort is being released to the public as the collection of ToxCast.[1)]

In vitro safety pharmacology profiling has opened the door to the identification of target–ADR pairs by common target–side effect linkage to different drugs, based on the principle described above. The data obtained from these studies revealed unknown off-targets and, in a significant number of drugs, pharmacological promiscuity. Importantly, it helped to develop *in silico* models [11] that extended the scope of ADR prediction during drug discovery beyond the capabilities of *in vitro* profiling. The integration of the experimental and *in silico* approaches flourish within the concept of the reductionist chemistry approach to drug discovery [12]. The new, large-scale capability of predictive safety profiling demands uniform ontology, which could be used broadly with clarity for various models and supports translation of preclinical findings into clinical ADRs. Today, the MedDRA (Medical Dictionary for Regulatory Activities) terms are broadly used for ADR annotation of targets and conveniently link their function to system organ classes with the benefit of clinical interpretation. Table 1.1 demonstrates this concept on a selected set of CNS targets, highlighting the diverse effects of agonists and antagonists. In this chapter, we will apply the above-described approach to marketed drugs to demonstrate its powerful translational capabilities, including applications for drug design, competitive intelligence, and possible drug repositioning.

1) ToxCast, http://epa.gov/ncct/toxcast/data.html.

Table 1.1 Selected CNS receptors potentially involved in psychoactive effects.

CNS receptor	Associated neurological/psychoactive effects (selection)	
	Agonism	**Antagonism**
5-HT_{1A}	Nervousness, agitation, miosis, hypothermia, cardiovascular regulation (hypotension and bradycardia)	May contribute to depression and suicidal ideation
5-HT_{2A}	Behavioral effects, smooth muscle contraction, hallucination	No relevant CNS side effects known
5-HT_7	May alter circadian rhythm, psychiatric disorders/schizophrenia might be a concern	No relevant CNS side effects known
CB1	Alteration of cognition and memory, sleep disturbance, drowsiness, sedation, locomotor dysfunction, bronchodilation, cardiovascular regulation (hypotension and bradycardia)	Emesis, depression, suicidal tendencies; the inverse agonist rimonabant may cause suicidal ideation
D_1	May induce dyskinesia, extreme arousal, flushing, nausea, vomiting, dizziness, locomotor activation	Tremor; depression, anxiety, and suicidal intent were observed with D_1 and D_5 antagonists; hypertension
D_{2L}	Drowsiness, dizziness, and nausea especially with the first dose and some psychosis may occur after long-term treatment; vasodilatation, ↓ heart rate; ↓ pituitary hormone secretions (e.g., prolactin)	Tardive dyskinesia (impairment of voluntary movement), akathisia (an inability to sit still or remain motionless), and other extrapyramidal effects (Parkinson-like syndrome)
D_3	Cognitive and emotional functions, psychosis, neurodegeneration, coordination, substance abuse, sedation, schizophrenia; it may induce hair loss (see pramipexole)	Dyskinesia (impairment of voluntary movement), akathisia (an inability to sit still or remain motionless), and other extrapyramidal effects (Parkinson-like syndrome)
D_5	No relevant CNS side effects known	Suicidal intent (observed with D_1 and D_5 antagonists)
GABA-A	Major receptor involved in inhibitory neurotransmission: psychological, neurological, sensory functions, sedation, movement disturbances, hallucinations, and potentially leading to tolerance	Mimics the symptoms of epilepsy, potential anxiogenics, and proconvulsants
GABA-A benzodiazepine	Somnolence, suppression of REM sleep or dreaming, impaired motor function, impaired coordination, impaired balance, dizziness, depression, anterograde amnesia (especially pronounced in higher doses), withdrawal and abuse risks	May cause seizures (strong black box warning)

(continued)

Table 1.1 (*Continued*)

CNS receptor	Associated neurological/psychoactive effects (selection)	
	Agonism	**Antagonism**
NMDA	Glycine site: may reduce negative and improve cognitive function in schizophrenics, cause seizures, neurotoxicity	PCP site: anesthetic properties, may induce psychosis (schizophrenia-like), hallucination, delirium and disoriented behavior, may cause seizures, neurotoxicity, ligands of the PCP receptor induce symptoms in humans that are virtually indistinguishable from schizophrenia; polyamine site: polyamine system is linked to suicidal ideation
OpD	Analgesia, sedation, physical dependence, emotional behavior, decrease of GI motility	No relevant CNS side effects known
OpK	Analgesia, sedation, hypotension, tachycardia, diuresis, dysphoria, dizziness, paresthesia and antipruritic effects (TRK-820), interaction with dopaminergic transmission, hallucination; full or partial agonists produce psychotomimetic effects, in the case of the mixed (partial) agonist/antagonist analgesic drugs (e.g., butorphanol, nalbuphine, pentazocine) the psychotomimesis is undesirable and serves to limit abuse potential	Selective kappa opioid antagonists explored for their effects in the treatment of a wide variety of areas including cocaine addiction, depression, and feeding behavior, and have been proposed as a treatment for psychosis and schizophrenia
OpM	Analgesia, sedation, physical dependence, bowel dysfunction, constipation, respiratory depression, modulation of cough reflex, development of tolerance and addiction risks	Selective peripheral antagonists are used to treat postoperative ileus and to reverse the effects of opioid agonists (e.g., naloxone, naltrexone, and nalmefene), may cause diarrhea

Adapted from Ref. [8].
CB1: cannabinoid 1; $D_{1,2L,3,5}$: dopamine 1, 2 (long form), 3, 5; GABA-A: gamma-aminobutyric acid A; NMDA: *N*-methyl aspartate; OpD, -K, -M: opioid delta, kappa, mu; PCP: phencyclidine; $5\text{-}HT_{1A,2A,7}$: serotonin 1A, 2A, 7.

1.2 Postmarketing Pharmacovigilance

ADRs (or their absence) are major contributors to the well-being of patients, compliance, and medical expenses [13–16]. They are mostly discovered during clinical trials; however, the full scope and impact of ADRs can be determined only by postmarketing monitoring and surveillance (e.g., FDA Adverse Event Reporting System (FAERS) [17]). FAERS is a public database containing reports on adverse drug reactions and medication errors submitted to the FDA. It is designed to align with the international safety reporting guidance issued by the International Conference on Harmonization (ICH) E2B(R3). The database contains over 4.6 million entries and is updated on a quarterly basis. The database provides ADRs associated with a particular drug with rich patient information, including age, gender, reason for hospitalization/doctor's visit, medication, and outcome. Although it gives information on the dosage, it lacks pharmacokinetic (PK) data; thus, determination of exposure and, more importantly, therapeutic index in a particular case is not possible. This is rectified by complex searchable databases such as the FDA, API, and Thomson-Reuters' Integrity or PharmaPendium,[2)] an online information repository that reviews drug safety issues by providing access to integrated preclinical, clinical, and postmarketing adverse effects together with PK data. Figure 1.1b is a screenshot from the FAERS profile of panitumumab (Vectibix) in PharmaPendium. The reported side effects are listed by preclinical and postmarketing appearance. As Vectibix affects a single protein kinase target, epidermal growth factor receptor (EGFR, HER1), it is presumed that all observed side effects are associated with this single target [18]. As expected, EGFR inhibitors would affect epidermal integrity and health (see Chapter 15); therefore, it is not surprising that panitumumab carries a box warning[3)] for severe dermatitis, clearly recorded by FAERS. The association of skin lesions with EGFR inhibition is further confirmed with all marketed small-molecule EGFR inhibitors (Figure 1.1a). Armed with this information, one can deselect small-molecule kinase inhibitors that carry EGFR as an off-target. Thus, this approach (termed reverse translation) is used to identify target–ADR associations and it is applied to the drug discovery process for early mitigation of off-target effects that would be a safety risk in the clinic [19].

As kinase inhibitors are relatively new in the clinic, their side effect profiles are relatively less well known. Pharmacovigilance is therefore of major importance to determine their ADR profiles and drug labeling (Table 1.2). The clinical introduction of monoclonal antibodies for kinase targets made it possible to link ADRs with well-defined therapeutic targets as these antibodies provide selectivity, which is a rare feature of small-molecule kinase inhibitors.

While FAERS is by far not perfect, it can provide a rich source of postmarketing information and supports identification of ADRs undetected during clinical trials. PharmaPendium[2)] gives access to the FAERS database and

2) http://thomsonreuters.com/integrity/; http://www.elsevier.com/online-tools/promo-page/pharmapendium/pbt_pp_adwordsgeneric_jan2014/home.
3) Vectibix, www.vectibix.com/.

(a)

ErbB1 (EGFR, HER1)

▸ Viewing by area affected
• View by name

	Preclinical Data view all 574	Clinical Data view all 3541	Post-Marketing Reports (AERS) view all 31788
⊞ Blood and lymphatic system disorders	24	139	3720
⊞ Cardiac disorders	4	118	2270
⊞ Skin and subcutaneous tissue disorders	60	609	7557
⊞ Vascular disorders	3	91	2765

(b)

Panitumumab

Adverse Effects / Toxicity :

▸ Viewing by area affected
• View by name

	Preclinical Data view all 112	Clinical Data view all 867	Post-Marketing Reports (AERS) view all 5252
⊞ Blood and lymphatic system disorders	1	14	809
⊞ Cardiac disorders	1	13	283
⊞ Congenital, familial and genetic disorders	1	no data	18
⊞ Ear and labyrinth disorders	no data	1	15
⊞ Endocrine disorders	1	no data	4
⊞ Eye disorders	3	47	168
⊞ Gastrointestinal disorders	6	132	1700
⊞ General disorders and administration site conditions	5	96	1357
⊞ Hepatobiliary disorders	1	12	158
⊞ Immune system disorders	no data	24	102
⊞ Infections and infestations	2	62	1255
⊞ Investigations	36	41	715
⊞ Metabolism and nutrition disorders	15	93	1111
⊞ Musculoskeletal and connective tissue disorders	no data	11	198
⊞ Neoplasms benign, malignant and unspecified (incl cysts and polyps)	1	3	530
⊞ Nervous system disorders	3	21	508
⊞ Pregnancy, puerperium and perinatal conditions	5	no data	no data
⊞ Psychiatric disorders	1	8	113
⊞ Renal and urinary disorders	1	4	284
⊞ Reproductive system and breast disorders	6	no data	28
⊞ Respiratory, thoracic and mediastinal disorders	1	69	963
⊞ Skin and subcutaneous tissue disorders	22	191	1515
⊞ Vascular disorders	no data	25	453

Figure 1.1 FAERS representation of side effects of epidermal growth factor receptor (EGFR, HER1, ErbB1) inhibitors. (a) Enhanced skin and subcutaneous ADR representation of marketed EGFR inhibitors (cetuximab, lapatinib ditosylate, and panitumumab) (not all ADRs shown). (b) FAERS profile of panitumumab (Vectibix) represents the typical high occurrence of skin and GI lesions associated with the inhibition of the therapeutic target. (Courtesy of PharmaPendium.)

allows the search for PK information that is essential to determine the therapeutic index for drugs [20]. The most reliable source of information on ADRs is obtained from drug labels, and the FDA ensures they are updated regularly.

Table 1.2 Kinases involved in cardiovascular risks: clinical evidence based on monoclonal antibody treatment.

Kinase target	Human safety (information based on FDA label)	Animal toxicity	Animal genetics – KO (OMIM)
ErbB2 (HER2)	Trastuzumab: black box for cardiomyopathy (supported by multi-KI lapatinib: warning for decrease in LVEF)	Trastuzumab: no cardiac toxicity in mice/monkeys; no TCR in adult monkey and human cardiac myocytes	Severe dilated cardiomyopathy, decreased contractility
EGFR (HER1)	Cetuximab: black box for cardiopulmonary arrest and/or sudden death (multi-KI erlotinib: warning for myocardial infarction/ischemia)	Cetuximab: no cardiac toxicity in mice/monkeys EKB-569 and AG-1478: significant changes in left ventricular wall thickness and cardiac function	Aortic valve disease and aortic stenosis
VEGFR2 (KDR)	Bevacizumab (anti-VEGF-A): warning for arterial thromboembolic events (ATEs) and hypertension (supported by multi-KI sunitinib: warning for cardiac toxicity/decrease in LVEF; supported by multi-KI sorafenib: warning for cardiac ischemia/infarction and hypertension)	Bevacizumab: no cardiac toxicity seen preclinically	Lack of VEGF(R)-deficient mouse models due to lethality
PDGFRa	Possibility for contributory factor for cardiac ADRs associated with certain KIs (current label data for dasatinib, sunitinib, and sorafenib); PDGFRs are expressed in cardiomyocytes	Depending on kinase spectrum	

Note that preclinical safety pharmacology evaluation did not signal cardiac toxicity; however, genetic evidence supported the observed side effects.

1.3 Polypharmacy and Pharmacological Promiscuity of Marketed Drugs

Marketed drugs are optimized molecules with two major requirements to be fulfilled: therapeutic efficacy and acceptable safety window at the prescribed dose [20]. Drug design can focus on a single molecular target or on a pathway with a defined phenotypic readout of the therapeutic effect. Most drugs belong to the first group, even when a combination of targets might be preferable for a therapeutic effect (e.g., for congestive heart failure). Remarkably "clean" compound profiles could be found with antihypertensive, cholesterol-lowering drugs, bisphosphonates, and several other groups of medicines (see Table 1.3 for antihypertensive drugs). In general, drugs for broad applications for non-life-threatening diseases should have a clean sheet of off-targets, particularly as they

Table 1.3 Lack of pharmacological promiscuity of antihypertensive drugs.

Drug	Off-targets found
Adrenergic receptor antagonists	
Alpha blockers	
Bunazosin	hERG
Prazosin	μ-Opioid
Terazosin	μ-Opioid
Beta blockers	
Atenolol	—
Propranolol	5-HT receptor family
Ca channel blockers	
Dihydropyridines	
Nifedipine	Adenosine receptors
Nitrendipine	PXR
ACE inhibitors	
Captopril	H1
Enalapril	—
Cilazapril	—
Angiotensin II receptor antagonists	
Candesartan	—
Losartan	PDE3
Irbesartan	PDE3

are often used in conjunction with other drugs for a different disease in the same patient population. According to the Center for Disease Control (CDC) statistics, about 37% of the over 60-year-old population use more than five prescription drugs [21]. Considering drug–drug interactions, possible cumulative effects of on- and off-targets, the most commonly used drugs in this patient population such as the above-mentioned cholesterol-lowering and antihypertensive drugs should be as safe as possible. As an example, patients who are taking a particular drug for hypertension might also need medication for psychiatric indications, such as depression. Many of the psychotropic agents have effects at adrenergic receptors that will have an additional effect on blood pressure [22] and might cause orthostatic hypotension, a serious issue in the elderly [23,24].

When exploring marketed databases, two classes of drugs, cancer treatments and antipsychotics, generally have a trend to be more promiscuous [25,26]. At present, the majority of small-molecule cancer drugs aim for inhibition of the highly conserved ATP binding site in the kinase family. Thus, binding to this site is likely to produce drugs with low selectivity between kinase targets and occasionally to non-kinase targets as well (see Figure 1.2).

Kinase inhibitors are new to clinical practice; thus, pharmacovigilance is of major importance to determine their long-term side effect profiles and provide information for correct drug labeling. As mentioned earlier, mAbs, but also the more specific allosteric kinase inhibitors, can give the best characterization of ADRs associated with a specific kinase target (as an example, Table 1.2 shows

	hERG	Ad1	Ad2A	Ad3	Alpha1A	Alpha2A	Alpha2B	Alpha2C	Beta1	Beta2	AT1	B2	CCKa	CCKb	D1	D2	D3
Vandetanib	<1	10	10	10			<1	1	10		10	10	10	10		10	10
Bosutinib	2	10	10	10		6	10	1	10	10	10	10	10	10	10	<1	6
Crizotinib	<1	10	10	9	<1		10	1	10	10	10		10	10	10	10	10
Sunitinib	<1	6	5	8	<1	9	5	2	6	8	4	3	7	10	5	1	2

	D4.4	ETa	GHS	H1	H2	H3	5HT1A	5HT2A	5HT2B	5HT2C	M1	M2	M3	MC3	Motilin	Y1	OpD	OpM	TP
Vandetanib		10	10	<1		2				10	10		10	10	10	10	10		
Bosutinib	10	10	4	10	2	<1	10	2		7	10	6		10	10	10	10		10
Crizotinib		10	14	10	4	10	10	2	<1	10	10	10	10	10	10	8	10	10	10
Sunitinib	<1	8	7	3		<1	7	<1	<1	2	2	7	2	8	7	7	2	5	9

	V1a	V2	AdT	DAT	NET	5HTT	BZD	Nic(ns)	NMDA	5HT3	AR_ago	PR_ago	PXR_ago	COX_1	COX_2	MAO_A	PDE3	PDE4D
Vandetanib	10	10	10	10	10	3	10	10	10	10	10	10	10	10	10	10	10	10
Bosutinib	5	10	10	9	10	10	10	10	10	10				10	10		10	10
Crizotinib	10	10	10	8	8	10	10	10		10	10	10	7	9	10	10	10	5
Sunitinib	10	5	5	3	2	<1	10	7	10	3	6	2		10	10	10	10	10

Figure 1.2 Non-kinase target-related promiscuity of selected kinase inhibitors vandetanib, bosutinib, crizotinib, and sunitinib. The non-kinase-related pharmacological promiscuity of the kinase inhibitors varies broadly and does not reflect on their kinase selectivity. Note that sunitinib (Sutent) is an extremely promiscuous kinase inhibitor. Red: $IC_{50} < 1\ \mu M$; yellow: $IC_{50} = 1–10\ \mu M$; green: $IC_{50} \geq 10\ \mu M$.

the drug labels of some mAb kinase inhibitors). A new generation of kinase inhibitors offers less promiscuity as they do not target the ATP binding pocket, but aim for allosteric modulator sites, for example, Akt inhibitors [27].

The other particularly promiscuous group of drugs is the family of antipsychotics [28]. We took several of the most commonly used antidepressants and annotated their on- and off-target hits (Figure 1.3). Adenosine, adrenergic, dopamine, histamine, serotonergic, muscarinic receptors, and neurotransmitter transporters DAT, NET, and SERT are those targets that are often encountered with these drugs. While it is considered that a combination of targets could be responsible for the antidepressant therapeutic effects, it is obvious that they could also exhibit psychiatric ADRs. For example, all SSRIs are labeled for suicidal intent and behavior in pediatric use [29] (see Chapter 20).

Specific off-target effects within a particular indication may strongly depend on the similarity between chemical structures of drugs associated with different therapeutic targets. As an example, we examined antihypertensive adrenergic receptor blockers, Ca channel blockers, angiotensin inhibitors, and ACE inhibitors (Table 1.3). Most of these drugs show high specificity of binding to the therapeutic target with the angiotensin II receptor blockers showing particularly good selectivity. None of these compounds carry any serious safety-related warnings. We investigated the side effect profile of the angiotensin receptor antagonist FAERS profiles and will use this example to highlight some shortcomings of the adverse reaction reporting systems. While the most common reported effects of angiotensin receptor inhibition include hypotension, dry mouth, excessive thirst, dizziness, and slow or irregular heartbeat, there are no major ADRs that would warrant warnings. However, the compiled ADR profile of these drugs (Figure 1.4) shows a large number of entries with particular emphasis on cardiovascular events. Over 16% of the entries are concerned with cardiac side effects, 18% of the reports are associated with vascular disorders, almost half of the "investigations" reported are related to cardiac and vascular effects, and finally 29% of nervous system disorders are CNS vascular events. This list of major ADRs suggests that this group of drugs or their metabolites seriously affect the cardiovascular system and generate safety issues. However, none of the drugs or their metabolites is promiscuous, and considering the major indications for these drugs (hypertension and congestive heart failure), we can attribute the above-mentioned cardiovascular events as symptoms of the treated diseases themselves, and with the exception of orthostatic hypotension and its consequences, others are not real ADRs. Thus, reports on adverse drug reactions are often biased by the disease the treatment is applied to and carry over many of the original symptoms. While this is a lesser issue during clinical trials, once released onto the market drugs lack the controlled environment of clinical trials; thus, the confidence in the reported ADRs is significantly diminished. This seems to be a general issue with the postmarketing reporting systems and should be taken into account by any pharmacovigilance analysis.

In the case of telmisartan, the observed cardiac disorders during clinical trials were about 7% of all registered ADRs, whereas FAERS reported 14%. One can argue that this can be due to the different, possibly more diverse and

DrugName	TradeName	Drug Class	THR	Ad1	Ad2A	Ad3	Alpha1A	Alpha2A	Alpha2B	Alpha2C	Beta1	Beta2	AT1	B2	CB1	CCKa	CCKb	D1	D2	D3	D4.4	ETa	GHS
Risperidone	Risperdal	AAP	21	10	10	10	<1	1	<1	<1	10		10	10	10	10	10	<1	<1	<1	<1	10	10
Olanzapine	Zyprexa	AAP	25	10	10	10	<1	4	1	<1	10	10	10	10	10	10	10	<1	<1	<1	<1	10	10
Aripiprazole	Abilify	AAP	27	10	10	10	3	3	2	<1	<1	<1	10	10	10	10	10		<1	<1		10	10
Trazodone	Desyrel	SARI	19	10	10	10	<1	<1	3	<1	10	10	10	10	10	10	10	10	3	2	1	10	10
Venlafaxine	Effexor	SNRI	9	10	10	10	10	10	10	10	10	10	10	10	5	10	10		10	10			10
Duloxetine	Cymbalta	SNRI	20	10	10	10	1	10	4	1	10		10	10	10	10	10		7	5			10
Citalopram	Celexa	SSRI	14	10	10	10	1	10	10	10	10	10	10	10	10	10	10	7	10	2	10	10	10
Sertraline	Zoloft	SSRI	16	10	10	10	1	10	3	3	10	10	10	10	10	10	10		10	10		10	10
Fluoxetine	Prozac	SSRI	17	10	10	10	5	10	4	10	10	10	10	10	3	10	10	10	8	10	10	10	10
Paroxetine	Paxil	SSRI	22	10	10	10	2	10	10	8	10	10	10	10	3	10	10	10	10	10	10	10	10
Amitriptyline	Elavil	TCA	30	10	10	10	<1	3	<1	<1	10	10	1	10	10	10	10	<1	<1	<1	<1	10	10
Nortriptyline	Sensoval	TCA	38	10	10	10	<1	9	<1	<1	10	5	10	10	10	10	10	<1	6	<1		10	10

DrugName	H1	H2	H3	5HT1A	5HT2A	5HT2B	5HT2C	M1	M2	M3	MC3	Motilin	Y1	OpD	OpK	OpM	TP	V1a	V2	AdT
Risperidone	<1	<1	10	1	<1	<1	<1	10	10		10	10	10	10	10	10	10	10	10	10
Olanzapine	<1	<1	10	4	<1	<1	<1	<1	<1	<1	10	10	10	10	10	10	10	10	10	10
Aripiprazole	<1		10			<1	1	10	10	10	10	10	10	10	10		10	10	10	10
Trazodone	1	10	10	<1	<1	<1	1	10	10	10	10	10	10	10	10	10	10	10	10	10
Venlafaxine	1		7	10	<1	10	10	10	10	10	10	10	10	10	10	10		10	10	10
Duloxetine	9		10		<1	10	10	10	10	10	10	5	10	10	2	10	10	10	10	10
Citalopram	2	<1	10	10	2	<1	4	10	8	10	10	10	10	10	10	10	10	10	10	10
Sertraline	10		10	10		9	5	10	10	10	7	10	10	10	<1		10	10	10	10
Fluoxetine	6	2	10	10	<1	6	<1	10	10	4	10	10	10	10	2	10	10	10	10	10
Paroxetine	10	4	10	10	4	10	10	2	1	<1	10	10	10	<1	1	2	10	10	10	10
Amitriptyline	<1	<1	10	4	<1	<1	<1	<1	<1	<1	10	10	10	10	1	10	10	10	10	10
Nortriptyline	<1		10	8	<1	<1	<1	<1	<1	<1	10	10	10	10	<1		10	10	10	10

DrugName	DAT	NET	5HTT	hERG	Ca2(L)	Ca2(N)	BZD	GABA A	Nic(ns)	NMDA	5HT3	AR	ERa	ERb	GR	PR	PXR	COX1	COX2	MAO A	PDE3	PDE4D
Risperidone	10	10	10	2	10	10	10		10	10	10	10	10	10	10	10		10	10	10	10	10
Olanzapine	10	10	10	11	10	10	10	10		10	2	10	10	10	10	10		10	7	10	10	10
Aripiprazole	4	8	<1	<1	10		10	10	10	10	10		10		10		10	10	10	10	2	10
Trazodone	10	10	<1	3	10	10	10	10	10	10	10	10	10	10	10	10		10	10	10	10	10
Venlafaxine	10	10	<1	10	10	10	10	10	10	10	10	10	10		10	10	10	10	10	10	10	10
Duloxetine	1	<1	<1	2	10		10	10	10	10	10	10	10		10	10	10	10	10	10	10	10
Citalopram	10	6	<1	3	10	10	10	10		10	10	10	10	10	10	10		10	10	10	10	10
Sertraline	<1	5	<1	2	10		10	10	10	10	10		10		10		10	10	10	10	10	10
Fluoxetine	10	2	<1	5	10	10	10	10	10	10	10	10	10	10	10	10		10	10	10	10	10
Paroxetine	1	<1	<1	3	2	10	10	10	10	10	10	10	10	10	10	10		10	10	10	10	10
Amitriptyline	10	<1	<1	3	10	10	10	10	10	10	9	10	10	10	10	10	10	10	10	10	10	10
Nortriptyline	3	<1	<1	3	10		10	10	10	10	10		10		10		10	10	10	10	10	8

Figure 1.3 The heat map demonstrates the high promiscuity of a group of frequently used antidepressants. SSRI: selective serotonin reuptake inhibitor; TCA: tricyclic antidepressant; SNRI: serotonin–norepinephrine reuptake inhibitor; SARI: serotonin antagonist and reuptake inhibitor; AAP: atypical antipsychotic. Red: $IC_{50} < 1\ \mu M$; yellow: $IC_{50} = 1–10\ \mu M$; green: $IC_{50} \geq 10\ \mu M$; THR = target hit rate, the percentage of targets with an IC_{50} of $<10\ \mu M$ (not all targets are shown).

‣ Viewing by area affected · View by name	Preclinical Data view all 577	Clinical Data view all 2994	Post-Marketing Reports (AERS) view all 30750
⊞ Blood and lymphatic system disorders	16	55	1547
⊞ Cardiac disorders	31	138	5008
⊞ Congenital, familial and genetic disorders	18	3	284
⊞ Ear and labyrinth disorders	no data	27	529
⊞ Endocrine disorders	15	no data	268
⊞ Eye disorders	3	26	1369
⊞ Gastrointestinal disorders	66	324	4277
⊞ General disorders and administration site conditions	19	240	9294
⊞ Hepatobiliary disorders	20	43	1440
⊞ Immune system disorders	no data	20	606
⊞ Infections and infestations	1	420	2705
⊞ Investigations	165	407	8175
⊞ Metabolism and nutrition disorders	65	104	3863
⊞ Musculoskeletal and connective tissue disorders	no data	171	3613
⊞ Mutagenicity	3	no data	no data
⊞ Neoplasms benign, malignant and unspecified (incl cysts and polyps)	6	6	1681
⊞ Nervous system disorders	21	362	7868
⊞ Pregnancy, puerperium and perinatal conditions	27	4	473
⊞ Psychiatric disorders	7	77	2176
⊞ Renal and urinary disorders	78	99	3694
⊞ Reproductive system and breast disorders	7	5	366
⊞ Respiratory, thoracic and mediastinal disorders	6	184	4268
⊞ Skin and subcutaneous tissue disorders	3	168	3321
⊞ Vascular disorders	no data	111	5585

Figure 1.4 A combined profile comprising representatives from the class of angiotensin II AT_1 receptor antagonists obtained from the FDA Adverse Event Reporting System. The case of angiotensin II antagonists demonstrates that reports on adverse drug reactions are often biased by the original symptoms of the disease the treatment is applied to. (Courtesy of PharmaPendium.)

significantly larger patient population. However, the same is true for vascular disorders, with 5% versus 12%, and for nervous system disorders, 7% compared with 24% of all reports. Accordingly, the label for telmisartan does not carry any warning for major cardiovascular adverse reactions, but correctly points to the possibility of orthostatic hypotension [30].

Drugs that are combinations of different active ingredients also cause a problem in the determination of target–ADR links. For example, local allergy medications have a combination of fexofenadine HCl and pseudoephedrine HCl [31]. This situation also occurs when several drugs are taken concomitantly and in FAERS only one is noted as the “suspect” drug. Thus, care should be taken of drug combinations when FAERS data are interpreted for target-related ADRs.

Finally, drugs withdrawn from the market provide valuable data for the reverse translation process. Drug withdrawals are based on the development of ADRs in the clinical setting that are life-threatening, cause unacceptable burden, or are difficult to manage [32]. The example we take is fenfluramine, an anorexiant that affects the serotonin transporter. Patients treated with fenfluramine developed cardiac valve disorders, a serious irreversible heart condition. FAERS registered 19,141 reports with 59% of the reports associated with cardiac disorders, an extraordinarily high incidence. When further investigated, 38% of the observed cardiac disorders revealed various cardiac valve anomalies (data from PharmaPendium).[4] Based on this observation, fenfluramine was withdrawn from the market and the otherwise rare ADR was later linked to the agonist effect of the major metabolite, norfenfluramine, at the 5-HT_{2B} receptor [33].

While this book highlights targets that we consider "antitargets" under various conditions, in this chapter we focus on information gathering (data mining) that would support claims for target–ADR links. We highlighted the importance of using clinical data for reverse translation to identify the targets that are associated with side effects and we use this information to set up predictive assays for hazard identification during the early phases of the drug discovery process. We demonstrated the importance of this method in the process of parallel optimization for therapeutic effects and mitigation of adverse reactions. Targets incorporated into the *in vitro* pharmacological profiling process are annotated with information obtained from clinical ADRs, which enables the cost-effective prediction of side effects of chemical structural classes or single molecules in the preclinical setting.

On the other hand, we have to be cautious with data interpretation from clinical observations. Cases from FAERS demonstrate the pitfalls that can be encountered if a statistical analysis of the data is conducted without taking into account important factors such as the patient population and their medical condition, other administered drugs, and off-label use of drugs. We demonstrated with the case of antihypertensive drugs that symptoms characteristic for a particular disease could mask the true ADR profile of a drug and we need to keep this in perspective by relying more on the ADRs reported from phase 3 clinical trials. However, be aware of the small chance of ADRs developing very slowly during chronic treatment, which would not be seen in the trials, or of rare alleles in the broad random patient population.

References

1 Kenakin, T. and Christopoulos, A. (2013) Signalling bias in new drug discovery: detection, quantification and therapeutic impact. *Nature Reviews. Drug Discovery*, **12**, 205–216.

2 Kalpaklioglu, F. and Baccioglu, A. (2012) Efficacy and safety of H1-antihistamines: an update. *Anti-Inflammatory & Anti-Allergy Agents in Medicinal Chemistry*, **11**, 230–237.

3 Kenakin, T.P. (2012) Biased signalling and allosteric machines: new vistas and challenges for drug discovery. *British Journal of Pharmacology*, **165**, 1659–1669.

4 Majure, D.T., Greco, T., Greco, M., Ponschab, M., Biondi-Zoccai, G., Zangrillo, A., and Landoni, G. (2013) Meta-analysis of randomized trials of effect of milrinone on mortality in cardiac surgery: an update. *Journal of*

4) PharmaPendium, www.pharmapendium.com/drugs.do;jsessionid=6874369FAAE8591CDA98D076CCC4AAA5#browse=1&lookup=1&hierarchical=1&type=d&name=Fenfluramine&alpha=al_9&query=fenfluramine.

Cardiothoracic and Vascular Anesthesia, **27**, 220–229.

5 Bair, S.M., Choueiri, T.K., and Moslehi, J. (2013) Cardiovascular complications associated with novel angiogenesis inhibitors: emerging evidence and evolving perspectives. *Trends in Cardiovascular Medicine*, **23**, 104–113.

6 Ortega, V.E., Hawkins, G.A., Moore, W.C., Hastie, A.T., Ampleford, E.J., Busse, W.W., Castro, M., Chardon, D., Erzurum, S.C., Israel, E., Montealegre, F., Wenzel, S.E., Peters, S.P., Meyers, D.A., and Bleecker, E.R. (2014) Effect of rare variants in ADRB2 on risk of severe exacerbations and symptom control during long-acting β agonist treatment in a multiethnic asthma population: a genetic study. *The Lancet Respiratory Medicine*, **2**, 204–213.

7 Roth, B.L. (2007) Drugs and valvular heart disease. *The New England Journal of Medicine*, **356**, 6–9.

8 Whitebread, S., Hamon, J., Bojanic, D. *et al.* (2005) *In vitro* safety pharmacology profiling: an essential tool for successful drug development. *Drug Discovery Today*, **10**, 1421–1433.

9 Hamon, J., Whitebread, S., Techer-Etienne, V., Le Coq, H., Azzaoui, K., and Urban, L. (2009) *In vitro* safety pharmacology profiling: what else beyond hERG? *Future Medicinal Chemistry*, **1**, 645–665.

10 Bowes, J., Brown, A.J., Hamon, J. *et al.* (2012) Reducing safety-related drug attrition: the use of *in vitro* pharmacological profiling. *Nature Reviews. Drug Discovery*, **11**, 909–922.

11 Azzaoui, K., Hamon, J., Faller, B., Whitebread, S., Jacoby, E., Bender, A., Jenkins, J.L., and Urban, L. (2007) Modeling promiscuity based on *in vitro* safety pharmacology profiling data. *ChemMedChem*, **2**, 874–880.

12 Nash, P.D. (2012) Why modules matter. *FEBS Letters*, **586**, 2572–2574.

13 Suh, D.C., Woodall, B.S., Shin, S.K., and Hermes-De Santis, E.R. (2000) Clinical and economic impact of adverse drug reactions in hospitalized patients. *Annals of Pharmacotherapy*, **34**, 1373–1379.

14 Sullivan, P.W., Valuck, R., Saseen, J., and MacFall, H.M. (2004) A comparison of the direct costs and cost effectiveness of serotonin reuptake inhibitors and associated adverse drug reactions. *CNS Drugs*, **18**, 911–932.

15 Gautier, S., Bachelet, H., Bordet, R., and Caron, J. (2003) The cost of adverse drug reactions. *Expert Opinion on Pharmacotherapy*, **4**, 319–326.

16 US FDA (2014) Preventable Adverse Drug Reactions: A Focus on Drug Interactions. ADRs: Prevalence and Incidence. Available at http://www.fda.gov/drugs/developmentapprovalprocess/developmentresources/druginteractionslabeling/ucm110632.htm (accessed December 2, 2014).

17 US FDA (2014) FDA Adverse Event Reporting System (FAERS): Latest Quarterly Data Files. Available at http://www.fda.gov/Drugs/GuidanceComplianceRegulatoryInformation/Surveillance/AdverseDrugEffects/ucm082193.htm (accessed December 2, 2014).

18 Hocking, C.M., Townsend, A.R., and Price, T.J. (2013) Panitumumab in metastatic colorectal cancer. *Expert Review of Anticancer Therapy*, **13**, 781–793.

19 Urban, L., Whitebread, S., Hamon, J., Mikhailov, D., and Azzaoui, K. (2011) Screening for safety-relevant off-target activities, in *Polypharmacology* (ed. U.-J. Peters), John Wiley & Sons, Inc., Hoboken, NJ.

20 Muller, P.Y. and Milton, M.N. (2012) The determination and interpretation of the therapeutic index in drug development. *Nature Reviews. Drug Discovery*, **11**, 751–761.

21 Gu, Q., Dillon, C.F., and Burt, V.L. (2010) Prescription drug use continues to increase: U.S. prescription drug data for 2007–2008. *NCHS Data Briefs*, 42, 1–8.

22 De Hert, M., Detraux, J., van Winkel, R., Yu, W., and Correll, C.U. (2011) Metabolic and cardiovascular adverse effects associated with antipsychotic drugs. *Nature Reviews Endocrinology*, **8**, 114–126.

23 Pepersack, T., Gilles, C., Petrovic, M., Spinnewine, A., Baeyens, H., Beyer, I., Boland, B., Dalleur, O., De Lepeleire, J., Even-Adin, D., Van Nes, M.C., Samalea-Suarez, A., and Somers, A. (Working Group Clinical Pharmacology,

Pharmacotherapy and Pharmaceutical Care; Belgian Society for Gerontology and Geriatrics) (2013) Prevalence of orthostatic hypotension and relationship with drug use amongst older patients. *Acta Clinica Belgica*, **68**, 107–112.

24 Woolcott, J.C., Richardson, K.J., Wiens, M.O., Patel, B., Marin, J., Khan, K.M., and Marra, C.A. (2009) Meta-analysis of the impact of 9 medication classes on falls in elderly persons. *Archives of Internal Medicine*, **169**, 1952–1960.

25 Hu, Y. and Bajorath, J. (2013) Compound promiscuity: what can we learn from current data? *Drug Discovery Today*, **18**, 644–650.

26 Ghoreschi, K., Laurence, A., and O'Shea, J.J. (2009) Selectivity and therapeutic inhibition of kinases: to be or not to be? *Nature Immunology*, **10**, 356–360.

27 Cox, K.J., Shomin, C.D., and Ghosh, I. (2011) tinkering outside the kinase ATP box: allosteric (type IV) and bivalent (type V) inhibitors of protein kinases. *Future Medicinal Chemistry*, **3**, 29–43.

28 Besnard, J., Ruda, G.F., Setola, V., Abecassis, K., Rodriguiz, R.M., Huang, X.P., Norval, S., Sassano, M.F., Shin, A.I., Webster, L.A., Simeons, F.R., Stojanovski, L., Prat, A., Seidah, N.G., Constam., D.B., Bickerton, G.R., Read, K.D., Wetsel, W.C., Gilbert, I.H., Roth, B.L., and Hopkins, A.L. (2012) Automated design of ligands to polypharmacological profiles. *Nature*, **492**, 215–220.

29 US FDA (2007) Antidepressant Use in Children, Adolescents, and Adults. Available at http://www.fda.gov/Drugs/DrugSafety/InformationbyDrugClass/ucm096273.htm (accessed December 2, 2014).

30 Center for Drug Evaluation and Research (CDER) (2012) Micardis (Telmisartan) Tablets. Detailed View: Safety Labeling Changes Approved by FDA. Available at http://www.fda.gov/Safety/MedWatch/SafetyInformation/ucm266672.htm (accessed December 2, 2014).

31 Mansfield, L.E. (2006) Once-daily immediate-release fexofenadine and sustained-release pseudoephedrine combination: a new treatment option for allergic rhinitis. *Expert Opinion on Pharmacotherapy*, **7**, 941–951.

32 US FDA (2014) How does FDA decide when a drug is not safe enough to stay on the market? Available at http://www.fda.gov/AboutFDA/Transparency/Basics/ucm194984.htm (accessed December 2, 2014).

33 Roth, B.L. (2007) Drugs and valvular heart disease. *The New England Journal of Medicine*, **356**, 6–9.

2
In Silico Prediction of Drug Side Effects

Michael J. Keiser

Established drugs are often not selective [1] and the prevalence of compound promiscuity reported within pharmacological databases ranges from 33 to 52% [1–3]. Yet this may be an unlooked-for boon, as exquisite selectivity is not always beneficial; for instance, the selective cyclooxygenase-2 (COX-2) inhibitors were withdrawn due to risk of cardiovascular events, whereas COX-1/2 inhibitors persist [4]. Likewise, no selective antipsychotic has made it to the market in 60 years despite concerted efforts; indeed, polypharmacology may underlie their efficacy [5]. In terms of safety, the notion of "selective synergy" [6] suggests that a drug with weak activity at multiple targets, whose therapeutic effect converges only where the targets are coexpressed within a diseased tissue or cell, might be safer than a compound that inactivates a single target globally.

Attempts to predict adverse drug reactions (ADRs) correspondingly now account for multitarget drug activity in the context of interacting networks of perturbation and biological effect that, taken together and stacked into layers of increasing complexity, comprise the drug response of a binding site, cell, tissue, organ, or patient in the clinic (Figure 2.1). Considering, for example, rosiglitazone's canonical target, peroxisome proliferator-activated receptor γ (PPARγ), which regulates PTGS2, SERPINE1, VEGFA, APOB, TSPO, MMP9, IL-6, CASP3, and CA2/4, we find effectors modulating cardiac function that may be relevant to the drug's observed association with myocardial infarction [7]. Is PPARγ itself an antitarget, and in what context? Or does rosiglitazone bind to additional off-targets that may potentiate its undesired effects?

Turning to efficacy, the broad profiles of multikinase inhibitors combat response to a host of growth factors exchanged among tumors and surrounding tissues that, left untreated, mutually stimulate angiogenesis and growth. Sunitinib, for instance, blocks the receptor kinases of VEGFR and PDGFR, which would otherwise trigger angiogenesis in endothelial cells and pericytes; the drug also inhibits c-Kit, Flt-3, RET, and CSF-1R [4]. Broad kinase profiles often seem a necessary evil, but Dar *et al.* [8] recently optimized initially unselective RET kinase inhibitors in kinome scans with a *Drosophila* model to

Antitargets and Drug Safety, First Edition. Edited by László Urbán, Vinod F. Patel, and Roy J. Vaz.

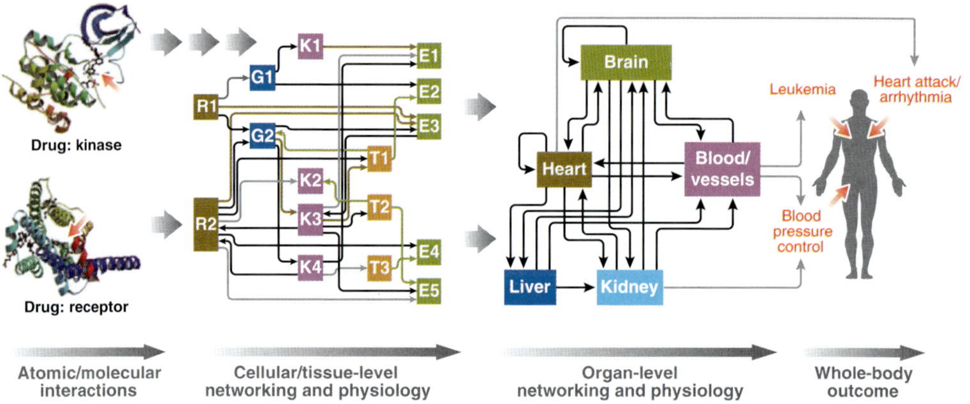

Figure 2.1 A schematic of the multiscale networks underlying a systems pharmacology approach to predicting drug action. Molecular interactions such as drug to receptor binding modulate the balance of cellular regulatory networks, which propagate changes to cellular and tissue physiologies and then to organ networks and whole-body outcomes. (Reprinted with permission from Ref. [7]; the drug–protein complexes are obtained from the Protein Data Bank (www.pdb.org) with PDB IDs 3QC4 and 2Y03.)

increase inhibition at certain kinases (Raf, Src) while avoiding it at others (mTor), in order to achieve well-tolerated polypharmacological compounds with 500 times better performance than vandetanib in human cell lines. A key innovation here was the discrimination of antitarget from target via appropriate use of a phenotypic model organism, and the insight that some targets are antitargets only in combination.

This quantitative systems pharmacology [9,10] viewpoint combines systems biology with computation and large-scale phenotypic and functional datasets to investigate how molecular interactions ultimately yield whole-body outcomes. Its application to the prediction of antitarget-mediated side effects is the focus of this chapter. In broad strokes, we first consider *in silico* methods to predict drug "off-target" activity from a chemocentric perspective and then turn to the analysis of off-targets as antitargets and the means by which we may associate specific side effects with them.

2.1
Large-Scale Prediction of Drug Activity

The discovery or design of selectively nonselective compounds, and the prediction of specific antitargets, requires a prospective organizing framework unless we are to rely solely on "polypharmacology by serendipity" [4]. Consequently, this section addresses current chemocentric computational methods, results, and challenges for the prediction of drug off-target activity.

2.1.1
Networks of Known and New Target Activity

There are many routes to adverse drug reactions, and our focus here is on those that arise from a drug's activity at unintended but specific antitargets. The requisite identification of a drug's full target profile is consequently a key challenge, especially as its off-targets may have little in common with its intended targets [11]. Databases such as DrugBank [12] and ChEMBL [13] report on a drug's canonical and research targets, respectively, but the histories of most drugs' characterizations are checkered ones, characterized by chance, so that substantial portions of secondary pharmacology may yet remain entirely overlooked.

2.1.1.1 Predicting Drug Off-Targets by Statistical Chemical Similarity

In a chemocentric approach to drug–target characterization, predictive methods draw on ligand associations long known to the literature but only more recently organized into coherent datasets. As these datasets have grown, so too has an extensive chemoinformatic literature exploring means to compare ligand pairs for similarity [14] and predict pharmacological profiles [15–19]. In one example, Izrailev and Farnum link targets solely by the most similar molecules between them [20]. Unlike metrics relying on the full distribution of ligand similarity between targets, this focus on the "average nearest neighbor" [20] detects similarity among small subsets of ligands that would otherwise be drowned out by the majority.

Similarity Ensemble Approach

A recent chemocentric method that has garnered some notoriety for its drug "off-target" predictions is the Similarity Ensemble Approach (SEA) [11,21–23]. Using statistics motivated by the extreme value distributions [24] underlying BLAST [25], this ligand-based approach returns to a logic that would be familiar to classical pharmacology, but does so on a scale undreamt of at that time. SEA takes an organic molecule, or a set of related molecules, and compares it with sets of ligands annotated to targets. The comparison with all features in the reference ligands, and with random expectation, is what is novel about the method. In the last seven years, SEA has predicted previously unknown targets for more than 200 drugs [21,23,26,27] and identified targets for small molecules active in phenotypic screens [28–30].

Many drug screening and profiling results in the literature and public databases are motivated by preexisting hypotheses of drug action. Whereas this practice substantially improves the chances of finding true positives in the screens, selection bias can omit unexpected biological side effect space. It is sensible to screen kinase inhibitors against other kinases, and selective transporter inhibitors against transporters, but off-target activities have been found crossing these boundaries [11,23]. Likewise, some of the most striking SEA predictions found new off-targets unrelated by sequence or structure to the canonical targets of the drug [21,23]. Thus, the anti-ribosomal emetine was predicted and found to bind to the α2 adrenergic receptor (α2 AR), the selective serotonin reuptake inhibitor (SSRI) Prozac to the β1 AR, and the HIV reverse transcriptase inhibitor Rescriptor to the histamine H4 receptor. Similarly, in a study over roughly a thousand off-target predictions, more than 25% of those confirmed crossed major target boundaries (i.e., the off-target was unrelated by sequence to any known target for the drug).

These networks fill in receptor–drug gaps left by incomplete testing or lack of public data (e.g., black edges in Figure 2.2). Whereas 38% of compounds in the public ChEMBL database are already reported to bind more than one target, only 2% cross target class boundaries [3], but the true number may be an order of magnitude larger. Although chemocentric networks do not share a fundamental underlying organization equivalent to the evolutionary theory that underpins bioinformatics, they nonetheless encode consistent information reflecting other

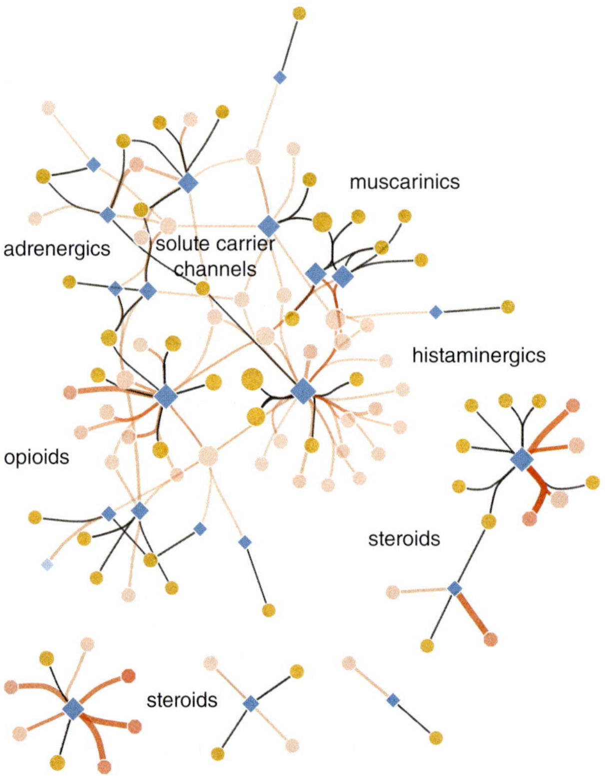

Figure 2.2 Network summarizing selected new associations among marketed drugs (gold circles), antitargets (cyan diamonds), and ADRs (red octagons) constructed from data in Supplementary Table S6 of Ref. [11]. Black edges mark new SEA drug-to-target predictions that were confirmed by full dose–response testing *in vitro*, while red edges link targets to ADRs. Red edge thickness increases with strength of target-to-ADR enrichment factor score. Opacity of red edges and red ADR nodes also increases with strength of ef score. Labels refer to the grouping of targets (blue diamonds) emerging from these associations.

bioactivity principles. Intriguingly, the topologies of predictive chemical similarity networks are stable to different ligand representations, and share the scale-free properties of their bioinformatics brethren [22].

Structure-Based Virtual Screens

The explicit modeling of drug to macromolecule binding interactions in virtual screens over large molecular target panels is another promising way to approach polypharmacological prediction. However, despite tremendous advance in transmembrane crystallography [31–42], many therapeutically important targets nonetheless remain recalcitrant to structural determination [7], constraining the full extension of structural approaches [43] such as docking [44,45], multitarget virtual screening [46–54], and structure-based pharmacophores [17,55,56]. The proposition of accurately profiling the pharmacopeia's thousands of therapeutic targets structurally thus remains daunting, though in combination with homology modeling [57–59] the field is advancing at a steamroller pace. For the purposes of this chapter, then, we maintain a focus on chemocentric approaches, which may achieve a wide breadth of target coverage, even if the predictions they yield are less informative of underlying interaction principles and thermodynamic considerations.

2.1.1.2 Representing Drugs Computationally for Rapid Comparison

A core ambition of systems pharmacology is to build comprehensive networks of known and new drug activity that span thousands of molecular targets, hundreds of thousands of ligands, and millions of candidate compounds. Consequently, techniques to calculate the off-target predictions discussed above must be scalable, widely applicable, and rapid; this section summarizes constituent methods derived from chemical informatics to computationally encode and rapidly compare bioactive molecules.

Molecular Descriptors (Fingerprints)

A small molecule has no primary sequence, nor is there a central dogma delineating biological information flow through its synthesis or structure. Consequently, the field encompasses disparate ways to encode bioactive small molecules computationally. A molecular descriptor, commonly called a fingerprint, represents a small molecule by encoding a portion of its structural or physical property patterns into a short series of "ON" and "OFF" bits. Fingerprints such as Daylight [60] or Scitegic's Extended Connectivity FingerPrint (ECFP) [22] encode a molecule's two-dimensional topology, such as its atom types and the bond connectivity among them. In contrast, Chemically Advanced Template Search (CATS) fingerprints [61,62] rely on physical properties such as counts of cations, anions, and hydrogen bond donors and acceptors, whereas ROCS [63,64], FEPOPS [65], and morphological similarity [66] incorporate three-dimensional shape. Moving aside from direct properties, affinity fingerprints [16,67] represent molecules indirectly, by their activity in high-throughput screens or other biological contexts.

Similarity Metrics

We compare fingerprint-encoded molecule pairs via similarity metrics. The most common metric is the Tanimoto coefficient (Tc) [68,69], which computes the number of ON bits in common between two fingerprints, compared with all the ON bits that could have matched between them. This is a variant of the Jaccard coefficient, which was used to calculate alpine flower population diversity in 1901 [70]. The Tc computes overall similarity between two molecules and is symmetric. In comparison, the Tversky index [71] is asymmetric, asking only whether one molecule is a substructure of another; if so, it can achieve a perfect score even when additional moieties on the second molecule remain unmatched. Any method using Tversky indices must then account for the directionality of the comparison. But which direction matters? Lacking any broader theoretical underpinnings, the specifics of the task at hand inform this choice.

Limitations and Opportunities

A fingerprint is an imperfect stand-in for a small molecule, as it collapses all of a molecule's information into a simple bit sequence in return for comparison speed. For knowledge-based fingerprints such as MDL keys [72], each bit denotes a chemical pattern or moiety that might make sense to a medicinal chemist. When a computer compares fingerprints, however, the similarity metric is ignorant of any bit's meaning and treats all equally, although the actual contribution of different chemical patterns to binding can vary greatly. Perhaps unsurprisingly, the performance of knowledge-based fingerprints often falls short of information-theoretic ones [73] such as ECFP, whose bits exhaustively encode algorithmic patterns that may not be intuitive.

Looking forward, the question of the best way to represent and encode a small molecule is far from solved. The first and perhaps most immediate critique of current approaches is their focus on two-dimensional (or topological) similarity. Turning the clock back to the late 1970s and early 1980s, a key pragmatic consideration favoring two dimensions was calculation space and speed; today the motivation is different. Whereas the calculation of similarity between pairs of small three-dimensional structures is now tractable, the enumeration of each molecule's conformational ensemble remains a source of error. Current techniques draw on millions of reference ligands, few of whose biologically competent conformations are known. Even were one to compute all possible low-energy conformations in solution for millions of ligands, the task remains to determine which conformations are relevant to macromolecular binding, and the sites vary. If this means we must evaluate and correct for hordes of irrelevant conformations (false positives) before encountering the few correct ones during each molecule-to-molecule comparison, it is inconvenient. If this means that we are not generating the correct binding-relevant conformations in the first place (false negatives), it is disastrous. Each of these challenges is amenable to correction, calculation, and careful planning; each is an opportunity.

2.1.2
Resources for Multiscale Inquiry

Quantitative systems pharmacology [9] bears little resemblance to its antecedents in chemical informatics, systems biology, and medical informatics of a decade ago. A primary factor in this transfiguration has been the advent and open availability of large databases annotating small-molecule bioactivities. Playing a role analogous to open genome browsers in bioinformatics, bioactivity databases and others now collating large-scale experimental results enable the interrogation of multiscale mechanisms [7], wherein we ask not only what targets a drug hits, but how this perturbation propagates across a cell, tissue, or entire biological system (Figure 2.1).

2.1.2.1 Ligands to Targets

In 2008, the European Molecular Biology Laboratory (EMBL) acquired the commercial StARlite database with support from the Wellcome Trust. Since then, the freely available and renamed ChEMBL database (www.ebi.ac.uk/chembl) [13] has undergone over 17 major releases under John Overington's chemogenomics group at the EMBL-EBI. ChEMBL (version 17) annotates 1.3 million distinct compounds across 9400 molecular targets via more than 12 million activity records derived from over 51 000 scientific publications. At this scale, it is feasible to statistically detect and correct for random and some forms of experimental error. This compilation complements long-standing commercial databases such as WOMBAT [74,75] and large though less curated public ones, including NCBI PubChem BioAssay, which consolidates publicly deposited assay results.

Table 2.1 lists several widely used and openly available pharmacological datasets organizing ligand structure and target information.

It is inevitable that even carefully curated databases will contain incorrect annotations, due to either faulty primary experiments or errors mining these data. In a plucky response, ChEMBL's active community and core team assiduously fix errors reported with each release. More generally, as the databases grow in size, the incidence of independent assays converging on the same small molecule to target pairs grows, reinforcing correct associations. An as-yet unresolved issue, however, is database fragmentation and the heavy lifting that will be required in the design and deployment of ontologies to consolidate them [10].

2.1.2.2 Perturbing Biological Systems (Phenotypes)

Moving further up the biological hierarchy, we encounter the prediction of system-wide drug outcomes and adverse drug reactions. A comprehensive computational model of a whole cell [76], much less of a tissue, is a substantial endeavor and one well beyond the remit of this chapter. Instead we take a pragmatic approach, asking what quantitative large-scale phenotypic readouts are amenable to a target-based analysis.

Table 2.1 Widely used data resources.

Resource or database	Type	URL
Chemical Effects in Biological Systems (CEBS)	ADR/Tox	cebs.niehs.nih.gov/
FDA Adverse Event Reporting System	ADR/Tox	http://www.fda.gov/Drugs/GuidanceComplianceRegulatoryInformation/Surveillance/AdverseDrugEffects/default.htm
SIDER	ADR/Tox	sideeffects.embl.de
Tox21 (Computational Toxicology Research Program)	ADR/Tox phenotypic, cell line	http://epa.gov/ncct/Tox21
Comparative Toxicogenomics Database	ADR/Tox, pharmacological	ctd.mdibl.org/
Human Interactome Database	Biological	interactome.dfci.harvard.edu/H_sapiens
Reactome	Biological	http://www.reactome.org/ReactomeGWT/entrypoint.html
European Bioinformatics Institute (EBI) ArrayExpress Archive	Functional genomic	http://www.ebi.ac.uk/microarray-as/ae/
Gene Expression Omnibus (GEO)	Functional genomic	www.ncbi.nlm.nih.gov/geo
The Gene Ontology	Functional genomic	www.geneontology.org
Genetic Association Database	Genomic	geneticassociationdb.nih.gov
Kyoto Encyclopedia of Genes and Genomes	Genomic	www.genome.jp/kegg
NCBI Database of Genotypes and Phenotypes (dbGaP)	Genomic, phenotypic	http://www.ncbi.nlm.nih.gov/gap/
International HapMap Project	Pharmacogenomic	hapmap.ncbi.nlm.nih.gov
Online Mendelian Inheritance in Man	Pharmacogenomic	www.ncbi.nlm.nih.gov/omim
The Pharmacogenomics Knowledgebase (PharmGKB)	Pharmacogenomic	www.pharmgkb.org
Psychoactive Drug Screening Program KiDB	Pharmacological	pdsp.med.unc.edu/kidb.php
ChEMBL	Pharmacological, ADR	https://www.ebi.ac.uk/chembl/
DrugBank	Pharmacological, ADR	www.drugbank.ca
Connectivity Map	Phenotypic, cell line	http://www.broadinstitute.org/genome_bio/connectivitymap.html
Library of Integrated Network-Based Cellular Signatures (LINCS)	Phenotypic, cell line	http://commonfund.nih.gov/lincs/
NCI-60 DTP Human Tumor Cell Line Screen	Phenotypic, cell line	http://dtp.nci.nih.gov/branches/btb/ivclsp.html
NCBI PubChem BioAssay	Phenotypic, pharmacological	www.ncbi.nlm.nih.gov/pcassay

Extended from and motivated by Bai *et al.* [10].

Ambitious efforts in genomics, proteomics, and metabolomics are fertile ground for the target-based analysis of drug activity [7]. In one example, a single-nucleotide polymorphism (SNP) in the coding region rs1799853 within cytochrome P540 2C9 affects warfarin metabolism and dosing [77]. This is no isolated case; pharmacogenomic markers play an important role in our understanding of drug action in terms of pharmacokinetics (e.g., warfarin–*CYP2C9*), pharmacodynamics (e.g., capecitabine–*DPD* [78]), and responsiveness (e.g., panitumumab–*k-RAS* [79]). The integration of systems pharmacology with proteomics and metabolomics is more recent but similarly promising. Proteomics quantifies states and levels of protein populations in biological samples of interest; to obtain sufficient tissue biopsies, many such studies have focused on target profiling [80] in human cancer cell lines [7], with and without compounds. Combining multiple approaches, a metabolomic study of amino acid levels in plasma detected higher glycine levels in patients who did not respond to the selective serotonin reuptake inhibitor citalopram; bringing genomics to bear, they consequently identified a SNP in the gene coding for glycine dehydrogenase associated with treatment outcome [81]. Other such efforts have linked aspirin response to the purine pathway [82].

Large-scale experimental perturbation readouts are particularly intriguing for their broad reach and potential to implicate unexpected and unlooked-for target mechanisms in a drug's action. In the pharmacogenomic association of warfarin with the cytochrome P450 SNP, computational prediction of warfarin's targets and metabolizing enzymes might narrow the field of genomic inquiry or help prioritize raw associations. The mechanism of the glycine dehydrogenase SNP's association with citalopram's therapeutic outcome is unknown, so a broader characterization of citalopram's target profile and of other drugs interacting with the glycine dehydrogenase pathway could, for instance, posit new mode of action hypotheses.

2.1.2.3 Functional and Biological Annotations (Diseases)

Whereas the direct phenotypic readouts described in the previous section have the virtues of clear quantification and a short mechanistic path linking a drug to its effect, they are not yet themselves disease states or adverse reactions. Pfizer and the CTD emphasized this distinction, differentiating "phenotypes" from "diseases" during their collaborative curation of 88 000 scientific articles comprising more than 2.5 million toxicogenomic interactions into a single dataset [83]. In this usage, "decreased blood pressure" is a phenotype, whereas "idiopathic orthostatic hypertension" is a disease. The latter is less well defined, yet it is what presents in the clinic, in ICD-9 codes (http://www.cdc.gov/nchs/icd/icd9.htm), and in the prescription of therapeutics. Ultimately, a "disease" or a drug's "side effect" is a whole-body function, and one that we would wish to predict ahead of time.

Functional annotation datasets organize relationships among abstract entities such as compounds, genes, proteins, pathways, diseases, and adverse drug reactions (Figure 2.1). If these entities are nodes in a network, the connecting edges are their relationships, such as "encodes-for" in "the gene ADRB1_HUMAN encodes-for the human β1 adrenergic receptor protein P08588" (www.uniprot.org) or "is-a-member-of" in the assertion "the protein P08588 is-a-member-of the "G alpha (s) signaling events" pathway (www.reactome.org). Such relationships, however, tend to be binary; whereas this is acceptable for concepts such as pathway membership, it limits our interpretation of links between proteins and disease states. For example, to what numerical extent does more pharmacological blocking of the β1 AR result in more effective treatment of hypertension? Does outcome scale proportionally with input (drug-based blocking of β1 AR), are there compensatory mechanisms, and is there a plateau effect? We can address these questions by direct experiment or perhaps literature survey, but they are not encoded explicitly in functional annotation databases, and this is a limitation.

Careful integration of complementary functional databases into hybrid models is one response to the conundrum of functional quantification. For instance, returning to the β1 AR, we see it is assigned to two pathways organized under "signal transduction" in Reactome [84], and we may extract the full circuitry of these extensively curated pathways and the connections among them into a network model. Context and metabolic associations may be extracted from the Kyoto Encyclopedia of Genes and Genomes (KEGG) [85] and MetaCyc [86], and we might then find it useful to narrow our network down to the genes and proteins most closely annotated to "signal transduction" (GO term #0007165) in the Gene Ontology (GO) [87]. Algorithms evaluating information flow, path discovery, or mean first passage time [88] may then highlight particularly important proteins within the hybrid network model. We could finally check genes encoding unexpected proteins against pharmacogenomic reports and SNPs from Online Mendelian Inheritance in Man (OMIM; www.omim.org), anchoring our inquiry in specific readouts and genetic–phenotypic associations. For instance, OMIM reports that already within the β1 AR encoding gene ADRB1 itself a SNP at location 10q25.3 modifies the efficacy of β-blocker drug response [89].

The above process is feasible, but admits multiple opportunities for error, whose effects can propagate in progressively wider oscillations across the model. In practice, it is now often easier and more reliable to replace at least some portion of the abstract model with concrete results from large phenotypic studies, as with the Connectivity Map [90], which consolidates a library of gene expression signatures arising in human cell lines exposed to drugs, in order to obtain whole-genome expression patterns. For the drugs and cell lines it profiles, Connectivity Map short-circuits a portion of the effort needed to link a drug to gene expression, replacing fused models drawn from qualitative biological annotations with quantitative data. As genomic, high-throughput screening, proteomic, and related technologies become more prevalent, they become ideal complements for quantitative systems pharmacology approaches, especially in the context of functional annotations.

2.1.2.4 Adverse Reactions as Drug-Induced Diseases

The treatment of a disease and the occurrence of an adverse reaction are both drug outcomes; in this sense, an adverse reaction may be thought of as a drug-induced disease. This framework is useful for analysis, because it allows us to draw on target predictions and phenotypic or biological datasets to posit new antitarget hypotheses. In contrast, antitargets are only partially characterized except in extreme cases (e.g., hERG-related K^+ channel, 5-HT_{2B} receptor, Table 2.2) [91], and multi-antitarget profiles languish mostly unaddressed. One way to identify new antitargets is to combine drug–target relationships with drug–ADR relationships so as to infer target–ADR links. This section addresses databases and methods linking drugs to ADRs.

Public databases such as the Side Effect Resource (SIDER) [93] and the CTD–Pfizer collection [83] aggregate drug–ADR and drug–disease associations from dispersed sources in the literature and package labels into human- and computer-readable formats. For instance, SIDER links clozapine to side effect terms; weight increased (4–56%), salivary hypersecretion (6–48%), and somnolence (25–46%), along with several others. Percentages are collated from studies or reports of ADR incidence within the label. However, the semi-automated curation of these data is imperfect, as illustrated by one of clozapine's serious side effects, agranulocytosis, which is incorrectly classified as an indication (as is "death") (March 2014; http://sideeffects.embl.de/drugs/2818). Digging down on the rationale for this association, "Because of a significant

Table 2.2 Frequently encountered antitargets.

Antitarget	Hit rate[a)] (%)	Associated adverse events
hERG channel	(60)	Arrhythmia
Serotonin 5-HT_{2B} receptor	14	Agonists: valvulopathy, pulmonary hypertension
Serotonin 5-HT_{2A} receptor	11	Agonists: cognition impairment, hallucination
α_{1A} Adrenergic receptor	10	Agonists: arrhythmia; antagonists: orthostatic hypotension
Dopamine D_2 receptor	9	Agonists: confusion, emesis; antagonists: orthostatic hypotension
Histamine H_1 receptor	6	Antagonists: weight gain, sedation, somnolence
α_{2A} Adrenergic receptor	6	Agonists: hypotension, sedation
Dopamine D_1 receptor	5	Antagonists: dyskinesia, tremor
M1–5 muscarinic receptors	5	Multiple cardiovascular and metabolic adverse effects, cognition impairment
μ-Opioid receptor	3	Agonists: sedation, respiratory depression, abuse potential

Adapted from Ref. [4]. Copyright 2013, American Chemical Society.

a) Hit rate: percentage of drug-like compounds that bind to this target with an $IC_{50} < 1\,\mu M$ in the BioPrint dataset, except for hERG [92].

risk of agranulocytosis, a potentially life-threatening adverse event, clozapine should be reserved for use in the treatment of severely ill schizophrenic patients" is cited as a sentence motivating it. This example illustrates both the strengths of ADR annotation datasets and their weaknesses; the task is analogous to the correct annotation of whether a drug is an agonist or antagonist at its molecular target in ligand–target datasets such as ChEMBL, which as yet relies primarily on manual supervision.

Correspondingly, the CTD–Pfizer dataset, built instead in a two-step process [83] of machine text mining followed by human curation, would be less likely to include links confusing adverse with intended effects but conversely may lack breadth of coverage. Furthermore, unlike SIDER's explicit focus on ADRs, this collection repurposes methods linking drugs to diseases to the task of linking drugs to ADRs within four primary toxicity profiles, CardioTox, NeuroTox, RenalTox, and HepatoTox. Annotations derive from text-mined phrases such as *"[DISEASE] induced by/caused by/due to/after [DRUG],"* for example, *"[OPTIC NEUROPATHY] caused by [AMIODARONE]"* [83]. While this is consistent with the notion of an ADR as a drug-induced disease, it lacks SIDER's prevalence data.

Aside from the literature, large "primary" datasets organize postmarketing reports of ADRs from the FDA's Adverse Event Reporting System (AERS) [94]. Its strength is scale and broad reach; its limitations arise from lack of curation and baseline data such as the number of people using a drug of interest [7]. To address this, Tatonetti *et al.* brought rigorous post-processing to bear, creating OFFSIDES and TWOSIDES datasets [95] enriched for statistically significant ADRs and drug–drug interactions. Upon release in March 2012, OFFSIDES contained nearly 439 000 drug–ADR associations for 1332 drugs and 10 097 adverse events, derived from the statistical analysis of more than 4 million primary FDA AERS reports. Tatonetti and coworkers have since complemented this approach with pharmacovigilance studies on nontraditional sources such as Google search histories [96]. These postmarketing analyses complement ones curated from the literature, as a source of confirmatory or novel signals from the worldwide "crowd" of patients and physicians. The trend is gaining traction with mobile device start-ups and the "quantified self" movement, wherein a phone's embedded sensors and logging capability (e.g., Google's Project Tango, https://www.google.com/atap/projecttango/) may soon generate vast datasets of individual's physical and mental states amenable to data mining for unexpected or clinically informative patterns.

2.2 Multiscale Models of Adverse Drug Reactions

Whereas we can often predict new drug "off-targets" computationally, this ability alone is not always sufficient for the direct prediction of drug side effects. Several antitargets and the side effects consequent to their modulation are well established, but open data resources compiling antitarget to side effect relationships are incomplete. Consequently, the discovery of new antitargets or quantification of interactions among established ones may benefit from computational or statistical inference. This section evaluates off-targets as antitargets, moves to methods inferring antitarget to side effect relationships, and concludes with a discussion of hybrid experimental–computational approaches to model and confirm side effect and phenotypic mechanisms in a hypothesis-free manner.

2.2.1 Inferring Adverse Reactions

2.2.1.1 From Off-Targets to Antitargets

The quantitative associations known between targets and adverse reactions can be at times surprisingly tenuous. We explored means to computationally incorporate biological and side effect datasets above (see Section 2.1.2.4), but this section starts from another perspective: that of a drug's off-target profile. This chemocentric view narrows the field of possible antitargets down to those predicted or known to bind the drug directly, making it possible to explore each target in the context of the drug's known side effects. As this approach builds from chemical structure to targets and thence to side effects, it complements the biological viewpoint, which proceeds instead from side effects back down to targets and structures.

A first means to identify antitargets is simply to ask which of a drug's off-targets might be consistent with its known side effects. Leveraging statistical patterns of atom and bond topology among small molecules, SEA (see Section 2.1.1.1) has uncovered multiple off-targets consistent with drug side effects [21,23]. The amebicide emetine, which can induce hypotension, tachycardia, and congestive heart failure, directly bound to the α_2 adrenergic receptor on *in vitro* testing [21]; methadone's unreported 1 μM muscarinic M3 binding was consistent with its side effects [21]; and Motilium, imported to stimulate lactation but banned by the FDA for cardiac arrest, bound to α_{1A} adrenergic receptors at 71 nM [23]. As mentioned earlier, the SSRIs Prozac and Paxil bound also to β_1 adrenergic receptors, consistent with the SSRI discontinuation syndrome and the sexual dysfunction they can induce [23]. This was borne out in a pilot study associating a human *ADRB1* SNP with SSRI-induced changes to heart rate and blood pressure [97], demonstrating a progression from *in silico* calculation to *in vitro* and pharmacogenomic testing.

Along these lines, multiple chemoinformatic approaches [7] now address specific antitarget prediction [98–100]. In some studies, groups have rediscovered overlooked antitargets and confirmed them by deep literature review, revealing relationships known to the literature but unknown to the datasets used to predict them [91,101–105]. More structurally oriented methods, using compounds and off-target sites or binding poses [106–109], provide an orthogonal viewpoint and new ways to model ADMET properties [110].

2.2.1.2 Systematic Antitarget Prediction and Testing

While it is feasible to manually determine which of a single drug's off-targets may contribute to its side effects, this route does not scale to the analysis of hundreds of drugs or adverse drug reactions. Correspondingly, pharma programs screen early compounds against predetermined antitarget panels, ranging from at least 15 "targets of most concern" (Pfizer) to 24 (Novartis) and 48 targets (Roche) [4]. In a joint effort among scientists from AstraZeneca, GlaxoSmithKline, Pfizer, and Novartis to evaluate safety and target hit rates, scientists identified a "minimal panel" of 44 antitargets [111]. These antitarget panels, comprised of well-characterized antitargets, lend themselves to virtual screening (see Section 2.1.1); the challenge is to link screening results and the antitargets themselves to direct predictions of adverse drug reactions.

A three-way collaboration with Novartis, UCSF, and a start-up put this question to the test by using SEA [21,23] to predict the associations of 656 marketed drugs against a 73-antitarget Novartis safety panel. This yielded 1239 novel off-target predictions that, when queried against Novartis' in-house knowledgebase, or experimentally tested via full dose–response determination, achieved a 48% positive predictive value without human supervision [11]. Intriguingly, 26% of the off-targets thereby discovered crossed traditional protein family boundaries from the drug's known targets.

The 151 newly confirmed off-targets discovered in the large-scale SEA panel (e.g., black edges in Figure 2.2) had 247 drug–target–ADR (DTA) links that were significant via a guilt-by-association metric. For instance, diphenhydramine was found to the bind dopamine transporter (DAT). DAT is associated with tremor, a side effect of this drug, with an enrichment factor (ef) of 2.02 (e.g., red edges in Figure 2.2). Similarly, the mid-nanomolar activity of azatadine at the M1 muscarinic receptor is consistent with its "dry mouth" ADR (ef = 2.45). Likewise, "abdominal pain upper" has been reported for 22 COX-1 inhibitors. As an illustration of ef scoring, this ADR occurred 2045 times with all drugs, while COX-1 binding occurred in 976 target–ADR pairs together with other ADRs. Given a total of 237 342 target–ADR pairs, the ef score for the pair ("abdominal pain upper" with "COX-1 binding") was 9.35. Thus, the observed count of this target–ADR pair was nearly 10 times higher than expected by chance. The p-value was 3.9×10^{-26}, supporting a significant association between COX-1 binding and the "abdominal pain upper" ADR. Overall, 116 of the DTAs were stronger by these criteria than was any previously known target for the drug in question, and many seemed sensible.

Perhaps the most compelling demonstration, however, of a drug–antitarget–ADR association is one *in vivo* or in an accepted *in vivo* biomarker. We tested the hypothesis that chlorotrianisene's novel potent COX-1 inhibition (160 nM) might play a role in its "abdominal pain upper" (epigastralgia) side effect, measured by inhibition of platelet aggregation, a COX-1 therapeutic biomarker. This effect is unreported for other synthetic estrogens, which instead promote platelet aggregation. Accordingly, chlorotrianisene inhibited platelet aggregation in whole human blood with a potency nearly indistinguishable from that of indomethacin [11]. This combination of *in silico* off-target prediction with ef ADR calculations demonstrated the potential to make specific drug–target–ADR predictions that could be confirmed *in vitro* and *ex vivo.*

2.2.1.3 Finding Side Effects sans Targets

In silico methods predicting drug side effects absent explicit antitargets also exist; their orthogonal perspective complements the methods described so far. One major class of techniques endeavors to predict a target or compound's overall binding promiscuity. Studies correlating compound physical properties, such as lipophilicity or molecular weight, with promiscuity have yielded contradictory results [4] and quantitative structure–activity relationship (QSAR) methods fare little better [10]. Correspondingly, efforts now focus on chemical structure-based promiscuity models [101,112] or, pragmatically, direct analysis of high-throughput screening profiles [104].

In a unique twist, Bork and coworkers ignored physical and structural molecular properties, instead developing a predictive method relating drugs by similarities in their package inserts [113]. From the resulting ADR similarity networks, they predicted and confirmed 13 cases of drugs binding to new off-targets. In one, a subnetwork of central nervous system (CNS) drugs clustered with the antiulcer drug rabeprazole, a proton pump inhibitor. They consequently found that rabeprazole also bound directly to two CNS targets, the dopamine D_3 (1.6 μM) and 5-HT_{1D} (7.6 μM) receptors. As rabeprazole reaches micromolar concentrations in plasma, it may be worthwhile to evaluate it for nervous system side effects [113]. Thus, analyzing patterns in side effect labels revealed new antitarget–drug relationships.

2.2.2 Forward Perturbation and Prediction of Mechanisms

A comprehensive mechanistic understanding of the interacting pathways, timescales, hierarchies [10], and distributions of drug action has predominantly eluded pharmacology; correspondingly, it is the elucidation of these "multiscale mechanisms" [7] that forms the central challenge of today's systems pharmacology efforts. As intimated in the previous sections, the sheer quantity of data and attendant techniques now emerging both confound the endeavor even as they fundamentally enable it. Methods relating side effects to antitargets are often correlative, literature-, or consensus-based, with causation addressed on a case-by-case basis. Returning instead to a concrete biological foundation, high-content and phenotypic screens under guided chemical and genetic perturbation can constructively focus our scope of inquiry.

2.2.2.1 Forward Synthetic Behavior in Cell and Whole-Organism Model Systems

Even toxicological biomarkers under routine use in clinical settings, such as serum ALT, AST, and bilirubin for liver toxicity, are in many cases neither sufficiently organ specific nor predictive of clinical drug toxicity [10]. Yet we have little access to *in vivo* mechanistic data at the patient level to address this, and no capability to generate such data under conditions of forward chemical or genetic perturbation despite the urgent need. Model systems in whole organisms and cell cultures are a first approximation, and can reveal novel pharmacological mechanisms conserved across species [8,29]. By combining computation with direct screens on whole cells, tissues, and organisms, we are returning to the phenotypic roots of pharmacology [114,115], albeit on a larger and more systematic scale.

Quantitatively "Fingerprinting" Compounds by Phenotype

High-content screens (HCSs) in whole cells are a promising source of quantitative datasets as described in Section 2.1.2.2. Cellular toxicity screening historically relied on single-parameter readouts of markers such as proliferation, mitochondrial activity, and membrane permeability; however, their predictive applicability to *in vivo* compound toxicity has been relatively poor [116]. In contrast, HCS data enable multiplex analysis, wherein disparate responses may be measured within a single run and cellular context [117]. By incorporating a compound's simultaneous effects on multiple parameters, these assays can achieve a higher level of cytotoxicity predictability [116].

From a high-throughput HCS perspective, any complex phenotype in a cell might be represented by a sufficiently large set of simpler morphological readouts [118]. During a screen, each compound acquires a "fingerprint" reflecting the ways in which it perturbs a compound-naïve cellular morphological baseline. Davies and coworkers [118] review several studies examining small-molecule HCSs, although the readouts in question are mostly cell integrity and toxicity. Even given information-rich HCS compound fingerprints encoding morphological or fluorescent readouts, however, the route to identifying new molecular targets driving the readout, much less those driving the overarching phenotype, often remains unclear.

A way around this is to computationally analyze similarity patterns across compound HCS readouts. Mitchison and coworkers [119,120] showed that drugs with common targets could be clustered by the phenotypes they induce, using only HCS data and unsupervised clustering algorithms. Similarly, by fluorescently staining cell cycle markers and observing "profiles" (or fingerprints) of how these stains changed in the presence of compounds, Feng and coworkers [121] achieved compound clustering consistent with known structural and bioactivity properties. They then predicted and confirmed that α-tubulin was a molecular target in common for three staining-profile-similar yet structurally distinct molecules (colchicine, quinoline, and pseudolarix acid B). Both of these stories leveraged compound-by-compound phenotypic fingerprints to transfer a target already known to one compound to its cluster neighbors. This required that least one relevant molecular target be known to one of the compounds in question.

Direct Target Prediction and Forward Synthetic Behavior

Identifying the molecular targets responsible for phenotypes in HCS and whole-organism screens is a core challenge, but it is one that ligand-based target prediction may at least partially address. A phenotypic screen for compounds with CNS activity illustrates the approach. Atypical antipsychotics have complex pharmacological profiles that encompass multiple aminergic GPCRs [5]. As with the prediction of side effects, the design of polypharmacological drugs is challenging because classical *in vitro* medicinal chemistry high-throughput binding screens are subject to artifacts, whereas deep assays at individual purified targets rarely scale.

In an approach starting instead with phenotype, Peterson, Kokel, and coworkers [30] used zebrafish as a model organism to identify compounds modulating CNS behavior via readouts of a single phenotype over time: response to a light pulse stimulus. After clustering the observed behavioral time course into "fingerprints," Laggner, Kokel, and coworkers used SEA [23] to directly predict molecular targets, such as the Kv1.2 channel and the β adrenergic receptors, for compounds with behavioral fingerprints unrelated to those of any known drug in the collection. The target predictions were confirmed *in vitro* via human protein assays and also *in vivo*, by "phenocopying" the original behavior in the zebrafish with an orthogonal ligand known to the same target but of disparate chemical structure. The zebrafish–CNS compounds bound to their predicted human targets at mid-to-high-nanomolar affinity, although especially potent cases such as a 5 nM binder to the human dopamine D4 receptor also arose [28].

A question naturally arising from the zebrafish study, however, is how often human receptors share this degree of pharmacology with those of other organisms. Likewise, could one confirm compound phenocopy results with genetic inactivations at the same targets to induce a chemical-genetic version of "synthetic behaviors" [122]? Motivated by double-mutant analysis and the use of genetic interaction maps [123–125] linking genotype to phenotype [126], we computationally predicted human molecular targets for compounds found to elevate feeding rates in a *Caenorhabditis elegans* phenotypic screen [29]. What is particularly salient about the work is that, of the predictions confirmed *in vitro*, not only were all targets successfully "phenocopied" within the worm, but the phenocopy compounds' feeding phenotypes were also epistatic with those of matching genetic inactivations, consistent with a mechanistic role for each target in feeding. This yielded four pathways modulating worm feeding whose targets are also present in humans [29]; indeed, SEA predictions on human pharmacological data had been the bridge from uncharacterized compound to molecular target. Exemplifying the exploratory power of this chemocentric approach, one prediction led to the discovery that the previously uncharacterized gene *gnrr-1* encodes for a worm protein with ligand pharmacology analogous to that of the human oxytocin receptor [29].

Taken together, the studies in zebrafish and in worm illustrate how direct *in silico* target prediction using human pharmacology can not only bridge the gap between species, but also directly augment experimental approaches to yield novel compound mechanism of action hypotheses. Where the phenotypic readout is desirable, this aids in drug discovery; where it is undesirable, it may be used to understand and avoid drug adverse reactions.

2.2.2.2 The Road Ahead

The early techniques sketched here barely scratch the surface of a comprehensive attempt to predict even those adverse drug reactions that are mediated by specific antitargets. The endeavor starts with atomic and molecular interactions yet must proceed onward and up through expanding networks of increasingly complex biological components to achieve the prediction of whole-body outcomes directly relevant to patients (e.g., Figure 2.1). It is little surprise then that our most successful generalized techniques so far eschew a stepwise, much less causative, progression through the intermediate layers of biological organization between drug and outcome.

The staggering becomes more tractable, however, when we focus on the most characterized antitargets and adverse reactions, but even here much remains to be done, particularly in elucidating the interplay among combinations of antitargets. Furthermore, the underlying selection of antitargets, while guided by our best understanding and experience of drug action, is one that remains deeply unsettling from the systems perspective, blinkered as we may be by the vagaries of historical testing. Yet these prospects, which confound a single-target view of drug action, nonetheless motivate a systematic and computational approach to it.

The topologies of networks that we encounter at different levels of chemical and biological organization share many properties and are hearteningly robust to our imperfect representations of their constituents [22,127]. Techniques both new [88,128,129] and venerable [130,131] quantify signal flow in network processing and path discovery, to better inform our biological understanding now that we can pair it with sufficiently large computer-readable datasets. Using Bayesian inference, we may now train belief networks on unbiased biological data to link genotype to phenotype [132–134] and soon both to pharmacology [135]. Nor as we tread this path are we alone – quantitative systems pharmacology analyses draw on deep interrogations of network topology and statistical modeling already underway in computer science, artificial intelligence, transportation optimization, power distribution, web search prioritization, social media, and beyond. Ever as we do so, of course, we must anchor our models in sound chemical, biological, and pharmacological foundations, so it is opportune that these too have seen rapid growth in experimental scale and resolution [7,10]. Linked with new quantitative methods and data, it is perhaps time for predictive pharmacology to come of age.

References

1 Mestres, J., Gregori-Puigjane, E., Valverde, S., and Sole, R.V. (2008) Data completeness – the Achilles heel of drug–target networks. *Nature Biotechnology*, **26**, 983–984.

2 Garcia-Serna, R. and Mestres, J. (2011) Chemical probes for biological systems. *Drug Discovery Today*, **16**, 99–106.

3 Hu, Y. and Bajorath, J. (2013) How promiscuous are pharmaceutically relevant compounds? A data-driven assessment. *AAPS Journal*, **15**, 104–111.

4 Peters, J.-U. (2013) Polypharmacology – foe or friend? *Journal of Medicinal Chemistry*, **56**, 8955–8971.

5 Roth, B.L., Sheffler, D.J., and Kroeze, W.K. (2004) Magic shotguns versus magic bullets: selectively non-selective drugs for mood disorders and schizophrenia. *Nature Reviews. Drug Discovery*, **3**, 353–359.

6 Keith, C.T., Borisy, A.A., and Stockwell, B.R. (2005) Multicomponent therapeutics for networked systems. *Nature Reviews. Drug Discovery*, **4**, 71–78.

7 Zhao, S. and Iyengar, R. (2012) Systems pharmacology: network analysis to identify multiscale mechanisms of drug action. *Annual Review of Pharmacology and Toxicology*, **52**, 505–521.

8 Dar, A.C., Das, T.K., Shokat, K.M., and Cagan, R.L. (2012) Chemical genetic discovery of targets and anti-targets for cancer polypharmacology. *Nature*, **486**, 80–84.

9 Sorger, P.K., Allerheiligen, S.R.B., Abernethy, D.R., Altman, R.B., Brouwer, K.L.R., Califano, A., David, Z., Argenio, D., Iyengar, R., Jusko, W.J., Lalonde, R., Lauffenburger, D.A., Shoichet, B., Stevens, J.L., Subramaniam, S., Graaf, P.V.D., Ward, R., and Ma, B. (2011) Quantitative and systems pharmacology in the post-genomic era: new approaches to discovering drugs and understanding therapeutic mechanisms. An NIH White Paper by the QSP Workshop Group, October 2011, NIH White Paper 0-47.

10 Bai, J.P.F. and Abernethy, D.R. (2013) Systems pharmacology to predict drug toxicity: integration across levels of biological organization. *Annual Review of Pharmacology and Toxicology*, **53**, 451–473.

11 Lounkine, E., Keiser, M.J., Whitebread, S., Mikhailov, D., Hamon, J., Jenkins, J.L., Lavan, P., Weber, E., Doak, A.K., Cote, S., Shoichet, B.K., and Urban, L. (2012) Large-scale prediction and testing of drug activity on side-effect targets. *Nature*, **486**, 361–367.

12 Wishart, D.S., Knox, C., Guo, A.C., Cheng, D., Shrivastava, S., Tzur, D., Gautam, B., and Hassanali, M. (2008) DrugBank: a knowledgebase for drugs, drug actions and drug targets. *Nucleic Acids Research*, **36**, D901–D906.

13 Overington, J. (2009) ChEMBL. An interview with John Overington, team leader, chemogenomics at the European Bioinformatics Institute Outstation of the European Molecular Biology Laboratory (EMBL-EBI). Interview by Wendy A. Warr. *Journal of Computer-Aided Molecular Design*, **23**, 195–198.

14 Willett, P. (2005) Searching techniques for databases of two- and three-dimensional chemical structures. *Journal of Medicinal Chemistry*, **48**, 4183–4199.

15 Nidhi, Glick, M., Davies, J.W., and Jenkins, J.L. (2006) Prediction of biological targets for compounds using multiple-category Bayesian models trained on chemogenomics databases. *Journal of Chemical Information and Modeling*, **46**, 1124–1133.

16 Bender, A., Jenkins, J.L., Glick, M., Deng, Z., Nettles, J.H., and Davies, J.W. (2006) "Bayes affinity fingerprints" improve retrieval rates in virtual screening and define orthogonal bioactivity space: when are multitarget drugs a feasible concept? *Journal of Chemical Information and Modeling*, **46**, 2445–2456.

17 Steindl, T.M., Schuster, D., Laggner, C., and Langer, T. (2006) Parallel screening: a novel concept in pharmacophore modeling and virtual screening. *Journal of Chemical Information and Modeling*, **46**, 2146–2157.

18 Schuffenhauer, A., Floersheim, P., Acklin, P., and Jacoby, E. (2003) Similarity metrics for ligands reflecting the similarity of the target proteins. *Journal of Chemical Information and Computer Sciences*, **43**, 391–405.

19 Horvath, D. and Jeandenans, C. (2003) Neighborhood behavior of *in silico* structural spaces with respect to *in vitro* activity spaces – a novel understanding of the molecular similarity principle in the context of multiple receptor binding profiles. *Journal of Chemical Information and Computer Sciences*, **43**, 680–690.

20 Izrailev, S. and Farnum, M.A. (2004) Enzyme classification by ligand binding. *Proteins*, **57**, 711–724.

21 Keiser, M.J., Roth, B.L., Armbruster, B.N., Ernsberger, P., Irwin, J.J., and Shoichet, B.K. (2007) Relating protein

pharmacology by ligand chemistry. *Nature Biotechnology*, **25**, 197–206.

22 Hert, J., Keiser, M.J., Irwin, J.J., Oprea, T.I., and Shoichet, B.K. (2008) Quantifying the relationships among drug classes. *Journal of Chemical Information and Modeling*, **48**, 755–765.

23 Keiser, M.J., Setola, V., Irwin, J.J., Laggner, C., Abbas, A.I., Hufeisen, S.J., Jensen, N.H., Kuijer, M.B., Matos, R.C., Tran, T.B., Whaley, R., Glennon, R.A., Hert, J., Thomas, K.L., Edwards, D.D., Shoichet, B.K., and Roth, B.L. (2009) Predicting new molecular targets for known drugs. *Nature*, **462**, 175–181.

24 Fréchet, M. (1927) Sur la loi de probabilité de l'écart maximum. *Annales de la Société Polonaise de Mathématique*, **6**, 93–116.

25 Altschul, S.F., Madden, T.L., Schaffer, A.A., Zhang, J., Zhang, Z., Miller, W., and Lipman, D.J. (1997) Gapped BLAST and PSI-BLAST: a new generation of protein database search programs. *Nucleic Acids Research*, **25**, 3389–3402.

26 DeGraw, A.J., Keiser, M.J., Ochocki, J.D., Shoichet, B.K., and Distefano, M.D. (2010) Prediction and evaluation of protein farnesyltransferase inhibition by commercial drugs. *Journal of Medicinal Chemistry*, **53**, 2464–2471.

27 Yadav, P.N., Abbas, A.I., Farrell, M.S., Setola, V., Sciaky, N., Huang, X.P., Kroeze, W.K., Crawford, L.K., Piel, D.A., Keiser, M.J., Irwin, J.J., Shoichet, B.K., Deneris, E.S., Gingrich, J., Beck, S.G., and Roth, B.L. (2011) The presynaptic component of the serotonergic system is required for clozapine's efficacy. *Neuropsychopharmacology*, **36**, 638–651.

28 Laggner, C., Kokel, D., Setola, V., Tolia, A., Lin, H., Irwin, J.J., Keiser, M.J., Cheung, C.Y., Minor, D.L., Jr., Roth, B.L., Peterson, R.T., and Shoichet, B.K. (2012) Chemical informatics and target identification in a zebrafish phenotypic screen. *Nature Chemical Biology*, **8**, 144–146.

29 Lemieux, G.A., Keiser, M.J., Sassano, M.F., Laggner, C., Mayer, F., Bainton, R.J., Werb, Z., Roth, B.L., Shoichet, B.K., and Ashrafi, K. (2013) *In silico* molecular comparisons of *C. elegans* and mammalian pharmacology identify distinct targets that regulate feeding. *PLoS Biology*, **11**, e1001712.

30 Kokel, D., Bryan, J., Laggner, C., White, R., Cheung, C.Y., Mateus, R., Healey, D., Kim, S., Werdich, A.A., Haggarty, S.J., Macrae, C.A., Shoichet, B., and Peterson, R.T. (2010) Rapid behavior-based identification of neuroactive small molecules in the zebrafish. *Nature Chemical Biology*, **6**, 231–237.

31 Cherezov, V., Rosenbaum, D.M., Hanson, M.A., Rasmussen, S.G., Thian, F.S., Kobilka, T.S., Choi, H.J., Kuhn, P., Weis, W.I., Kobilka, B.K., and Stevens, R.C. (2007) High-resolution crystal structure of an engineered human β2-adrenergic G protein coupled receptor. *Science*, **318**, 1258–1265.

32 Kolb, P., Rosenbaum, D.M., Irwin, J.J., Fung, J.J., Kobilka, B.K., and Shoichet, B.K. (2009) Structure-based discovery of beta2-adrenergic receptor ligands. *Proceedings of the National Academy of Sciences of the United States of America*, **106**, 6843–6848.

33 Zhang, C., Srinivasan, Y., Arlow, D.H., Fung, J.J., Palmer, D., Zheng, Y., Green, H.F., Pandey, A., Dror, R.O., Shaw, D.E., Weis, W.I., Coughlin, S.R., and Kobilka, B.K. (2012) High-resolution crystal structure of human protease-activated receptor 1. *Nature*, **492**, 387–392.

34 Granier, S. and Kobilka, B. (2012) A new era of GPCR structural and chemical biology. *Nature Chemical Biology*, **8**, 670–673.

35 Granier, S., Manglik, A., Kruse, A.C., Kobilka, T.S., Thian, F.S., Weis, W.I., and Kobilka, B.K. (2012) Structure of the delta-opioid receptor bound to naltrindole. *Nature*, **485**, 400–404.

36 Shoichet, B.K. and Kobilka, B.K. (2012) Structure-based drug screening for G-protein-coupled receptors. *Trends in Pharmacological Sciences*, **33**, 268–272.

37 Kruse, A.C., Hu, J., Pan, A.C., Arlow, D.H., Rosenbaum, D.M., Rosemond, E., Green, H.F., Liu, T., Chae, P.S., Dror, R.O., Shaw, D.E., Weis, W.I., Wess, J., and Kobilka, B.K. (2012) Structure and dynamics of the M3 muscarinic

acetylcholine receptor. *Nature*, **482** 552–556.

38 Haga, K., Kruse, A.C., Asada, H., Yurugi-Kobayashi, T., Shiroishi, M., Zhang, C., Weis, W.I., Okada, T., Kobilka, B.K., Haga, T., and Kobayashi, T. (2012) Structure of the human M2 muscarinic acetylcholine receptor bound to an antagonist. *Nature*, **482**, 547–551.

39 Kruse, A.C., Ring, A.M., Manglik, A., Hu, J., Hu, K., Eitel, K., Hubner, H., Pardon, E., Valant, C., Sexton, P.M., Christopoulos, A., Felder, C.C., Gmeiner, P., Steyaert, J., Weis, W.I., Garcia, K.C., Wess, J., and Kobilka, B.K. (2013) Activation and allosteric modulation of a muscarinic acetylcholine receptor. *Nature*, **504**, 101–106.

40 Ring, A.M., Manglik, A., Kruse, A.C., Enos, M.D., Weis, W.I., Garcia, K.C., and Kobilka, B.K. (2013) Adrenaline-activated structure of beta2-adrenoceptor stabilized by an engineered nanobody. *Nature*, **502**, 575–579.

41 Kobilka, B. (2013) The structural basis of G-protein-coupled receptor signaling (Nobel Lecture). *Angewandte Chemie (International Edition in English)*, **52**, 6380–6388.

42 Shukla, A.K., Manglik, A., Kruse, A.C., Xiao, K., Reis, R.I., Tseng, W.C., Staus, D.P., Hilger, D., Uysal, S., Huang, L.Y., Paduch, M., Tripathi-Shukla, P., Koide, A., Koide, S., Weis, W.I., Kossiakoff, A.A., Kobilka, B.K., and Lefkowitz, R.J. (2013) Structure of active beta-arrestin-1 bound to a G-protein-coupled receptor phosphopeptide. *Nature*, **497**, 137–141.

43 Kellenberger, E., Muller, P., Schalon, C., Bret, G., Foata, N., and Rognan, D. (2006) sc-PDB: an annotated database of druggable binding sites from the Protein Data Bank. *Journal of Chemical Information and Modeling*, **46**, 717–727.

44 Shoichet, B.K., Stroud, R.M., Santi, D.V., Kuntz, I.D., and Perry, K.M. (1993) Structure-based discovery of inhibitors of thymidylate synthase. *Science*, **259**, 1445–1450.

45 Hermann, J.C., Ghanem, E., Li, Y., Raushel, F.M., Irwin, J.J., and Shoichet, B.K. (2006) Predicting substrates by docking high-energy intermediates to enzyme structures. *Journal of the American Chemical Society*, **128**, 15882–15891.

46 Jenwitheesuk, E., Horst, J.A., Rivas, K.L., Van Voorhis, W.C., and Samudrala, R. (2008) Novel paradigms for drug discovery: computational multitarget screening. *Trends in Pharmacological Sciences*, **29**, 62–71.

47 Carrieri, A., Perez-Nueno, V.I., Lentini, G., and Ritchie, D.W. (2013) Recent trends and future prospects in computational GPCR drug discovery: from virtual screening to polypharmacology. *Current Topics in Medicinal Chemistry*, **13**, 1069–1097.

48 Irwin, J.J., Shoichet, B.K., Mysinger, M.M., Huang, N., Colizzi, F., Wassam, P., and Cao, Y. (2009) Automated docking screens: a feasibility study. *Journal of Medicinal Chemistry*, **52**, 5712–5720.

49 Xie, L., Wang, J., and Bourne, P.E. (2007) *In silico* elucidation of the molecular mechanism defining the adverse effect of selective estrogen receptor modulators. *PLoS Computational Biology*, **3**, e217.

50 Kinnings, S.L., Liu, N., Buchmeier, N., Tonge, P.J., Xie, L., and Bourne, P.E. (2009) Drug discovery using chemical systems biology: repositioning the safe medicine Comtan to treat multi-drug and extensively drug resistant tuberculosis. *PLoS Computational Biology*, **5**, e1000423.

51 Rollinger, J.M., Schuster, D., Danzl, B., Schwaiger, S., Markt, P., Schmidtke, M., Gertsch, J., Raduner, S., Wolber, G., Langer, T., and Stuppner, H. (2009) *In silico* target fishing for rationalized ligand discovery exemplified on constituents of *Ruta graveolens*. *Planta Medica*, **75**, 195–204.

52 Aronov, A.M., Munagala, N.R., Kuntz, I.D., and Wang, C.C. (2001) Virtual screening of combinatorial libraries across a gene family: in search of inhibitors of *Giardia lamblia* guanine phosphoribosyltransferase. *Antimicrobial Agents and Chemotherapy*, **45**, 2571–2576.

53 Cai, J., Han, C., Hu, T., Zhang, J., Wu, D., Wang, F., Liu, Y., Ding, J., Chen, K., Yue, J., Shen, X., and Jiang, H. (2006) Peptide

deformylase is a potential target for anti-*Helicobacter pylori* drugs: reverse docking, enzymatic assay, and X-ray crystallography validation. *Protein Science*, **15**, 2071–2081.

54 Muller, P., Lena, G., Boilard, E., Bezzine, S., Lambeau, G., Guichard, G., and Rognan, D. (2006) *In silico*-guided target identification of a scaffold-focused library: 1,3,5-triazepan-2,6-diones as novel phospholipase A2 inhibitors. *Journal of Medicinal Chemistry*, **49**, 6768–6778.

55 Langer, T. and Hoffmann, R.D. (2001) Virtual screening: an effective tool for lead structure discovery? *Current Pharmaceutical Design*, **7**, 509–527.

56 Rella, M., Rushworth, C.A., Guy, J.L., Turner, A.J., Langer, T., and Jackson, R.M. (2006) Structure-based pharmacophore design and virtual screening for novel angiotensin converting enzyme 2 inhibitors. *Journal of Chemical Information and Modeling*, **46**, 708–716.

57 Eswar, N., John, B., Mirkovic, N., Fiser, A., Ilyin, V.A., Pieper, U., Stuart, A.C., Marti-Renom, M.A., Madhusudhan, M.S., Yerkovich, B., and Sali, A. (2003) Tools for comparative protein structure modeling and analysis. *Nucleic Acids Research*, **31**, 3375–3380.

58 Fan, H., Irwin, J.J., Webb, B.M., Klebe, G., Shoichet, B.K., and Sali, A. (2009) Molecular docking screens using comparative models of proteins. *Journal of Chemical Information and Modeling*, **49**, 2512–2527.

59 Pieper, U., Webb, B.M., Barkan, D.T., Schneidman-Duhovny, D., Schlessinger, A., Braberg, H., Yang, Z., Meng, E.C., Pettersen, E.F., Huang, C.C., Datta, R.S., Sampathkumar, P., Madhusudhan, M.S., Sjolander, K., Ferrin, T.E., Burley, S.K., and Sali, A. (2011) ModBase, a database of annotated comparative protein structure models, and associated resources. *Nucleic Acids Research*, **39**, D465–D474.

60 James, C., Weininger, D., and Delany, J. (1992–2005) *Daylight Theory Manual*, Daylight Chemical Information Systems, Inc., Mission Viejo, CA.

61 Fechner, U., Franke, L., Renner, S., Schneider, P., and Schneider, G. (2003) Comparison of correlation vector methods for ligand-based similarity searching. *Journal of Computer-Aided Molecular Design*, **17**, 687–698.

62 Schneider, G., Neidhart, W., Giller, T., and Schmid, G. (1999) "Scaffold-hopping" by topological pharmacophore search: a contribution to virtual screening. *Angewandte Chemie (International Edition in English)*, **38**, 2894–2896.

63 Rush, T.S., 3rd, Grant, J.A., Mosyak, L., and Nicholls, A. (2005) A shape-based 3-D scaffold hopping method and its application to a bacterial protein–protein interaction. *Journal of Medicinal Chemistry*, **48**, 1489–1495.

64 OpenEye Scientific Software (2004) ROCS (Rapid Overlay of Chemical Structures), version 2.0, OpenEye Scientific Software, Santa Fe, NM.

65 Jenkins, J.L., Glick, M., and Davies, J.W. (2004) A 3D similarity method for scaffold hopping from known drugs or natural ligands to new chemotypes. *Journal of Medicinal Chemistry*, **47**, 6144–6159.

66 Jain, A.N. (2000) Morphological similarity: a 3D molecular similarity method correlated with protein–ligand recognition. *Journal of Computer-Aided Molecular Design*, **14**, 199–213.

67 Kauvar, L.M., Higgins, D.L., Villar, H.O., Sportsman, J.R., Engqvist-Goldstein, A., Bukar, R., Bauer, K.E., Dilley, H., and Rocke, D.M. (1995) Predicting ligand binding to proteins by affinity fingerprinting. *Chemistry & Biology*, **2**, 107–118.

68 Willett, P. (1987) *Similarity and Clustering in Chemical Information Systems*, Research Studies Press/Wiley, Letchworth, UK, xii + 254 pp.

69 Brown, R.D. and Martin, Y.C. (1996) Use of structure–activity data to compare structure-based clustering methods and descriptors for use in compound selection. *Journal of Chemical Information and Computer Sciences*, **36**, 572–584.

70 Jaccard, P. (1901) Étude comparative de la distribution florale dans une portion

des Alpes et des Jura. *Bulletin de la Société Vaudoise des Sciences Naturelles*, **37**, 547–579.

71 Tversky, A. (1977) Features of similarity. *Psychological Reviews*, **84**, 327–352.

72 Durant, J.L., Leland, B.A., Henry, D.R., and Nourse, J.G. (2002) Reoptimization of MDL keys for use in drug discovery. *Journal of Chemical Information and Computer Sciences*, **42**, 1273–1280.

73 Hert, J., Willett, P., Wilton, D.J., Acklin, P., Azzaoui, K., Jacoby, E., and Schuffenhauer, A. (2004) Comparison of fingerprint-based methods for virtual screening using multiple bioactive reference structures. *Journal of Chemical Information and Computer Sciences*, **44**, 1177–1185.

74 Olah, M., Mracec, M., Ostopovici, L., Rad, R., Bora, N., Hadaruga, N., Olah, I., Banda, M., Simon, M., Mracec, T.I., and Oprea, T.I. (2004) WOMBAT: World of Molecular Bioactivity, in *Chemoinformatics in Drug Design* (ed. T.I. Oprea), Wiley-VCH Verlag GmbH, Weinheim, pp. 223–239.

75 Olah, M., Rad, R., Ostopovici, L., Bora, A., Hadaruga, N., Hadaruga, D., Moldovan, R., Fulias, A., Mracec, M., and Oprea, T.I. (2007) WOMBAT and WOMBAT-PK: bioactivity databases for lead and drug discovery, in *Chemical Biology: From Small Molecules to Systems Biology and Drug Design* (eds S.L. Schreiber, T.M. Kapoor, and G. Wess), Wiley-VCH Verlag GmbH, Weinheim, pp. 760–786.

76 Karr, J.R., Sanghvi, J.C., Macklin, D.N., Gutschow, M.V., Jacobs, J.M., Bolival, B., Jr., Assad-Garcia, N., Glass, J.I., and Covert, M.W. (2012) A whole-cell computational model predicts phenotype from genotype. *Cell*, **150**, 389–401.

77 Aithal, G.P., Day, C.P., Kesteven, P.J., and Daly, A.K. (1999) Association of polymorphisms in the cytochrome P450 CYP2C9 with warfarin dose requirement and risk of bleeding complications. *Lancet*, **353**, 717–719.

78 Ishikawa, T., Sekiguchi, F., Fukase, Y., Sawada, N., and Ishitsuka, H. (1998) Positive correlation between the efficacy of capecitabine and doxifluridine and the ratio of thymidine phosphorylase to dihydropyrimidine dehydrogenase activities in tumors in human cancer xenografts. *Cancer Research*, **58**, 685–690.

79 Amado, R.G., Wolf, M., Peeters, M., Van Cutsem, E., Siena, S., Freeman, D.J., Juan, T., Sikorski, R., Suggs, S., Radinsky, R., Patterson, S.D., and Chang, D.D. (2008) Wild-type KRAS is required for panitumumab efficacy in patients with metastatic colorectal cancer. *Journal of Clinical Oncology*, **26**, 1626–1634.

80 Rix, U., Remsing Rix, L.L., Terker, A.S., Fernbach, N.V., Hantschel, O., Planyavsky, M., Breitwieser, F.P., Herrmann, H., Colinge, J., Bennett, K.L., Augustin, M., Till, J.H., Heinrich, M.C., Valent, P., and Superti-Furga, G. (2010) A comprehensive target selectivity survey of the BCR-ABL kinase inhibitor INNO-406 by kinase profiling and chemical proteomics in chronic myeloid leukemia cells. *Leukemia*, **24**, 44–50.

81 Ji, Y., Hebbring, S., Zhu, H., Jenkins, G.D., Biernacka, J., Snyder, K., Drews, M., Fiehn, O., Zeng, Z., Schaid, D., Mrazek, D.A., Kaddurah-Daouk, R., and Weinshilboum, R.M. (2011) Glycine and a glycine dehydrogenase (GLDC) SNP as citalopram/escitalopram response biomarkers in depression: pharmacometabolomics-informed pharmacogenomics. *Clinical Pharmacology and Therapeutics*, **89**, 97–104.

82 Yerges-Armstrong, L.M., Ellero-Simatos, S., Georgiades, A., Zhu, H., Lewis, J.P., Horenstein, R.B., Beitelshees, A.L., Dane, A., Reijmers, T., Hankemeier, T., Fiehn, O., Shuldiner, A.R., and Kaddurah-Daouk, R. (2013) Purine pathway implicated in mechanism of resistance to aspirin therapy: pharmacometabolomics-informed pharmacogenomics. *Clinical Pharmacology and Therapeutics*, **94**, 525–532.

83 Davis, A.P., Wiegers, T.C., Roberts, P.M., King, B.L., Lay, J.M., Lennon-Hopkins, K., Sciaky, D., Johnson, R., Keating, H., Greene, N., Hernandez, R., McConnell, K.J., Enayetallah, A.E., and Mattingly, C.J. (2013) A CTD–Pfizer collaboration:

manual curation of 88 000 scientific articles text mined for drug–disease and drug–phenotype interactions. *Database: The Journal of Biological Databases and Curation*, **2013**, bat080–bat080.

84 Vastrik, I., D'Eustachio, P., Schmidt, E., Gopinath, G., Croft, D., de Bono, B., Gillespie, M., Jassal, B., Lewis, S., Matthews, L., Wu, G., Birney, E., and Stein, L. (2007) Reactome: a knowledge base of biologic pathways and processes. *Genome Biology*, **8**, R39.

85 Kanehisa, M. and Goto, S. (2000) KEGG: Kyoto Encyclopedia of Genes and Genomes. *Nucleic Acids Research*, **28**, 27–30.

86 Caspi, R., Altman, T., Dreher, K., Fulcher, C.A., Subhraveti, P., Keseler, I.M., Kothari, A., Krummenacker, M., Latendresse, M., Mueller, L.A., Ong, Q., Paley, S., Pujar, A., Shearer, A.G., Travers, M., Weerasinghe, D., Zhang, P., and Karp, P.D. (2012) The MetaCyc database of metabolic pathways and enzymes and the BioCyc collection of pathway/genome databases. *Nucleic Acids Research*, **40**, D742–D753.

87 Ashburner, M., Ball, C.A., Blake, J.A., Botstein, D., Butler, H., Cherry, J.M., Davis, A.P., Dolinski, K., Dwight, S.S., Eppig, J.T., Harris, M.A., Hill, D.P., Issel-Tarver, L., Kasarskis, A., Lewis, S., Matese, J.C., Richardson, J.E., Ringwald, M., Rubin, G.M., and Sherlock, G. (2000) Gene Ontology: tool for the unification of biology. The Gene Ontology Consortium. *Nature Genetics*, **25**, 25–29.

88 Berger, S.I., Ma'ayan, A., and Iyengar, R. (2010) Systems pharmacology of arrhythmias. *Science Signaling*, **3**, ra30.

89 Mason, D.A., Moore, J.D., Green, S.A., and Liggett, S.B. (1999) A gain-of-function polymorphism in a G-protein coupling domain of the human beta1-adrenergic receptor. *The Journal of Biological Chemistry*, **274**, 12670–12674.

90 Lamb, J., Crawford, E.D., Peck, D., Modell, J.W., Blat, I.C., Wrobel, M.J., Lerner, J., Brunet, J.P., Subramanian, A., Ross, K.N., Reich, M., Hieronymus, H., Wei, G., Armstrong, S.A., Haggarty, S.J., Clemons, P.A., Wei, R., Carr, S.A., Lander, E.S., and Golub, T.R. (2006) The Connectivity Map: using gene-expression signatures to connect small molecules, genes, and disease. *Science*, **313**, 1929–1935.

91 Scheiber, J., Chen, B., Milik, M., Sukuru, S.C., Bender, A., Mikhailov, D., Whitebread, S., Hamon, J., Azzaoui, K., Urban, L., Glick, M., Davies, J.W., and Jenkins, J.L. (2009) Gaining insight into off-target mediated effects of drug candidates with a comprehensive systems chemical biology analysis. *Journal of Chemical Information and Modeling*, **49**, 308–317.

92 Urban, L. (2012) Translational value of early target-based safety assessment and associated risk mitigation. 4th Annual Predictive Toxicology Summit, February 15–17, 2012, London.

93 Kuhn, M., Campillos, M., Letunic, I., Jensen, L.J., and Bork, P. (2010) A side effect resource to capture phenotypic effects of drugs. *Molecular Systems Biology*, **6**, 343.

94 US FDA (2014) Adverse Event Reporting System (AERS), US FDA, Silver Spring, MD.

95 Tatonetti, N.P., Ye, P.P., Daneshjou, R., and Altman, R.B. (2012) Data-driven prediction of drug effects and interactions. *Science Translational Medicine*, **4**, 125ra31.

96 White, R.W., Tatonetti, N.P., Shah, N.H., Altman, R.B., and Horvitz, E. (2013) Web-scale pharmacovigilance: listening to signals from the crowd. *Journal of the American Medical Informatics Association*, **20**, 404–408.

97 Thomas, K.L., Ellingrod, V.L., Bishop, J.R., and Keiser, M.J. (2010) A pilot study of the pharmacodynamic impact of SSRI drug selection and beta-1 receptor genotype (ADRB1) on cardiac vital signs in depressed patients: a novel pharmacogenetic approach. *Psychopharmacology Bulletin*, **43**, 11–22.

98 Ekins, S. (2004) Predicting undesirable drug interactions with promiscuous proteins *in silico*. *Drug Discovery Today*, **9**, 276–285.

99 Zakharov, A.V., Lagunin, A.A., Filimonov, D.A., and Poroikov, V.V. (2012) Quantitative prediction of

antitarget interaction profiles for chemical compounds. *Chemical Research in Toxicology*, **25**, 2378–2385.
100 Klabunde, T. and Evers, A. (2005) GPCR antitarget modeling: pharmacophore models for biogenic amine binding GPCRs to avoid GPCR-mediated side effects. *ChemBioChem*, **6**, 876–889.
101 Bender, A., Scheiber, J., Glick, M., Davies, J.W., Azzaoui, K., Hamon, J., Urban, L., Whitebread, S., and Jenkins, J.L. (2007) Analysis of pharmacology data and the prediction of adverse drug reactions and off-target effects from chemical structure. *ChemMedChem*, **2**, 861–873.
102 Scheiber, J. and Jenkins, J.L. (2009) Chemogenomic analysis of safety profiling data. *Methods in Molecular Biology*, **575**, 207–223.
103 Scheiber, J., Jenkins, J.L., Sukuru, S.C., Bender, A., Mikhailov, D., Milik, M., Azzaoui, K., Whitebread, S., Hamon, J., Urban, L., Glick, M., and Davies, J.W. (2009) Mapping adverse drug reactions in chemical space. *Journal of Medicinal Chemistry*, **52**, 3103–3107.
104 Azzaoui, K., Hamon, J., Faller, B., Whitebread, S., Jacoby, E., Bender, A., Jenkins, J.L., and Urban, L. (2007) Modeling promiscuity based on *in vitro* safety pharmacology profiling data. *ChemMedChem*, **2**, 874–880.
105 Rognan, D. (2010) Structure-based approaches to target fishing and ligand profiling. *Molecular Informatics*, **29**, 176–187.
106 Kitchen, D.B., Decornez, H., Furr, J.R., and Bajorath, J. (2004) Docking and scoring in virtual screening for drug discovery: methods and applications. *Nature Reviews. Drug Discovery*, **3**, 935–949.
107 Schmidtke, P., Le Guilloux, V., Maupetit, J., and Tuffery, P. (2010) fpocket: online tools for protein ensemble pocket detection and tracking. *Nucleic Acids Research*, **38**, W582–W589.
108 Ballester, P.J. and Mitchell, J.B. (2010) A machine learning approach to predicting protein–ligand binding affinity with applications to molecular docking. *Bioinformatics*, **26**, 1169–1175.
109 Chang, R.L., Xie, L., Xie, L., Bourne, P.E., and Palsson, B.O. (2010) Drug off-target effects predicted using structural analysis in the context of a metabolic network model. *PLoS Computational Biology*, **6**, e1000938.
110 Schneider, G. and Fechner, U. (2005) Computer-based *de novo* design of drug-like molecules. *Nature Reviews. Drug Discovery*, **4**, 649–663.
111 Bowes, J., Brown, A.J., Hamon, J., Jarolimek, W., Sridhar, A., Waldron, G., and Whitebread, S. (2012) Reducing safety-related drug attrition: the use of *in vitro* pharmacological profiling. *Nature Reviews. Drug Discovery*, **11**, 909–922.
112 Perez-Nueno, V.I. and Ritchie, D.W. (2012) Identifying and characterizing promiscuous targets: implications for virtual screening. *Expert Opinion on Drug Discovery*, **7**, 1–17.
113 Campillos, M., Kuhn, M., Gavin, A.C., Jensen, L.J., and Bork, P. (2008) Drug target identification using side-effect similarity. *Science*, **321**, 263–266.
114 Ahlquist, R.P. (1948) A study of the adrenotropic receptors. *The American Journal of Physiology*, **153**, 586–600.
115 Lands, A.M., Arnold, A., McAuliff, J.P., Luduena, F.P., and Brown, T.G., Jr. (1967) Differentiation of receptor systems activated by sympathomimetic amines. *Nature*, **214**, 597–598.
116 Rausch, O. (2006) High content cellular screening. *Current Opinion in Chemical Biology*, **10**, 316–320.
117 Korn, K. and Krausz, E. (2007) Cell-based high-content screening of small-molecule libraries. *Current Opinion in Chemical Biology*, **11**, 503–510.
118 Bender, A., Young, D.W., Jenkins, J.L., Serrano, M., Mikhailov, D., Clemons, P.A., and Davies, J.W. (2007) Chemogenomic data analysis: prediction of small-molecule targets and the advent of biological fingerprints. *Combinatorial Chemistry & High Throughput Screening*, **10**, 719–731.
119 Mitchison, T.J. (2005) Small-molecule screening and profiling by using automated microscopy. *ChemBioChem*, **6**, 33–39.

120 Perlman, Z.E., Slack, M.D., Feng, Y., Mitchison, T.J., Wu, L.F., and Altschuler, S.J. (2004) Multidimensional drug profiling by automated microscopy. *Science*, **306**, 1194–1198.

121 Young, D.W., Bender, A., Hoyt, J., McWhinnie, E., Chirn, G.W., Tao, C.Y., Tallarico, J.A., Labow, M., Jenkins, J.L., Mitchison, T.J., and Feng, Y. (2008) Integrating high-content screening and ligand–target prediction to identify mechanism of action. *Nature Chemical Biology*, **4**, 59–68.

122 Hopkins, A.L. (2012) Introduction: the case for polypharmacology, in *Polypharmacology in Drug Discovery* (ed. J.-U. Peters), John Wiley & Sons, Inc., Hoboken, NJ.

123 Kapitzky, L., Beltrao, P., Berens, T.J., Gassner, N., Zhou, C., Wüster, A., Wu, J., Babu, M.M., Elledge, S.J., Toczyski, D., Lokey, R.S., and Krogan, N.J. (2010) Cross-species chemogenomic profiling reveals evolutionarily conserved drug mode of action. *Molecular Systems Biology*, **6**, 451–1451.

124 Beltrao, P., Ryan, C., and Krogan, N.J. (2012) *Comparative Interaction Networks: Bridging Genotype to Phenotype*, vol. 751 (ed. O.S. Soyer), Springer, New York.

125 Roguev, A., Bandyopadhyay, S., Zofall, M., Zhang, K., Fischer, T., Collins, S.R., Qu, H., Shales, M., Park, H.O., Hayles, J., Hoe, K.L., Kim, D.U., Ideker, T., Grewal, S.I., Weissman, J.S., and Krogan, N.J. (2008) Conservation and rewiring of functional modules revealed by an epistasis map in fission yeast. *Science*, **322**, 405–410.

126 Fraser, J.S., Gross, J.D., and Krogan, N.J. (2013) From systems to structure: bridging networks and mechanism. *Molecular Cell*, **49**, 222–231.

127 Yildirim, M.A., Goh, K.I., Cusick, M.E., Barabasi, A.L., and Vidal, M. (2007) Drug–target network. *Nature Biotechnology*, **25**, 1119–1126.

128 Ma'ayan, A., Jenkins, S.L., Neves, S., Hasseldine, A., Grace, E., Dubin-Thaler, B., Eungdamrong, N.J., Weng, G., Ram, P.T., Rice, J.J., Kershenbaum, A., Stolovitzky, G.A., Blitzer, R.D., and Iyengar, R. (2005) Formation of regulatory patterns during signal propagation in a mammalian cellular network. *Science*, **309**, 1078–1083.

129 Maslov, S. and Sneppen, K. (2002) Specificity and stability in topology of protein networks. *Science*, **296**, 910–913.

130 Dijkstra, E.W. (1959) A note on two problems in connexion with graphs. *Numerische Mathematik*, **1**, 269–271.

131 Kruskal, J.B. (1956) On the shortest spanning subtree and the traveling salesman problem. *Proceedings of the American Mathematical Society*, **7**, 48–50.

132 Schadt, E.E., Lamb, J., Yang, X., Zhu, J., Edwards, S., Guhathakurta, D., Sieberts, S.K., Monks, S., Reitman, M., Zhang, C., Lum, P.Y., Leonardson, A., Thieringer, R., Metzger, J.M., Yang, L., Castle, J., Zhu, H., Kash, S.F., Drake, T.a., Sachs, A., and Lusis, A.J. (2005) An integrative genomics approach to infer causal associations between gene expression and disease. *Nature Genetics*, **37**, 710–717.

133 Chen, Y., Zhu, J., Lum, P.Y., Yang, X., Pinto, S., MacNeil, D.J., Zhang, C., Lamb, J., Edwards, S., Sieberts, S.K., Leonardson, A., Castellini, L.W., Wang, S., Champy, M.-F., Zhang, B., Emilsson, V., Doss, S., Ghazalpour, A., Horvath, S., Drake, T.a., Lusis, A.J., and Schadt, E.E. (2008) Variations in DNA elucidate molecular networks that cause disease. *Nature*, **452**, 429–435.

134 Schadt, E.E. (2009) Molecular networks as sensors and drivers of common human diseases. *Nature*, **461**, 218–223.

135 Schadt, E.E., Friend, S.H., and Shaywitz, D.A. (2009) A network view of disease and compound screening. *Nature Reviews. Drug Discovery*, **8**, 286–295.

3
Translational Value of Preclinical Safety Assessment: System Organ Class (SOC) Representation of Off-Targets

Mateusz Maciejewski, Eugen Lounkine, Andreas Hartmann, Steven Whitebread, and László Urbán

3.1
Introduction

Identification of targets associated with adverse reactions is an important element of drug discovery. Early safety assessment is largely based on finding "off-targets" that are hit by drug candidates [1,2]. These off-target effects can be mitigated by applying structure–activity relationship (SAR) methods during lead optimization to prevent the development of adverse drug reactions (ADRs) in the clinic. As described in Chapter 1, this involves profiling lead compounds at identified targets that are associated with specific ADRs. Although this process starts with a relatively simple and inexpensive *in vitro* profiling ("secondary pharmacology"), correct interpretation of the data is a major task and is often difficult. One essential factor in this process is the translation of simple biochemical or functional data into a prediction of adverse events. The first step requires integration of *in vitro* pharmacological data with physicochemical and ADME properties to understand the performance of the assays and assure the quality of the data [3]. Poor solubility and permeability could have a significant effect on assay performance, and the presence or absence of metabolizing enzymes might provide conflicting results. As the major role of early safety assessment is to predict side effects, pharmacokinetic/pharmacodynamic (PK/PD) evaluation is necessary for clinical interpretation [4]. Once these steps are completed, *in vivo* preclinical confirmation of the predictions can take place. In this chapter, we highlight the importance of correct translation of target-based ADR prediction into the clinical symptoms that are considered during preclinical and clinical regulatory and safety assessments. Thus, we explore the appropriate translation of mode of action (MoA) into symptoms classified in system organ class (SOC) [5]. First, we will address the necessary ontology to provide a solid basis for this concept.

Antitargets and Drug Safety, First Edition. Edited by László Urbán, Vinod F. Patel, and Roy J. Vaz.

3.2
Terminology: Medicinal Dictionary for Regulatory Activities (MedDRA)

> "In the late 1990s, the International Conference on Harmonisation of Technical Requirements for Registration of Pharmaceuticals for Human Use (ICH) developed MedDRA, a rich and highly specific standardised medical terminology to facilitate sharing of regulatory information internationally for medical products used by humans. ICH's powerful tool, MedDRA is available to all for use in the registration, documentation and safety monitoring of medical products both before and after a product has been authorised for sale. Products covered by the scope of MedDRA include pharmaceuticals, biologics, vaccines and drug–device combination products. Today, its growing use worldwide by regulatory authorities, pharmaceutical companies, clinical research organisations and health care professionals allows better global protection of patient health."[1)]

The above paragraph is the introduction taken from the ICH MedDRA website, which outlines the content and the aim of this broadly used dictionary. In short, it provides the ontology necessary for the evaluation of adverse reactions of drugs; it is searchable and allows grouping of medically meaningful terms to facilitate analysis of safety data.

MedDRA is well structured and identifies different levels of terminology that are arranged in a hierarchical manner. The highest level represents the SOCs, which closely represent medicinal disciplines and define organ-based classification of symptoms and biomarker behavior:

Blood and lymphatic system disorders
Cardiac disorders
Congenital, familial, and genetic disorders
Ear and labyrinth disorders
Endocrine disorders
Eye disorders
Gastrointestinal disorders
General disorders and administration site conditions
Hepatobiliary disorders
Immune system disorders
Infections and infestations
Injury, poisoning, and procedural complications
Investigations
Metabolism and nutrition disorders
Musculoskeletal and connective tissue disorders
Neoplasms benign, malignant, and unspecified (including cysts and polyps)

1) ICH MedDRA, http://www.meddra.org/how-to-use/support-documentation/english (last accessed August 7, 2014).

Nervous system disorders
Pregnancy, puerperium, and perinatal conditions
Psychiatric disorders
Renal and urinary disorders
Reproductive system and breast disorders
Respiratory, thoracic, and mediastinal disorders
Skin and subcutaneous tissue disorders
Surgical and medical procedures
Vascular disorders

When compounds are assessed for safety during the optimization phase of drug discovery, the panels of assays are selected to represent targets associated with ADRs assigned to SOCs. For example, targets known to be linked to any kind of hepatotoxicity would be uniformly listed under hepatobiliary disorders. The bile salt export pump (BSEP) is one of these targets, and its inhibition will trigger further exploration of hepatotoxicity [6]. This way, all targets can be associated with SOCs and a target–ADR network can be generated [7,8].

Figure 3.1 demonstrates target association with blood and lymphatic disorders. The color code represents whether the agonist (blue) or antagonist (red) modality would be responsible for the SOC effects. This level represents a broad selection of targets (see Figure 3.1 for details) that once hit could cause ADRs in a particular system organ class. The hierarchical structure of MedDRA allows further classification of target–ADR relationships at descending, more descriptive levels that provide means for better identification of side effects and dissection of targets within the same SOC.

The next level in MedDRA is the "High level group term" (HLGT), which refines ADR definition to disease groups. An example of this refinement is represented by "coagulopathies and bleeding diathesis," which is one of the HLGTs belonging to the "blood and lymphatic disorders" SOC (Figure 3.1). This level is more descriptive in terms of related pathomechanisms and streamlines the targets listed for the complete SOC. As such, it gives guidance in experimental design of safety pharmacology investigations toward a more defined mode of action. Many times targets associated with "High level group terms" and "High level terms" (here it is represented by coagulopathy alone) overlap, like in our example: KDR, P2RX1, PTGDR, and PTGER2.

The lowest level we consider for target–MedDRA term association is the "Preferred term" (PT) exemplified by "thrombotic microangiopathy." We demonstrate that the kinase insert domain receptor (KDR) is involved in this particular condition based on the clinical data obtained from the KDR kinase inhibitor monoclonal antibody (mAb), bevacizumab[2] [9], further confirmed by reports on small-molecule KDR inhibitors such as sunitinib [10] (Figure 3.2). It is relatively common that PTs are associated with multiple targets (see Figure 3.1). Most of

2) Bevacizumab (Avastin®), www.avastin.com/patient.

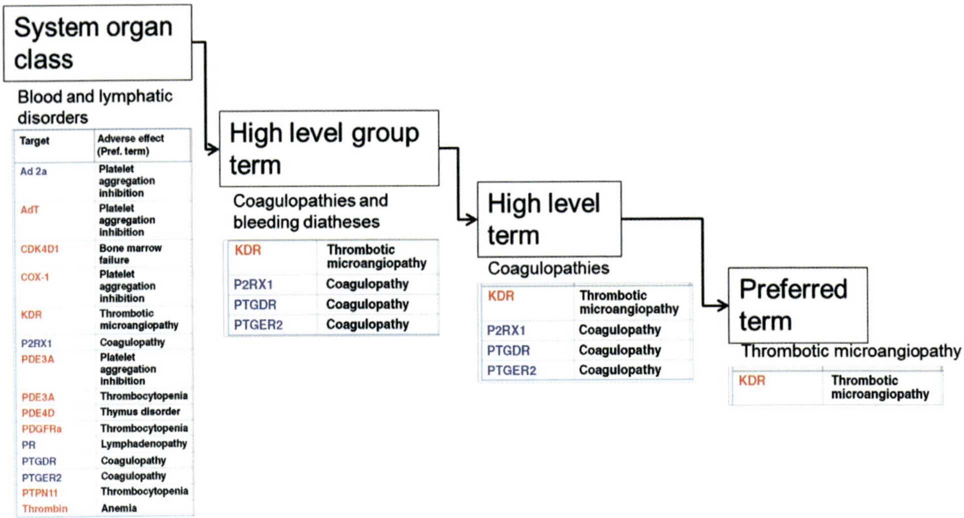

Figure 3.1 Targets associated with possible ADRs in a particular organ class. Classification provides clear guidance for downstream investigation of effects in the preclinical regulatory toxicology assessment. Red color represents antagonist effects and blue color represents agonist effects at the targets. Safety pharmacology and histopathology investigations should be focused on this organ class in case a drug candidate has high affinity to any of the listed targets. This approach can be used to speed up *in vivo* toxicology profiling (see the text for further details). Ad2a: adenosine 2A receptor; AdT: adenosine transporter; CDK4D1: cyclin-dependent kinase 4D1; COX-1: cyclooxygenase-1 enzyme; KDR (VEGFR): vascular endothelial growth factor; P2RX1: purinoceptor; PDE3A: phosphodiesterase-1 enzyme; PDE4D: phosphodiesterase 4D enzyme; PR: progesterone receptor; PTGDR: prostanoid, prostaglandin D_2 receptor; PTPN11: protein tyrosine phosphatase N11.

the well-documented target–ADR associations are supported by the FDA post-marketing Adverse Event Reporting System (FAERS).[3]

The lowest level of the MedDRA hierarchy is the "Lowest level term" (LLT), which represents highly specific adverse events. We do not consider this term in our target–ADR association terminology. The reason for this is the limited precision of target–ADR association, particularly when it is used for ADR prediction of a drug candidate at early stages of drug discovery.

3.2.1
Correct Use of MedDRA Terminology at Different Phases of Drug Discovery

It is imperative to match targets with the right terms in MedDRA. This is an important matter, as different terms at the same level of MedDRA are more appropriate to describe biological effects at various stages of drug discovery.

3) FAERS, http://www.fda.gov/Drugs/GuidanceComplianceRegulatoryInformation/Surveillance/AdverseDrugEffects/default.htm.

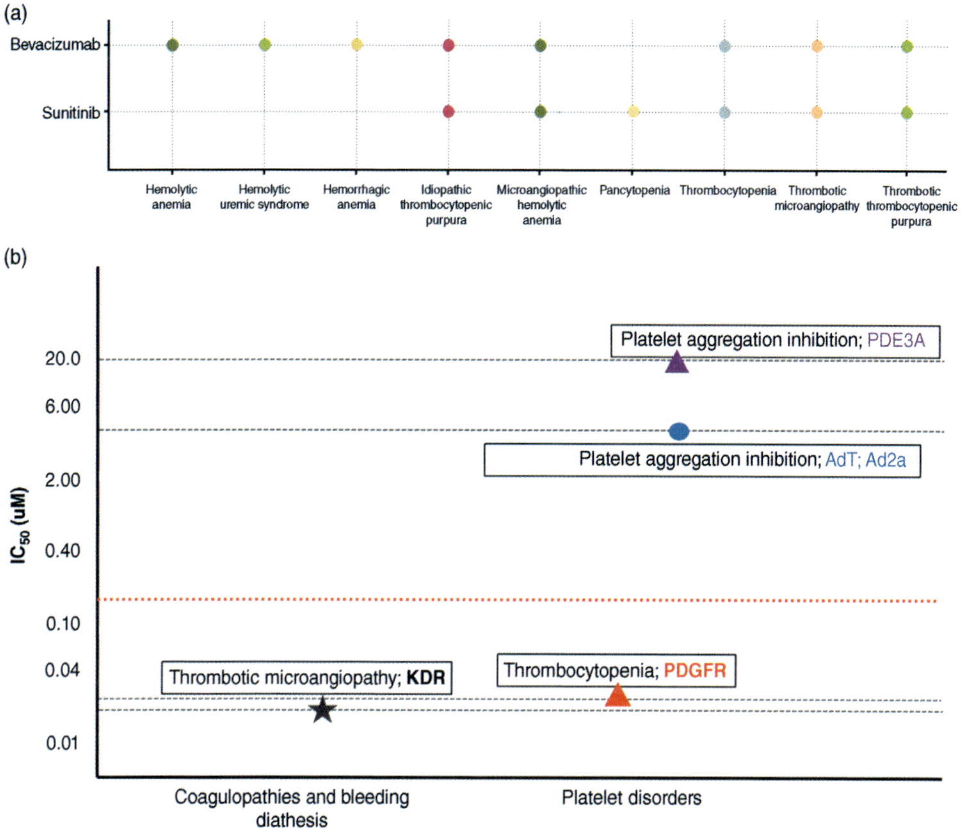

Figure 3.2 Association of ADRs with targets: reverse translation of side effects. Demonstration of "Preferred term" characteristics of two protein kinase inhibitors (both acting at the VEGFR), bevacizumab (mAb) and sunitinib (small-molecule inhibitor), in thrombotic angiopathy. (a) Postmarketing ADR profile of sunitinib and bevacizumab obtained from the FAERS. Note the significant overlap of ADRs recorded for the two drugs. Total number of case reports for bevacizumab is 30 748 and for sunitinib is 17 075. (b) Thrombotic angiopathic ADRs of sunitinib reported in FAERS (a) are linked to targets associated with these ADRs hit by sunitinib in the *in vitro* safety pharmacology assessment. The *y*-axis represents IC_{50} values for sunitinib at the targets. In addition to KDR, more target hits were discovered, which could further contribute to thrombotic diathesis (PDGFR: platelet-derived growth factor receptor; Ad2a: adenosine 2A receptor; AdT: adenosine transporter; KDR (VEGFR): vascular endothelial growth factor; PDE3A: phosphodiesterase-1 enzyme). However, with the exception of PDGFR, the potency of sunitinib at these targets was significantly less than the required therapeutic free plasma concentration measured at C_{max} (represented by the dotted red line).

MedDRA allows term selection and supports the flexibility required for this task. Use of terminology that is definitive in terms of clinical diagnosis might be unsuitable for early safety assessment, as the precision of prediction does not allow it (i.e., selection of PT, the lowest level in MedDRA) in the absence of any clinical data. For example, the PT positive or negative cardiac inotropy is a relevant marker of a predicted off-target effect, such as PDE3 inhibition [11,12]. However, at the stage of clinical candidate selection one would not use the term congestive heart failure, which could be exacerbated by blocking PDE3 and describes a well-defined diagnosis. Preference toward positive cardiac inotropic effect (increased contraction of cardiac muscle) versus exacerbation of congestive heart failure demonstrates that while PDE3 inhibition would in general increase cardiac inotropy with the possible outcome of worsening congestive heart failure, at the stage of early safety assessment only the hazard can be identified (positive inotropy) but not the level of risk, which needs the integration of PDE3 inhibition data with other characteristics of the drug candidate, including epidemiology of the targeted patient population. Therefore, in our evaluation we distinguish between biological effects and clinical phenotype. The effects of PDE3 inhibition (e.g., the therapeutic target of milrinone [13]) could be explained as positive inotropy (biological effect), which could contribute to the acceleration of congestive heart failure, or contribute to its development at an effective concentration (clinical phenotype). In this case, the consensus PT is positive inotropy. On the other hand, in some cases a concrete disease should be used as the preferred term, such as cardiac valvulopathy in conjunction with the agonist effects of drugs at the 5-HT_{2B} receptor [14]. In this case, the biological effect is fibrosis, which would affect several organs, in particular any serous membranes, and produce adhesions. However, the major risk is the development of cardiac valve enlargement and rigidity, which makes the valves dysfunctional [14]. Here, we use the life-threatening condition as the PT that directly led to withdrawal of several drugs[4),5)] from the market.

3.2.2
Determination of Symptoms Associated with a Target

A single off-target may produce various effects in different organs, as we discussed earlier for 5-HT_{2B} agonism. It is well recognized that the major effect is cardiac valvular disease, but it is less obvious that serous membrane adhesions will significantly enhance the incidence of pleurisy and abdominal pain (Table 3.1). It is common that the same biological effect initiated or supported with the activation, inactivation, or modulation of a target manifests in different phenotype, depending on the cell type. Antihistamines will produce anti-allergic effects in the periphery, while they are associated with somnolence and dizziness in the central nervous system (CNS) [15], as briefly discussed in Chapter 1.

Figure 3.3 demonstrates the effects of 5-HT_3 channel (and the endothelin-1 receptor) activation and antagonism as it translates to various phenotypes in

4) http://www.fda.gov/Drugs/DrugSafety/PostmarketDrugSafetyInformationforPatientsandProviders/ucm179871.htm.

5) http://www.fda.gov/Drugs/DrugSafety/PostmarketDrugSafetyInformationforPatientsandProviders/ucm143341.htm.

Table 3.1 Transformation of an antitarget effect into clinical phenotype determined by organ class: demonstration of different effects of 5-HT_{2B} activation in various organs and associated ADRs.

Target	Molecular effect (pharmacology)	Pathway	Pathological effect	ADR phenotype by SOC
5-HT_{2B}	Receptor activation	Fibroblast proliferation and transformation (fibrosis)	Adhesion of serous membranes	Pleurisy, abdominal pain
5-HT_{2B}	Receptor activation	Fibroblast proliferation and transformation (fibrosis)	Deformation of cardiac valves	Cardiac valvular disease

The same molecular effect within the same pathway causes different pathologies in the peritoneum and pleura than in the cardiac valve, with distinct clinical phenotypes.

different organs. Adverse reactions also depend on the modality of the target effect, as demonstrated by 5-HT_3. Activation of the 5-HT_3 channel is associated with tachycardia in the heart [16] and nausea/vomiting in the gastrointestinal (GI) system [17]. On the other hand, antagonists would not have any serious effect on the 5-HT_3 channels in the heart, but could cause ischemic colitis, constipation, and associated abdominal discomfort in the GI tract [18]. Furthermore, headache and dizziness would be the result of antagonist effect in the

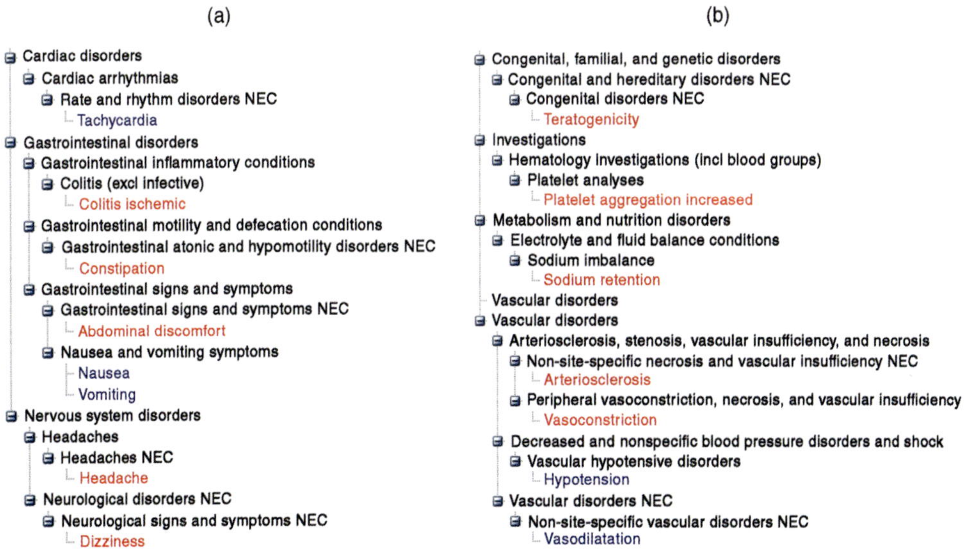

Figure 3.3 MedDRA terms associated with activation or inhibition of the 5-HT_3 ion channel (a) and endothelin-A receptor (b). These examples demonstrate the variety of SOC representation of a single target. Also, the importance of modality of the interaction with the targets is highlighted. Red color represents antagonist effects and blue color represents agonist effects at the "preferred term" level.

CNS [16]. This case demonstrates the diversity of side effects associated with a single off-target unintended for a particular indication. *In vivo* safety pharmacology studies can be employed downstream to further investigate if any of the above-mentioned phenotypes would manifest close to the clinical conditions. A more complex picture could develop with pharmacologically promiscuous compounds, when several off-targets are hit, and their coexpression in various organs could be synergistic or antagonistic as well. This aspect can be easily revealed by applying *in vitro* pharmacological profiling [1,2] and *in silico* methods [5] that identify off-targets. Once this has been established, one can look up the associated ADRs at the SOC level. Figure 3.2 gives an example of the application of this method. Sunitinib, a nonselective protein kinase inhibitor used for the indication of renal and gastrointestinal solid tumors (GISTs), hits many kinase and non-kinase targets, including vascular endothelial growth factor receptor 1–3 (VEGFR1–3), platelet-derived growth factor receptor (PDGFR), and c-KIT and RET proto-oncogenes, which are linked to increase in blood pressure and decreased left ventricular ejection fraction [19]. It is likely that these targets, when inhibited, all contribute to the observed ADRs to a different extent. Mice undergoing sunitinib treatment suffered the same conditions with supporting histopathology of mitochondrial injury and cardiomyocyte apoptosis [20]. Verapamil, on the other hand, blocks both hERG and L-type calcium channels, which have opposite effects in the generation of cardiomyocyte action potentials. Thus, the Ca current will neutralize the hERG-induced rapid delayed rectifier current (I_{Kr}) and prevents prolongation of the action potential depolarization and triangulation [21].

The same off-target molecule could be linked differently to other targets or participate in different pathways, and could be further modified by changes in pathways during pathological conditions. It is well documented that hERG inhibition in diabetic patients is more likely to increase the incidence of arrhythmias [22]. Clinical data support that the "Parkinsonian heart" is more susceptible for 5-HT_{2B} agonist-induced cardiac valvular disease than a healthy heart [23].

3.3 Data Interpretation: Modifying Factors

3.3.1 Access to Organs

When off-targets associated with clinical candidates are linked with organ-specific ADRs, one has to consider access to the specific organ. This can be influenced by physiological/physical barriers or by organ-specific targets. The barrier effect is most obvious with the CNS targets, as mentioned previously, in conjunction with neurological effects of antihistamines [15]. In general, tissue distribution of drugs is influenced by their water or lipid solubility. The route of administration can also alter access of a drug to different organs. In case of drugs applied by inhalation or by ocular application, the local therapeutic concentration may be achieved without significant systemic exposure.

Prediction of side effects should be reconsidered under these conditions and the risk assessment needs to be adjusted accordingly. In this approach, however, off-target effects might also be enhanced in the target organ (e.g., allergic skin reactions to ointments).

Conversely, some drugs accumulate in specific organs, which may provide an advantage, and hence tools are used to increase accumulation in particular tissues for better therapeutic benefit and less exposure to other organs where the drug may cause harm. Best examples are isotope-labeled ligands, which damage cells in an organ-specific manner [24].

3.3.2
Off-Target Promiscuity: Target Interactions (Synergies and Antagonism)

Compounds that engage in multiple potent off-target interactions are likely to have more effects, thus more ADRs. When the off-target effects manifest in the same organ, they can either synergize or antagonize with each other. This can significantly modify the ADRs, by either reducing or eliminating them, as we saw in the case of verapamil, when the hERG and Ca channel effects basically neutralized their individual effects [21], or enhance the development of the adverse reaction by their effect on a particular pathway. The latter can happen when 5-HT_{2B} activation and the activation of the serotonin transporter (SERT) are off-target effects for the same drug, as in the case of norfenfluramine [25].

It is also important to emphasize that the same targets will represent diverse effects in different organs. Thus, once an off-target hit is identified, safety pharmacology observations should consider this aspect. For example, VMAT-2 inhibition could manifest in hypotension, tremor, suicidal ideation, and depression.

3.4
Conclusions

As we presented in this chapter, association of targets with ADRs by SOC classification is of high importance in preclinical drug discovery for several reasons. First, this method will provide a uniform ontology for identifying target–ADR associations with well-defined clinical relevance, which provides a safety hazard signal, and can guide the design of safety pharmacology experiments to focus on confirmation/rejection of phenotypic translation of the detected off-target effect. Therefore, careful selection of terms is important for appropriate guidance and risk prediction. Overemphasizing clinical symptoms and diseases associated with off-target effects in the absence of clinical data is of no benefit and could lead to inappropriate, overreactive preclinical and clinical safety assessment. In short, the approach that we outlined provides a "handshake" between early safety assessment and preclinical safety investigations, using the MedDRA terminology as the essential element.

Clarity of ADR predictions also guides decision making for mitigation processes. ADRs that are tolerated within a defined indication should not trigger extensive efforts to modify the structure of compounds that are already well optimized for their intended therapeutic effect. On the other hand, off-targets that are associated with life-threatening effects need to be strongly mitigated, and their safety window should be calculated prior to clinical trials.

We have demonstrated a practical approach that allows establishing a link between targets (off-targets) and MedDRA terms in SOC with the consideration of therapeutic concentrations of the selected drug. Integration of these data provides a high confidence in predicting side effects when a particular off-target is affected by a drug candidate; hence, it can aid mitigation of off-targets and selection of the right clinical candidate.

References

1 Bowes, J., Brown, A.J., Hamon, J., Jarolimek, W., Sridhar, A., Waldron, G., and Whitebread, S. (2012) Reducing safety-related drug attrition: the use of *in vitro* pharmacological profiling. *Nature Reviews. Drug Discovery*, **11**, 909–922.

2 Whitebread, S., Hamon, J., Bojanic, D., and Urban, L. (2005) *In vitro* safety pharmacology profiling: an essential tool for drug development. *Drug Discovery Today*, **10**, 1421–1433.

3 Urban, L., Valentin, J.-P., Kaitin, K.I., and Wang, J. (2014) Current social, clinical, and scientific environment of pharmaceutical R&D, in *Predictive ADMET: Integrated Approaches in Drug Discovery and Development* (eds J. Wang and L. Urban), John Wiley & Sons, Inc., Hoboken, NJ.

4 Muller, P.Y. and Milton, M.N. (2012) The determination and interpretation of the therapeutic index in drug development. *Nature Reviews. Drug Discovery*, **11**, 751–761.

5 Urban, L., Maciejewski, M., Lounkine, L., Whitebread, S., Jenkins, J.L., Hamon, J., Fekete, A., and Muller, P.Y. (2014) Translation of off-target effects: prediction of ADRs by integrated experimental and computational approach. *Toxicology Research*. doi: 10.1039/C4TX00077C.

6 Dawson, S., Stahl, S., Paul, N., Barber, J., and Kenna, J.G. (2012) *In vitro* inhibition of the bile salt export pump correlates with risk of cholestatic drug-induced liver injury in humans. *Drug Metabolism and Disposition*, **40**, 130–138.

7 Csermely, P., Korcsmáros, T., Kiss, H.J., London, G., and Nussinov, R. (2013) Structure and dynamics of molecular networks: a novel paradigm of drug discovery. A comprehensive review. *Pharmacology & Therapeutics*, **138**, 333–408.

8 Kuhn, M., Campillos, M., Letunic, I., Jensen, L.J., and Bork, P. (2010) A side effect resource to capture phenotypic effects of drugs. *Molecular Systems Biology*, **6**, 343.

9 Eremina, V., Jefferson, J.A., Kowalewska, J., Hochster, H., Haas, M., Weisstuch, J., Richardson, C., Kopp, J.B., Kabir, M.G., Backx, P.H., Gerber, H.P., Ferrara, N., Barisoni, L., Alpers, C.E., and Quaggin, S.E. (2008) VEGF inhibition and renal thrombotic microangiopathy. *The New England Journal of Medicine*, **358**, 1129–1136.

10 Buckley, F.D., Preston, G., Meiklejohn, D.J., and Adamson, D. (2014) Sunitinib-associated thrombotic microangiopathy: a significant risk. *Clinical Oncology*, **26**, 515.

11 Smith, C.J., Huang, R., Sun, D., Ricketts, S., Hoegler, C., Ding, J.Z., Moggio, R.A., and Hintze, T.H. (1997) Development of decompensated dilated cardiomyopathy is associated with decreased gene expression and activity of the milrinone-sensitive cAMP phosphodiesterase PDE3A. *Circulation*, **96**, 3116–3123.

12 Thompson, P.E., Manganiello, V., and Degerman, E. (2007) Re-discovering PDE3 inhibitors – new opportunities for a long neglected target. *Current Topics in Medicinal Chemistry*, 7, 421–436.

13 Hilleman, D.E. and Forbes, W.P. (1989) Role of milrinone in the management of congestive heart failure. *DICP*, **23**, 357–362.

14 Roth, B.L. (2007) Drugs and valvular heart disease. *The New England Journal of Medicine*, **356**, 6–9.

15 Kalpaklioglu, F. and Baccioglu, A. (2012) Efficacy and safety of H1-antihistamines: an update. *Anti-Inflammatory & Anti-Allergy Agents in Medicinal Chemistry*, **11**, 230–237.

16 Goodin, S. and Cunningham, R. (2002) 5-HT_3-receptor antagonists for the treatment of nausea and vomiting: a reappraisal of their side effect profile. *The Oncologist*, 7, 424–436.

17 Chandrakala, R., Vijayashankara, K., Kumar, K.K., and Sarala, N. (2008) Ondansetron induced fatal ventricular tachycardia. *Indian Journal of Pharmacology*, **40**, 186–187.

18 Fayyaz, M. and Lackner, J.M. (2008) Serotonin receptor modulators in the treatment of irritable bowel syndrome. *Journal of Therapeutics and Clinical Risk Management*, **4**, 41–48.

19 Chu, T.F., Rupnick, M.A., Kerkela, R., Dallabrida, S.M. *et al.* (2007) Cardiotoxicity associated with sunitinib. *Lancet*, **370**, 2011–2019.

20 Harris, K., Aylott, M., Cui, Y., Louttit, J.B., McMahon, N.C., and Sridhar, A. (2013) Comparison of electrophysiological data from human-induced pluripotent stem cell-derived cardiomyocytes to functional preclinical safety assays. *Toxicological Sciences*, **134**, 412–426.

21 Honda, M., Kiyokawa, J., Tabo, M., and Inoue, T. (2011) Electrophysiological characterization of cardiomyocytes derived from human induced pluripotent stem cells. *Journal of Pharmacological Sciences*, **117**, 149–159.

22 Hreiche, R., Plante, I., David, L.P., Simard, C., Turgeon, J., and Drolet, B. (2009) Impact of glucose concentration on cardiac ventricular repolarization under I_{Kr}/I_{Ks} blocking agents. *Journal of Molecular and Cellular Cardiology*, **47**, 210–220.

23 Iodice, V., Low, D.A., Vichayanrat, E., and Mathias, C.J. (2011) Cardiovascular autonomic dysfunction in MSA and Parkinson's disease: similarities and differences. *Journal of the Neurological Sciences*, **310**, 133–138.

24 Pacini, F., Brilli, L., and Marchisotta, S. (2009) Targeted therapy in radioiodine refractory thyroid cancer. *Quarterly Journal of Nuclear Medicine and Molecular Imaging*, **53**, 520–525.

25 Rothman, R.B. and Baumann, M.H. (2002) Therapeutic and adverse actions of serotonin transporter substrates. *Pharmacology & Therapeutics*, **95**, 73–88.

4
Pathological Conditions Associated with the Disturbance of the 5-HT System

Daniel Hoyer

4.1
Introduction

Epidemics of ergotism since the Middle Ages have killed thousands of people and mutilated many more, centuries before serotonin and its receptors and transporters were identified. Ergot alkaloids were responsible for these horrible mutilations and deaths, mediated primarily but not exclusively by 5-hydroxytryptamine (5-HT) receptors, located both in vascular beds in limbs and more centrally. In the early twentieth century, chemists such as Stoll and Hofmann at Sandoz in Basel isolated ergots and synthesized natural and new ergot alkaloids and peptides, including LSD, and this was the beginning of the rich and complex 5-HT pharmacology. About 95% of 5-HT (serotonin) is produced in the gut, in intestinal enterochromaffin cells; in the brain, the raphe nuclei are the principal source of 5-HT. 5-HT and its receptors/transporters [1–5] represent one of the most complex neurotransmitter systems that is targeted by many successful drugs. As such the field has also seen a number of major market withdrawals, starting with LSD, which in the 1960s was developed for the treatment of psychosis/schizophrenia, and was withdrawn due to its prominent hallucinogenic effects [4,6–8]. 5-HT acts on several classes of targets such as G-protein-coupled receptors (GPCRs; 5-HT_{1-7} receptor families, except 5-HT_3), ligand-gated ion channels (5-HT_3 receptor family), and transporters (5-HT transporter). With the subtypes, there are about 15 different receptors, many of which are the targets of drugs. The 5-HT transporter is targeted by the SSRIs (selective serotonin reuptake inhibitors), an important class of antidepressants as well as other less selective drugs (tricyclics and tetracyclics), and several amphetamine-like releasers that were used to treat obesity. The metabolizing enzymes monoamine oxidases A and B (MAO A and B) are the targets of old antidepressant, known as MAO inhibitors. The 5-HT system represents a complex set of targets for which many drugs have been developed, and this chapter will only skim the surface of the numerous compounds, whether they are marketed, have been withdrawn, or are very close to registration. There are five receptor subtypes in the 5-HT_1 receptor family: 5-HT_{1A} agonists are generally anxiolytics/antidepressants,

Antitargets and Drug Safety, First Edition. Edited by László Urbán, Vinod F. Patel, and Roy J. Vaz.

although some newer additions include antipsychotics that have 5-HT_{1A} activity. 5-$HT_{1B/1D}$ agonists represent another breakthrough class of antimigraine compounds: the triptans, of which sumatriptan was the first in class. The triptans are generally well tolerated, although caution needs to be used in patients with coronary diseases, as vasoconstriction can become prominent and the combination triptans/SSRIs is not recommended due to a risk of 5-HT syndrome. There is no 5-HT_{1E} or 5-HT_{1F} ligand on the market, although 5-HT_{1F} receptors had been targeted for the treatment of migraine. There are three subtypes of 5-HT_2 receptors: 5-HT_{2A} antagonism is present in a number of antipsychotics, the most prominent being clozapine, which was the first and still is the most efficacious atypical antipsychotic. Clozapine was temporarily withdrawn from the market due to agranulocytosis, which can be fatal, but is reversible in most cases. Clozapine, thanks to a couple of prominent clinicians, made it back to the market for a specific population of patients: blood cell counts must be monitored closely. Agranulocytosis is not a class effect, as it is not shared by any other 5-HT_2 antagonist and/or antipsychotic. What is, however, prominent with a number of antipsychotics, including olanzapine, risperidone, and others, is weight gain and the risk of type 2 diabetes, which limits the use of many of these antipsychotics. The 5-HT_{2A} receptor is the target of another class of drugs, such as LSD, psilocybin, mescaline, or DOI, all of which produce prominent hallucinations. On the other hand, a few compounds, which have also 5-HT_{2A} affinity (e.g., lisuride), lack the hallucinogenic component; this peculiarity is explained by what is now known as biased signaling. The 5-HT_{2B} receptor is not voluntarily targeted by established drugs; however, different classes of compounds display 5-HT_{2B} receptor agonism, which results in cardiac regurgitation, valvulopathies, and pulmonary hypertension. These effects are common to some 5-HT releasers such as fenfluramine, dexfenfluramine, benfluorex, and their active metabolite norfenfluramine (all used as appetite suppressants and eventually withdrawn from the different markets between 1997 and 2009 for the latter). MDMA (ecstasy) also shares this property, as well as some antiparkinsonian and/or anti-prolactin principles such as pergolide or cabergoline, which have eventually also been withdrawn or have a very strong black box labeling, respectively. Finally, some ergolines such as ergotamine or DHE display some level of 5-HT_{2B} agonism and should be used with caution. A few drugs have also 5-HT_{2B} agonism (e.g., lisuride), but lack the cardiac component; this peculiarity is explained by what is now known as biased signaling (a progress made possible by the crystallization of the 5-HT_{2B} receptor and the new insight into structure biology). The 5-HT_{2C} receptor is the target of many drugs, including the fenfluramine-like compounds, and there is little evidence for adverse events; the latest addition is lorcaserin, a 5-HT_{2C} agonist developed to treat obesity.

5-HT_3 receptors are ligand-gated channels (five subtypes, but the most prominent target is the 5-$HT_{3A/3B}$ heteropentamer). 5-HT_3 receptor antagonists such as ondansetron, tropisetron, and granisetron have been originally developed for the treatment of chemotherapy-induced emesis, and as such represented a paradigm shift in accompanying the treatment of a number of cancers. One of the prominent side effects of 5-HT_3 receptor antagonists is constipation, which was specifically targeted with alosetron for the treatment of IBS (irritable bowel syndrome) with diarrhea; after a number of serious adverse events due to occlusion, alosetron was withdrawn from the market but eventually reintroduced with a severe warning (black box): the compound can only be prescribed for IBS with diarrhea in a specific female patient population, and is clearly contraindicated in IBS with constipation.

The 5-HT_4 receptor was a very promising target also for the treatment of IBS with constipation. Tegaserod was developed as a 5-HT_4 agonist, since it increases transit in the gut; as such 5-HT_4 agonists have a major side effect that is diarrhea; however, tegaserod had apparently produced a number of cardiac events and deaths and thus was withdrawn from the market. The compound is still available for compassionate use, although the cause of the side effects was never established; it does not seem to be a class effect, as other 5-HT_4 agonists are safe (except for diarrhea). Another 5-HT_4 agonist, cisapride, had previously been withdrawn; it was used for similar indications, but had a marked arrhythmogenic (QTc) effect. There is no 5-HT_5 or 5-HT_6 ligand on the market, although a number of antidepressants or antipsychotics have 5-HT_6 antagonism. There is no selective 5-HT_7 ligand in the clinic; however, there are a number of antipsychotics and antidepressants with 5-HT_7 antagonism, such as asenapine, amisulpride, lurasidone, and the recently approved vortioxetine. Finally, the 5-HT transporter is the target of many antidepressants, the best known being fluoxetine, but there are many others such as citalopram, paroxetine, and escitalopram, collectively known as the SSRIs, some NA/5-HT uptake blockers (SNRIs) such as reboxetine, and still the older tricyclic antidepressants that target the DA transporter as well. The major issue with SSRIs is their use in adolescents: there is a strong warning that such drugs may trigger suicidal ideations and eventually suicide. Another issue with SSRIs is their combination with triptans that may result in exacerbation of the 5-HT syndrome. The 5-HT transporter was also the target of fenfluramine and related compounds that were used as appetite suppressants, but had to be withdrawn because of off-target activity at the 5-HT_{2B} receptor leading to valvulopathies and death; the same applies to ecstasy (MDMA).

4.2 From "St. Anthony's Fire" to Ergot Alkaloids, the Serotonin Syndrome, and Modern 5-HT Pharmacology

Ergot alkaloids represent the basis of modern 5-HT chemistry and pharmacology: when Sandoz decided to enter the pharmaceutical field, Stoll and Hofmann started working on mainly natural compounds, including these alkaloids [7,9–11]. In 1918, Stoll isolated ergotamine, the first chemically pure ergot alkaloid, which found widespread therapeutic use in obstetrics and internal medicine. It was known from the German physician Lonitzer since 1582 that ergot was used by midwives for quickening childbirth, although many stillbirths did result from that treatment. Later, it was used to stop postpartum bleeding. In 1935, the oxytocic principle ergonovine was discovered in four separate laboratories. Since then, the study of ergot alkaloids resulted in the elucidation of their structures and total syntheses and preparation of valuable therapeutics such as ergotamine, DHE, Hydergine, and many others, and of course in 1938/1943 the famous LSD [6]. 5-HT was discovered in the 1930s and its receptor in the 1950s [11b]. How did that chemobiology journey start? "Epidemics of ergotism occurred frequently in the Middle Ages. They were a source of inspiration for artists (see the tryptic of Matthias Grunewald in Colmar or some paintings of Hieronymus Bosch) and were popularly known as 'St. Anthony's Fire', resulting in gangrene, neurological diseases and death. It was caused by eating rye bread contaminated with the fungus *Claviceps purpurea*. In 1582 it was described that a delivery could be hastened by administering a few spurs of the secale cornutum. The dosage was, however, very inaccurate resulting in frequent uterine ruptures. The nickname of the preparation of 'pulvis ad partum' was changed to 'pulvis ad mortem'. Therefore, after 1828 the ergot alkaloids were no longer used during delivery but only as a measure to prevent postpartum haemorrhage. From 1875 onwards many derivatives of ergot alkaloids were found. Dudley and Moir isolated ergometrine in 1932. It proved to have a very specific uterotonic action. However, because of severe and unpredictable side effects and the instability of the drug, ergometrine is not the drug of choice for either the prevention or the treatment of postpartum hemorrhage" [12]. "Epidemics of '*convulsive* ergotism' were widespread east of the Rhine in Europe due to consumption of grain contaminated with ergot . . . West of the Rhine, consumption of ergot-contaminated food caused epidemics of *gangrenous* ergotism. The clinical features of convulsive ergotism—muscle twitching and spasms, changes in mental state, hallucinations, sweating, and fever lasting for several weeks—suggest . . . overstimulation of the CNS (i.e., the serotonin syndrome) . . . Ergots produced by different strains of *Claviceps purpurea*, . . . may have different ergot alkaloid compositions. An alkaloid, present in high concentrations in ergots from east of the Rhine, may have caused convulsive ergotism at a circulating concentration insufficient to produce peripheral ischemia. The serotonin syndrome may, therefore, have been a public-health problem long before it was recognized as a complication of modern psychopharmacology. In the present days, ergotism is an uncommon vasospastic disorder, . . . normally caused by the antimigraine drug ergotamine and results in peripheral ischemia. However, in the past ergotism occurred in epidemics of two main clinical forms: a vasospastic gangrenous form, similar to present-day sporadic ergotism, and a 'convulsive' form. The convulsive form disappeared nearly a century ago as a result of public-health measures" [13]; however, as recently as 1977 there was still an epidemic in Ethiopia. *Claviceps* comes in many different species and can produce three major classes of compounds in various proportions: clavine alkaloids, D-lysergic acid and its derivatives, and ergopeptines/ergopeptides. The serotonin syndrome as experienced in the Middle Ages and today may well be different: it is clear that the massive vasoconstriction can be mediated by adrenergic and 5-HT receptors, whereas some of the hallucinations described may come from LSD and its mimics. At present, the serotonin syndrome relates primarily to a combination of direct vascular effects and those produced by 5-HT released from platelets and in the CNS (e.g., in certain drug combinations with SSRIs). *Claviceps* is still used to produce intermediates for the synthesis of a number of ergoline-like chemicals. The life and achievements of Albert Hofmann have been much celebrated (e.g., his 100th birthday in Basel [10b]) as has the discovery of LSD been celebrated. Hofmann has summarized his complex relationship with LSD, mescaline, and psilocybin [8,14] compounds found in various mushrooms that shamans in Central and South America have used over centuries for various "treatments." LSD, as we know now, stimulates selectively 5-HT_{2A} receptors as do other hallucinogens; however, we also know from modern structural biology that some 5-HT_{2A} agonists do not produce hallucinations; this phenomenon is known as pathway selectivity [15–18]. Thus, all 5-HT_{2A} agonists do not produce hallucinations, but given that 5-HT_{2A} receptor activation does constrict a number of vessels and results in hypertension, there is no real interest in that mechanism of action.

The hallucinations and mental state changes induced by LSD and other hallucinogens have been amply described, including in Hofmann's account on his ride on the bike back home after having inadvertently ingested some compound following a resynthesis in 1943; another account comes from the Beatles in "Lucy in the Sky with Diamonds." The compound was initially used to treat psychosis and even today there are still some clinical psychiatrists who test the effects of LSD in volunteers and patients, although the compound has obviously been withdrawn from the market in the early 1960s.

4.3 Appetite-Reducing Agents, Fenfluramine, and Other 5-HT Releasers

The biggest recent issue in 5-HT drug-mediated adverse events, the *New England Journal of Medicine* calls it quite rightly scandal, was the discovery that a number of compounds targeting the 5-HT (fenfluramine and related compounds), but also the dopamine systems [18b], were producing cardiac valvular disease (mitral and aortic valvulopathies, or cardiac valve regurgitation) and pulmonary hypertension [19–23]. These effects are mediated by 5-HT_{2B} receptor activation [24,25]. In spite of the existing mechanistic knowledge [19,26] of the causes for pulmonary arterial hypertension (PAH) and cardiac valve disease since 1999–2000, one of these compounds (benfluorex) was only withdrawn from the European market in 2009 and banned by the European Commission in 2010. Starting in the 1970s, fenfluramine was used initially alone, and then in combination with phentermine (known as Fen-Phen) as an anorexigenic principle. The actual Fen-Phen combination has never been approved in the United States, yet was massively prescribed (18 million prescriptions in 1996!).

Later, dexfenfluramine made it to the market, with the same indication, but predictably had similar major side effects [27]. Benfluorex, which has only been withdrawn recently (especially from the French market), was never approved by the FDA and produces the same metabolite as the fenfluramines, norfenfluramine that has potent and efficacious 5-HT$_{2B}$ agonist activity [28–31].

The 5-HT$_{2B}$ receptor is present in the interstitial cells of the heart valves and in endothelial cells of pulmonary arteries; it is understood that chronic stimulation of this receptor leads to fibrosis in the heart valves and increases mitogenic signaling on pulmonary artery endothelial cells and other fibroblasts. Fenfluramine, dexfenfluramine, and benfluorex, all of which produce the same active metabolite norfenfluramine, a potent 5-HT$_{2B}$ agonist, have been used as appetite suppressants until the two first drugs were withdrawn from the world markets in 1997. Benfluorex continued to be prescribed in certain countries until 2009. Norfenfluramine, the active metabolite of all three anorexigens, is a 5-HT and NE releaser, but also an agonist at all three 5-HT$_2$ receptors. Therefore, it is not surprising that norfenfluramine may also produce some profound central effects such as hallucinations, as it is a potent 5-HT$_{2A}$ receptor agonist, like LSD and other hallucinogenic compounds. It is also a potent 5-HT$_{2C}$ agonist; probably this feature is responsible for the anorectic effects of the fenfluramine and related compounds. This ultimately led to the development of lorcaserin, a selective 5-HT$_{2C}$ agonist, to treat weight gain due to food intake, but devoid of 5-HT$_{2B}$ activity.

Bryan Roth and coworkers [28] have investigated the effects of a number of compounds suspected to induce valvular disease on all 5-HT receptors: (−)-, (+)-, and racemic fenfluramine; its metabolites (−)-, (+)-, and racemic norfenfluramine; ergotamine; methysergide and its metabolite methylergonovine; and a few negative controls. Norfenfluramine, ergotamine, and methylergonovine all had high affinities for the cloned human serotonin 5-HT$_{2B}$ receptor and were partial to full agonists. Subsequently, additional compounds were found to be agonists at 5-HT$_{2B}$ receptors, for example, pergolide, cabergoline, and MDMA (ecstasy [4,32]). The immediate conclusion was that 5-HT$_{2B}$ agonism was to be avoided in any medication (see above); as a result of these findings, the fenfluramines and the antiparkinsonian pergolide were taken off the market. Cabergoline used for hyperprolactinemic disorders, but not Parkinson's disease in the United States, remains available [33–37]. Interestingly, bromocriptine is a 5-HT$_{2B}$ receptor antagonist. Lisuride does not produce valvulopathies, as it has very little affinity for 5-HT$_{2B}$ receptors [38]. Non-ergoline D$_2$ receptor agonists (e.g., ropinirole and pramipexole) have no record of producing valvular disease; thus, D$_2$ receptors are not involved in these adverse events. It may be argued at length whether MDMA/ecstasy is dangerous or not; however, based on its brain neurotoxicity combined with possible effects in heart disease, its use is clearly not recommended. There are cases of people that have been exposed to gram quantities of ecstasy, and indeed cardiac valve disease has been linked to ecstasy use!

Such data have been amply discussed and publicized in early 2000 and in general the pharmaceutical industry has put in place 5-HT$_{2B}$ receptor screens to avoid the development of further 5-HT$_{2B}$ receptor agonists [39]. The recent crystallization of the 5-HT$_{1B}$ and 5-HT$_{2B}$ receptors has confirmed the initial finding and allowed now to rationalize the interactions of these compounds with the receptor's orthosteric binding pocket (and some accessory binding site for the ergolines [40,41]). Thus, some antimigraine ergolines such as DHE and ergotamine act as 5-HT$_{2B}$ agonists, although the antimigraine activity is mediated by 5-HT$_{1B}$ receptors. On the other hand, all the triptans tested have low affinity at 5-HT$_{2B}$ receptors and do not fit well into the 5-HT$_{2B}$ orthosteric pocket, in contrast to norfenfluramine and some of the ergolines. Thus, the cardiovascular effects (PAH) and valvulopathies of the fenfluramine analogues are due to fibrosis induced by chronic 5-HT$_{2B}$ receptor stimulation in the heart and pulmonary artery (benfluorex was administered three times, 150 mg/day, chronically). In retrospective studies, it was found that valvular disease was present in patients without previous heart condition following approximately 300 days of active treatment.

Benfluorex (Servier) was originally approved in 1974, but started to be actively promoted in 1997 when fenfluramine and its analogues were taken off the market. In France, benfluorex was prescribed as an adjuvant to overweight diabetic patients, although the compound had little effect on diabetes, but certainly helped reducing body mass [42]. Servier also made sure that benfluorex was not associated with the other class of fenfluramines, in spite of similar mode of action and indeed the same active metabolite. In fact, a good deal of prescriptions were not for diabetic patients, but simply for people who wanted to lose weight; it is estimated that 1.5–2 million patients/year were prescribed benfluorex in France. Pharmacovigilance started checking actively on benfluorex since the 1990s when the Fen-Phen disaster was revealed. In addition, the French authorities knew from 2003–2005 of the risk of PAH and valvular disease linked to benfluorex (similar to Fen-Phen). The risk of both PAH and valvular heart disease was found to be increased in the "Regulate" study [43], which eventually led to the withdrawal. Until then, the status quo prevailed in France, although the compound had been voluntarily withdrawn in other European countries from 2003–2005 onward. Even more astonishing, the French authorities had supported market approval of two generics of benfluorex (by Mylan and Qualimed, both companies had the same address) as late as October 2009, only to be withdrawn in November 2009! One wonders how the compound could have been proposed as a generic at that time by any drug producer, and how regulatory authorities could have accepted the dossier when all the alarms had been raised around this class of compounds since at least 2000 and reiterated frequently [28,44–46]. These aspects have been amply discussed [42,47–54] and many newspaper reports can be accessed on the Web.

4.4 Gastrointestinal and Antiemetic Indications, the 5-HT$_3$/5-HT$_4$ Receptor Links

5-HT$_3$ and 5-HT$_4$ receptors are prominently expressed in the gastrointestinal tract and have been the subject of intense research [1,55–58]. The first classification of 5-HT receptors comes from Gaddum and Picarelli [11b] from the work performed in the guinea pig ileum, which distinguished 5-HT_D and 5-HT_M receptors [1,2], 5-HT_D being the G-protein-coupled receptors (e.g., 5-HT_2 but others as well) whereas 5-HT_M represented the 5-HT_3 receptors. About 30 years later, after considerable efforts, IBS became the target of 5-HT_4 receptor agonists such as tegaserod [58–62] and the 5-HT_3 antagonist alosetron [63,64]. Cisapride, another 5-HT_4 agonist, was voluntarily withdrawn in 2003 due to ventricular tachyarrhythmias but remained accessible via a limited access program (FDA). Cisapride was not indicated for IBS, but was found effective in short bowel syndrome; it had significant effects on hERG channels, in contrast to tegaserod and other 5-HT_4 agonists.

5-HT_3 antagonists such as ondansetron, tropisetron, or granisetron had been developed with success in the United Kingdom and Switzerland for the treatment of chemotherapy-induced emesis [1,65–67]. This was a major breakthrough that helped many patients to complete their treatment, whereas before these compounds were available, compliance was a major issue in chemotherapy treatment due to the terrible side effects of very prominent emesis and vomiting. It was known that 5-HT_3 antagonists were producing constipation due to slowing of bowel movement [68], whereas 5-HT_4 agonists were accelerating bowel movement and producing diarrhea. Thus, tegaserod was developed for the treatment of IBS with constipation and then also for chronic idiopathic constipation [69–75], whereas alosetron was developed for IBS with diarrhea [63,64,76–79]; alosetron may also have positive effects in visceral pain, which is a major issue in this patient population. Unfortunately, both compounds had to be withdrawn from the market.

Tegaserod was withdrawn from the market because of a higher incidence of cardiac adverse events and several deaths as revealed in a meta-analysis: 13 subjects experienced ischemic cardiovascular events (myocardial infarction, stroke, and unstable angina pectoris) compared with only one case in the placebo study. In 2007, FDA reviewed the data of 29 studies that included 11 614 patients treated with tegaserod and 7031 treated with placebo. The patients treated with tegaserod had a higher incidence of myocardial infarction, stroke, or angina than those who were treated with placebo (0.1% versus 0.01%). A public health advisory was released by FDA in March 2007, and tegaserod was taken off the market by Novartis. In July 2007, FDA announced that it is permitting restricted use of tegaserod under an investigational new drug (IND) protocol to treat IBS-C and chronic idiopathic constipation in women younger than 55 and who meet specific guidelines. The compound has never been registered in the male population. In spite of numerous attempts to understand the mechanism of the cardiac events, the investigations remained inconclusive [80–82], as reviewed recently by FDA (UCM281532, November 2011). There have been speculations that 5-HT_1 receptors may have mediated the cardiac effects of tegaserod; however, tegaserod had no contractile activity on the isolated coronary arteries from pigs (30 μM), nonhuman primates (10 μM), and humans (30 μM), whereas it produced minimal contractile response in canine coronary arteries at 5–10 μM not different from vehicle [82,83]. In other words, the ischemic cardiovascular events observed in the clinic remain unexplained, but are not 5-HT_4 receptor mediated. Other 5-HT_4 agonists or mixed 5-HT_4 agonists/5-HT_3 antagonists are in the pipeline (velusetrag [84–86]) or have been approved in other countries (e.g., mosapride), although clinical studies in IBS are very difficult to complete. Recruiting enough patients with IBS has always been a major issue, and the initial indication may include chronic idiopathic constipation, constipation-predominant irritable bowel syndrome, gastroparesis, or other functional motility diseases.

Alosetron was withdrawn from the market in November 2000, as during post-marketing surveillance, the Food and Drug Administration received reports of 84 cases of ischemic colitis (including 2 deaths). Also, 113 cases of serious complications of constipation (including 2 deaths) were associated with the use of alosetron from March 2000 to March 2002 [87–90]. It is to be mentioned here that ischemic colitis is rather common in the IBS population, and it should be checked carefully at baseline [91]. It is also possible that some of the occlusion occurred in patients who may have suffered from both forms of IBS, and it is understandable that IBS with constipation should under no circumstance be treated with a compound that causes constipation. Eventually, after a careful analysis alosetron was allowed back on the market under very strict conditions, that is, with a black box warning; it can only be prescribed by practitioners who are enlisted in a special program and the patients need to fill acknowledgment forms (see NDA 21-107): "Alosetron is approved only for women with severe, diarrhea-predominant irritable bowel syndrome who: have chronic irritable bowel syndrome symptoms (generally lasting for 6 months or longer), had anatomic or biochemical abnormalities of the gastrointestinal tract excluded, and have not responded adequately to conventional therapy. Diarrhea-predominant irritable bowel syndrome is severe if it includes diarrhea and one or more of the following: frequent and severe abdominal pain and discomfort, frequent bowel urgency or fecal incontinence, disability or restriction of daily activities due to irritable bowel syndrome." There is currently no other 5-HT_3 receptor antagonist approved in IBS and constipation is a target-related side effect that needs to be monitored closely.

4.5
Antipsychotics and the 5-HT_2/Dopamine D_2 Link (and Many Other 5-HT Receptors)

Clozapine was the first real atypical antipsychotic discovered at Wander, later Sandoz in 1959 [92–95], that is devoid of the classical side effects of the typical antipsychotics such as chlorpromazine and haloperidol, especially catalepsy, as seen in rodents and it was used a screening model. Extrapyramidal side effects (EPS), dystonic reactions, drug-induced parkinsonism, akathisia, and tardive dyskinesia can make treatment intolerable for patients, leading to subjective distress, diminished function, stigma, and nonadherence. EPS can be seen in up to 40% of treated patients. Interestingly, some leading figures in psychiatry suggested that, since clozapine was not inducing catalepsy or EPS, it was not a neuroleptic, therefore the name atypical neuroleptic [96]. The side effects of "typicals" are due to excessive blockade of dopamine D_2/D_3 receptors (the ceiling is set at about 80% as seen in PET studies) and are present in most typical antipsychotics, whereas they are absent in the "atypicals." Clozapine at therapeutic doses appears to occupy a much lower proportion of striatal D_2/D_3 receptors (60% or so) than typical antipsychotics such as haloperidol. Similar receptor occupancy can be seen with quetiapine; however, there are exceptions, such as aripiprazole that occupies up to 90% of striatal D_2/D_3 receptors [96] and yet has no EPS liability. In addition, it is believed that the multiple 5-HT receptors at which clozapine interacts are beneficial, especially 5-HT_{2A}. The concept of striatal binding is being debated; what is, however, clear is that clozapine is an inverse 5-HT_{2A} agonist, which is able to increase DA in prefrontal cortex and hippocampus. This is the basis for the development of more selective 5-HT_{2A} antagonists such as pimavanserin [97–102]. Second-generation antipsychotics are used to treat schizophrenia spectrum disorders, bipolar disorders, dementia, psychotic depression, autism, developmental disorders, and, to a lesser extent, individuals with conditions such as delirium, aggressive behavior, personality disorders, and posttraumatic stress disorder, although the primary approval in general was schizophrenia.

Clozapine has notable side effects, the most prominent being agranulocytosis; this was discovered in one of the first large-scale studies in Finland and resulted in eight deaths, which lead to a temporary withdrawal from the markets where it was registered. However, when switching clozapine-treated patients to the existing typical neuroleptics, it was noted that many of these patients relapsed; therefore, the compound remained available for compassionate use [96]. Thanks to relentless efforts of a few leading clinical psychiatrists [92–94], which demonstrated superiority of clozapine over chlorpromazine and positive effects in treatment-resistant patients, the compound was officially reintroduced where it was already used: in German-speaking countries, Scandinavia, and China, in addition to being successfully submitted and registered in the United States in 1990 and the rest of the world (Japan was a long-time exception before it became registered). The cause for agranulocytosis is unclear.

Clozapine comes with a black label; thus, clozapine is reserved for "the treatment of severely ill patients with schizophrenia who fail to show an acceptable response to adequate courses of standard antipsychotic drug treatment." White blood levels and absolute neutrophil counts are closely monitored at baseline and must continue to be monitored: doses must be reduced in case of granulocytopenia or leukopenia, or discontinued if they become severe, and then monitoring continues until normal levels are attained again and treatment can be gradually reinstated following a very detailed protocol. Agranulocytosis is reversible upon treatment cessation in most cases. In principle, clozapine is not given first line, although the latter depends very much upon country and prescribing habits. The compound has a specific distribution system, which includes blood monitoring. There is a dose-dependent incidence of seizure with clozapine; thus, there is a warning for patients that are susceptible. There is a risk of myocarditis especially at the beginning of treatment, as well as a few other cardiovascular/respiratory side effects. There is an increased mortality in patients with dementia-related psychosis that is not specific to clozapine; however, clozapine is contraindicated in this patient population. (FDA ALERT [6/16/2008]: FDA is notifying healthcare professionals that both conventional and atypical antipsychotics are associated with an increased risk of mortality in elderly patients treated for dementia-related psychosis.)

Another major issue with clozapine, which, however, is common to many of the second-generation antipsychotics, such as risperidone, olanzapine, quetiapine, aripiprazole, and ziprasidone, is the high propensity to metabolic side effects, with weight gain, hyperglycemia, and hyperlipidemia. Their "use has been associated with reports of dramatic weight gain, diabetes [even acute metabolic decompensation, e.g., diabetic ketoacidosis (DKA)], and an atherogenic lipid profile [increased low-density lipoprotein (LDL) cholesterol and triglyceride levels and decreased high-density lipoprotein (HDL) cholesterol]" [103]. This may lead to reduced compliance among patients and carries the risk of increased cardiovascular and metabolic side effects, especially type 2 diabetes. The reasons for metabolic effects of many antipsychotics are not clear at this stage and require careful monitoring.

There are debates about the general use of the term atypical antipsychotic, since some of the second-generation antipsychotics do not fare as well as clozapine in a number of symptoms or dimensions, although indeed they are devoid of major EPS. However, there is much more to be achieved in schizophrenia, especially about negative symptoms, depression, and cognitive impairment. What is remarkable is that clozapine improves some of these aspects, although modestly, but was eventually submitted and registered for its capacity to reduce the rate of suicide risk that is significant in those patients [100,104–106]. Thus, clozapine is indicated for "reducing the risk of recurrent suicidal behavior in patients with schizophrenia or schizoaffective disorder who are judged to be at risk of re-experiencing suicidal behavior." This is remarkable as many psychotropic drugs come with a label about increased suicide risk or fail to be registered because of such potential, as has happened several times in the last decade.

4.6
Antimigraine Medications of Old and New and the 5-$HT_{1B/1D}$ Receptors

The great breakthrough in the migraine field was the identification of sumatriptan as a new and selective 5-$HT_{1B/1D}$ receptor agonist for the treatment of acute migraine [107–109], although at the time the compound was profiled primarily at 5-HT_1-like receptors in various vessel preparations [110–114]. The second-generation triptans, except for naratriptan, were developed based on 5-$HT_{1B/1D}$ receptor screening, for example, almotriptan, frovatriptan, rizatriptan, eletriptan, and zolmitriptan [115]. However, the triptans are not the first drugs to target the 5-$HT_{1B/1D}$ receptor. "Over the past decade the various triptan derivatives have been accepted as the most effective available agents for relieving migraine attacks. Prior to that, for a period of half a century, ergotamine was the only 'specific' available for this purpose. In 1918, Stoll had isolated it from the various alkaloids present in extracts of the sclerotia of the fungus *Claviceps purpurea* (ergot), which grow on rye and, to a lesser extent, on other grasses. By 1925 ergotamine was beginning to be used to treat migraine attacks. However, as ergotamine was present in extracts of ergot, which had been used to treat migraine first in Italy in 1862, and then by Edward Woakes (1868) in England, and after him by Albert Eulenburg in Germany (1883), the drug had actually come into unrecognized use for the disorder more than half a century before ergotamine itself was known to exist" [13]. The effects of ergotamine and DHE on migraine are largely mediated by 5-$HT_{1B/1D}$ receptors [1,116–118]. All these compounds are effective in the treatment of acute migraine [119], and it was presumed that the effect on migraine is essentially vascular [120], although a neurogenic and inflammatory component is not ruled out. The side effects of the triptans are clearly less pronounced than those of DHE or ergotamine (especially since the latter have been at times used subchronically, with the possible appearance of ergotism [121]). Sumatriptan and the other triptans are clearly indicated and restricted for acute use; some patients may show cardiovascular side effects (see below for contraindications and warnings), especially in the coronary tree and/or chest pain that may occur more frequently in the presence of a pre-existing cardiac condition; interestingly, vascular 5-$HT_{1B/1D}$ receptors are rarely constricting in healthy tissue [1,116], yet will show marked constriction, for example, in coronary arteries from animals or patients suffering from coronary heart disease or with an incidence of atherosclerosis; thus, caution needs to be exercised.

Contraindications:

- History of coronary artery disease or coronary vasospasm.
- Wolff–Parkinson–White syndrome or other cardiac accessory conduction pathway disorders.
- History of stroke, transient ischemic attack, or hemiplegic or basilar migraine.
- Peripheral vascular disease.
- Ischemic bowel disease.
- Uncontrolled hypertension.
- Recent (within 24 h) use of another 5-HT_1 agonist (e.g., another triptan) or an ergotamine-containing medication.
- Current or recent (past 2 weeks) use of monoamine oxidase A inhibitor.
- Hypersensitivity to sumatriptan (angioedema and anaphylaxis seen).
- Severe hepatic impairment.

Warnings:

- Myocardial ischemia/infarction and prinzmetal's angina: perform cardiac evaluation in patients with multiple cardiovascular risk factors.
- Arrhythmias: discontinue sumatriptan if occurs.
- Chest/throat/neck/jaw pain, tightness, pressure, or heaviness: generally not associated with myocardial ischemia; evaluate for coronary artery disease in patients at high risk.
- Cerebral hemorrhage, subarachnoid hemorrhage, and stroke: discontinue sumatriptan if occurs.
- Gastrointestinal ischemia and infarction events, peripheral vasospastic reactions: discontinue sumatriptan if occurs.
- Medication overuse headache: detoxification may be necessary.
- Serotonin syndrome: discontinue sumatriptan if occurs.
- Seizures: use with caution for patients with epilepsy or a lowered seizure threshold.

There is potential for the 5-HT syndrome to develop when SSRIs and triptans are combined. "FDA ALERT [7/2006]: Potentially Life-Threatening Serotonin Syndrome with Combined Use of SSRIs or SNRIs and Triptan Medications. There is the potential for life-threatening serotonin syndrome (a syndrome of changes in mental status, autonomic instability, neuromuscular abnormalities, and gastrointestinal symptoms) in patients taking 5-hydroxytryptamine receptor agonists (triptans) and selective serotonin reuptake inhibitors (SSRIs) or selective serotonin/norepinephrine reuptake inhibitors (SNRIs) concomitantly . . . This information is based on reports of serotonin syndrome occurring in patients treated with triptans and SSRIs/SNRIs, and the biological plausibility of such a reaction in persons receiving two serotonergic medications. The FDA recommends that patients treated concomitantly with a triptan and an SSRI/SNRI be informed of the possibility of serotonin syndrome (which may be more likely to occur when starting or increasing the dose of an SSRI, SNRI, or triptan) and be carefully followed." This may also occur in combination with MAO inhibitors or tricyclic antidepressants. In spite of these side effects that are shared by many triptans, and are indeed target related, the new concept of 5-$HT_{1B/1D}$ agonism to treat migraine has had a major impact on patients, who before the advent of triptans had to suffer in the silence and obscurity of their bedroom until the end of the crisis, if they were not prepared to take ergotamine or DHE or other pain medications.

4.7
Antidepressants/Anxiolytics Acting at 5-HT and Other Transporters

Many "new" antidepressants, of which the most famous is paroxetine, target primarily the 5-HT transporter: they are collectively known as SSRIs. There are many more compounds belonging to the same class, for example, paroxetine, citalopram, escitalopram, and others, which are more or less selective for the 5-HT transporter. Fluoxetine is indicated in "Major Depressive Disorder (MDD), Obsessive Compulsive Disorder (OCD), Bulimia Nervosa, Panic Disorder, Depressive episodes associated with Bipolar I Disorder, taken with olanzapine, Treatment Resistant Depression (depression that has not gotten better with at least 2 other treatments), taken with olanzapine." Then, there are those antidepressants that target both the 5-HT and the NA transporter, known as SNRIs (e.g., duloxetine or venlafaxine). Further, there are triple target antidepressants that in addition to 5-HT and NA target the DA transporter or even a combination of various receptors and transporters (vilazodone, vortioxetine, and others). It would appear that the field has been going full circle since the original antidepressants better known as tricyclics (and some tetracyclics) have been developed about 50–60 years ago, at the time the identity of the targets was not known, but they clearly act on all three monoamine transporters. There is another class of "older" compounds, for example, the MAO inhibitors, which will not be addressed here. More recent antidepressants target a combination of 5-HT/NA transporters and various 5-HT receptors. The reason for a revival in this "polypharmacy" is that although a role of the 5-HT transporter in depression is well recognized some patients respond better to multitarget compounds, and it has been realized that very selective compounds may not do the job. Occasional but prominent side effects of SSRIs are sexual dysfunction and suicidal ideation (especially in younger patients and adolescents). "*Suicidal thoughts or actions: Fluoxetine and other antidepressant medicines may increase suicidal thoughts or actions* in some children, teenagers, or young adults within the *first few months of treatment or when the dose is changed*. Depression or other serious mental illnesses are the most important causes of suicidal thoughts or actions. Watch for these changes and call your healthcare provider right away if you notice: New or sudden changes in mood, behavior, actions, thoughts, or feelings, especially if severe. Pay particular attention to such changes when fluoxetine is started or when the dose is changed. Keep all follow-up visits with your healthcare provider and call between visits if you are worried about symptoms" (FDA UCM406910). There are also risks of pulmonary hypertension for children born to mothers who have been treated by SSRIs during their pregnancy. "FDA ALERT [7/2006]: Increased Risk of Neonatal Persistent Pulmonary Hypertension. A recently published case-control study has shown that infants born to mothers who took selective serotonin reuptake inhibitors (SSRIs) after the 20th week of pregnancy were 6 times more likely to have persistent pulmonary hypertension (PPHN) than infants born to mothers who did not take antidepressants during pregnancy (see SSRI drug names at the bottom of this sheet). The background risk of a woman giving birth to an infant affected by PPHN in the general population is estimated to be about 1 to 2 infants per 1000 live births. Neonatal PPHN is associated with significant morbidity and mortality. The FDA is updating the prescribing information for all SSRIs with this new information. The FDA is also accruing data from additional sources pertaining to the potential association between SSRIs and neonatal PPHN." Furthermore, there is potential for the 5-HT syndrome to develop when SSRIs and triptans (5-$HT_{1B/1D}$ agonists in migraine) are combined (see triptans above). "Serotonin syndrome symptoms may include mental status changes (e.g., agitation, hallucinations, coma), autonomic instability (e.g., tachycardia, labile blood pressure, hyperthermia), neuromuscular aberrations (e.g., hyperreflexia, incoordination), and/or gastrointestinal symptoms (e.g., nausea, vomiting, diarrhea). The onset of symptoms usually occurs within minutes to hours of receiving a new or a greater dose of a serotonergic medication." Such combinations are not recommended. Serotonin does increase ejaculatory latency and delay orgasm; SSRIs may be prescribed off-label to treat premature ejaculation. On the other hand, all SSRIs prolong ejaculatory latency especially paroxetine, and that may also explain the negative side effects described by patients treated with SSRIs with respect to reduced libido and sexual function. Again, in spite of these possible side effects, SSRIs have changed the life of a generation of patients, keeping in mind that drugs are used to treat symptoms or syndromes, under expert medical advice: they are not mere lifestyle additions.

4.8 Conclusions

There are many drugs affecting the 5-HT system on the market and on the streets that whether by design (more recently) or serendipitously (in the early 1900s) target many 5-HT receptors, its transporters, or metabolizing enzymes. The contribution to public health need no demonstration: think of clozapine and the second-generation antipsychotics in schizophrenia or in suicide prevention, the triptans in headaches/migraines, the SSRIs and combinations thereof as antidepressants, the 5-HT_3 antagonists as treatment for chemotherapy-induced emesis, 5-HT_3/5-HT_4 ligands to treat IBS (although with less success due to side effects), or lorcaserin to treat weight gain. There is more to come; the 5-HT field has not been fully exploited yet, as structural biology may help to design better compounds.

On the other hand, a number of drugs have shown significant adverse event, starting indeed with clozapine that produces agranulocytosis or more generally the antipsychotics that induce severe weight gain and thus may lead to diabetic and cardiovascular complications. We have amply discussed not only the issue related to the use and abuse of fenfluramines and related compounds, but also how the increased knowledge of their mechanism of action has led to the withdrawal of such compounds from the market or at least the issuing of severe warnings where patients have little other treatment options. The immediate attention raised toward 5-HT_{2B} agonism has been generally well implemented in drug screening and the awareness of the side effects is high. One can argue that some withdrawals were precipitated such as that of tegaserod, where no mechanism of action could be deduced and link to mediation may even be questioned, but since there is no incentive to continue with tegaserod, we will probably never know. Other withdrawals, for example, alosetron, were reversed under the condition that the drug and patient population are carefully monitored (as is the case with clozapine) and the prescribers are well educated and trained.

With the exceptions of the ergots inducing ergotism in the middle ages, the first compound to show real side effects was LSD, which, as we know now, produces hallucinations by activating a given pathway through the 5-HT_{2A} receptor (other 5-HT_{2A} agonists with different biased agonism do not produce hallucinations), at a time the notion of 5-HT receptors was extremely vague and the target of LSD unsuspected. It was initially developed and marketed for the treatment of psychosis, and subsequently withdrawn because of the hallucinogenic potential and its real value on the street market. Some argue that LSD still has value for the treatment of some forms of psychotic syndromes, and this research is going on. However, it is clear that one would not develop a drug that acts as an agonist at the 5-HT_{2A} receptor, or at the 5-HT_{2B} receptor for that matter. On the other hand, 5-HT_{2C} agonists, if selective enough, will have value. The SSRIs have been transformative in the depression field in spite of side effects, thanks to some individuals such as Ray Fuller [122–125] who championed fluoxetine at a time Lilly and other pharmaceutical companies were not convinced about its utility in depression. SSRIs may affect sexuality in a negative way and in some patients may increase suicidality, especially in the adolescent population; therefore, prescriptions have to be carefully monitored, but this should be common standard with all drugs. Another champion is Herb Meltzer who relentlessly supported 5-HT research in neuropsychiatry, a strong supporter of clozapine [92], especially when it was first withdrawn from the market. Later, Herb was the one who kept pushing until Novartis agreed to test and eventually registered clozapine for the prevention of suicide [100]. One of his mentees, Bryan Roth, has made significant contributions to the field by alerting about the fibrotic/cardiac valve pathologies mediated by 5-HT_{2B} receptor activation, and continues to contribute significantly to the understanding of the mechanisms of action of many drugs, whether main or side effects, and more generally to the understanding of the structural biology of the 5-HT receptors and many other receptor–ligand complexes. There are many aspects of the large 5-HT drugstore that have not been covered, due to space limitation and possibly biases of the author.

References

1 Hoyer, D., Clarke, D.E., Fozard, J.R., Hartig, P.R., Martin, G.R., Mylecharane, E.J., Saxena, P.R., and Humphrey, P.P.A. (1994) International Union of Pharmacology classification of receptors for 5-hydroxytryptamine (serotonin). *Pharmacological Reviews*, **46**, 157–203.

2 Hoyer, D., Hannon, J.P., and Martin, G.R. (2002) Molecular, pharmacological and functional diversity of 5-HT receptors. *Pharmacology, Biochemistry and Behavior*, **71**, 533–554.

3 Hannon, J. and Hoyer, D. (2008) Molecular biology of 5-HT receptors.

Behavioural Brain Research, **195**, 198–213.
4 Berger, M., Gray, J.A., and Roth, B.L. (2009) The expanded biology of serotonin. *Annual Review of Medicine*, **60**, 355–366.
5 Mengod, G., Cortes, R., Vilaro, M.T., and Hoyer, D. (2010) Distribution of 5-HT receptors in the central nervous system. *Handbook of Behavioral Neurobiology of Serotonin*, **21**, 123–138.
6 Hofmann, A. (1975) Discovery of LSD and subsequent investigations of related magic drugs of Mexico. *Lloydia: Journal of Natural Products*, **38**, 532–1532.
7 Hofmann, A. (1978) Historical view on ergot alkaloids. *Pharmacology*, **16**, 1–11.
8 Hofmann, A. (1994) Notes and documents concerning the discovery of LSD. *Agents and Actions*, **43**, 79–81.
9 Stoll, A. and Hofmann, A. (1938) Partial synthesis of ergobasine, a natural ergot alkaloid as well as optical antipodes (3rd announcement on ergot alkaloids). *Hoppe-Seyler's Zeitschrift für Physiologische Chemie*, **251**, 155–163.
10 (a) Stoll, A. and Hofmann, A. (1943) Alkaloid of the ergotoxine group: ergocristine, ergokryptine and ergocornine (7th announcement on ergot alkaloids). *Helvetica Chimica Acta*, **26**, 1570–1603; (b) Giger, R.K.A. and Engel, G. (2006) Albert Hofmann's pioneering work on ergot alkaloids and its impact on the search of novel drugs at Sandoz, a predecessor company of Novartis – dedicated to Dr. Albert Hofmann on the occasion of his 100th birthday. *Chimia*, **60**, 83–87.
11 (a) Stoll, A. and Hofmann, A. (1943) Dihydro derivative of natural levorotatory ergot alkaloids (9th announcement on ergot alkaloids). *Helvetica Chimica Acta*, **26**, 2070–2081; (b) Gaddum, J.H. and Picarelli, Z.P. (1957) Two kinds of tryptamine receptor. *British Journal of Pharmacology and Chemotherapy*, **12**, 323–328.
12 Van Dongen, J.J. and de Groot, R. (1995) History of ergot alkaloids from ergotism to ergotamine. *Obstetrics and Gynecology*, **60**, 109–116.
13 Eadie, M.J. (2003) Convulsive ergotism: epidemics of the serotonin syndrome? *Lancet Neurology*, **2**, 429–434.
14 Hofmann, A. (1979) How LSD originated. *Journal of Psychedelic Drugs*, **11**, 53–60.
15 Roth, B.L., Choudhary, M.S., Khan, N., and Uluer, A.Z. (1997) High-affinity agonist binding is not sufficient for agonist efficacy at 5-hydroxytryptamine (2A) receptors: evidence in favor of a modified ternary complex model. *Journal of Pharmacology and Experimental Therapeutics*, **280**, 576–583.
16 Roth, B.L., Willins, D.L., Kristiansen, K., and Kroeze, W.K. (1999) Activation is hallucinogenic and antagonism is therapeutic: role of 5-HT_{2A} receptors in atypical antipsychotic drug actions. *Neuroscientist*, **5**, 254–262.
17 Roth, B.L. (2011) Irving Page Lecture: 5-HT_{2A} serotonin receptor biology: interacting proteins, kinases and paradoxical regulation. *Neuropharmacology*, **61**, 348–354.
18 (a) Lee, H.M. and Roth, B.L. (2012) Hallucinogen actions on human brain revealed. *Proceedings of the National Academy of Sciences of the United States of America*, **109**, 1820–1821; (b) Horvath, J., Fross, R.D., Kleiner-Fisman, G. *et al.* (2004) Severe multivalvular heart disease: a new complication of the ergot derivative dopamine agonists. *Movement Disorders*, **19**, 656–662.
19 Connolly, J.M., Bakay, M.A., Fulmer, J.T., Gorman, R.C., Gorman, J.H., Oyama, M.A., and Levy, R.J. (2009) Fenfluramine disrupts the mitral valve interstitial cell response to serotonin. *American Journal of Pathology*, **175**, 988–997.
20 Dahl, C.F., Allen, M.R., Urie, P.M., and Hopkins, P.N. (2008) Valvular regurgitation and surgery associated with fenfluramine use: an analysis of 5743 individuals. *BMC Medicine*, **6**, 34.
21 Droogmans, S., Cosyns, B., D'Haenen, H., Creeten, E., Weytjens, C., Franken, P.R., Scott, B., Schoors, D., Kemdem, A., Close, L., Vandenbossche, J.L., Van Bechet, S., and Camp, G. (2007) Possible association between 3,4-methylenedioxymethamphetamine abuse

and valvular heart disease. *American Journal of Cardiology*, **100**, 1442–1445.
22 (a) Droogmans, S., Roosens, B., Cosyns, B., Degaillier, C., Hernot, S., Weytjens, C., Garbar, C., Caveliers, V., Pipeleers-Marichal, M., Franken, P.R., Bossuyt, A., Schoors, D., Van Lahoutte, T., and Camp, G. (2009) Dose dependency and reversibility of serotonin-induced valvular heart disease in rats. *Cardiovascular Toxicology*, **9**, 134–141; (b) Droogmans, S., Roosens, B., Cosyns, B., Degaillier, C., Hernot, S., Weytjens, C., Garbar, C., Caveliers, V., Pipeleers-Marichal, M., Franken, P.R., Lahoutte, T., Van Schoors, D., and Camp, G. (2009) Cyproheptadine prevents pergolide-induced valvulopathy in rats: an echocardiographic and histopathological study. *American Journal of Physiology: Heart and Circulatory Physiology*, **296**, H1940–H1948.
23 Droogmans, S., Van Cosyns, B., and Camp, G. (2011) Benfluorex: the last chapter of drug-induced valvular heart disease? *European Journal of Echocardiography*, **12**, 263–264.
24 Rothman, R.B. and Baumann, M.H. (2009) Appetite suppressants, cardiac valve disease and combination pharmacotherapy. *American Journal of Therapeutics*, **16**, 354–364.
25 Rothman, R.B. and Baumann, M.H. (2009) Serotonergic drugs and valvular heart disease. *Expert Opinion on Drug Safety*, **8**, 317–329.
26 Jian, B., Xu, J., Connolly, J., Savani, R.C., Narula, N., Liang, B., and Levy, R.J. (2002) Serotonin mechanisms in heart valve disease I – serotonin-induced up-regulation of transforming growth factor-beta 1 via G-protein signal transduction in aortic valve interstitial cells. *American Journal of Pathology*, **161**, 2111–2121.
27 Shively, B.K., Roldan, C.A., Gill, E.A., Najarian, T., and Loar, S.B. (1999) Prevalence and determinants of valvulopathy in patients treated with dexfenfluramine. *Circulation*, **100**, 2161–2167.
28 Rothman, R.B., Baumann, M.H., Savage, J.E., Rauser, L., McBride, A., Hufeisen, S.J., and Roth, B.L. (2000) Evidence for possible involvement of 5-HT_{2B} receptors in the cardiac valvulopathy associated with fenfluramine and other serotonergic medications. *Circulation*, **102**, 2836–2841.
29 Hajjo, R., Grulke, C.M., Golbraikh, A., Setola, V., Huang, X.P., Roth, B.L., and Tropsha, A. (2010) Development, validation, and use of quantitative structure–activity relationship models of 5-hydroxytryptamine (2B) receptor ligands to identify novel receptor binders and putative valvulopathic compounds among common drugs. *Journal of Medicinal Chemistry*, **53**, 7573–7586.
30 Hutcheson, J.D., Setola, V., Roth, B.L., and Merryman, W.D. (2011) Antagonism of the 5-HT_{2B} receptor prevents TGF-beta1 effects in aortic valve fibroblasts. *FASEB Journal*, **25**, 177.5.
31 Hutcheson, J.D., Setola, V., Roth, B.L., and Merryman, W.D. (2011) Serotonin receptors and heart valve disease – it was meant 2B. *Pharmacology & Therapeutics*, **132**, 146–157.
32 (a) Setola, V., Hufeisen, S.J., Grande-Allen, K.J., Vesely, I., Glennon, R.A., Blough, B., Rothman, R.B., and Roth, B.L. (2003) 3,4-Methylenedioxymethamphetamine (MDMA, “ecstasy”) induces fenfluramine-like proliferative actions on human cardiac valvular interstitial cells *in vitro*. *Molecular Pharmacology*, **63**, 1223–1229; (b) Setola, V., Dukat, M., Glennon, R.A., and Roth, B.L. (2005) Molecular determinants for the interaction of the valvulopathic anorexigen norfenfluramine with the 5-HT_{2B} receptor. *Molecular Pharmacology*, **68**, 20–33.
33 Van Camp, G., Flamez, A., Cosyns, B., Weytjens, C., Muyldermans, L., Van Zandijcke, M., De Sutter, J., Santens, P., Decoodt, P., Moerman, C., and Schoors, D. (2004) Treatment of Parkinson's disease with pergolide and relation to restrictive valvular heart disease. *Lancet*, **363**, 1179–1183.
34 Antonini, A. and Poewe, W. (2007) Fibrotic heart-valve reactions to dopamine-agonist treatment in

Parkinson's disease. *Lancet Neurology*, **6**, 826–829.

35 Simonis, G., Fuhr-Mann, J.T., and Strasser, R.H. (2007) Meta-analysis of heart valve abnormalities in Parkinson's disease patients treated with dopamine agonists. *Movement Disorders*, **22**, 1936–1942.

36 Zanettini, R., Antonini, A., Gatto, G., Gentile, R., Tesei, S., and Pezzoli, G. (2007) Valvular heart disease and the use of dopamine agonists for Parkinson's disease. *New England Journal of Medicine*, **356**, 39–46.

37 Rasmussen, V.G., Poulsen, S.H., Dupont, E., Ostergaard, K., Safikhany, G., and Egeblad, H. (2009) Heart abnormalities in Parkinson patients after discontinuation or continuation of ergot-derived dopamine agonists: a treatment-blinded echocardiographic study. *Journal of Heart Valve Disease*, **18**, 463–469.

38 Hofmann, C., Penner, U., Dorow, R., Pertz, H.H., Jahnichen, S., Horowski, R., Latte, K.P., Palla, D., and Schurad, B. (2006) Lisuride, a dopamine receptor agonist with 5-HT_{2B} receptor antagonist properties: absence of cardiac valvulopathy adverse drug reaction reports supports the concept of a crucial role for 5-HT_{2B} receptor agonism in cardiac valvular fibrosis. *Clinical Neuropharmacology*, **29**, 80–86.

39 Huang, X.P., Setola, V., Yadav, P.N., Allen, J.A., Rogan, S.C., Hanson, B.J., Revankar, C., Robers, M., Doucette, C., and Roth, B.L. (2009) Parallel functional activity profiling reveals valvulopathogens are potent 5-hydroxytryptamine (2B) receptor agonists: implications for drug safety assessment. *Molecular Pharmacology*, **76**, 710–722.

40 Wacker, D., Wang, C., Katritch, V., Han, G.W., Huang, X.P., Vardy, E., McCorvy, J.D., Jiang, Y., Chu, M.H., Siu, F.Y., Liu, W., Xu, H.E., Cherezov, V., Roth, B.L., and Stevens, R.C. (2013) Structural features for functional selectivity at serotonin receptors. *Science*, **340**, 615–619.

41 Wang, C., Jiang, Y., Ma, J.M., Wu, H.X., Wacker, D. *et al.* (2013) Structural basis for molecular recognition at serotonin receptors. *Science*, **340**, 610–614.

42 Vincent, L., Guardiola, B., Tsouderos, Y., and Canet, E. (2011) Mediator: who's to blame? *Lancet*, **377**, 2003.

43 Derumeaux, G., Ernande, L., Serusclat, A., Servan, E., Investigators, R.T. *et al.* (2012) Echocardiographic evidence for valvular toxicity of benfluorex: a double-blind randomised trial in patients with type 2 diabetes mellitus. *PLoS One*. doi: 10.1371/journal.pone.0038273.

44 Roth, B.L. (2007) Dopamine agonists and valvular heart disease – reply. *New England Journal of Medicine*, **356**, 1679–1680.

45 Roth, B.L. (2007) Focus on research – drug and valvular heart disease. *New England Journal of Medicine*, **356**, 6–9.

46 Cavero, I. and Guillon, J.M. (2014) Safety pharmacology assessment of drugs with biased 5-HT_{2B} receptor agonism mediating cardiac valvulopathy. *Journal of Pharmacological and Toxicological Methods*, **69**, 150–161.

47 Boutet, K., Frachon, I., Jobic, Y., Gut-Gobert, C., Leroyer, C., Carlhant-Kowalski, D., Sitbon, O., Simonneau, G., and Humbert, M. (2009) Fenfluramine-like cardiovascular side-effects of benfluorex. *European Respiratory Journal*, **33**, 684–688.

48 Etienne, Y., Jobic, Y., Frachon, I., Fatemi, M., Castellant, P., and Quintin-Roue, I. (2011) Mitral and aortic valvular disease associated with benfluorex use. *Journal of Heart Valve Disease*, **20**, 348–350.

49 Frachon, I., Etienne, Y., Jobic, Y., Le Gal, G., Humbert, M., and Leroyer, C. (2010) Benfluorex and unexplained valvular heart disease: a case-control study. *PLoS One*. doi: 10.1371/journal.pone.0010128.

50 Frachon, I., Etienne, Y., Jobic, Y., Le Gal, G., Lacut, K., Humbert, M., and Leroyer, C. (2010) Benfluorex and unexplained valvular heart disease: a case-control study. *Fundamental & Clinical Pharmacology*, **24**, 6.

51 Frachon, I. (2011) Benfluorex (Mediator®), our vigilance in question. *Presse Medicale*, **40**, 459–461.

52 Nicot, P., Frachon, I., and Hill, C. (2013) About the settlement of litigations

concerning the harm caused by benfluorex (Mediator®). *Presse Medicale*, **42**, 411–418.
53 Savale, L., Chaumais, M.C., Cottin, V., Bergot, E., Frachon, I., Prevot, G. *et al.* (2012) Pulmonary hypertension associated with benfluorex exposure. *European Respiratory Journal*, **40**, 1164–1172.
54 Mullard, A. (2011) Mediator scandal rocks French medical community. *Lancet*, **377**, 890–892.
55 Buchheit, K.H., Gamse, R., Giger, R., Hoyer, D., Klein, F., Kloppner, E., Pfannkuche, H.J., and Mattes, H. (1995) The serotonin 5-HT_4 receptor. 1. Design of a new class of agonists and receptor map of the agonist recognition site. *Journal of Medicinal Chemistry*, **38**, 2326–2330.
56 Gaster, L.M. and King, F.D. (1997) Serotonin 5-HT_3 and 5-HT_4 receptor antagonists. *Medicinal Research Reviews*, **17**, 163–214.
57 Jones, B.J. and Blackburn, T.P. (2002) The medical benefit of 5-HT research. *Pharmacology, Biochemistry and Behavior*, **71**, 555–568.
58 Gershon, M.D. and Tack, J. (2007) The serotonin signaling system: from basic understanding to drug development for functional GI disorders. *Gastroenterology*, **132**, 397–414.
59 Ford, A.C., Brandt, L.J., Young, C., Chey, W.D., Foxx-Orenstein, A.E., and Moayyedi, P. (2009) Efficacy of 5-HT_3 antagonists and 5-HT_4 agonists in irritable bowel syndrome: systematic review and meta-analysis. *American Journal of Gastroenterology*, **104**, 1831–1843.
60 Buchheit, K.H., Gamse, R., Giger, R., Hoyer, D., Klein, F., Kloppner, E., Pfannkuche, H.J., and Mattes, H. (1995) The serotonin 5-HT_4 receptor. 2. Structure–activity studies of the indole carbazimidamide class of agonists. *Journal of Medicinal Chemistry*, **38**, 2331–2338.
61 Rivkin, A. (2003) Tegaserod maleate in the treatment of irritable bowel syndrome: a clinical review. *Clinical Therapeutics*, **25**, 1952–1974.
62 Giger, R., Mattes, H., and Pfannkuche, H.J. (2007) Case history on tegaserod (Zelnorm®/Zelmac®). *Annual Reports in Medicinal Chemistry*, **42**, 195.
63 Clayton, N.M., Sargent, R., Butler, A., Gale, J., Maxwell, M.P., Hunt, A.A.E., Barrett, V.J., Cambridge, D., Bountra, C., and Humphrey, P.P.A. (1999) The pharmacological properties of the novel selective 5-HT_3 receptor antagonist, alosetron, and its effects on normal and perturbed small intestinal transit in the fasted rat. *Neurogastroenterology and Motility*, **11**, 207–217.
64 Mayer, E.A. and Bradesi, S. (2003) Alosetron and irritable bowel syndrome. *Expert Opinion on Pharmacotherapy*, **4**, 2089–2098.
65 Milne, R.J. and Heel, R.C. (1991) Ondansetron – therapeutic use as an antiemetic. *Drugs*, **41**, 574–595.
66 Freeman, A.J., Cunningham, K.T., and Tyers, M.B. (1992) Selectivity of 5-HT_3 receptor antagonists and antiemetic mechanisms of action. *Anti-Cancer Drugs*, **3**, 79–85.
67 Hesketh, P.J. (2000) Comparative review of 5-HT_3 receptor antagonists in the treatment of acute chemotherapy-induced nausea and vomiting. *Cancer Investigation*, **18**, 163–173.
68 Sanger, G.J. and Wardle, K.A. (1994) Constipation evoked by 5-HT_3-receptor antagonism – evidence for heterogeneous efficacy among different antagonists in guinea-pigs. *Journal of Pharmacy and Pharmacology*, **46**, 666–670.
69 (a) Camilleri, M. (2001) Management of the irritable bowel syndrome. *Gastroenterology*, **120**, 652–668; (b) Camilleri, M. (2009) Is adequate relief fatally flawed or adequate as an end point in irritable bowel syndrome? *American Journal of Gastroenterology*, **104**, 920–922; (c) Camilleri, M. (2013) Current and future pharmacological treatments for diarrhea-predominant irritable bowel syndrome. *Expert Opinion on Pharmacotherapy*, **14**, 1151–1160.
70 Jones, B.W., Moore, D.J., Robinson, S.M., and Song, F. (2002) A systematic review of tegaserod for the treatment of irritable bowel syndrome. *Journal of Clinical*

Pharmacy and Therapeutics, **27**, 343–352.

71 Hasler, W.L. and Schoenfeld, P. (2004) Safety profile of tegaserod, a 5-HT_4 receptor agonist, for the treatment of irritable bowel syndrome. *Drug Safety*, **27**, 619–631.

72 Patel, S., Berrada, D., and Lembo, A. (2004) Review of tegaserod in the treatment of irritable bowel syndrome. *Expert Opinion on Pharmacotherapy*, **5**, 2369–2379.

73 Sandham, D.A. and Pfannkuche, H.J. (2006) Recent advances in gastrointestinal prokinetic agents. *Annual Reports in Medicinal Chemistry*, **41**, 211–219.

74 McLaughlin, J. and Houghton, L.A. (2006) The rationale, efficacy and safety evidence for tegaserod in the treatment of irritable bowel syndrome. *Expert Opinion on Drug Safety*, **5**, 313–327.

75 Evans, B.W., Clark, W.K., Moore, D.J., and Whorwell, P.J. (2007) Tegaserod for the treatment of irritable bowel syndrome and chronic constipation. *Cochrane Database of Systematic Reviews*, **4** (Art. No.: CD003960). doi: 10.1002/14651858.CD003960.pub3.

76 Lewis, J.H. (2010) Alosetron for severe diarrhea-predominant irritable bowel syndrome: safety and efficacy in perspective. *Expert Review of Gastroenterology & Hepatology*, **4**, 13–29.

77 Bleser, S. (2011) Alosetron for severe diarrhea-predominant irritable bowel syndrome: improving patient outcomes. *Current Medical Research and Opinion*, **27**, 503–512.

78 Spiller, R.C. (2011) Targeting the 5-HT_3 receptor in the treatment of irritable bowel syndrome. *Current Opinion in Pharmacology*, **11**, 68–74.

79 Cremonini, F., Nicandro, J.P., Atkinson, V., Shringarpure, R., Chuang, E., and Lembo, A. (2012) Randomised clinical trial: alosetron improves quality of life and reduces restriction of daily activities in women with severe diarrhoea-predominant IBS. *Alimentary Pharmacology & Therapeutics*, **36**, 437–448.

80 Pfannkuche, H.J. and Dennis, E. (2004) Tegaserod-induced myocardial infarction: case report and hypothesis – an alternative viewpoint. *Pharmacotherapy*, **24**, 1649–1650.

81 Chan, K.Y.Y., de Vries, R., Leijten, F.P.J., Pfannkuche, H.J., van den Bogaerdt, A.J., Danser, A.H.J., and MaassenVanDenBrink, A. (2009) Functional characterization of contractions to tegaserod in human isolated proximal and distal coronary arteries. *European Journal of Pharmacology*, **619**, 61–67.

82 Higgins, D.L., Ero, M.P., Loeb, M., Kersey, K., Hopkins, A., and Beattie, D.T. (2012) The inability of tegaserod to affect platelet aggregation and coronary artery tone at supratherapeutic concentrations. *Naunyn-Schmiedeberg's Archives of Pharmacology*, **385**, 103–109.

83 Weber, E., Hamel, C.T., Bernhard, M., and Pfannkuche, H.J. (2006) Tegaserod has no potential for vasoconstriction or impairment of vasodilatation in isolated human and non-human primate mesenteric arteries. *Gastroenterology*, **130**, A489.

84 Goldberg, M., Li, Y.P., Johanson, J.F., Mangel, A.W., Kitt, M., Beattie, D.T., Kersey, K., and Daniels, O. (2010) Clinical trial: the efficacy and tolerability of velusetrag, a selective 5-HT_4 agonist with high intrinsic activity, in chronic idiopathic constipation – a 4-week, randomized, double-blind, placebo-controlled, dose-response study. *Alimentary Pharmacology & Therapeutics*, **32**, 1102–1112.

85 Long, D.D., Armstrong, S.R., Beattie, D.T., Choi, S.K. *et al.* (2012) Discovery, oral pharmacokinetics and *in vivo* efficacy of velusetrag, a highly selective HT_4 receptor agonist that has achieved proof-of-concept in patients with chronic idiopathic constipation. *Bioorganic & Medicinal Chemistry Letters*, **22**, 6048–6052.

86 Shin, A., Camilleri, M., Kolar, G., Erwin, P., West, C.P., and Murad, M.H. (2014) Systematic review with meta-analysis: highly selective 5-HT_4 agonists (prucalopride, velusetrag or naronapride) in chronic constipation. *Alimentary*

Pharmacology & Therapeutics, **39**, 239–253.

87 Chang, L., Tong, K., and Ameen, V. (2010) Ischemic colitis and complications of constipation associated with the use of alosetron under a risk management plan: clinical characteristics, outcomes, and incidences. *American Journal of Gastroenterology*, **105**, 866–875.

88 Lucak, S. (2012) Irritable bowel syndrome and ischemic colitis: evidence supporting the increased use of alosetron. *Therapeutic Advances in Gastroenterology*, **5**, 215–218.

89 Thompson, C.A. (2013) FDA's advisers recommend updating alosetron's REMS. *American Journal of Health-System Pharmacy*, **70**, 1365–1366.

90 Tong, K., Nicandro, J.P., Shringarpure, R., Chuang, E., and Chang, L. (2013) A 9-year evaluation of temporal trends in alosetron postmarketing safety under the risk management program. *Therapeutic Advances in Gastroenterology*, **6**, 344–357.

91 Mosli, M., Parfitt, J., and Gregor, J. (2013) Retrospective analysis of disease association and outcome in histologically confirmed ischemic colitis. *Journal of Digestive Diseases*, **14**, 238–243.

92 Kane, J.M., Honigfeld, G., Singer, J., and Meltzer, H. (1988) Clozapine in treatment-resistant schizophrenics. *Psychopharmacology Bulletin*, **24**, 62–67.

93 Kane, J.M., Honigfeld, G., Singer, J., and Meltzer, H. (1989) Clozapine for the treatment-resistant schizophrenic – results of a US multicenter trial. *Psychopharmacology*, **99**, S60–S63.

94 Kane, J., Honigfeld, G., Singer, J., and Meltzer, H. (1988) Clozapine for the treatment-resistant schizophrenic – a double-blind comparison with chlorpromazine. *Archives of General Psychiatry*, **45**, 789–796.

95 Krupp, F., Hippius, H., Meltzer, H.P., Kane, J.M., Gerlach, J. *et al.* (1992) Clozapine – the atypical antipsychotic – discussion. *British Journal of Psychiatry*, **160**, 60–64.

96 Grunder, G., Hippius, H., and Carlsson, A. (2009) The 'atypicality' of antipsychotics: a concept re-examined and re-defined. *Nature Reviews. Drug Discovery*, **8**, 197–202.

97 Meltzer, H.Y. (1992) Treatment of the neuroleptic-nonresponsive schizophrenic patient. *Schizophrenia Bulletin*, **18**, 515–542.

98 Meltzer, H.Y. (2004) What's atypical about atypical antipsychotic drugs? *Current Opinion in Pharmacology*, **4**, 53–57.

99 Meltzer, H.Y. (2013) Update on typical and atypical antipsychotic drugs. *Annual Review of Medicine*, **64**, 393–406.

100 Meltzer, H.Y., Alphs, L., Green, A.I., Altamura, A.C. *et al.* (2003) Clozapine treatment for suicidality in schizophrenia – International Suicide Prevention Trial (InterSePT). *Archives of General Psychiatry*, **60**, 82–91.

101 Meltzer, H.Y. and Roth, B.L. (2013) Lorcaserin and pimavanserin: emerging selectivity of serotonin receptor subtype-targeted drugs. *Journal of Clinical Investigation*, **123**, 4986–4991.

102 Abbas, A. and Roth, B.L. (2008) Pimavanserin tartrate: a 5-HT_{2A} inverse agonist with potential for treating various neuropsychiatric disorders. *Expert Opinion on Pharmacotherapy*, **9**, 3251–3259.

103 Barrett, E., Blonde, L., Clement, S., Davis, J. *et al.* (American Diabetes Association; American Psychiatric Association; American Association of Clinical Endocrinologists; North American Association for the Study of Obesity) (2004) Consensus development conference on antipsychotic drugs and obesity and diabetes. *Obesity Research*, **12**, 362–368.

104 Meltzer, H.Y. and Fatemi, H. (1995) Suicide in schizophrenia: the effect of clozapine. *Clinical Neuropharmacology*, **18**, S18–S24.

105 Meltzer, H.Y., Li, Z., Kaneda, Y., and Ichikawa, J. (2003) Serotonin receptors: their key role in drugs to treat schizophrenia. *Progress in Neuro-Psychopharmacology & Biological Psychiatry*, **27**, 1159–1172.

106 Alphs, L., Anand, R., Islam, M.Z., Meltzer, H.Y., Kane, J.M., Krishnan, R.

et al. (2004) The International Suicide Prevention Trial (InterSePT): rationale and design of a trial comparing the relative ability of clozapine and olanzapine to reduce suicidal behavior in schizophrenia and schizoaffective patients. *Schizophrenia Bulletin*, **30**, 577–586.
107 Goadsby, P.J. (1998) Serotonin 5-$HT_{1B/1D}$ receptor agonists in migraine – comparative pharmacology and its therapeutic implications. *CNS Drugs*, **10**, 271–286.
108 Goadsby, P.J. (2007) Emerging therapies for migraine. *Nature Clinical Practice Neurology*, **3**, 610–619.
109 Lipton, R.B., Bigal, M.E., and Goadsby, P.J. (2004) Double-blind clinical trials of oral triptans vs other classes of acute migraine medication – a review. *Cephalalgia*, **24**, 321–332.
110 Humphrey, P.P.A., Feniuk, W., Perren, M.J., Beresford, I.J.M., Skingle, M., and Whalley, E.T. (1990) Serotonin and migraine. *Annals of the New York Academy of Sciences*, **600**, 587–600.
111 Humphrey, P.P.A., Feniuk, W., Marriott, A.S., Tanner, M.R. *et al.* (1991) Preclinical studies on the antimigraine drug, sumatriptan. *European Neurology*, **31**, 282–290.
112 Humphrey, P.P.A., Hartig, P., and Hoyer, D. (1993) A proposed new nomenclature for 5-HT receptors. *Trends in Pharmacological Sciences*, **14**, 233–236.
113 Connor, H.E., Stubbs, C.M., Feniuk, W., and Humphrey, P.P.A. (1992) Effect of sumatriptan, a selective 5-HT_1-like receptor agonist, on pial vessel diameter in anesthetized cats. *Journal of Cerebral Blood Flow and Metabolism*, **12**, 514–519.
114 Feniuk, W. and Humphrey, P.P.A. (1992) The development of a highly selective 5-HT_1 receptor agonist, sumatriptan, for the treatment of migraine. *Drug Development Research*, **26**, 235–240.
115 Humphrey, P.P.A. (2008) The discovery and development of the triptans, a major therapeutic breakthrough. *Headache*, **48**, 685–687.
116 Schoeffter, P. and Hoyer, D. (1989) How selective is GR-43175 – interactions with functional 5-HT_{1A}, 5-HT_{1B}, 5-HT_{1C} and 5-HT_{1D} receptors. *Naunyn-Schmiedeberg's Archives of Pharmacology*, **340**, 135–138.
117 Hoyer, D., Schoeffter, P., and Gray, J.A. (1989) A comparison of the interactions of dihydroergotamine, ergotamine and GR 43175 with 5-HT_1 receptor subtypes. *Cephalalgia*, **9**, 340–341.
118 Tfelt-Hansen, P., Saxena, P.R., Dahlof, C., Pascual, J., Lainez, M., Henry, P., Diener, H.C., Schoenen, J., Ferrari, M.D., and Goadsby, P.J. (2000) Ergotamine in the acute treatment of migraine – a review and European consensus. *Brain*, **123**, 9–18.
119 Ferrari, M.D., Goadsby, P.J., Roon, K.I., and Lipton, R.B. (2002) Triptans (serotonin, 5-$HT_{1B/1D}$ agonists) in migraine: detailed results and methods of a meta-analysis of 53 trials. *Cephalalgia*, **22**, 633–658.
120 Humphrey, P.P.A. and Goadsby, P.J. (1994) The mode of action of sumatriptan is vascular – a debate. *Cephalalgia*, **14**, 401–410.
121 Meyler, W.J. (1996) Side effects of ergotamine. *Cephalalgia*, **16**, 5–10.
122 Fuller, R.W. (1991) Role of serotonin in therapy of depression and related disorders. *Journal of Clinical Psychiatry*, **52**, 52–57.
123 Fuller, R.W., Hemrickluecke, S.K., and Snoddy, H.D. (1994) Effects of duloxetine, an antidepressant drug candidate, on concentrations of monoamines and their metabolites in rats and mice. *Journal of Pharmacology and Experimental Therapeutics*, **269**, 132–136.
124 Fuller, R.W. and Marshall, W.S. (1965) Treatment of depression. *Lancet*, **2**, 640.
125 Robertson, D.W. and Fuller, R.W. (1991) Progress in antidepressant drugs. *Annual Reports in Medicinal Chemistry*, **26**, 23–32.

Section 2
Hepatic Side Effects

Antitargets and Drug Safety, First Edition. Edited by László Urbán, Vinod F. Patel, and Roy J. Vaz.

5
Drug-Induced Liver Injury: Clinical and Diagnostic Aspects*

John R. Senior

5.1
Introduction

This chapter is divided into four main sections. This section deals with introductory and general comments, and isoniazid hepatitis as an example, Section 5.2 provides a discussion of postmarketing concerns, Section 5.3 deals with new development issues, and Section 5.4 provides closing comments and research opportunities.

It is pertinent first to ask the following question:

> Is it a toxic drug? Or an especially susceptible patient?

We must remember and accept that drugs have different effects on different people, both for intended beneficial effects on a targeted organ or receptor and for possibly adverse effects on unintended, off-target sites. These adverse effects, here called "antitarget" effects, may occur. The latter term is relatively new, appearing first in a published title only as recently as 2005 [1]. It refers to a receptor, enzyme, or other biological site for a drug action that leads to undesirable or adverse side effects when the site is affected. Perhaps we should consider extending that definition to an especially susceptible person.

The problems facing those who develop new drugs and those who later prescribe them are quite different. Drugs are developed and selected to induce beneficial and not harmful effects in patients to whom the drug is meant to be prescribed, recommended, or sold. It is not enough just to develop new drugs that are safe for most or nearly all of the people, because the very same dose of

*Although the material discussed here is based largely on experiences since 1995 as a medical reviewer and since 2000 as a consultant in hepatology at the FDA, the opinions expressed do not necessarily reflect regulatory positions or policies of the agency. The author received no special funding for preparing this chapter and has no conflicts of interest.

Antitargets and Drug Safety, First Edition. Edited by László Urbán, Vinod F. Patel, and Roy J. Vaz.

the very same drug may be quite safe, well tolerated, and effective for most patients, but quite toxic to a few. Not just the number of effects, but their severity and consequences, time course, and degree of causal likelihood should be considered. Just a few patients who show serious adverse effects, even if rare, may negate moderate benefits to many. This balance may determine whether or not a drug remains available in the market. It is also easy to appreciate why liver injury is so often seen after exposure to a drug, for the liver receives something over a quarter of the cardiac output of blood, including both portal venous and hepatic arterial flow, and metabolizes xenobiotic nonendogenous compounds as well as many endogenous materials. Therefore, liver cells are exposed to the fresh metabolites that may cause injury or perturbation by a variety of mechanisms that are still being explored by basic scientists, including many authors of other chapters in this book. The liver is of course not the only antitarget for adverse drug effects, but has been a principal one [2], perhaps because of its metabolism of drugs and compounds. Severe hepatotoxicity was the leading cause for withdrawing approved drugs from the market previously, before cardiovascular problems supplanted it.

The liver is unique among our major internal organs in having the remarkable ability to regenerate even after quite drastic resection or damage to two-thirds or even more of its volume, regrowing quickly to its original size and function, and then stopping, as so well summarized in 1967 by Dr. Nancy Bucher in her excellent two-part review [3,4]. A very recent update on liver regeneration was written by Itoh and Miyajima [5]. The unique ability of the liver, among all our vital internal organs, to regrow rapidly after injury has been known for a very long time, as recalled to us by the story of Prometheus [6]. The ancient Greeks were onto something, in naming the liver "hēpar" (after hēpaomai, which means "to repair oneself"); they clearly understood the liver's capability to regenerate.

Short of full regeneration, hepatic cells often appear to be able to adapt and change their functioning, becoming tolerant to drugs initially injurious. They may show hepatocellular necrosis or apoptosis first, and then little or no adverse effect when re-exposed to drug [7].

5.1.1
Postmarketing Hepatotoxicity versus Hepatotoxicity in Development

Although the focus of this book is on identifying and excluding from development new compounds that are likely to be toxic to the liver, a persisting major problem is the often rare but serious hepatotoxicity that occurs after marketing in certain individual patients, a phenomenon termed "idiosyncrasy," for lack of better understanding of its mechanisms or causes. The often-used distinction between "dose-related" and "idiosyncratic" drug reactions is not absolute. There are very few drugs at the extreme ends of the Zimmerman [8] "spectrum of hepatotoxicity," shown as Figure 1.1 in his texts of 1978 and 1999 [9].

Most adverse drug reactions manifest features of both (see Figure 5.1). It is overly simplistic to state that some drugs are predictably and reproducibly "true"

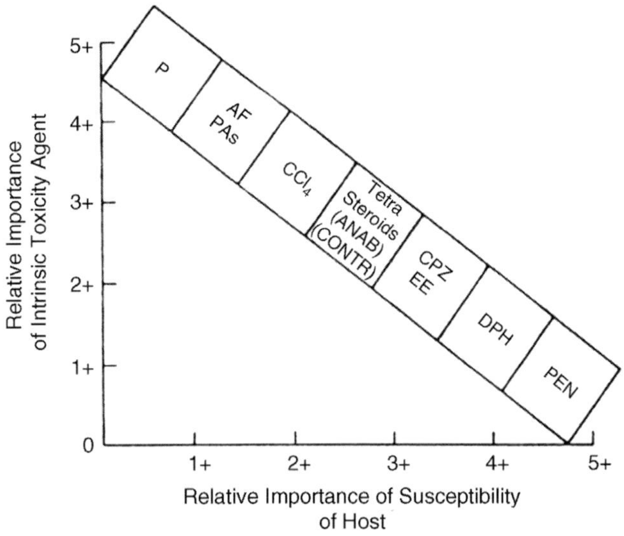

Figure 5.1 Relative importance of the intrinsic toxicity of a chemical agent and susceptibility of an exposed individual in production of hepatic injury. P, elemental phosphorous; AF, aflatoxins; PAs, pyrrolizidine alkaloids; CCl_4, carbon tetrachloride; Tetra, tetracycline; ANAB and CONTRA, anabolic and contraceptive steroids; CPZ, chlorpromazine; EE, erythromycin estolate; DPH, diphenylhydantoin, phenytoin; PEN, penicillin.

hepatotoxins because of properties that cause dose-related liver injury, whereas others show none of those features and effects depend only upon undefined idiosyncrasies of the person to whom the drug is given. Although there are many forms of chemically induced liver injury, idiosyncrasy of the host is responsible for many of the cases of serious hepatotoxicity currently seen in new drugs after approval for marketing. The term means "one's own mixing together" (idios = one's self + syn = together + krasis = mixture, a word of Greek derivation) and implies that each human is somewhat different from others despite many common characteristics.

5.1.2
Isoniazid – If It Were Newly Discovered, Would It Be Approved Today?

Hydrazine derivatives of pyridine carbonic acids have been known for more than 100 years, dating to 1912 when two graduate chemistry students in Prague [10] synthesized isonicotinyl hydrazide, known as isoniazid and abbreviated INH. Isonicotinic acid is the 4-isomer of nicotinic acid (vitamin B_3, 3-carboxypyridine). Free hydrazine is a toxic, flammable, and unstable substance used for rocket fuel and for emergency power in F-16 fighter jets. Nicotinic acid, vitamin B_3, was called niacin (= nicotinic acid vitamin) to distinguish it from the addicting plant alkaloid nicotine, found by Jean Nicot in tobacco, but also in other

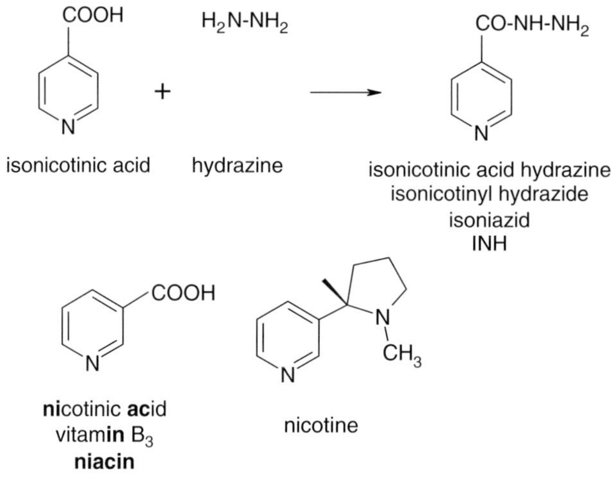

Figure 5.2 Chemical structures of key compounds mentioned.

plants such as green pepper, eggplant, and tomato (see Figure 5.2). It is also toxic (lethal dose for 50% of humans is 0.5 mg/kg, 100 times the toxicity in rats).

In 1936, Gerhard Domagk in Germany, after researching many compounds, discovered sulfanilamide as the first antibacterial agent. He was awarded the Nobel Prize in 1939, but the Nazi regime would not allow him to accept it. He later did so in 1947 but without the monetary award. In 1944, Schatz and Waksman discovered streptomycin to be active against tuberculosis [11], a first pharmaceutical alternative to the regimen of sanatorium rest and fresh air, leading to another Nobel Prize, for Waksman in 1952. Domagk kept on working and searched among many compounds for activity against tuberculosis. In 1950, he found active thiosemicarbazones [12] and isoniazid, an orally administrable compound found to be more active against tuberculosis by Grunberg and Schnitzer [13].

INH was first used for treatment of tuberculosis in June 1951 by Selikoff and Robitzek [14] at Sea View Hospital on Staten Island, NY, as cited by Lapp *et al.* [15], who wrote that “A new drug is with us in the treatment of tuberculosis. It is a synthetic chemical of known composition, relatively non-toxic, cheap, and simple to prepare.” INH use spread rapidly in 1952 in North America and Europe [16], because it could be given orally.

An early case of serious liver injury with jaundice was published in 1953 [17]. The later story of clinical liver effects of INH has been well summarized at the LiverTox website [18], with 363 references. INH became used mainly to prevent tuberculosis. For treating active disease it had been found that INH alone was insufficient, and combinations of two or more drugs (such as pyrazinamide, *para*-aminosalicylic acid, rifampin, ethambutol, and streptomycin) were needed to prevent emergence of resistance. Sporadic reports of a few deaths in patients taking just isoniazid appeared in the 20 years after it was first used to treat tuberculosis, sometimes complicated by underlying disease, administration of other antitubercular therapy, but in some cases isoniazid alone appeared capable of causing liver injury and sometimes killing susceptible patients [19–22].

Two notable studies were carried out in the early 1970s. First was a Public Health study of 13 838 patients at 26 United States health clinics from July 1971 to November 1972 [23,24]. Black *et al.* reported [23] that 224 of the 13 838 patients (1.6%) were suspected to have INH-caused hepatitis on clinical grounds, but no routine testing of serum enzymes was done consistently. Of that number they assessed 87 as probably INH-induced hepatitis, another 76 possibly related, 18 due to other liver disease, 20 as not hepatitis, and 23 with insufficient data to decide. They then added another 27 cases from other hospitals (with no known total exposed) to make up 114 cases probably induced by INH, to characterize the syndrome. There were 7 deaths from the 87 Public Health group and 6 from the 27 added patients, totaling 13 fatal cases from the 114 probably induced by INH (1.1%). The clinical picture of probably INH-induced hepatitis was chemically and histologically not distinguishable from viral hepatitis but was more likely to occur among elderly patients. Fatal outcome was more likely if INH therapy was prolonged for more than 2 months.

Later analysis of the large Public Health study by Kopanoff *et al.* [24] reported 8 deaths, 7 in Baltimore of 3196 patients (0.2%), among 25 cases of INH-induced hepatitis (0.8%). Six of the seven Baltimore cases were female, five black and one white, and the seventh a white male. One death occurred in Cincinnati, out of 709. No deaths and 64 cases (0.6%) of probably INH-induced hepatitis occurred among 9933 patients from the other 24 cities.

The second study [25] was smaller and more controlled, done at the Eastern State Hospital (a psychiatric hospital) in Williamsburg, VA, of 358 patients in 1971–1972. Of them, 218 were reactive to tuberculin and were treated with isoniazid 300 mg/day as prophylaxis against tuberculosis and 140 nonreactive patients were followed but not treated with INH. In that more carefully monitored study of the psychiatric patients, 201 of the 218 patients given INH completed at least 4 weeks of a planned year of observation with regular monthly testing of serum aspartate aminotransferase (AST) and total bilirubin (TBL), as did 107 of the 140 untreated patients. Frozen sera were sent to the Center for Disease Control in Atlanta, but neither were analyzed immediately nor influenced clinical management. Weekly records were kept of symptoms and medications. Chemistry results were not known until after the treatment year. In 22 of the 173 patients (12.7%) who completed a year, AST elevations were >30 mU/ml, taken as the upper limit of normal (ULN). Three (see Figure 5.3) showed elevated TBL >3 mg/dl in addition to AST elevations from 14.6 to 30.7 times the ULN – what we would now consider Hy's law cases if caused by INH and not cholestatic!

None of the patients receiving INH had any clinical symptoms during treatment and all three with highest abnormalities recovered to normal levels of bilirubin by the end of their treatment despite continuing the INH, and did not progress to liver failure. Note that the older patient (M61b) showed delayed rise

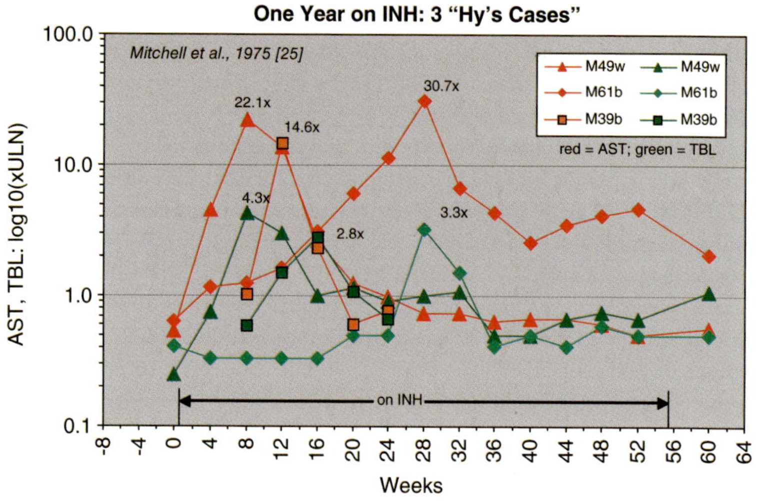

Figure 5.3 The *x*–*y* plot of $\log_{10}$ values of liver tests over time.

in AST and persisting but lesser elevations, although his bilirubin had returned to normal when the AST subsided.

These findings then confirmed what had been shown beautifully at New York Hospital in 1969 by Scharer and Smith [20] – that INH alone could cause acute liver injury, with fairly frequent elevations in serum transaminases, but less common liver dysfunction with bilirubin elevations. Patients showing worrisome abnormalities did not usually progress to liver failure or death. In very large studies, with many thousands of patients observed, some deaths could occur, particularly if patients were not closely followed. These were important lessons for a valuable drug that prevented tuberculosis!

The issues were argued back and forth, but a large study by Nolan *et al.* [26] of 11 141 patients treated with INH to prevent tuberculosis in Seattle–King County from January 1989 through December 1995 did much to resolve the debate. They also observed another 1427 patients with active tuberculosis treated with combination regimens. Patients were seen in clinic monthly, given medication refills, and were reminded at each visit to take note of and report symptoms of liver toxicity, but were not monitored with serum tests. Only 11 of the 11 141 patients on INH prophylaxis (0.10%) had symptoms leading to findings of elevated serum hepatocellular enzyme activities (peak AST: 303–1160 U/l). Among them, eight also showed elevated bilirubin (2.8–10.6 mg/dl), and one was hospitalized. None developed liver failure or died, and all recovered without sequelae. Among the 1427 patients treated with multiple antitubercular drugs for active disease, there were 15 (1.05%) who showed hepatotoxic effects. They attributed these results to including mostly (80%) only younger patients <35 years of age and using clinical symptoms to trigger investigation rather than serum enzyme tests.

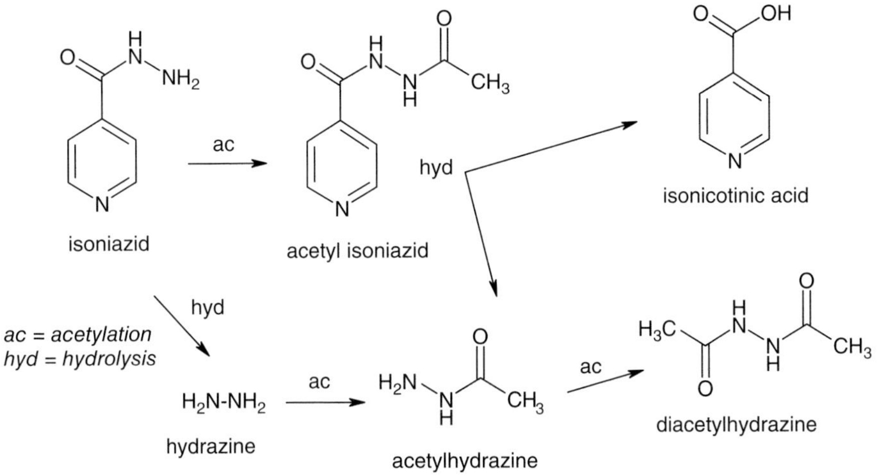

Figure 5.4 Chemical structures of isoniazid derivatives.

Mitchell *et al.* had postulated [25] that people who showed rapid acetylation rates might be at higher risk of developing hepatitis from isoniazid, whose principal metabolite was acetyl isoniazid [27], competitively inhibited by other substrates [28], and that acetylation was polymorphic [29]. However, this was challenged by several other investigators, leading to the current consensus that slow acetylators may be at higher risk [30–32].

As may be seen, it is necessary to consider not only the first step of INH acetylation, but also its subsequent hydrolysis that can generate even more toxic secondary metabolites, such as acetylhydrazine and even free hydrazine (see Figure 5.4). Rapid acetylation to harmless, nontoxic diacetylhydrazine is protective, so slow acetylators may be at greater risk.

This example illustrates what could have been a major problem, if it were judged by current standards and criteria. There were many "Hy's law" cases that today might be ominous for a new drug, but over that earlier time it became evident that isoniazid was doing far more good than harm, and that it could be used safely. We can only speculate on what the answer might be to the question posed at the beginning of this section.

5.2
Special Problems of Postmarketing Hepatotoxicity

There are major differences between pre- and postmarketing strategies for dealing with hepatotoxicity. Clinical studies may include hundreds or even thousands of subjects, but after marketing, hundreds of thousands or millions of patients may be given or take the drug, enormously increasing the likelihood of seeing a relatively rare but serious adverse event. In addition, patients to whom the drug is prescribed after approval or perhaps taken without prescription may be less carefully selected than subjects who had met protocol restrictions of controlled studies before marketing, and may be less carefully followed. Adverse drug reactions are often missed or never reported if they occur, or if reported too frequently are not well enough described for making accurate diagnosis of the probable cause. Errors of both omission (false-negative, beta errors) and nonspecificity (false-positive, alpha errors) are common in postmarketing reports.

During clinical development, in controlled trials under protocols, subjects chosen for participation are usually observed for liver cell injury by scheduled monitoring of serum enzyme activities that are quite sensitive for detecting early injury. In the postmarketing use of approved drugs, the focus is on efficacy, whether the drug administered produces beneficial effects, and monitoring is usually poorly done or not at all. Even if elevated serum enzymes are found, they may not be well investigated to determine the severity and cause of the findings, or the results not reported. Consequently, adverse, off-target effects are too often missed, not detected, and underreported, creating a large type 2 (beta, false-negative) error, and no reliable assessment of the incidence of the problem is possible. In clinical trials, where routine monitoring is done, there is more likely a type 1 (alpha) error in which modest elevations of serum enzyme activities are taken as important but represent false-positive findings that would resolve without treatment or interruption of treatment, due to the frequent process of hepatic adaptation.

5.2.1 Voluntary Monitoring after Approval for Marketing

In some cases, findings of modest liver injury during controlled clinical trials may lead to labeling recommendations for periodic monitoring of serum aminotransferase activity to detect early hepatocellular injury. This has often turned out to be ineffective because it is dependent on cooperation of patients and their physicians, both of whom grow weary of receiving repeatedly negative test results, because what is being looked for is rare, and may not occur for some time, so that the vast majority of test results are negative. This leads to quitting the monitoring, which consequently cannot be effective. Alternatively, waiting for patients to report symptoms such as nausea, fatigue, or jaundice may cause such delay that really serious liver toxicity by then may be irreversible even if the drug is stopped. No universally satisfactory alternative to routine monitoring has been found as yet. Theoretically, patients under treatment should be closely observed, and even early and mild symptoms investigated thoroughly, but this is extremely difficult to enforce. This situation has been a driving factor for seeking predictive biomarkers.

5.2.2 Prediction of Serious, Dysfunctional Liver Injury

Unfortunately, there are not as yet any biomarkers that reliably predict which individual will develop progressively severe liver injury from a drug. This is especially difficult because of the rarity of serious effects leading to disability, life-threatening illness, death, or need for transplantation. Only observation over time currently is effective in finding an individual who can neither tolerate nor adapt to the drug, and the only treatment is to stop administration of the drug to those persons. Because of the quite common ability of many patients to adapt to a new drug after showing transient or nonprogressive liver injury from it, negative rechallenge results are not convincing proof of susceptibility to serious drug-induced liver injury (DILI). Positive rechallenge, on the other hand, is powerful evidence of such susceptibility, but is dangerous unless patients are very closely watched. Not all prescribing physicians in medical practice are experts in liver disorders, and their ability to recognize, investigate, and diagnose the problem is quite variable. Lack of reporting, or inadequate reporting of necessary details, is too common, and no reliable estimate of the incidence of drug-induced liver injury can be made from the spontaneous and often isolated, delayed reports that reach publication or official recognition.

5.2.3 Severity of Liver Injury Is Not Measured by Aminotransferase Elevations

It is important to appreciate that severity of drug-induced injury to the liver varies from mild asymptomatic injury detectable only by elevated serum aminotransferase or other biomarkers without symptoms or functional disturbance of the liver to acute liver failure and death or need for transplantation. Activities of serum enzymes, released from injured hepatocytes, are not valid measures of the severity of adverse liver effect, which is really dependent on how much of the whole organ is not injured and still able to function well. The level of serum activity of enzymes released from injured cells depends upon the rapidity and extent of the injury and is a useful indicator of the *urgency to investigate* the patient to determine the course and cause of the abnormal findings. The only tests commonly and routinely done that truly measure a liver function are the serum bilirubin concentration (measures ability of liver to clear plasma of bilirubin, conjugate it with glucuronide, and excrete it into bile) and the prothrombin time or its derived international normalized ratio (INR; measures ability of the liver to synthesize and regulate the level of a key coagulation protein). Serum albumin concentration is too insensitive to be useful for acute cases. Other tests of liver functions may be done in special cases, but *regulation of serum aminotransferase activity is not a liver function, so activities of biomarker enzymes in serum should not be called "liver function tests."*

5.2.4 Attempts to Standardize Terminology

International conferences were held in 1974 and 1978 at the Fogarty International Center of the National Institutes of Health (NIH) in Bethesda, MD, on standardization of liver and biliary disease nomenclature [33] and detection of drug-induced hepatotoxicity [34]. At the latter conference, it was the consensus (not data-based, but opinions of experts) that elevations of serum enzyme activities were "markedly abnormal" if more than three times the upper limit of the normal range (>3× ULN). This concept was carried forward to the first 1982 version[1)] of the National Cancer Institute Common Toxicity Criteria at which a slightly lower cutoff of >2.5× ULN was taken as distinguishing mildly from moderately severe toxicity (grade 1 from grade 2). The Common Toxicity Criteria were revised in 1998 (version 2) and 2006 (version 3), at which time the listing was greatly expanded and the name changed to Common Terminology Criteria for Adverse Events (CTCAE) and the cutoff between grades 1 and 2 was raised slightly to 3× ULN.

The CTCAE are again in revision for version 5, expected in 2015, but continue to use the concepts of earlier versions. Standard liver tests, such as serum enzyme activities of alanine and aspartate aminotransferases (ALT and AST) and alkaline phosphatase (ALP), as well as concentration of TBL, are graded by how much they are elevated above the ULNs. Grades of severity are assigned, depending on how much elevated: grade 1, mild and not requiring intervention, from >1 to 3× ULN for ALT and AST, from >1 to 2.5× ULN for ALP, and from >1 to 1.5× ULN for bilirubin. Grade 2 denotes moderate severity, for up to 5× ULN for the three enzymes and up to 3× ULN for bilirubin. Grade 3 elevations are taken as severe, with need for or extension of hospitalization, disability but not immediately threatening to life, for enzyme elevations from >5 to 20× ULN or bilirubin elevations from >3 to 10× ULN. Grade 4 enzyme elevations of >20× ULN or bilirubin elevations of >10× ULN are classified as immediately life-threatening and requiring urgent intervention. Grade 5 is used for fatal outcomes, not applicable to these serum tests. These grades were not based on data analyses but on opinions from unidentified committees. Unfortunately, no definition of *normal* was made, and the range of normal was left to local laboratories to define, which has led to wide variation in the putative normal ranges. Even greater than differences in methods used to measure enzyme activity are differences in people who are assumed to be normal because they do not appear ill but may have undiagnosed diseases.

5.2.5
What Is the "Normal" Range, or the "Upper Limit of Normal"?

The word *normal* has many meanings. Two that are most pertinent to this discussion are the statistical term meaning frequent or common, and the medical term meaning well or healthy, not diseased. After marketing, major interest is whether the findings in a given patient should raise concern about a possible disease being present. In clinical practice, the medical view should be used, certainly to assess individual cases. An approach to the question was taken by

1) National Cancer Institute: Common Toxicity Criteria 1982 and 1998; Common Terminology Criteria for Adverse Events 2003 and 2009.

Dr. Daniele Prati [35] who studied prospective first-time blood donors in Milan, ruling out those who had asymptomatic chronic hepatitis C, excessive use of alcohol, obesity, skeletal or cardiac muscle damage, concurrent medications, or other possibilities, concluding from 3927 volunteers that healthy normal upper limit of serum ALT normal for men was 30 U/l (U = μmol/min) and for women was 19 U/l. She also reported median values of the tests for healthy men and women as 13 and 9 U/l, respectively. These are much lower ULNs than found by statistical methods that ignore elevations caused by disease, age, and gender. There are no known clinical implications for having lowered serum enzyme activities.

5.2.6 Diagnostic Test Evaluation

Evaluation of diagnostic tests for distinguishing diseased from nondiseased persons was advanced greatly in 1966 by the much-cited paper of Thomas Vecchio [36]. It introduced the idea of "positive predictive value" and "negative predictive value" of the test result. *It is unfortunate that Vecchio used the word "predictive" for a single test result, without knowing what the results were before or might be afterward.* However, he emphasized a critical point that has been overlooked too often, which was the prevalence of the sought disease in the population considered and tested (see Figure 5.5). For occurrence of a new finding, onset of drug-induced liver injury at a future time, the term *incidence* is better.

It is evident that evaluation of such a test looks very good indeed, when results from equal numbers of people with or without the disease are compared. However, when the results of such a very well "validated" test are applied to seeking a relatively rare event in a population where only 1 per 1000 develops disease (compare results above), a very different conclusion would be reached about the value of a positive test result (Figure 5.6).

Obviously, a positive test that is nearly always wrong is not useful, and the value of test result must consider incidence of new events or prevalence of existing problems.

"Validated" on Common Events

test result	SDILI present	none	total count	"value"
positive	47,500 TP	2,500 FP	50,000 P	0.95 looks good
negative	2,500 FN	47,500 TN	50,000 N	0.95 looks good
incidence	50,000 *50%*	50,000 *50%*	100,000 tested	
	sensitivity *95%*	*specificity,* *95%*	*accuracy,* *95%*	

Figure 5.5 Validation for common (50% incidence) events.

Looking for a Rare Event

test result	SDILI present	none	total count	"value"
positive	95 TP	4,995 FP	5,090 P	0.0187 98.1% wrong
negative	5 FN	94,950 TN	94,910 N	0.9999 who cares ?
incidence	100 *0.1%*	99,900 *99.9%*	100,000	
	sensitivity *95%*	*specificity,* *95%*	*accuracy,* *95%*	

Figure 5.6 Poor positive test value for rare (1/1000) event incidence.

5.2.7 Determination of the Likely Cause of Liver Abnormalities

The most notable deficiency in postmarketing reports of liver injuries possibly caused by a drug or chemical is lack of proof of causality. We have come to realize that almost any drug may cause at least some transient injury to the hepatocytes of at least a few people, and that the range of the injury is from minimal, asymptomatic, slow leakage of enzymes from the injured cells into circulating plasma all the way to liver failure. Although those leaked enzymes do not have any useful function in the plasma and are simply proteins awaiting proteolytic degradation, their enzymatic activity can be coaxed out by addition of cofactors and substrates for some days before they are degraded and inactivated. We also have come to appreciate that not only hepatocytes but other types of liver cells may also be injured, and that the patterns of injury are diverse, mimicking almost all types of liver diseases. Consequently, it is not possible to diagnose injuries as drug-induced, actually caused by the drug, on liver biopsy. At best it may be said that patterns of histological findings are "compatible with" or "possibly related to" the drug effect. Proof of causality is not yet possible by any single biomarker. Diagnosis of drug–cause requires obtaining extra supplemental clinical information to rule out to a reasonable degree of likelihood other possible causes. At present, this cannot be done by serum chemistries alone, but requires medical differential diagnosis. It remains unfortunate that drug-induced liver injury is still a "diagnosis of exclusion" that requires medical expertise. It seems a waste of effort to pursue minor forms of liver injury that produce no symptoms or loss of true functions of the liver, to chase after transient serum enzyme increases. That effort should be put on observation and investigation of potentially serious cases of DILI that lead to clinical illness, inability to work, hospitalization, or worse.

At present, diagnosis of the cause of liver injury is still a medical art and cannot be done accurately by biomarkers or nonphysicians. It is not sufficient to use the weaker and almost meaningless terms of "associated with" or "related to" to a drug if what is meant is that the drug actually caused the liver problem. Admittedly, it is difficult to determine the likelihood of causality, whether the drug or something else really was of the probable cause for liver injury caused by drugs.

5.2.8 Treatment and Management of DILI in Practice

Treatment is dependent on correct diagnosis; wrong diagnosis leads to wrong treatment. If the injury is mild and transient, no treatment may be required, and administration of the drug may be continued, if it is having a beneficial effect. If the injury is worsening, it is wise to interrupt treatment until the course over time is clearer, and to be cautious in restarting the drug. If the injury becomes serious, the drug must be stopped. There are no known antidotes that are generally useful, so the difficult burden of deciding whether or not to stop drug administration falls upon the prescribing physician. Serious DILI may come rapidly, and is unpredictable. Despite this, detection and recognition of DILI is often missed and unreported even if found. Mild DILI is often asymptomatic, detectable only by testing serum for high activity of enzymes such as ALT, AST, and ALP.

5.3 Special Problems for New Drug Development

As mentioned earlier, the problem of avoiding serious DILI from potential new drugs is a major concern of pharmaceutical companies engaged in the very competitive and costly process of developing new drugs. Testing for safety in human subjects taking part in controlled clinical trials requires large numbers of study sites and subjects. This makes it possible to start applying the test questions mentioned in Section 5.1: "How many? How much? How soon? How likely?" It is very difficult to find out exactly how many patients have been prescribed a drug after approval for marketing, how many actually took what dose for how long, how many had what side effects or when, or even if they did whether it was reported. Controlled clinical trials provide an opportunity to do so, because all subjects need to be accounted for, routine observation with mandatory reporting is done, and records are kept. Opportunity is available to obtain some idea of the incidence of adverse effects and to determine whether they are mild, moderate, or severe; when they occur after administering the drug; and to investigate the serious cases for probable cause (which may not be the drug). We shall consider each of these four simple questions in following sections.

5.3.1 How Many?

The incidence of adverse effects is a useful and important issue that is difficult or even impossible to determine with any reliability after marketing. Only during controlled trials when subjects are carefully selected, followed, data recorded, and analyzed can some idea of how often abnormalities occur (incidence), at which doses of medications in which populations, that is, the incidence of the problem, be obtained. The need to obtain a quick bird's-eye view of all the subjects in one study was a force for developing our eDISH program [37], acronym for evaluation of drug-induced serious hepatotoxicity. The term "serious" refers to cases with liver dysfunction sufficient to cause clinical disability, to require or prolong hospitalization, or to cause death or need for transplantation. More will be said about eDISH later. It should be noted that eDISH provides only raw estimates of how many subjects had how much elevation of peak serum ALT activity and total bilirubin concentration in the initial x–y log–log plot of ALT values on the abscissa and TBL on the ordinate. Further analyses for time course of individual subjects and probable causality by supplemental clinical narrative information must be done to reach conclusions.

5.3.2
How Much?

The severity of drug-induced liver injury may be suspected but not proved by the fairly sensitive but not specific serial measurement of serum ALT activity. Because of its high sensitivity, few cases are missed, so the false-negative (beta, type 2) error is very low. But not all elevations of ALT are due to drug-induced injury, and must be distinguished from other possible causes such as viral infections, skeletal or cardiac muscle injury, and other liver diseases. Without considering the other possible causes, which requires differential diagnosis, grossly high false-positive (alpha, type 1) error rates occur. This is addressed by the inclusion of serum TBL concentration, a true liver function test, because only the liver clears bilirubin from the plasma, conjugates it with glucuronide, and excretes it into the bile. Most of the bilirubin originates from red blood cell turnover that releases the iron-containing, tetrapyrrolic red pigment heme [38] that is then oxidized by ring opening, salvage of the Fe^{2+}, and production of biliverdin, and then reduced to bilirubin and transported bound to serum albumin [39] to the liver sinusoids where it enters hepatocytes and is carried by intracellular proteins for conjugation [40].

It is not a liver function to regulate the activities of serum enzymes that themselves have no function in plasma, but only had some function inside the cells from which they were released because of injury to those cells. The clinical severity of liver disorders depends upon how well the *uninjured* hepatocytes can function after loss of some by injury. It is wrong to conclude that extent of injury determines remaining function rather than still functioning uninjured cells. True functions unique and specific to the liver include the clearance of bilirubin from the plasma and synthesis and regulation of proteins such as the coagulation factors (namely prothrombin) and albumin. The plasma albumin, the principal protein of plasma, is in the range of 100–150 g, and changes rather slowly, so it is not a sensitive indicator of acute liver injury. *It is wrong to assess severity of liver dysfunction by grading elevations of serum ALT values.*

5.3.3 How Soon?

The time between first administration of a drug and the hepatic response to it is extremely variable, ranging from days to months. It probably depends on just what mechanism may be causing the injury, an interesting field of research that is still underway, depending on what metabolites are produced and the host responses to them. There is a vast amount of basic science study underway that will be important to understanding the latency between drug administration and antitarget effect observable. Some of this is covered in the other chapters of this book, and more will come.

5.3.4 How Likely?

This is one of the most difficult issues facing developers of new drugs. It goes back to the opening question of whether an observed antitarget or adverse effect such as liver injury was caused by the drug or by some peculiarity of the person receiving it. As stated above, it is not enough to say "associated with" because the effect was seen and the drug was given. The somewhat stronger term of "related to" implies some cause is suspected, but not convincingly. To state that the effect was drug-induced means that other causes have been excluded, which requires work to consider what all of those causes might be, and what needs to be done to exclude them, for we do not yet have any test or procedure to make a positive diagnosis of drug-induced liver injury. That diagnosis remains one of exclusion. Routine study protocols do not usually specify all possible causes of adverse effects, nor what must be done to make or exclude their likelihood as an explanation for the findings. This is a process of medical differential diagnosis, learned and practiced by physicians as students, and then over many years of experience improved if not perfected. It is a skill and art unique to medical scientists and not usually included in the training and experience of basic scientists in the fields of chemistry, toxicology, pharmacology, or statistics that play such important roles in new drug development. It has been a field of consultation activity for 15 years at the FDA for this writer, from which much has been learned and continues to be. It is perhaps better to address the questions before approval of new drugs for use in medical practice, because more detailed and better information is available, rather than try to collect information from busy practitioners after approvals.

5.3.5 Compared with What?

A fundamental issue is whether a given subject under observation should be compared with a group of normal people, however that may be determined, or to him/herself, in looking for drug effects. This has come into prominent consideration for evaluating many new treatments proposed for chronic hepatitis C, where many or most of the patients treated and studied will show abnormalities before treatment starts, and then often show a reduction in disease activity when the viral infection is suppressed. This effect may lead to a new and lower "baseline" level of serum enzyme activity with which to compare later effects during treatment. If serum ALT rises without viral load increase, it may indicate possible drug toxicity. It may be preferable to establish the individual patient's own baseline for liver injury and dysfunction biomarkers, rather than comparing them with a hypothetical normal population. This issue has been discussed very recently by Dr. Leonard Seeff, an established expert in viral hepatitis C [37], who pointed out that it is time to rethink the current acceptance of "normal" ranges provided by machine vendors or local laboratories and consider using changes in each person's own "baseline" to evaluate drug effects.

5.3.6 ROC Curves

It has become very popular to evaluate tests with receiver operating characteristic (ROC) curves, based on comparing test sensitivity (true-positive results) on the ordinate with the complement of specificity (false-positive results) on the abscissa. The origin of this method dates back to World War II when it was very important to evaluate signals of radar reflection to distinguish approaching enemy planes from flocks of geese or other harmless results that would lead to the unnecessary "scrambling" of defensive aircraft, wasting precious fuel. It was later applied to psychology and radiology, and now to many areas of medicine. An example of such a curve is shown in Figure 5.7, in which the point at the maximal distance from the diagonal line of no discrimination is at (0.05, 0.95), indicating (1 − specificity) of 5% (or specificity of 95%) and sensitivity of 95%. The area under the ROC curve is 0.982, a very high value (Figure 5.7). The best point for a perfect test would be at (0.00, 1.00) and has an area under it of 1.000, indicating that all diseased persons were detected and no undiseased people were wrongly classified. Such perfection has not been achieved with available tests, and there is a well-known trade-off between seeking higher sensitivity at the cost of lower specificity, so the cutoff value separating positive from negative test results must be chosen to optimize it.

Unfortunately, prevalence and incidence are not considered in ROC curves, and therefore they should not be applied to detection of rare events if "validated" or "qualified" on common ones. Even if the same 95% sensitivity and 95% specificity are "validated" by comparing equal numbers of patients with the disease sought (here serious drug-induced liver injury) and those without disease, but applied to screening for rare events, mischief is done. *ROC curves are the same for both common and rare events; they should not be used to validate new tests if neither incidence nor prevalence is considered.*

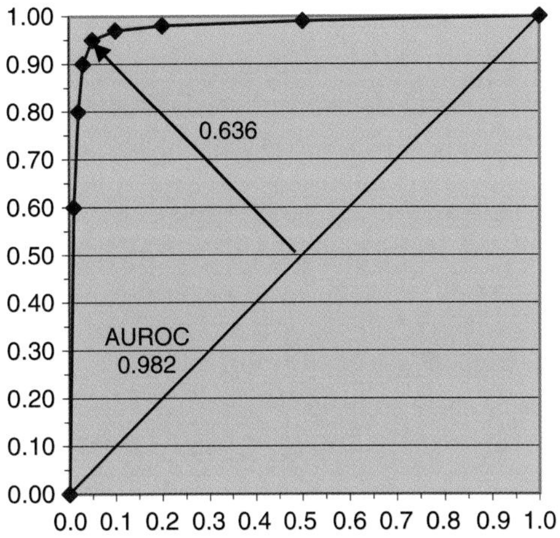

Figure 5.7 A ROC curve for a very good hypothetical biomarker.

5.3.7
eDISH: Especially for Controlled Trials

We have developed an in-house program for evaluating serum liver tests during clinical trials, plotting peak values of serum ALT activity and TBL concentration for all subjects in a given study during their time of observation.[2] This program has been used at the FDA by reviewers and consultants since 2004 when it was first applied to a study of 3922 patients randomized in about equal numbers to either an experimental drug (X) or a control agent (C). The symbols are plotted as peak observed $\log_{10}$ x–y values for each subject.

These graphs were developed as an aid to medical reviewers, to help them visualize very quickly the elevations of serum ALT (abscissa) and TBL (ordinate). The data were obtained from new drug applications and plotted according to a software program written in SAS/IntrNet code by our research statistician Dr. Ted Guo (Figure 5.8). Arbitrary cutoff levels of 3× ULN for ALT and 2× ULN for TBL were chosen, in keeping with 1978 Fogarty conference [34], as being "markedly abnormal," and with concepts of Dr. Hyman Zimmerman concerning ALT as an indicator of acute hepatocellular injury to the liver and bilirubin concentration as a measure of reduction in overall liver function.

The program was intended for internal FDA use, was not published openly, but was very quickly copied by many pharmaceutical companies who wished to evaluate their own data before submitting them for review and possible approval. The second step of eDISH programming is to point to an individual symbol on the first x–y plot to obtain all the liver test data for that single subject for the

2) Guo, T., Senior, J., and Gelperin, K. (2005) How a SAS/IntrNet tool was created at the FDA for the detection of potential drug-induced liver injury using data with CDISC standards. Unpublished personal communication.

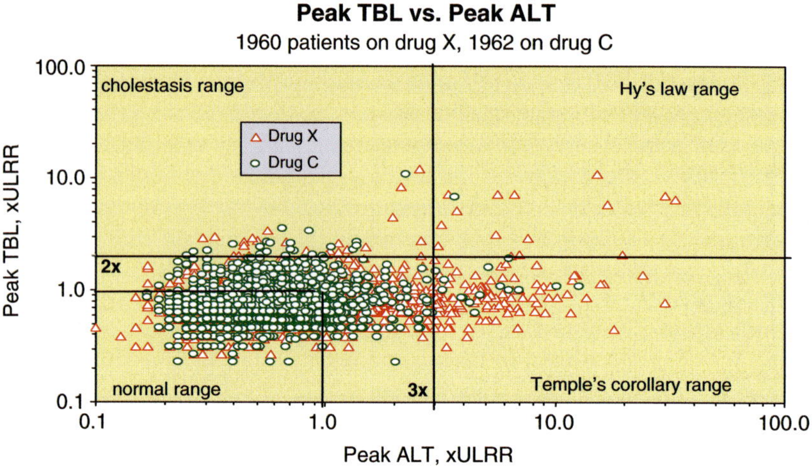

Figure 5.8 An eDISH plot#1 (peak ALT, TBL) for 3922 clinical trial subjects.

entire period of observation, including ALT, AST, ALP, and TBL values, all plotted in terms of ULN multiples. This time course made it quite simple to see if the hepatocellular injury preceded the rise in bilirubin or not. If the latter, some other cause for the bilirubin retention had to be sought. The third step in the eDISH program was to request a clinical narrative report describing alternative possible explanations for the abnormal findings, to aid in the medical differential diagnosis and an estimate of how likely the leading possible causes might be.

This allowed a clinical idea of what might have been the probable cause, more likely than all others combined (for an estimate of 51–75%), a very likely cause (>75–95%), or an almost certain cause (>95%). These numbers were not exact, and were based on the judgment of the medical analyst. The value of the eDISH program to academic consultants to the pharmaceutical industry has been cited by Watkins *et al.* [41,42].

A frequent misuse of the eDISH program and concepts followed when statisticians of some companies began to refer to "chemical Hy's law cases" for subjects whose peak values of ALT and TBL placed them in the right upper quadrant of the first graph. This is wrong, for the diagnosis of a Hy's law case absolutely requires that it be "drug-induced, hepatocellular, and with visible jaundice." It demands medical diagnosis of causality, and ruling out all other causes than the drug, and not principally cholestatic in presentation. *It is wrong to "label" a case as Hy's law based only on serum chemistry findings.*

5.3.8
Test Validation and Qualification

Considerable recent thought has been devoted to how best to verify, validate, and qualify new tests and biomarkers for use in detecting and diagnosing findings of interest such as drug-induced liver injury and many other problems. These words all refer to processes or acts that may be done to establish the test methods as reliable and true, conceptually well related to the problem being evaluated and applicable in clinical use, but their definitions and meanings are often confused. This thinking has been captured in two publications from the US Food and Drug Administration [43,44]. Not included, however, appears to have been the idea of how important specificity is, or the importance of considering the incidence or prevalence when assessing the value of a positive test result validated on common findings when used to screen for rare findings (see Section 5.2.6).

5.4 Closing Considerations

The bulk of this book is devoted to many erudite chapters by basic scientists who focus on new drug development, and who have been very successful in recent years of avoiding or terminating new drugs that cause too much liver injury in comparison with their benefits.

The raising of awareness among FDA reviewers, industry scientists, and consultants to both from academic venues has also been effective in that no drug has been approved by the FDA since the end of 1997 that later had to be withdrawn because of hepatotoxicity.

5.4.1 A Handful of "Do Nots"

Shown earlier in italics are five warnings recently presented at the same conference and emphasized again here as terms that we believe should not be used, inviting comments in disagreement or opposition. The contexts are listed for the five points:

(Section 5.2.3): . . . *regulation of serum aminotransferase activity is not a liver function, so activities of biomarker enzymes in serum should not be called "liver function tests."*

(Section 5.2.6): *It is unfortunate that Vecchio used the word "predictive" for a single test result, without knowing what the results were before or might be afterward.*

(Section 5.3.2): *It is wrong to assess severity of liver dysfunction by grading elevations of serum ALT values.*

(Section 5.3.6): *ROC curves are the same for both common and rare events; they should not be used to validate new tests if neither incidence nor prevalence is considered.*

(Section 5.3.7): *It is wrong to "label" a case as Hy's law based only on serum chemistry findings.*

These "do nots" are offered as examples of fairly frequent misuse of terms, not just to be semantically pure or as examples of nitpicking, but as instances where the terms we use reflect our sometimes less-than-careful thinking. We accept that objecting to this type of terminology may be disputed, and welcome debate on the issues raised.

5.4.2
Need to Standardize ALT Measurement and Interpretation of Normal Ranges

It is now more than 60 years since the then-medical-student Arthur Karmen announced [45] his discovery of a rapid new spectrophotometric assay of serum activity of the enzyme glutamic–oxaloacetic transaminase (SGOT, now called aspartate aminotransferase) released into the circulation from ischemically injured myocardial tissue. Full details of his method followed in January 1955 [46], which led to a revolution in clinical chemistry by reducing the time needed to obtain results from days of tedious paper chromatography to 5 min in a spectrophotometer, and many awards for Dr. Karmen. His mentors, Drs. John LaDue and Felix Wróbleski, quickly used the method to show that serum glutamic–pyruvic transaminase (SGPT, now called alanine aminotransferase) was useful in diagnosing liver injury to hepatocytes [47]. Despite passage of six decades, we still do not have any international standard for how to measure the activity of serum ALT, nor how best to define the range of normal. An early step in advancing research in the field would be to call together the influential policy makers to agree on exactly how it should be measured, and what should be its range of normal.

5.4.3
Research Opportunities

The power, usefulness, and value of the concepts embodied in the eDISH program now have become evident, and it is time to consider development of "eDISH2" to improve any deficiencies and increase the power of the program to learn more about liver disease. We envision two immediate improvements: (1) ability to reset lines separating nearly normal from elevated values for both ALT and TBL, and (2) ability to use the pretreatment and screening values for measurement of both to establish individual baselines, for comparison with later values after drug treatment is started. The programs do not contain data but can process data, including confidential data in FDA files after submissions for approval and company data developed by expenditures for clinical trials. Previous efforts have focused on points (subjects) in the right upper quadrant, as cases to be investigated further that may represent Hy's law cases. New work could well be undertaken to examine the other three quadrants for insights into causes for innocent and reversible ALT elevations, causes for TBL rise without ALT increase, and the large group of normal or near-normal values to obtain detailed descriptions of the type of distributions and reasons therefor. The great power of the computer to process numbers rapidly, combined with the human ability of quick pattern recognition, has been the mainstay of the eDISH success.

Standardization of how best to measure serum ALT activity and what data should be used to validate the healthy normal range are obvious candidates for appropriate research and international consensus.

Another promising area of research might be application of the insights of the late Rev. Thomas Bayes [48] whose logic has led to an appreciation two-and-a-half centuries later that medical differential diagnosis is perhaps a Bayesian process, and that it might be possible to use the stupendous power of computers to streamline and standardize the now artful skill of diagnostic inquiry. It is an area of interest now [49]. If it were possible to reconcile the conflicting opinions and approaches to diagnosing DILI, debated between adherants of the RUCAM (Roussel Uclaf Causality Assessment Method) developed in France 20–25 years ago [50,51] and the proponents of expert consensus [52], it would help resolve a sticky wicket.

We shall see.

References

1 Klabunde, T. and Evers, A. (2005) GPCR antitarget modeling: pharmacophore models for biogenic amine binding GCPRs to avoid GCPR-mediated side effects. *ChemBioChem*, **6** (5), 876–889.

2 Schuster, D., Laggner, C., and Langer, T. (2005) Why drugs fail – a study on side effects in new chemical entities. *Current Pharmaceutical Design*, **11** (27), 3545–3559.

3 Bucher, N.L. (1967) Experimental aspects of hepatic regeneration. *The New England Journal of Medicine*, **277** (13), 686–696.

4 Bucher, N.L. (1967) Experimental aspects of hepatic regeneration (concluded). *The New England Journal of Medicine*, **277** (14), 738–746.

5 Itoh, T. and Miyajima, A. (2014) Liver regeneration by stem/progenitor cells. *Hepatology*, **59** (4), 1617–1626.

6 Chen, T.S. and Chen, P.S. (1994) The myth of Prometheus and the liver. *Journal of The Royal Society of Medicine*, **87** (12), 754–755.

7 Strubelt, O., Siegers, C.P., Völpel, M., and Younes, M. (1979) Studies on the mechanism of paracetamol protection against paracetamol hepatotoxicity. *Toxicology*, **12** (2), 121–133.

8 Zimmerman, H.J. (1968) The spectrum of hepatotoxicity. *Perspectives in Biology and Medicine*, **12** (1), 135–161.

9 Zimmerman, H.J. (1978) *Hepatotoxicity: The Adverse Effects of Drugs and Other Chemicals on the Liver*, 1st edn, Appleton-Century-Crofts; Zimmerman, H.J. (1999) *Hepatotoxicity: The Adverse Effects of Drugs and Other Chemicals on the Liver*, 2nd edn, Lippincott Williams & Wilkins.

10 Meyer, H. and Mally, J. (1912) On hydrazine derivatives of pyridine carbonic acids. *Monatshefte für Chemie und verwandte Teile anderer Wiesenscheffe*, **33** (4), 393–414 (in German).

11 Schatz, A. and Waksman, S.A. (1944) Effect of streptomycin and other antibiotic substances upon *Mycobacterium tuberculosis* and related organisms. *Proceedings of the Society for Experimental Biology and Medicine*, **57** (2), 244–248.

12 Domagk, G. (1950) Investigations on the antituberculosis activity of the thiosemicarbazones *in vitro* and *in vivo*. *American Review of Tuberculosis*, **61** (1), 8–19.

13 Grunberg, E. and Schnitzer, R.J. (1952) The effect of hydrazine derivatives of

isonicotinic acid on infection of mice with *M. tuberculosis* var. *bovis*. *The Yale Journal of Biology and Medicine*, **24** (5), 359–365.

14 Selikoff, I.J. and Robitzek, E.H. (1952) Tuberculosis chemotherapy with hydrazine derivatives of isonicotinic acid. *Diseases of the Chest*, **21** (4), 385–438.

15 Lapp, A.D., Black, G.A., and O'Rafferty, J.N. (1952) Isonicotinic acid hydrazide in pulmonary tuberculosis. *Canadian Medical Association Journal*, **67** (6), 619–623.

16 British Tuberculosis Association (1952) Isoniazid in pulmonary tuberculosis. *Lancet*, **2** (6723), 19–21.

17 Randolph, H. and Joseph, S. (1953) Toxic hepatitis with jaundice occurring in a patient treated with isoniazid. *The Journal of the American Medical Association*, **157** (1), 38–40.

18 LiverTox (2013) Isoniazid. Edited by J.H. Hoofnagle and staff; 7 pages of text including background, summary, five case reports, and 363 references. Available at www.livertox.nih.gov (accessed November 26, 2014).

19 Cohan, R., Kalser, M., and Thompson, R.V. (1961) Fatal hepatic necrosis secondary to isoniazid therapy. *The Journal of the American Medical Association*, **176**, 877–879.

20 Scharer, L. and Smith, J.P. (1969) Serum transaminase elevations and other hepatic abnormalities in patients receiving isoniazid. *Annals of Internal Medicine*, **71** (6), 1113–1120.

21 Garibaldi, R.A., Drusin, R.E., Ferebee, S.H., and Gregg, M.B. (1972) Isoniazid-associated hepatitis. Report of an outbreak. *The American Review of Respiratory Disease*, **106** (3), 357–365.

22 Maddrey, W.C. and Boitnott, J.K. (1973) Isoniazid hepatitis. *Annals of Internal Medicine*, **79** (1), 1–12.

23 Black, M., Mitchell, J.R., Zimmerman, H.J., Ishak, K.G., and Epler, G.R. (1975) Isoniazid-associated hepatitis in 114 patients. *Gastroenterology*, **69** (2), 289–302.

24 Kopanoff, D.E., Snider, D.E., Jr., and Caras, G.J. (1978) Isoniazid-related hepatitis: a U.S. Public Health Service cooperative surveillance study. *The American Review of Respiratory Disease*, **117** (6), 991–1001.

25 Mitchell, J.R., Long, M.W., Thorgeirsson, U.P., and Jollow, D.J. (1975) Acetylation rates and monthly liver function tests during one year of isoniazid preventative therapy. *Chest*, **68** (2), 181–190.

26 Nolan, C.M., Goldberg, S.V., and Buskin, S.E. (1999) Hepatotoxicity associated with isoniazid preventive therapy. A 7-year survey from a public health tuberculosis clinic. *The Journal of the American Medical Association*, **281** (11), 1014–1018.

27 Hughes, H.B. (1953) On the metabolic fate of isoniazid. *The Journal of Pharmacology and Experimental Therapeutics*, **109** (4), 444–452.

28 Johnson, W.J. (1954) Biological acetylation of isoniazid. *Nature*, **174** (4433), 744–745.

29 Evans, D.A. (1964) Acetylation polymorphisms. *Proceedings of the Society for Experimental Biology and Medicine*, **57**, 508–511.

30 Huang, Y.S., Chern, H.D., Su, W.J., Wu, J.C., Lai, S.L., Yang, S.Y., Chang, F.Y., and Lee, S.D. (2002) Polymorphisms of the *N*-acetyltransferase 2 gene as a susceptibility risk factor for antituberculosis drug-induced hepatitis. *Hepatology*, **35** (4), 883–889.

31 Singla, N., Gupta, D., Birbian, N., and Singh, J. (2014) Association of NAT2, GST and CYP2E1 polymorphisms and anti-tuberculosis drug-induced hepatotoxicity. *Tuberculosis*, **94** (3), 293–298.

32 Huang, Y.S. (2014) Recent progress in genetic variation and risk of antituberculosis drug-induced liver injury. *Journal of the Chinese Medical Association*, **77** (4), 169–173.

33 Leevy, C.M., Popper, H., and Sherlock, S. (1975) Diseases of the liver and biliary tract. Standardization of nomenclature, diagnostic criteria and diagnostic methodology. Proceedings No. 22, DHEW Publication No. NIH 76-725, Fogarty International Center, Bethesda, MD, U.S. Government Printing Office, Washington, DC.

34 Davidson, C.S., Leevy, C.M., and Chamberlayne, E.C. (1979) Guidelines for the detection of hepatotoxicity due to drugs and chemicals, NIH Publication 79-313, U.S. Department of Health, Education, and Welfare, Public Health Service, National Institutes of Health.

35 Prati, D., Taioli, E., Zanella, A., DellaTorre, E., Butelli, S., DelVecchio, L., Vianello, L., Zanuso, F., Mozzi, F., Milani, S., Conte, D., Colombo, M., and Sirchia, G. (2002) Updated definitions of healthy ranges for serum alanine aminotransferase levels. *Annals of Internal Medicine*, **137** (1), 1–10.

36 Vecchio, T.J. (1966) Predictive value of a single diagnostic test in unselected populations. *The New England Journal of Medicine*, **274** (21), 1171–1173.

37 Seeff, L.B. (2014) Subjects with active liver disease need special observation. Presented at Training/Education, Drug-Induced Liver Injury Annual Program, March 30, University of Maryland, College Park, MD. Available at www.aasld.org (accessed November 26, 2014).

38 Schmid, R. (1972) Bilirubin metabolism in man. *The New England Journal of Medicine*, **287** (14), 703–709.

39 Ostrow, J.D. and Schmid, R. (1963) The protein-binding of C14-bilirubin in human and murine serum. *The Journal of Clinical Investigation*, **42** (8), 1286–1299.

40 Arias, I.M. (2012) Liver function from Y to Z. *The Journal of Clinical Investigation*, **122** (8), 2763–2764.

41 Watkins, P.B., Desai, M., Berkowitz, S.D., Peters, G., Horsmans, Y., Larrey, D., and Maddrey, W. (2011) Evaluation of drug-induced serious hepatotoxicity (eDISH): application of this data organization approach to phase III clinical trials of rivaroxaban after total hip or knee replacement surgery. *Drug Safety*, **34** (3), 243–252.

42 Shen, X., Yuan, Z., Mei, J., Zhang, Z., Guo, J., Wu, Z., Wu, J., Zhang, H., Pan, J., Huang, W., Gong, Yuan, D., Xiao, P., Wang, Y., Shuai, Y., Lin, S., Pan, Q., Zhou, T., Watkins, P.B., and Wu, F. (2014) Anti-tuberculosis drug-induced liver injury in Shanghai: validation of Hy's Law. *Drug Safety*, **37** (1), 43–51.

43 Woodcock, J., Buckman, S., Goodsaid, F., Walton, M.K., and Zineh, I. (2011) Qualifying biomarkers for use in drug development: a U.S. Food and Drug Administration overview. *Expert Opinion on Medical Diagnostics*, **5** (5), 369–374.

44 Food and Drug Administration (2014) Guidance for Industry and FDA Staff: Qualification Process for Drug Development Tools, 32 pp. Available at http://www.fda.gov/downloads/Drugs/GuidanceComplianceRegulatory-Information/Guidances/UCM230597.pdf (accessed November 26, 2014).

45 LaDue, J.S., Wróbleski, F., and Karmen, A. (1954) Serum glutamic oxaloacetic transaminase activity in human acute transmural myocardial infarction (Letter). *Science*, **120** (3117), 497–499.

46 Karmen, A. (1955) A note on the spectrophotometric assay of glutamic–oxaloacetic transaminase in human blood serum (Appendix). *The Journal of Clinical Investigation*, **24** (1), 131–133.

47 LaDue, J.S. and Wróbleski, F. (1956) Serum glutamic pyruvic transaminase SGP-T in hepatic disease: a preliminary report. *Annals of Internal Medicine*, **45** (5), 801–811.

48 Price, R. (1763) An essay towards solving a problem in the doctrine of chances. *Philosophical Transactions of the Royal Society of London*, **53**, 370–418 (by the late Rev. Mr. Bayes, communicated by Mr. Price in a letter to John Canton, MA, FRS).

49 Douali, N., Csaba, H., De Rop, J., Papageorgiou, E.I., and Jaulent, M.C. (2014) Diagnosis support system based on clinical guidelines: comparison between case-based fuzzy cognitive maps and Bayesian networks. *Computer Methods and Programs in Biomedicine*, **113** (1), 133–143.

50 Danan, G. and Benichou, C. (1993) Causality assessment of adverse reactions to drugs. I. A novel model based on the conclusions of international consensus meetings: application to drug-induced liver injuries. *Journal of Clinical Epidemiology*, **46** (11), 1323–1330.

51 Benichou, C., Danan, G., and Flahault, A. (1993) Causality assessment of adverse

reactions to drugs. II. An original model for validation of drug causality assessment methods: case reports with positive rechallenge. *Journal of Clinical Epidemiology*, **46** (11), 1331–1336.

52 Rockey, D.C., Seeff, L.B., Rochon, J., Freston, J., Chalsani, N., Bonacini, M., Fontana, R., and Hayashi, P.H. (US Drug-Induced Liver Network) (2010) Causality assessment in drug-induced liver injury using a structured expert opinion process: comparison to the Roussel-Uclaf causality assessment method. *Hepatology*, **55** (6), 2117–2126.

6
Mechanistic Safety Biomarkers for Drug-Induced Liver Injury

Daniel J. Antoine

6.1
Introduction

An adverse drug reaction (ADR) can be defined as "an appreciably harmful or unpleasant reaction, resulting from an intervention related to the use of a medicinal product, which predicts hazard from future administration and warrants prevention or specific treatment, or alteration of the dosage regimen, or withdrawal of the product" [1]. ADRs are both a leading cause of hospital admissions in the developed world and a major cause of drug attrition in the pharmaceutical industry. The financial burden of ADRs to both these sectors is great, and as the incidence of ADRs has increased in the last 10 years, and is projected to grow further, this is an area of health care that requires effective strategies to counter this growth. Within the pharmaceutical industry, ADRs are a major concern, with 30% of compound attrition in drug development being due to ADRs [2]. The estimated cost of a new chemical entity from discovery to market was projected at around $1billion in 2003 [3] and is now thought to be around $1.8 billion, with a large part of this expenditure being due to attrition of other prospective compounds at various stages of the pipeline.

Clinical studies have defined the proportions of ADRs caused by different classifications of drugs and also which organs are most prevalently targeted by ADRs [4,5]. The consensus among these studies is that the reporting of ADRs may be underestimating the true incidence of ADRs, and hence the impact on hospitals may be greater than estimated. In 2004, Pirmohamed *et al.* undertook a study of hospital admissions to two NHS hospitals in the northwest of England over a 6-month period. This study showed that 6.5% of admissions were classified as ADRs, and the projected national cost to the NHS of ADRs was £466 million [5]. However, this study did exclude certain groups of patients – women with obstetric or gynecological problems and pediatric patients. Wu *et al.* looked at hospital admissions over a 10-year period to all NHS hospitals. This study showed ADRs to be responsible for 0.9% of the admissions, a 76.8% increase in admissions during the study time, and an in-hospital mortality rate increase of 10% (4.3–4.7%) [4]. A major contributor to the costs associated with ADRs is

Antitargets and Drug Safety, First Edition. Edited by László Urbán, Vinod F. Patel, and Roy J. Vaz.

the shortcomings of current clinically used biomarkers and this establishes the need for novel biomarkers of ADRs that can be used to improve clinical assessment and direct treatment.

Drug-induced liver injury (DILI) represents both a significant ADR for currently used medicines and a significant impediment to the development of new therapies. It is a major human health concern as it is a leading cause of patient morbidity and mortality. It has been widely cited that of the 10 000 documented human medicines, more than 1000 are associated with liver injury [6]. The overall incidence of DILI in the general population has been estimated to range from 10 to 15 cases per 100 000 patient years, with the incidence of DILI resulting from an individual drug used in clinical practice ranging from 1 in 10 000 to 1 in 1 000 000 patient years [7,8]. Although DILI accounts for <1% of the hospitalized patients presenting to hospital with jaundice [7,9], it is an adverse event that most frequently results in regulatory action leading to black box warnings or removal of a drug from the market. In the clinic, DILI accounts for more than 50% of acute liver failure cases, and improved detection of DILI before overt liver failure occurs has been the subject of intense investigation [6].

Drug attrition due to DILI occurs in all phases of the development pipeline, from preclinical testing to clinical trials to the marketplace. In cases where the frequency is high in either animal species or in humans, DILI is considered "intrinsic" in that it is assumed to result from direct hepatocellular damage [10]. However, another concerning manifestation of DILI, termed "idiosyncratic," occurs very rarely in susceptible individuals exposed to therapeutic doses [7].

Due to the low incidence and multiple contributing factors, currently, a confident diagnosis of DILI in man can only be attained once other possible causes of liver injury have been excluded, which may delay discontinuation of the offending drug. When DILI is suspected in a patient treated with multiple medications, it may be impossible to confidently identify the specific drug responsible and this may force the physician to unnecessarily stop medications, potentially placing the patient at increased risk from the disease(s) being treated. Furthermore, it is almost impossible to identify which patients are susceptible to DILI before they develop it. Therefore, there is a need to develop new and improved DILI biomarkers that can either confidently establish the diagnosis of DILI or identify the specific drug causing DILI and predict the course of patients (adapt, survive, and develop liver failure).

The presentation of DILI (clinical and histological) can mimic most types of naturally occurring liver diseases. Idiosyncratic hepatocellular liver injury is generally the DILI of greatest concern because it can develop quickly and be life-threatening before the development of jaundice. Regardless of type, detection of DILI relies upon a small number of routine laboratory tests. However, there is a lack of specificity and sensitivity in currently utilized markers, which leads to poor prediction of toxicity risk for individual patients or patient populations. The assessment of the potential for new chemical entities to elicit clinical hepatotoxicity is heavily dependent on the histopathological evaluation of hepatotoxicity endpoints in preclinical species coupled with the quantitative assessment of circulating enzymes that are enriched in hepatic tissue [11,12]. However, when clinical trials are performed, current preclinical testing regimens at best successfully correlate with clinical adverse hepatic events in about 50% of cases [13]. In addition, liver biopsies are not routinely taken from clinical trial subjects or patients with overt DILI, leading to incomplete assessment of the mechanisms of injury for a given drug.

The lack of qualified mechanistic biomarkers has resulted in a significant challenge to investigate the true extent and diagnosis of DILI [14]. The development and qualification of sensitive and specific hepatic biomarkers that hold translation between preclinical and clinical studies is urgently required to accelerate the pace of drug development. Improved DILI biomarkers may additionally enable patient and/or DILI-specific treatment stratification for marketed therapeutics. Moreover, the potential for novel biomarkers to provide enhanced understanding of the fundamental mechanisms that result in clinical DILI is becoming increasingly recognized.

The US National Institute of Health (NIH) defined a biomarker (e.g., oligonucleotide, protein, or metabolite) in 2001 as a characteristic that is objectively measured and evaluated as an indicator of normal biological process, a pathogenic process, or a pharmacological response to a therapeutic intervention [15]. Biomarkers are classified by the US Food and Drug Administration (FDA) as exploratory, probable valid, and known valid. A valid biomarker is further defined as a biomarker that is measured in an analytical test system with well-established performance characteristics and for which there is an established scientific framework or a body of evidence that elucidates the physiological, toxicological, pharmacological, or clinical significance of the test result [16]. Since then recommendations have been set to avoid confusion: the term "validation" should refer to the technical characterization and documentation of methodological performances, and the term "qualification" should refer to the evidentiary process of linking a biomarker to a clinical endpoint or biological process [17].

However, the development and clinical integration of potential hepatic biomarkers over the past 60 years has revealed only a limited number of candidates [12]. This concept is perhaps not so surprising given the fact that less focus has been placed on the science of drug safety and the rigorous guidelines we impose on the validation and biological qualification of a potential DILI biomarker [11,17] compared with drug efficacy [18]. Furthermore, the delayed qualification and ultimate scientific acceptance of a potential DILI biomarker has been hindered by what has been previously thought of as the competing interest between the various stakeholders. Safety assessment within drug development has traditionally focused on reliable clinical–preclinical concordance. Low baseline variability, specificity, and rapid analysis are sought after by clinicians and the ability to provide an enhanced mechanistic understanding about toxicological processes is required by the academic community. Public–private consortia were developed to meet this goal and these consist of leading academic groups, large pharmaceutical companies, small–medium enterprises, and clinical units of excellence such as the Predictive Safety Testing Consortium (PSTC) (www.c-path.org/pstc.cfm) and the Safer and Faster Evidence-Based Translation (SAFE-T) consortium (www.imi-safe-t.eu). These consortia efforts, coupled with feedback and representation from regulatory authorities as external members and advisors, provide an opportunity for collaborative efforts to aid the identification, validation, and qualification of novel translation safety biomarkers (TSBM) for DILI [17].

6.2
Drug-Induced Toxicity and the Liver

DILI can be inherent to the drug itself or idiosyncratic (rare, attributed to the individual with multiple potential underlying susceptibility factors and unknown causes). The first-pass exposure to drugs administered orally and the high capacity for xenobiotic metabolism are considered significant reasons why the liver is a target for drug toxicity and this aspect has been widely reviewed [19]. Toxic metabolites can be generated and accumulated within hepatocytes as a result of oxidation–reduction (phase I), conjugation (phase II), and the saturation of transporter (phase III) reactions that normally serve to remove or detoxify xenobiotics [19,20]. The metabolic capacity of the liver coupled to the portal blood supply and the resident immune system contribute to hepatic susceptibility to drug toxicity.

The most frequent cause of DILI in the Western world is acetaminophen (APAP, paracetamol) overdose, which accounted for 38 000 emergency hospital admissions in the financial year 2010–2011 in England alone [21]. Between 1998 and 2007, almost half (46%) of reported cases of acute liver failure had been attributed to APAP, with DILI resulting from other drugs accounting for 11% [22]. APAP hepatotoxicity has been widely studied and is reproducible in animal models. Therefore, due to difficulties in studying clinical idiosyncratic DILI in animal models, APAP hepatotoxicity represents an excellent paradigm to identify new biomarkers and to understand mechanisms of clinically induced liver stress in the exploratory setting, which has a clear clinical significance [23,24]. The biochemical basis of APAP hepatotoxicity is well defined through cytochrome P450 (CYP2E1, 1A2, and 2D6)-mediated reactive metabolite formation (*N*-acetyl-*p*-benzoquinone imine) and hepatic GSH depletion [25,26]. Covalent adduction to cellular proteins then propagates injury through a number of mechanisms, including oxidative stress, which ultimately leads to hepatocyte necrosis and sterile inflammation [27,28] and has been recently reviewed [23].

Clinically, antidote treatment with acetylcysteine (AC) is time consuming and results in significant bed occupancy in hospitals (around 47 000 bed days per year in England). Furthermore, adverse reactions to AC are common in around half of the patients. The majority of APAP overdose patients present to hospital early, soon after overdose and before acute liver injury (ALI) can be diagnosed, or confidently excluded, using current blood-based biomarkers such as alanine aminotransaminase (ALT) [29,30]. Therefore, decisions regarding the initiation of antidote treatment are predominately based on the dose of APAP ingested and a timed blood APAP concentration [31]. This time delay coupled with the early clinical uncertainty of the presence of liver injury prevents treatment being individualized, potentially leading to patients being overtreated with a time-consuming and potentially harmful antidote or undertreated, with increased risk of ALI.

Novel biomarkers that detect ALI at the earliest possible time point are required both from the viewpoint of idiosyncratic hepatotoxicity and for detecting toxicity and patient stratification of risk resulting from APAP [32]. Moreover, given the multistep and multicellular processes of DILI, panels of biomarkers that have potential to provide insights into the underlying mechanistic basis of ALI are increasingly being recognized as fundamental to efforts in translational research and patient treatment stratification.

6.3 Current Status of Biomarkers for the Assessment of DILI

To date, only a relatively small number of blood-based tests are used to assess DILI in human, whereas the assessment of DILI in preclinical drug development is heavily dependent upon hepatic histological interpretation [11]. These tests primarily consist of the determination of serum total bilirubin (TBL) concentration and the activity of the enzymes alkaline phosphatase (ALP), aspartate aminotransferase (AST), and alanine aminotransferase (ALT). Elevations in the activity of these enzymes may indicate injury to biliary cells or hepatocytes, whereas elevations of TBL concentration represent declining hepatic function (Figure 6.1) [12]. Although the assay of ALT has become the primary screening tool to detect DILI, it is not without its problems. Changes in enzyme activities are not specific for DILI and can occur in a number of disease processes, including viral hepatitis, fatty liver disease, and liver cancer [33]. Elevations in aminotransferases are also not unique to liver injury since increases in ALT and AST in circulation can also result from myocardial damage, muscle damage, or extreme exercise. Elevations in ALP are not specific for biliary injury as the marker may also be attributed to hyperthyroidism or bone disease. Also, the methods used to quantify ALT activity have not been standardized and a robust definition of normal reference ranges have not been agreed upon; these ranges inevitably depend upon the population group defined as normal and assay measurements will vary between laboratories. Although ALT activity is regarded as generally sensitive for detecting liver injury when it occurs, it is not sensitive with respect to time/kinetics. Furthermore, ALT activity has often been described as having little prognostic value due to the fact that an ALT elevation represents probable injury to the liver after it has occurred. From a regulatory point of view, elevations in ALT activity are also worrisome with respect to establishing liver safety during drug treatment. However, frequent and relatively

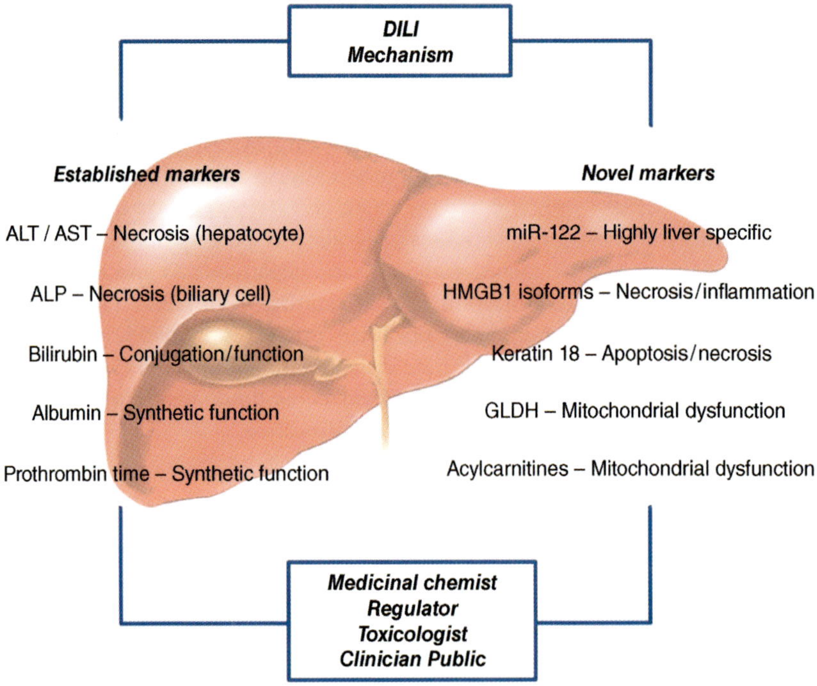

Figure 6.1 Experimental mechanism-based biomarkers that can be used alongside currently used clinical chemistry standards to inform the medical chemist, regulator, toxicologist, clinician, and the public to improve the safer use of existing drugs and the development of safe medicines. Novel translational biomarkers that reflect the mechanistic basis of DILI are fundamental to efforts in translational research.

large elevations in ALT activity are associated with treatments that do not pose a clinical liver safety issue, such as heparins and tacrine [34,35]. The challenge is to identify or assess current biomarkers (on their own or in combination) that can distinguish between benign elevations in ALT activity and the potential for a serious DILI outcome.

ALT activity is often combined with the liver-specific assessment of TBL as part of Hy's law (Table 6.1). Zimmerman first noted that a patient who presents with jaundice as a result of hepatocellular DILI has at least a 10% chance of developing ALF, regardless of which drug has caused the hepatocellular injury [36]. Hy's law is currently the only accepted regulatory model to assess significant, acute DILI [18,37,38]. Staff at the FDA have developed a liver safety data management tool called eDISH (evaluation of drug-induced serious liver injury), which involves data visualization by plotting the peak serum ALT versus the peak serum TBL for each subject in a clinical trial [38]. Although eDISH has revolutionized the standardization and transparent means of displaying and organizing relevant liver safety data from a clinical trial, it remains limited by its reliance on Hy's law. TBL most likely rises once there has been a substantial loss

Table 6.1 Criteria determining the potential for serious drug-induced liver injury with "Hy's law".

Hepatocellular injury	ALT or AST >3× upper limit of normal (ULN)
Hepatic impairment	TBL >2× ULN with no initial findings of cholestasis (ALP elevation)
Exclusion of other causes	No underlying condition, for example, hepatitis A, B, or C, existing liver disease, or the presence of another potential DILI-causing factor

of functioning hepatocytes, placing the patient in danger of liver failure. Therefore, serum TBL in this setting is not a biomarker that predicts severe toxicity potential, but instead a confirmation that severe hepatotoxicity has occurred. An ideal biomarker would predict the liver safety of the drug (and the patient) before the injury progresses to the point of TBL elevation. Therefore, the diagnosis of a Hy's law case is often delayed and death of the patient may still occur despite discontinuation of the drug even after relatively subtle liver signals [18]. This highlights the need for improvement and modification to Hy's law criteria that novel biomarkers can fulfill. Due to the difficulties in defining a true Hy's law case, defined by these biochemical characteristics, an international expert working group of clinicians and scientists reviewed current terminology and diagnostic criteria for DILI based on currently used clinical chemistry parameters to enable uniformed criteria to define a case as DILI and to characterize the spectrum of clinical patterns encompassing it [39]. Currently, a liver biopsy is still the definitive form of diagnosis. Consequently, with the exception of APAP (APAP adducts, *N*-acetylcysteine), there is no specific noninvasive diagnosis, treatment, or prevention of DILI except for the early withdrawal of a drug in the case of suspected DILI. Therefore, there has been a considerable effort to identify and develop new biomarkers that can inform the mechanistic basis of DILI and provide potential measures for patient management.

6.4 Novel Investigational Biomarkers for DILI

The identification and eventual qualification of sensitive and specific DILI biomarkers that hold translation between preclinical and clinical studies is urgently required for improved safety screening in drug development and sensitive clinical diagnosis of DILI for patient treatment stratification. An added benefit of novel biomarkers would be to provide enhanced understanding of the fundamental mechanisms that result in clinical DILI.

Significant resource has recently been directed toward the qualification of new DILI biomarkers and a number of public–private consortia have been developed, namely, the Predictive Safety Testing Consortium in the United States and the Safer and Faster Evidence-Based Translation consortium in Europe, which are currently funding prospective clinical and preclinical DILI biomarker studies [17]. To synergise efforts and minimize the overlap, these consortia collaborate closely in what has been described as a highly efficient scientific "meta-consortium" on a global scale [40].

The strategies for biomarker discovery broadly fall into two categories: unbiased and targeted analyses. Unbiased approaches driven by omic technologies to integrate biological samples are excellent mechanisms to identify novel biomarkers and develop testable theories and have been reviewed with a specific focus on hepatotoxicity [41,42]. Furthermore, efforts have been reported to describe their utility to define proteomic profiles that relate to idiosyncratic hepatotoxicity [43]. However, these strategies are very important, but are often scientifically challenging because of the paucity of well-defined clinical samples for a particular drug and because of the heterogeneous sample sets and disease manifestations. It is to be noted that the alternative is to use model systems to investigate target analytes in biofluids as biomarkers where the chemistry of the drug/molecule reflects the internal biology of the cell/organ and where it is possible to investigate the mechanism of appearance from the cell into the biological matrix and its further clearance. This concept forms the basis of the Innovative Medicines Initiative MIP-DILI (Mechanism-Based Integrated Systems for the Prediction of Drug-Induced Liver Injury) consortium (www.mip-dili.eu). In this chapter, we focus on specific mechanism-based biomarkers that have shown evidence of utility in both preclinical and clinical DILI studies and are of interest to aforementioned biomarker and modeling consortia.

Important and noteworthy progress has been made in the development of biomarkers for renal drug safety evaluation [44,45], which have been qualified for use by various regulatory authorities and the lessons learnt from these efforts can also apply to the liver. In particular, the concept has arisen that new biomarkers are used to complement existing ones and not to replace them to inform the medicinal chemist, clinician, toxicologist, regulator, and the public. Novel biomarkers of DILI that have shown clinical utility will be discussed. These novel biomarkers have enhanced sensitivity and specificity for liver injury or offer mechanistic insights into the pathogenic processes that result in DILI.

6.4.1 Glutamate Dehydrogenase (GLDH)

GLDH is an enzyme present in matrix-rich mitochondria (liver) and not in cristae-rich mitochondria (cardiac and skeletal muscle). It is important to note that while GLDH is also expressed in the brain and in kidney, its release from these tissues enters the cerebrospinal fluid and tubular lumen, respectively, rather than the blood [46,47]. GLDH is a key enzyme in amino acid oxidation and urea production that is highly conserved across species, making it an attractive biomarker candidate [48]. It is considered relatively liver specific and provides an indicator of leakage of mitochondrial contents into the circulation [12]. GLDH localization within the liver is regional, with higher concentrations present in the centrilobular area, the region of metabolic activation and site of tissue damage during APAP toxicity. GLDH use as a DILI biomarker is well documented and appears more sensitive and indicative of DILI than other cytosolic enzymes [49]. A recent study in rats subjected to multiple liver injury modalities indicated that GLDH increases were up to 10-fold greater and 3-fold more persistent than ALT elevations [50]. As GLDH is localized to the mitochondrial matrix and due to its relative large size (330 kDa), release of GLDH into the circulation is delayed during hepatocellular necrosis compared with cytosolic enzymes such as the aminotransferases. This property may contribute to the increased specificity of GLDH to indicate hepatocellular necrosis. GLDH is additionally elevated in acute liver injury models as it is elevated in blood in both preclinical models and clinical cases of DILI and liver impairment [49,51,52], highlighting its potential as a translational biomarker. Circulating GLDH has also been shown to rise in healthy volunteers treated with heparins and cholestyramine, treatments that are not associated with clinically important liver injury [35,53] and specific recommendations have been made when drawing conclusions on data regarding the sample type and specimen preparation [54]. Measurement of GLDH alone may or may not be useful in distinguishing benign elevations in ALT from those that are portent of severe DILI potential.

6.4.2
Acylcarnitines

Due to the fact that most large enzymes used to investigate mitochondrial dysfunction track changes in ALT activity [51], a promising approach to the identification of biomarkers of injury that are useful at earlier time points may involve metabolomics. In general, metabolic intermediates are much smaller than proteins and more likely to cross cell membranes and enter blood before the development of injury. In 2009, Chen *et al.* [55] measured increased levels of acylcarnitines in serum from APAP-treated mice. Acylcarnitines are derivatives of long-chain fatty acids that are required for transport of these fatty acids into mitochondria for β-oxidation. First, a coenzyme A (CoA) group is attached in a reaction catalyzed by acyl-CoA synthetase. The CoA group is then displaced by carnitine through the action of carnitine palmitoyltransferase I (CPT I), forming an acylcarnitine that can enter the mitochondrial matrix through facilitated diffusion with the help of a carnitine-acylcarnitine translocase (CACT). Because acylcarnitines are broken down within mitochondria by carnitine palmitoyltransferase II (CPT II) and β-oxidation, mitochondrial dysfunction may result in their accumulation. It has been shown that increases in these fatty acid–carnitine conjugates rise in the serum of mice treated with APAP (mitochondrial-dependent hepatocyte death) but not with mice treated with furosemide (which has been shown to cause liver injury without primarily affecting mitochondrial function) [56]. Therefore, circulating acylcarnitines have potential as specific biomarkers of mitochondrial dysfunction. It is important to note that acylcarnitines have been shown to not to be elevated in patients with APAP overdose [56]. This is most likely due in part to the standard-of-care treatment *N*-acetylcysteine. However, it might be useful to measure acylcarnitines in other forms of liver injury or APAP patients that present to the "hospital front door" prior to the treatment with AC [29,30,32].

6.4.3
High-Mobility Group Box-1 (HMGB1)

HMGB1 is a chromatin binding protein that is passively released by cells undergoing necrosis where it acts as a damage-associated molecular pattern (DAMP) molecule by linking cell death to the activation of an immune response by targeting Toll-like receptors and the receptor for advanced glycation end products (RAGE) [57–59]. HMGB1 has activity at the intersection between infectious and sterile inflammation. It is also actively secreted as a cytokine by innate immune cells in a hyperacetylated form [60,61] and its biological function is highly dependent upon and is regulated by posttranslational redox modifications of three key cysteine residues [62,63]. Furthermore, a recently defined nomenclature has been developed to identify these functional relevant isoforms [64]. Acetylation of lysine residues is also important for the active release of HMGB1 from immune cells and for its release in cell death mechanisms such as pyroptosis [60,61,65,66]. HMGB1 is an informative and early serum indicator of cell death processes in preclinical models of APAP poisoning [67,68] and in the clinic [29,30]. Circulating levels of total and acetylated HMGB1 displayed different temporal profiles, which in mouse models of APAP toxicity correlate with the onset of necrosis and inflammation, respectively [67]. Serum levels of total HMGB1 correlate strongly with ALT activity and prothrombin time in patients with established acute liver injury following APAP overdose [69]. The prognostic utility of acetylated HMGB1 has also been demonstrated in clinical DILI. In patients with established acute liver injury following APAP overdose, elevations in acetylated HMGB1 associate with a poor prognosis and outcome [69]. Elevations in serum HMGB1 and a secondary rise in acetylated HMGB1 were also observed during treatment of healthy volunteers with heparins, suggesting that these measurements alone may not reliably identify serious injury potential and further investigation is required [35].

6.4.4
Keratin 18 (K18)

K18 is a type I intermediate filament protein expressed in epithelial cells and is responsible for cell structure and integrity [70]. Caspase-mediated cleavage of K18 is an early event in cellular structural rearrangement during apoptosis [71]. Caspases 3, 7, and 9 have been implicated in the cleavage of K18 at the C-terminal DALD/S motif. Full-length K18 is released passively during necrotic cell death, whereas fragmented K18 is released with apoptosis [72]. The use of immunoassays directed toward the recognition of caspase-cleaved K18 (apoptosis) and full-length K18 (necrosis) has been reported clinically as biomarkers for the therapeutic drug monitoring of chemotherapeutic agents and for the quantification of apoptosis during liver disorders such as nonalcoholic steatohepatitis (NASH) and hepatitis C infection [73,74] and mutations in K18 predispose toward acute liver failure and hepatotoxicity [75,76]. Circulating necrosis K18 and apoptosis K18 have been shown to represent indicators of hepatic necrotic and apoptotic events in a mouse model of APAP-induced liver injury [67] and during heparin-induced hepatocellular injury in man [35]. The prognostic utility of K18 has also been demonstrated in clinical DILI and acute liver injury [69,77]. In patients with established acute liver injury following APAP overdose, elevations in absolute levels of necrosis K18 associate with a poor prognosis Kings College Criteria (KCC)) and outcome and a total percentage of K18 attributed to apoptosis is associated with improved survival [69]. Interestingly, in the first blood sample taken at the point of admission following APAP overdose, when currently used markers of liver injury remained within the normal range and prior to antidote treatment, K18 (and also miR-122 and HMGB1) was significantly elevated in the group of patients who subsequently went on to develop liver injury and also even in patients who presented less than 8 h postoverdose [29]. Furthermore, the values of K18, HMGB1, and miR-122 at presentation correlated with the peak ALT activity and peak INR recorded during the hospital admission. Interestingly, these data are also supported by a recently published case report highlighting that life-threatening hepatotoxicity following APAP overdose could have potentially been avoided if these biomarkers had been measured [30]. These data demonstrate for the first time in man that these novel biomarkers represent more sensitive biomarkers of DILI in a temporal sense compared with currently used indicators and can be used to aid treatment stratification and identify risk.

6.4.5 MicroRNA-122 (miR-122)

MicroRNAs are small noncoding RNAs, approximately 22–25 nucleotides in length, that predominantly serve to negatively regulate posttranscriptional gene expression. Circulating microRNAs are stable and provide disease state biomarkers spanning diverse therapeutic areas and have been associated with a wide range of tissue-specific toxicities [78]. Many microRNA species show a high degree of organ specificity and cross-species conservation that make them attractive candidates as translational safety biomarkers [79]. MicroRNA-122 (miR-122) represents 75% of the total hepatic miRNA content and exhibits exclusive hepatic expression. miR-122 has been shown to be a serum biomarker of APAP-induced ALI in mice, which was more sensitive with respect to dose and time than ALT [80]. The improved tissue specificity of miR-122 versus ALT is supported by the observation that clinical ALT elevations associated with muscle injury are not accompanied by concomitant elevations in miR-122 [81]. MicroRNA-122 has also been previously shown to serve as a clinical indicator of heparin-induced hepatocellular necrosis [35]. Moreover, as observed in mice, miR-122 is elevated in blood following APAP overdose in man and correlates strongly with ALT activity in patients with established acute liver injury. Furthermore, miR-122 has been shown to represent a more sensitive biomarker of APAP hepatotoxicity in humans compared with currently used clinical chemistry parameters [30,52]. In these investigations, elevated miR-122 was observed in patients that present to hospital with normal liver function test values but then later develop acute liver injury compared with those that did not develop acute liver injury following APAP overdose. Furthermore, lessons from healthy volunteer studies have also shown that increases in serum livers of miR-122 are associated with individuals that develop liver injury despite taking the therapeutic dose and that miR-122 rise at time points 24 h before ALT activity [82]. In these APAP overdose studies, miR-122 correlated strongly with peak ALT levels [83]. Interestingly, serum miR-122 levels in APAP-induced acute liver injury patients who satisfied KCC for liver transplantation were higher than those who did not satisfy KCC. However, this did not reach statistical significance, potentially due to small patient numbers [83]. Further prospective and longitudinal biomarker studies in acute liver injury patients will be required to determine whether miR-122 can provide added clinical prognostic value. The translational value of miR-122 as a sensitive circulating biomarker has also been demonstrated in an APAP overdose model in zebra fish [84]. This represents an important observation for translational research and data interpretation given the increasing utility of this organism for earlier drug development studies. Despite the advantages of miR-122, future efforts should be coordinated with developed cross-laboratory validated methods for miRNA isolation and quantification as well as for developing a consensus on normalization standards [85].

6.5 Conclusions and Future Perspectives

The following are the key questions related to the development of new mechanistic biomarkers for DILI in man:

- Can new biomarkers sensitively identify DILI when it occurs with enhanced specificity?
- Are new biomarkers translational between preclinical models and man?
- Can we use new biomarkers to report clinical mechanisms of DILI?
- Can new biomarkers be used to predict patient prognosis or stratify treatment?
- Do new investigational biomarkers distinguish benign transaminase elevations from serious DILI to build on "Hy's law?"
- What are the hurdles that could prevent clinical adoption?

Recently, significant progress has been made and clinical utility has been shown regarding "mechanism-based" biomarkers such as acylcarnitines, HMGB1, K18, and GLDH and highly liver-specific markers such as miR-122.

These biomarkers have been shown to be translational, can report DILI sensitively when it occurs, shed light on mechanistic aspects of clinical DILI, and can predict patient prognosis. However, the vast majority of clinical data to date have been obtained from studies of APAP-induced liver injury and have not been assessed in rare cases of idiosyncratic DILI. Moreover, a clear knowledge gap still exists regarding the identification and development of biomarkers that predict serious DILI and reflect hepatic regenerative processes. Therefore, it will become increasingly important to utilize appropriate and well-annotated tissue banks. Important efforts from the US-based DILIN [86] and the Spanish Hepatotoxicity Registry [87] have been collecting serum and urine from all subjects in their registry and where possible to make a comprehensive histological evaluation against which new biomarkers can be compared [88]. However, these subjects are enrolled only after the diagnosis of DILI is established; the utility of the biospecimens collected will probably be limited to studies of biomarkers for diagnosis and management of DILI. The qualification of biomarkers that will predict individual subject susceptibility, or that can accurately and safely assess the liver liability of a new drug in development, will require the collection of biospecimens before the start of treatment and during treatment prior to the onset of clinically overt DILI. This effort will require adoption of standardized liver safety databases as well as standardized protocols for biospecimen collection and storage and the initiation of large prospective clinical trials, involving diverse disease populations and treatment with many different drugs. This should now become a high priority within the pharmaceutical industry.

The lessons learnt from the preclinical qualification of renal safety biomarkers have demonstrated that no single biomarker will be the solution and that a panel approach of novel biomarkers alongside a more intelligent use of currently used biomarkers represents the way forward to inform all stakeholders. Moreover, novel translational biomarkers that reflect the mechanistic basis of DILI are fundamental to efforts in translational research. However, despite significant progress in preclinical renal injury biomarker qualification, to date, clinical biomarker qualification has not been accomplished; however, prospective clinical studies are ongoing to achieve this. Defining the context of use for novel biomarkers in man represents an important area of collaborative research interest. Understanding reference ranges for these novel markers in preclinical species and their evaluation in diverse healthy human populations and liver disease cohorts is an important area of investigation and question to address. Further areas of research focus should also be targeted toward the generation of robust cross-species bioanalytical assays that are standardized or point of care tests in parallel with a comprehensive understanding of cross-species differences in biomarker expression, mechanisms of release and clearance, distribution, and kinetics. It is also important to understand the cost-effectiveness of a new biomarker and the added value when moving from an experimental tool to the clinical settling, defining whether a biomarker is fit for purpose or what purpose is it fit for in the context of DILI. In addition, understanding what is the right biomarker to assay and at what particular time for an individual patient or at what stage during drug development is also a critical research question to move forward the development and qualification of experimental DILI biomarkers.

The qualification of novel DILI biomarkers will require application to biospecimens obtained from many different patient populations treated with many different drugs, both those that cause clinically important DILI and those that cause elevations in traditional liver chemistries but do not cause clinically important liver injury. It is important that pharmaceutical companies start now to archive samples and link these specimens to the relevant liver safety data. Ideally, liver safety data management tools should be standardized across the industry to facilitate the precompetitive collaborations on biomarker validation and qualification, such as eDISH [38]. As formal biomarker validation and qualification will be a lengthy and challenging process, these proposed biomarkers are likely to retain their exploratory status for some time. A more intelligent use of currently used markers in the meantime can bridge the gap between novel biomarkers being used in the experimental context to formal qualification.

Serum ALT activity is the primary method to assess acute liver injury associated with drugs. Although not formally qualified against human histology for DILI, ALT has been widely "qualified" as a DILI biomarker by its extensive use and ease of measurement. Despite there are several limitations associated with ALT activity, it can still be an important biomarker of DILI if understood and used properly. This is the topic of Ref. [37] where Senior proposes new interpretations relating to ALT activity and suggests how they might lend themselves to better general use and that suitable revisions in guidance, teaching approaches, and clinical practice will need to reflect this. A number of key points were raised and have been built upon to gain a better understanding of serum ALT activity as a biomarker of DILI [37,89].

In summary, DILI is a complex multicellular and multimechanism disease; therefore, it is logical that a battery of complimentary biomarkers (both genetic and circulating) that reflect specific cellular processes and predisposition to DILI are required, which have been investigated in prospective studies of DILI in the first instance to compliment the use of current markers.

References

1 Edwards, I.R. and Aronson, J.K. (2000) Adverse drug reactions: definitions, diagnosis, and management. *Lancet*, **356** (9237), 1255–1259.

2 Kola, I. and Landis, J. (2004) Can the pharmaceutical industry reduce attrition rates? *Nature Reviews. Drug Discovery*, **3** (8), 711–715.

3 DiMasi, J.A., Hansen, R.W., and Grabowski, H.G. (2003) The price of innovation: new estimates of drug development costs. *Journal of Health Economics*, **22** (2), 151–185.

4 Wu, T.Y. *et al.* (2010) Ten-year trends in hospital admissions for adverse drug reactions in England 1999–2009. *Journal of the Royal Society of Medicine*, **103** (6), 239–250.

5 Pirmohamed, M. *et al.* (2004) Adverse drug reactions as cause of admission to hospital: prospective analysis of 18 820 patients. *BMJ*, **329** (7456), 15–19.

6 Lee, W.M. (2003) Drug-induced hepatotoxicity. *New England Journal of Medicine*, **349** (5), 474–485.

7 Sgro, C. *et al.* (2002) Incidence of drug-induced hepatic injuries: a French population-based study. *Hepatology*, **36** (2), 451–455.

8 Meier, Y. *et al.* (2005) Incidence of drug-induced liver injury in medical inpatients. *European Journal of Clinical Pharmacology*, **61** (2), 135–143.

9 Vuppalanchi, R., Liangpunsakul, S., and Chalasani, N. (2007) Etiology of new-onset jaundice: how often is it caused by idiosyncratic drug-induced liver injury in the United States? *The American Journal of Gastroenterology*, **102** (3), 558–562.

10 Corsini, A. *et al.* (2012) Current challenges and controversies in drug-induced liver injury. *Drug Safety*, **35** (12), 1099–1117.

11 Moggs, J. *et al.* (2012) Investigative safety science as a competitive advantage for Pharma. *Expert Opinion on Drug Metabolism and Toxicology*, **8** (9), 1071–1082.

12 Antoine, D.J. *et al.* (2009) Mechanism-based bioanalysis and biomarkers for hepatic chemical stress. *Xenobiotica*, **39** (8), 565–577.

13 Olson, H. *et al.* (2000) Concordance of the toxicity of pharmaceuticals in humans and in animals. *Regulatory Toxicology and Pharmacology*, **32** (1), 56–67.

14 Aithal, G.P., Rawlins, M.D., and Day, C.P. (1999) Accuracy of hepatic adverse drug reaction reporting in one English health region. *BMJ*, **319** (7224), 1541.

15 Biomarkers Definitions Working Group (2001) Biomarkers and surrogate endpoints: preferred definitions and conceptual framework. *Clinical Pharmacology and Therapeutics*, **69** (3), 89–95.

16 Ratner, M. (2005) FDA pharmacogenomics guidance sends clear message to industry. *Nature Reviews. Drug Discovery*, **4** (5), 359.

17 Matheis, K. *et al.* (2011) A generic operational strategy to qualify translational safety biomarkers. *Drug Discovery Today*, **16** (13–14), 600–608.

18 Watkins, P.B. (2011) Drug safety sciences and the bottleneck in drug development. *Clinical Pharmacology and Therapeutics*, **89** (6), 788–790.

19 Park, B.K. *et al.* (2005) The role of metabolic activation in drug-induced hepatotoxicity. *Annual Review of Pharmacology and Toxicology*, **45**, 177–202.

20 Park, B.K. *et al.* (2011) Drug bioactivation and protein adduct formation in the pathogenesis of drug-induced toxicity. *Chemico-Biological Interactions*, **192** (1–2), 30–36.

21 NHS, H.E.S. (2011) http://www.hesonline.nhs.uk/Ease/servlet/ContentServer?siteID=1937 (last accessed January 2014.

22 Lee, W.M. *et al.* (2008) Acute liver failure: summary of a workshop. *Hepatology*, **47** (4), 1401–1415.

23 Williams, C.D. and Jaeschke, H. (2012) Role of innate and adaptive immunity during drug-induced liver injury. *Toxicology Research*, **1**, 161–170.

24 Kaplowitz, N. (2005) Idiosyncratic drug hepatotoxicity. *Nature Reviews. Drug Discovery*, **4** (6), 489–499.

25 Mitchell, J.R. *et al.* (1973) Acetaminophen-induced hepatic necrosis: I. Role of drug metabolism. *Journal of Pharmacology and Experimental Therapeutics*, **187** (1), 185–194.

26 Mitchell, J.R. *et al.* (1973) Acetaminophen-induced hepatic necrosis: IV. Protective role of glutathione. *Journal of Pharmacology and Experimental Therapeutics*, **187** (1), 211–217.

27 Jollow, D.J. *et al.* (1973) Acetaminophen-induced hepatic necrosis: II. Role of covalent binding *in vivo*. *The Journal of Pharmacology and Experimental Therapeutics*, **187** (1), 195–202.

28 Potter, W.Z. *et al.* (1973) Acetaminophen-induced hepatic necrosis: 3. Cytochrome P-450-mediated covalent binding *in vitro*. *Journal of Pharmacology and Experimental Therapeutics*, **187** (1), 203–210.

29 Antoine, D.J. *et al.* (2013) Mechanistic biomarkers provide early and sensitive detection of acetaminophen-induced acute liver injury at first presentation to hospital. *Hepatology*, **58** (2), 777–787.

30 Dear, J.W. *et al.* (2014) Early detection of paracetamol toxicity using circulating liver

microRNA and markers of cell necrosis. *British Journal of Clinical Pharmacology*, **77** (5), 904–905.

31 Ferner, R.E., Dear, J.W., and Bateman, D.N. (2011) Management of paracetamol poisoning. *BMJ*, **342**, d2218.

32 Dear, J.W. and Antoine, D.J. (2014) Stratification of paracetamol overdose patients using new toxicity biomarkers: current candidates and future challenges. *Expert Review of Clinical Pharmacology*, 7 (2), 181–189.

33 Ozer, J. *et al.* (2008) The current state of serum biomarkers of hepatotoxicity. *Toxicology*, **245** (3), 194–205.

34 Watkins, P.B. *et al.* (1994) Hepatotoxic effects of tacrine administration in patients with Alzheimer's disease. *The Journal of the American Medical Association*, **271** (13), 992–998.

35 Harrill, A.H. *et al.* (2012) The effects of heparins on the liver: application of mechanistic serum biomarkers in a randomized study in healthy volunteers. *Clinical Pharmacology and Therapeutics*, **92** (2), 214–220.

36 Zimmerman, H.J. (1968) The spectrum of hepatotoxicity. *Perspectives in Biology and Medicine*, **12** (1), 135–161.

37 Senior, J.R. (2012) Alanine aminotransferase: a clinical and regulatory tool for detecting liver injury – past, present, and future. *Clinical Pharmacology and Therapeutics*, **92** (3), 332–339.

38 Watkins, P.B. *et al.* (2011) Evaluation of drug-induced serious hepatotoxicity (eDISH): application of this data organization approach to phase III clinical trials of rivaroxaban after total hip or knee replacement surgery. *Drug Safety*, **34** (3), 243–252.

39 Aithal, G.P. *et al.* (2011) Case definition and phenotype standardization in drug-induced liver injury. *Clinical Pharmacology and Therapeutics*, **89** (6), 806–815.

40 Zhang, X. *et al.* (2011) Involvement of the immune system in idiosyncratic drug reactions. *Drug Metabolism and Pharmacokinetics*, **26** (1), 47–59.

41 Coen, M. (2010) A metabonomic approach for mechanistic exploration of pre-clinical toxicology. *Toxicology*, **278** (3), 326–340.

42 Van Summeren, A. *et al.* (2012) Proteomics in the search for mechanisms and biomarkers of drug-induced hepatotoxicity. *Toxicology In Vitro: An International Journal Published in Association with BIBRA*, **26** (3), 373–385.

43 Bell, L.N. *et al.* (2012) Serum proteomic profiling in patients with drug-induced liver injury. *Alimentary Pharmacology & Therapeutics*, **35** (5), 600–612.

44 Bonventre, J.V. *et al.* (2010) Next-generation biomarkers for detecting kidney toxicity. *Nature Biotechnology*, **28** (5), 436–440.

45 Vaidya, V.S. *et al.* (2010) Kidney injury molecule-1 outperforms traditional biomarkers of kidney injury in preclinical biomarker qualification studies. *Nature Biotechnology*, **28** (5), 478–485.

46 Feldman, B.F. (1989) Cerebrospinal fluid, in *Clinical Biochemistry of Domestic Animals* (ed. J. Kaneko), Academic Press, San Diego, pp. 835–865.

47 Stonard, M.D. (1996) Assessment of nephrotoxicity, in *Animal Clinical Chemistry* (ed. G.O. Evans), Taylor & Francis, London, pp. 87–89.

48 Schmidt, E.S. and Schmidt, F.W. (1988) Glutamate dehydrogenase: biochemical and clinical aspects of an interesting enzyme. *Clinica Chimica Acta; International Journal of Clinical Chemistry*, **173** (1), 43–55.

49 Schomaker, S. *et al.* (2013) Assessment of emerging biomarkers of liver injury in human subjects. *Toxicological Sciences*, **132** (2), 276–283.

50 O'Brien, P.J. *et al.* (2002) Advantages of glutamate dehydrogenase as a blood biomarker of acute hepatic injury in rats. *Laboratory Animals*, **36** (3), 313–321.

51 McGill, M.R. *et al.* (2012) The mechanism underlying acetaminophen-induced hepatotoxicity in humans and mice involves mitochondrial damage and nuclear DNA fragmentation. *The Journal of Clinical Investigation*, **122** (4), 1574–1583.

52 Antoine, D.J. *et al.* (2013) Mechanistic biomarkers provide early and sensitive detection of acetaminophen-induced acute

liver injury at first presentation to hospital. *Hepatology*, **58** (2), 777–787.
53 Singhal, R., Harrill, A.H., Menguy-Vacheron, F., Jayyosi, Z., Benzerdjeb, H., and Watkins, P.B. (2014) Benign elevations in serum aminotransferases and biomarkers of hepatotoxicity in healthy volunteers treated with cholestyramine. *British Journal of Clinical Pharmacology*, **15**, 42.
54 Jaeschke, H. and McGill, M.R. (2013) Serum glutamate dehydrogenase: biomarker for liver cell death or mitochondrial dysfunction? *Toxicological Sciences*, **134** (1), 221–222.
55 Chen, C. *et al.* (2009) Serum metabolomics reveals irreversible inhibition of fatty acid beta-oxidation through the suppression of PPARalpha activation as a contributing mechanism of acetaminophen-induced hepatotoxicity. *Chemical Research in Toxicology*, **22** (4), 699–707.
56 McGill, M.R. *et al.* (2014) Circulating acylcarnitines as biomarkers of mitochondrial dysfunction after acetaminophen overdose in mice and humans. *Archives of Toxicology*, **88** (2), 391–401.
57 Scaffidi, P., Misteli, T., and Bianchi, M.E. (2002) Release of chromatin protein HMGB1 by necrotic cells triggers inflammation. *Nature*, **418** (6894), 191–195.
58 Wang, H. *et al.* (1999) HMG-1 as a late mediator of endotoxin lethality in mice. *Science*, **285** (5425), 248–251.
59 Yang, H. *et al.* (2013) The many faces of HMGB1: molecular structure–functional activity in inflammation, apoptosis, and chemotaxis. *Journal of Leukocyte Biology*, **96** (6), 865–873.
60 Nystrom, S. *et al.* (2013) TLR activation regulates damage-associated molecular pattern isoforms released during pyroptosis. *The EMBO Journal*, **32** (1), 86–99.
61 Lu, B. *et al.* (2012) Novel role of PKR in inflammasome activation and HMGB1 release. *Nature*, **488** (7413), 670–674.
62 Yang, H. *et al.* (2012) Redox modification of cysteine residues regulates the cytokine activity of high mobility group box-1 (HMGB1). *Molecular Medicine (Cambridge, Mass.)*, **18** (1), 250–259.
63 Venereau, E. *et al.* (2012) Mutually exclusive redox forms of HMGB1 promote cell recruitment or proinflammatory cytokine release. *The Journal of Experimental Medicine*, **209** (9), 1519–1528.
64 Antoine, D.J. *et al.* (2014) A systematic nomenclature for the redox states of high mobility group box (HMGB) proteins. *Molecular Medicine (Cambridge, Mass.)*, **20** (1), 135–137.
65 Bonaldi, T. *et al.* (2003) Monocytic cells hyperacetylate chromatin protein HMGB1 to redirect it towards secretion. *The EMBO Journal*, **22** (20), 5551–5560.
66 Lu, B. *et al.* (2014) JAK/STAT1 signaling promotes HMGB1 hyperacetylation and nuclear translocation. *Proceedings of the National Academy of Sciences of the United States of America*, **111** (8), 3068–3073.
67 Antoine, D.J. *et al.* (2009) High-mobility group box-1 protein and keratin-18, circulating serum proteins informative of acetaminophen-induced necrosis and apoptosis *in vivo*. *Toxicological Sciences*, **112** (2), 521–531.
68 Antoine, D.J. *et al.* (2010) Diet restriction inhibits apoptosis and HMGB1 oxidation and promotes inflammatory cell recruitment during acetaminophen hepatotoxicity. *Molecular Medicine*, **16** (11–12), 479–490.
69 Antoine, D.J. *et al.* (2012) Molecular forms of HMGB1 and keratin-18 as mechanistic biomarkers for mode of cell death and prognosis during clinical acetaminophen hepatotoxicity. *Journal of Hepatology*, **56** (5), 1070–1079.
70 Ku, N.O. *et al.* (2007) Keratins let liver live: mutations predispose to liver disease and crosslinking generates Mallory–Denk bodies. *Hepatology*, **46** (5), 1639–1649.
71 Caulin, C., Salvesen, G.S., and Oshima, R.G. (1997) Caspase cleavage of keratin 18 and reorganization of intermediate filaments during epithelial cell apoptosis. *Journal of Cell Biology*, **138** (6), 1379–1394.
72 Schutte, B. *et al.* (2004) Keratin 8/18 breakdown and reorganization during

apoptosis. *Experimental Cell Research*, **297** (1), 11–26.

73 Wieckowska, A. *et al.* (2006) *In vivo* assessment of liver cell apoptosis as a novel biomarker of disease severity in nonalcoholic fatty liver disease. *Hepatology*, **44** (1), 27–33.

74 Cummings, J. *et al.* (2008) Preclinical evaluation of M30 and M65 ELISAs as biomarkers of drug induced tumor cell death and antitumor activity. *Molecular Cancer Therapeutics*, **7** (3), 455–463.

75 Ku, N.O. *et al.* (1996) Susceptibility to hepatotoxicity in transgenic mice that express a dominant-negative human keratin 18 mutant. *The Journal of Clinical Investigation*, **98** (4), 1034–1046.

76 Strnad, P. *et al.* (2010) Keratin variants predispose to acute liver failure and adverse outcome: race and ethnic associations. *Gastroenterology*, **139** (3), 828–835.

77 Bechmann, L.P. *et al.* (2010) Cytokeratin 18-based modification of the MELD score improves prediction of spontaneous survival after acute liver injury. *Journal of Hepatology*, **53** (4), 639–647.

78 Starkey Lewis, P.J. *et al.* (2012) Serum microRNA biomarkers for drug-induced liver injury. *Clinical Pharmacology and Therapeutics*, **92** (3), 291–293.

79 Zen, K. and Zhang, C.Y. (2012) Circulating microRNAs: a novel class of biomarkers to diagnose and monitor human cancers. *Medicinal Research Reviews*, **32** (2), 326–348.

80 Wang, K. *et al.* (2009) Circulating microRNAs, potential biomarkers for drug-induced liver injury. *Proceedings of the National Academy of Sciences of the United States of America*, **106** (11), 4402–4407.

81 Zhang, Y. *et al.* (2010) Plasma microRNA-122 as a biomarker for viral-, alcohol-, and chemical-related hepatic diseases. *Clinical Chemistry*, **56** (12), 1830–1838.

82 Thulin, P. *et al.* (2013) Keratin-18 and microRNA-122 complement alanine aminotransferase as novel safety biomarkers for drug-induced liver injury in two human cohorts. *Liver International*. doi: 10.1111/liv.12322.

83 Starkey Lewis, P.J. *et al.* (2011) Circulating microRNAs as potential markers of human drug-induced liver injury. *Hepatology*, **54** (5), 1767–1776.

84 Vliegenthart, A.D. *et al.* (2014) Retro-orbital blood acquisition facilitates circulating microRNA measurement in zebrafish with paracetamol hepatotoxicity. *Zebrafish*, **11** (3), 219–226.

85 Sharkey, J.W., Antoine, D.J., and Park, B.K. (2012) Validation of the isolation and quantification of kidney enriched miRNAs for use as biomarkers. *Biomarkers*, **17** (3), 231–239.

86 Hoofnagle, J.H. (2004) Drug-Induced Liver Injury Network (DILIN). *Hepatology*, **40** (4), 773.

87 Andrade, R.J. *et al.* (2006) Outcome of acute idiosyncratic drug-induced liver injury: long-term follow-up in a hepatotoxicity registry. *Hepatology*, **44** (6), 1581–1588.

88 Kleiner, D.E. *et al.* (2014) Hepatic histological findings in suspected drug-induced liver injury: systematic evaluation and clinical associations. *Hepatology*, **59** (2), 661–670.

89 Antoine, D.J. *et al.* (2013) Are we closer to finding biomarkers for identifying acute drug-induced liver injury? *Biomarkers in Medicine*, **7** (3), 383–386.

7
In Vitro Models for the Prediction of Drug-Induced Liver Injury in Lead Discovery

Frederic Moulin and Oliver Flint

7.1
Introduction

The term drug-induced liver injury (DILI) is used to broadly describe all insults to the liver caused by prescription and over-the-counter medications, herbs, or dietary supplements [1]. Today, DILI is still the leading cause of death from acute liver failure in the United States and the most frequent reason for the refusal to approve or postmarketing withdrawal of a therapeutic agent [2].

The clinical picture of drug-induced hepatotoxicity is diverse (Table 7.1), even for a single drug in different patients. Manifestations range from mild, asymptomatic changes in serum transaminases to fulminant hepatic failure, a rare but life-threatening complication often leading to liver transplantation. Although asymptomatic rises in transaminases are common with many medications, the more severe forms of DILI are fortunately rare, occurring with a frequency between 1 in 1000 and 1 in 10 000. The rarity of these severe toxic occurrences and the lack of common mechanism of injury have led to the distinction developed by Dr. Zimmerman between the predictable adverse hepatic effects of a few chemicals called "intrinsic toxicity" and the low-frequency events typically recorded postmarketing and termed "idiosyncratic hepatotoxicity" [3] for which the extent of liver injury appears critically dependent on some patient-specific conditions.

Idiosyncratic reactions are characterized by a latency period, ranging from 5 to 90 days from the initial ingestion of the causative agent, and are frequently fatal once the reaction has started if the drug is not promptly discontinued. Rechallenge typically leads to more severe reactions regardless of the intensity of the initial toxicity. In contrast, intrinsic toxicants such as acetaminophen injure the hepatic parenchymal cells in a dose-related fashion, showing that the amount of administered drug is a stronger determinant of the liver damage than the host's response to the insult. This dichotomy is overly simplified, and the true potential of any chemical to injure the liver forms a spectrum between the two poles.

Antitargets and Drug Safety, First Edition. Edited by László Urbán, Vinod F. Patel, and Roy J. Vaz.

Table 7.1 Clinicopathological presentation and proposed mechanisms of DILI [4].

Phenotype	Histology	Proposed mechanism
Acute fatty liver with lactic acidosis	Microvesicular hepatic steatosis and/or other tissue involvement (didanosine and fialuridine)	Severe acute mitochondrial injury
Acute hepatic necrosis	Collapse and necrosis of liver parenchyma (isoniazid, aspirin, and niacin)	Reactive metabolite and/or immune activation
Autoimmune-like hepatitis	Plasma cells and interface hepatitis with detectable autoantibodies (nitrofurantoin and minocycline)	Adduct formation and autoimmunity
Bland cholestasis	Balloon hepatocytes with minimal inflammation (anabolic steroids)	Inhibition of bile salt export pump or other biliary transporters
Cholestatic hepatitis	Balloon hepatocytes with inflammation and predominance of elevated serum alkaline phosphatase levels (phenytoin and amoxicillin–clavulanate)	Immune-mediated and/or reactive metabolite
Fibrosis/cirrhosis	Hepatic collagenization with minimal inflammation (methotrexate and amiodarone)	Stellate cell activation/chronic endothelial cell injury
Nodular regeneration	Microscopic or macroscopic liver nodules (azathioprine and oxaliplatin)	Chronic injury to endothelial cells
Immunoallergic hepatitis	Skin rash, fever, and eosinophilia (trimethoprim–sulfamethoxazole)	Drug hypersensitivity/allergy
Nonalcoholic fatty liver	Macrosteatosis and microsteatosis, hepatocyte ballooning, and periportal inflammation (tamoxifen)	Chronic mitochondrial injury or altered lipid metabolism
Sinusoidal obstruction syndrome	Inflammation with obliteration of central veins (busulfan)	Severe, acute endothelial cell injury
Vanishing bile duct syndrome	Paucity of interlobular bile ducts (amoxicillin–clavulanate, sulfonamides)	Immune-mediated cholangiocyte injury

Idiosyncratic toxicities are, by their rarity, difficult to observe within the limited number of participants in clinical studies and there are few, if any, applicable animal models to anticipate their occurrences. Hence, these reactions are often only detected after broad exposure of a large patient population to the drug, and the consequences in terms of human health, scientific progress, and drug discovery costs are often catastrophic.

Currently, we do not have biomarkers or protocols to identify, before drug administration, which person will face life-threatening DILI or any test capable of conclusively demonstrating that someone's hepatic injury was caused by a specific agent [1]. No antidotes or treatments are available for DILI other than the immediate discontinuation of the causative agent, and in an age of polypharmacy, even this simple step is not always easy to implement. The monitoring of serum transaminases at regular intervals for detection of liver injury is a standard procedure in most clinical trials. Unfortunately, increases in serum alanine aminotransferase (ALT) and aspartate aminotransferase (AST) activities are poor predictors of the extent and origin of liver damage. They can be caused by many pathologies such as fatty liver disease, fluctuations in chronic viral hepatitis, undiagnosed hepatic problems, or sometimes transient physiological changes that lead to no apparent clinical consequence. Therefore, clinical investigators face the daunting task of trying to recognize a condition that can mimic any known liver disease, has many different mechanisms or manifestations, and whose severity and progression are extremely variable, ranging from transient, asymptomatic rises in serum enzymes to massive liver necrosis, acute liver failure, and death [2].

Complicating human risk assessment, the timing between observable changes in liver function tests and potential evolution toward liver failure is also variable. For example, during the EXTEND clinical trials of ximelagatran, elevation of liver function tests greater than three times the upper limit of normal was recorded in several patients only after the end of the 35 days of drug treatment. In one case, these effects further evolved into severe liver injury, prompting cancellation of the study and subsequent removal of the drug from the European market [5]. Thus, the monitoring of liver functions every few weeks during clinical development might not be sufficient to ensure patient's safety and the lack of specificity of these biomarkers in trying to detect rare but potentially lethal events results in many false safety signals and can lead to the premature termination of novel therapeutic agents.

In an attempt to limit the impact of unrecognized toxicity in new therapeutic candidates, both the North American and European health authorities require the conduct of multiple animal tests before humans can be exposed to a new molecular entity [6]. Such a process is based on the assumption that the animal models and study designs employed in the preclinical investigation of a drug candidate's safety are predictive of the human hazards. In 1990, the pharmaceutical industry attempted to evaluate the relevance of *in vivo* toxicology studies to human risks by pooling preclinical and clinical information on drug-induced toxicity. Twelve companies sent preclinical and clinical data to the International Life Sciences Institute to examine how well adverse events detected in animal safety studies could forecast clinical toxicity for specific target organs. The results of this collaboration were later reported by Olson *et al.* [7]. Although the overall concordance of animal to human toxicities was 71%, this number proved variable across different organ systems. Multispecies preclinical studies were only able to predict 55% of the drugs associated with human DILI and rodent studies alone, even with dosing periods of 2 or more months at maximum tolerated doses, were only predictive 7% of the time. Hepatic toxicity was the fourth most common adverse reaction reported, yet it leads to the second highest rate of program termination, perhaps because of the poor confidence of clinical investigators in the ability of preclinical toxicology studies to guarantee patient safety.

Several important factors hinder the ability of animal models to predict human hepatic adverse events. First, preclinical safety studies typically include doses of test articles that are orders of magnitude greater than those used in patients. Dose–response relationships are complex and toxicity findings from high doses can mask adverse effects that might predominate at clinical exposures. In addition, the dose–response relationship for idiosyncratic DILI (iDILI) is at best difficult to define in humans [8], and it seems questionable to expect an improvement of this situation across species and wide dosing ranges. Second, *in vivo* studies examine the response of standard laboratory animals to a chemical. The same response may or may not occur in humans because of genetic differences between the species. Even when the animals manifest some form of the toxicity mechanism, a single homogeneous animal strain cannot be expected to model the range of responses that could be observed in the heterogeneous patient population. Hence, a mild elevation of liver function tests in preclinical studies is unable to confidently ascertain whether patients will simply adapt and normalize their liver enzymes after a few doses, or will instead evolve toward acute liver failure and the need for transplantation. Finally, we must recognize the limitations of our current biomarkers of liver injury. The first clinical manifestations of DILI in both humans and animals are usually rises in plasma ALT and AST enzyme levels and the interpretation of modest or transient elevations remains very ambiguous [9].

Nonetheless, the frequently reported background of mild cytosolic protein leakage into the circulation suggests some ability of the DILI agents to directly injure hepatic cells, whereas the transient nature of the changes points to adaptive mechanisms overcoming the toxicity in most patients. Retrospective studies have highlighted the propensity of lipophilic drugs administered at a daily dose of more than 50 mg/day to cause DILI compared with less lipophilic agents given at a lower daily dose [8,10]. Because chemicals given in large oral doses often result in high intrahepatic concentrations and lipophilic drugs are known to require greater metabolism for elimination from the body, these observations pointed toward metabolism being involved in the pathogenesis of idiosyncratic liver damage. Unfortunately, structure–activity models combining the daily dose of a chemical, its polarity, and the extent of hepatic metabolism have been unable to adequately predict the DILI risk of many problematic drugs. Although it is generally accepted that the mechanisms contributing to the mild injury are likely contributors to the more severe effects, it is also clear that unexplained genetic and environmental factors, as well as differences in the adaptive processes and the immune response, determine which patients will progress toward acute liver failure [11]. The challenge facing the drug discovery community today is the identification of these factors and the design of screening strategies to avoid the use of problematic drugs in the rare susceptible individual while allowing the therapeutic benefits to the larger patient population even in the presence of mild, transient transaminase elevation. Unfortunately, such an effort would require an understanding of the drug-specific (metabolism, transport, and elimination) and patient-specific (cell death, innate immune response, repair, and regeneration) pathways determinant of both common, mild and rare, severe idiosyncratic hepatotoxicity that is beyond our current knowledge [12].

The drug-related perturbations contributing to the initial insults are currently better understood than the patient-specific processes determining the evolution of DILI. Six mechanisms arising from the interaction of parent molecules and/or their metabolites with biochemical processes in the hepatocytes have been linked to the onset of iDILI [13]. The current screening strategy for hepatotoxicity during lead optimization consists broadly in recognizing the ability of some candidate molecules to participate in one or more of these processes and selecting them out of the discovery pipeline as early as possible.

- High-energy reactions involving cytochrome P450 enzymes can produce chemically reactive intermediates that bind to intracellular proteins and disrupt cell metabolism leading to a decline in ATP levels, loss of ionic gradients, and finally plasma membrane swelling and rupture [11,14,15].
- Inhibition of carrier proteins at the canalicular membrane or within the cytoplasm can disrupt the liver's ability to synthesize and transport bile, causing cholestasis. The intracellular accumulation of toxic bile acids can then cause secondary injury to the hepatocytes themselves [16–18].
- Binding of reactive species formed during biotransformation to cellular proteins can also create foreign structures large enough to be targeted by the immune system. When the adducted proteins migrate to the cell surface or are released into the blood, they can initiate antibody production or direct cytolytic T-cell responses against hepatocytes. The secondary cytokine release also causes inflammation and may initiate neutrophil-mediated hepatotoxicity [19].
- Drugs can damage cellular mitochondria, disrupting fatty acid oxidation and energy production. Disabling the respiratory chain enzymes or interfering with the mitochondrial DNA creates oxidative stress. The resulting anaerobic metabolism produces lactic acidosis and triglyceride accumulation, frequently in the form of microvesicular steatosis or steatohepatitis [20].
- Activation of proapoptotic and intracellular stress response pathways can initiate programmed cell death and the release of endogenous damage-associated molecular patterns (DAMPs), which in turn activate receptors on immune cells. The sterile inflammation produced in response amplifies liver injury [21].
- Finally, nonparenchymal cells within the liver may also be the target of drug injury or serve as modulators of an adverse reaction. Kupffer cells, for example, can release cytokines that amplify injury, and stellate cells produce fibrosis [22]. Chemotherapeutic agents have been shown to injure sinusoidal endothelial cells, a process that can lead to veno-occlusive disease [23].

Since these mechanisms center around the physiology of the liver parenchymal cells, various human *in vitro* models have been proposed to predict and study the hepatic effects of therapeutic candidates. Although this area of research has made tremendous progress since the identification of the tissue model's limitations for risk assessment [24], we still do not have *in vitro* assays capable of predicting with confidence the risk of clinical DILI in patients. Nonetheless, *in vitro* models have become an integral part of the drug discovery process, enabling the early identification of undesirable properties, the investigation of toxicity mechanisms at the cellular level for interspecies extrapolation, and the design of follow-up assays to prevent the reoccurrence of DILI in structurally related backup candidates. This chapter reviews the most common and validated *in vitro* techniques used for these purposes as well as some of the experimental strategies hoping to address the limitations of today's methodology.

7.2 Simple Systems for the Detection and Investigation of Hepatic Toxicants

The liver comprises two categories of cells: parenchymal and nonparenchymal. The hepatocytes, the sole cell type of the parenchymal fraction, account for 60% of the total liver cell population and 80% of the organ volume, and perform the majority of the drug-metabolizing functions [25]. In the basic structural unit of the liver, the hepatic lobule, plates of parenchymal cells radiate from the periportal region toward the central vein, draining the blood supply from the gastrointestinal tract through the liver capillaries back toward the abdominal vena cava [26,27]. This directionality of flow creates chemical gradients that impact cell maturation, matrix chemistry, endogenous substrate utilization, oxygen tension, gene expression, and xenobiotic clearance mechanisms [28]. The plate-like arrangement of the parenchyma in single- or double-cell thick layers and the high permeability of the endothelium lining the sinusoids maximize the contact of the cell's basal membrane with blood. In addition, the apical portions of two adjacent hepatocytes form a narrow lumen, which is the site of bile secretion. These luminal domains combine throughout the length of the hepatic plates, forming a network of bile canaliculi that carry the bile in a direction opposite to the blood flow toward the portal triad.

Thus, hepatocytes support two countercurrent flow systems: the synthesis and secretion of bile and the uptake, processing, and secretion of sinusoidal blood components. To perform these functions, the cells exhibit a marked polarization with distinct luminal and basolateral domains segregated by tight junctions [29]. The combination of functional differences linked to chemical gradients and the marked cell polarity have significantly complicated the development of *in vitro* models to replicate the complete functionalities of a liver lobule.

7.2.1 Primary Hepatocytes

The liver is the major source of biotransformation for ingested chemicals, and the metabolic pathways involved are frequently qualitatively and/or quantitatively different in laboratory animals and humans. For this reason, cultures of primary human and animal hepatocytes have been for many years the gold standard for *in vitro* testing of metabolism and enzyme induction or inhibition and for examining interspecies and interindividual differences in hepatic biotransformation of drug candidates [30,31]. Primary cultures of hepatocytes have also been extensively applied to the investigation and prediction of hepatotoxicity.

7.2.1.1 Cells

Hepatocytes are highly differentiated epithelial cells rich in mitochondria and lysosomes, as well as endoplasmic reticulum where many of the enzymes involved in the biotransformation of foreign chemicals are synthesized and anchored [32]. Primary hepatocytes are isolated from fresh human liver by collagenase digestion, frequently from organ donations when a suitable recipient cannot be located in a timely fashion. The collagenase perfusion disrupts the bonds between cells in the liver and allows the collection of single-cell suspensions that are further purified by centrifugation. Although the perfusion protocols are now well established [33–35], the preparation of human primary hepatocytes still requires extensive experience and a real-time network connecting surgeons to those who isolate the cells, as human tissue availability is unpredictable. The continuous increase in demand for human liver cells coupled with the technical challenges of isolation supported the creation of several commercial entities specialized in the collection and supply of primary hepatocytes from human and laboratory animals.

With the progress of cryopreservation methods in the last 10 years, it is now possible to order vials of frozen hepatocytes from well-characterized donors directly from online commercial suppliers and use the cells for testing purposes in a manner very similar to fresh primary hepatocytes.

7.2.1.2 Cell Culture Conditions

Primary hepatocytes are exposed to test articles essentially in three different ways: in suspension shortly after isolation, as a monolayer on collagen-coated plates, or in sandwich cultures under Matrigel. Each one of these culture techniques improves some aspects of hepatic cellular functions at the cost of increasing model complexity, which reduces in proportion the throughput of assays and the reproducibility of results.

Suspensions of hepatocytes are the easiest method for high-throughput metabolism studies. Investigators have demonstrated that cells in suspension provide a generally more accurate estimate of internal clearance rate when compared with conventional monolayer cultures [36]. This is attributed to the decrease in CYP P450 activity occurring during the attachment period required by the monolayer system. Unfortunately, this method of cell culture is only usable for short incubation periods as the absence of contact with the extracellular matrix and cell membrane components causes a rapid loss of hepatocyte polarity, structure, and ultimately plasma membrane integrity. Drug-induced hepatotoxicity frequently develops over several hours and the decrease in viability resulting from the suspension culture confounds the recognition of drug-induced adverse cellular events.

The most common primary hepatocyte culture method for toxicology studies involves plating the cells on a rigid collagen substratum and allowing them to form a monolayer across the bottom of the culture plate wells. The cells are then exposed for 24–48 h to increasing concentrations of test articles and the compounds are ranked by the concentration required to decrease by 50% the indicator of cell viability selected as the endpoint. Using this technique, assays can be adapted to high-throughput profiling on robotic platforms and potentially screen hundreds of discovery compounds per week as long as measurements and cell culture conditions are purposefully kept simple.

Unfortunately, monolayers of primary hepatocytes undergo major changes in cell morphology and expression of liver-specific genes in a process referred to as dedifferentiation [37,38]. This process has been linked to the dysregulation of key hepatic transcription factors [39] resulting from damages to cell surface receptors, cellular junctions, and membrane architecture sustained during the isolation procedure [40]. Hepatocyte dedifferentiation remains a severe limitation for toxicological studies. The drastic changes in intracellular metabolism, cell-to-cell interactions, and membrane structures following the switch toward a proliferative state alter the response to chemicals and limit the predictive value of the primary hepatocyte culture models for hepatotoxicity.

7.2.1.3 **Toxicity Endpoints**

The methods used for the evaluation of cell viability can be classified into two categories: functional assays that measure some aspect of the cell physiology and expression assays that record changes in gene transcription via mRNA or protein synthesis. The functional assays rely on measurement of one or more cytotoxic indicators, including loss of membrane integrity (e.g., LDH release and membrane-impermeable DNA stain), apoptosis (e.g., increase in caspase-1 or caspase-3 activity), loss of critical macromolecules or reactive molecule scavengers (e.g., ATP or glutathione), increased formation of reactive oxygen species, mitochondrial inhibition (e.g., tetrazolium salt assays and Alamar blue assay), antiproliferative effects (e.g., inhibition of DNA or protein synthesis), and excretion of proinflammatory cytokines (i.e., IL-1). Xu *et al.* have reported the predictivity of these cytotoxicity assays when applied to the discrimination between 325 severe and moderate human hepatotoxic drugs and 286 therapeutic agents with no report of clinical DILI [41]. Their results are presented in Table 7.2. Clearly, the cytotoxic assays were unable to identify a large fraction of the known hepatotoxicants and, even when used in combination, fell significantly short of the predictivity of preclinical *in vivo* studies. However, the drugs that tested positive in the assays had a high probability of also having shown hepatotoxicity in the clinic. By collecting several biochemical endpoints on each compound, a more complete toxicity profile could be obtained and the rate of false-positive and false-negative results reduced without the requirement for multiple replicates of the same experiment [42].

Many authors have questioned the exclusive use of cytotoxicity endpoints for the prediction of liver injury. As a common final manifestation of toxicity, cell

Table 7.2 Predictivity of drug-induced human hepatotoxicity by cytotoxicity assays [41].

Functional assay	Sensitivity	Specificity
DNA synthesis	10	92
Protein synthesis	4	97
Glutathione depletion	19	85
Superoxide induction	1	97
Caspase-3 induction	5	95
Membrane integrity	2	99
Cell viability (mitochondrial activity/ATP)	10	92
Viability or GSH or DNA synthesis	25	83

death clearly identifies undesirable properties in a molecule. However, the weak sensitivity of the cytotoxic assays suggests that cell death alone may not be the most appropriate measure of all the possible mechanisms leading to clinical hepatotoxicity. Indeed, the list of intracellular pathways associated with DILI includes mechanisms that do not cause direct cell lethality while still impairing cellular physiology. Hence, a variety of pre-lethal mechanistic assays have been developed to study the impact of chemicals on liver parenchymal cell functions, such as lipid accumulation, bile synthesis and transport, capture of reactive intermediates, mitochondrial membrane activity, response to oxidative stress, or intracellular calcium homeostasis [43,44]. Most of these assays are not currently in formats allowing high-throughput screening of drug candidates with multiple endpoints, and thus are reserved for the investigation of toxicity mechanisms once hepatotoxicity has been identified. However, progress in the area of high-content screening and the development of dyes capable of reporting from one well multiple cellular endpoints at once suggest that in the future pre-lethal toxicity assays may become an integral part of drug candidate optimization [45].

Finally, the rapid progress of molecular biology techniques is promoting the investigation of cellular pathways involved in the adaptive response to cellular injury, such as changes in cell division, upregulated detoxification, and enhanced expression of survival factors. Although new information appears regularly in the scientific literature, the complexity of the systems governing changes in gene expression and protein activity in response to cellular stress is staggering and the field of toxicogenomics has not yet produced comprehensive gene signatures or usable biomarkers of hepatic adverse events for *in vitro* models. Nonetheless, these methods have started to be described for lead optimization [46] and the investigation of toxicity mechanisms where they can provide testable hypothesis quickly [47,48].

7.2.1.4 **Limitations of Hepatocyte Cultures**

Although primary hepatocytes offer significant functional benefits, their routine use for toxicological studies also suffers from several issues. First, primary human, dog, or monkey hepatocytes or the tissues from which they can be isolated are in scarce supply, since they require terminal surgery for collection. As mentioned earlier, commercial suppliers have become an important source of primary cells, particularly those of human origin, and it is possible to order primary hepatocytes directly online (www.bioreclamationivt.com). The advances in cryopreservation of liver cells have abolished the necessity of using the hepatocytes within a few hours of isolation and enabled the conduct of multiple experiments with well-characterized cells obtained from a single donor. However, this new convenience comes with a severe drawback: the cost of the cells. Fresh and cryopreserved commercially provided human hepatocytes are expensive, and this factor often limits the size of the assay's validation sets and the number of replicates within an experiment. To improve cost effectiveness, assays conducted on primary hepatocytes are usually reserved for the later stages of lead optimization, when the number of potential candidates has been significantly reduced by prior, less expensive screening methods.

Furthermore, it is difficult to replicate experiments conducted with primary hepatocytes. The cells are the product of the genetic make-up of the donors, their lifestyle and health status, whatever medication affected their livers in life, and whether organ collection was conducted pre- or postmortem. One can expect a fair amount of homogeneity from laboratory animals, but not from the human donors. This effect is particularly problematic during lead optimization campaigns over several months as the results obtained for some candidates on one batch of cells may not be comparable with data collected for subsequent molecules on hepatocytes from different donors. Even in preclinical species, the choice of strain and sex, the conditions of cell isolation, and the methods of cell purification can vary between investigators and over time. Although the systematic use of cryopreserved hepatocytes from a single supplier can alleviate some of these issues, the lots have a finite number of vials and one may not be able to purchase the needed amount of cells from a single preferred donor.

Finally, primary hepatocyte cultures are not miniature livers. Hepatic parenchymal cells begin losing architecture, viability, and drug-metabolizing capacities within a few hours of isolation [49]. Although several types of culture systems have been developed to extend the life span of isolated hepatocytes, none of these systems can completely restore liver-specific function to the levels seen *in vivo*. Frequently, the effects of dedifferentiation are minimized by limiting the duration of drug incubation, and the cells are exposed to concentrations several orders of magnitude greater than the therapeutic exposures to compensate for the longer clinical dosing period. Unfortunately, these supratherapeutic concentrations can trigger routes of metabolism or mechanisms of toxicity without clinical relevance and undermine the predictivity of the toxicity assays. In addition, the absence of other cell types in the culture precludes the modeling of toxicity mechanisms that depend on interactions with nonparenchymal cells and the immune system.

Despite these problems, primary cultures of adult human hepatocytes remain the current standard for *in vitro* hepatic metabolism and toxicology studies, and set the standard against which all other models of hepatotoxicity are judged.

7.2.2
Liver-Derived Cell Lines

The scarce supply and cost of fresh human tissues have encouraged the establishment of permanent human cell lines for the study of liver functions. Cells derived from liver tumors are popular *in vitro* models for their unlimited life span, stable phenotype, low-cost availability, and easy handling. These qualities also make them convenient *in vitro* models for lead optimization screening. Unfortunately, most hepatocarcinoma cells show very weak and/or incomplete expression of drug-metabolizing pathways compared with primary hepatocytes or human livers, likely due to well-described differences in gene transcription patterns [39,50]. Among the numerous hepatic cell lines available today, two have been more extensively applied to the investigation of DILI: the HepG2 and HepaRG lines.

7.2.2.1 HepG2

The HepG2 line was generated in 1977 from hepatic tissues of a 15-year-old male patient with a well-differentiated hepatocellular carcinoma. These cells express many liver-specific genes, secreting a variety of plasma and acute-phase proteins, and have been extensively described over 30 years of use. A subclone called HepG2/C3A was further selected for its ability to switch from a fast-growing, fetal phenotype to a more differentiated phenotype as the cell density in the culture increases [51]. HepG2 (ATCC® HB-8065) and HepG2/C3A (ATCC® CRL-10741) cells can be purchased from the American Type Culture Collection (Manassas, VA). Since these cells are well differentiated and display many of the biochemical functions of normal liver parenchymal cells, they are commonly used by pharmaceutical companies to screen new chemical entities for cytotoxicity in the early lead generation phase [41,52–54].

Unfortunately, even in differentiated state, HepG2 cells demonstrate very limited biotransformation capacity. The metabolic enzymes they do express are present in considerably lower amounts than those found in a normal adult liver [39,50], and this lack of expression affects particularly the reactions involved in the oxidative metabolism of drugs and xenobiotics. The ability of HepG2 cells to respond to enzyme inducers is very poor in terms of enzyme activity, except for the nonhepatic isoform CYP1A1. In a study of gene expression and induction capabilities, Gerets *et al.* [52] showed that the largest difference in the number of differentially expressed probes was found between primary human hepatocytes and HepG2 cells after exposure to three different known cytochrome P450 inducers. Almost every phase I and II xenobiotic metabolism gene present on the microarray was significantly less expressed in HepG2 compared with primary hepatocytes. The low CYP450 system functionality restricts the use of HepG2 cells to the evaluation of parent molecule toxicity and completely prevents them from anticipating the cellular effects of metabolites.

7.2.2.2 HepaRG

New cellular models have also been investigated to address the problem of low metabolic activity observed in HepG2 cells. Among them, the HepaRG cells, a human liver carcinoma line [55] that matures into a mix of hepatocyte- and biliary-like cells, appears to retain drug metabolism capacity and gene expression patterns of primary human hepatocytes without the interdonor variability or decrease in functions with time in culture characteristic of that model [56]. HepaRG cells originate from the liver tumor of a female patient suffering from hepatocarcinoma and are currently commercialized by Biopredic International (Saint-Gregoire, France).

HepaRG cells have a stable karyotype, a high proliferative capacity in growth phase, and have demonstrated consistency and reproducibility of results across experiments. After differentiation from low-density seeded cultures, the cells form typical colonies exhibiting a morphology similar to hepatocytes in primary culture with a dense cytoplasm, one or two nuclei, and bile canaliculus-like structures surrounded by flattened epithelial cells resembling cholangiocytes [55]. Jossé *et al.* showed that expression of transcripts encoding CYP1A2, 2B6, 3A4, and 2E1, as well as phase II enzymes, membrane transporters (OATP1 and BSEP), and nuclear receptors involved in the induction of metabolism, remained stable for up to 4 weeks [57]. Their study confirmed that the HepaRG cells were much more sensitive than HepG2 cells to the toxicity of aflatoxin B1 (AFB1), a prototypical hepatic toxicant requiring bioactivation by CYP3A4 [58], and that sensitivity was comparable to primary human hepatocytes. Similarly, HepaRG cells have been shown to undergo oxidative stress following exposure to chlorpromazine [59] and do generate reactive metabolites and toxicity following acetaminophen exposure [60]. Still, the absolute expression of liver-specific genes remains generally lower in HepaRG cells than in primary human hepatocytes and they represent the phenotype of a single donor and therefore cannot account for the diversity of metabolic pathways encountered in the general patient population [61].

The ability of HepG2, HepaRG, and primary human hepatocytes to predict drug-induced liver injury has been compared by exposing cells for 72 h to increasing concentrations of 21 reference compounds (16 hepatotoxic and 5 nonhepatotoxic) selected from prior publications [45]. The primary endpoint was cytotoxicity measured by electrical impedance, and dose–response curves were generated for all test articles. In that study, the three *in vitro* models showed a specificity of 100%, underscoring the low incidence of false-positive results afforded by cell culture systems. However, the ability to identify well-recognized hepatotoxic drugs remained well below the desirable range (>80%). Cryopreserved human hepatocytes provided the highest sensitivity, ranging from 31 to 44%, depending on donors, followed by the HepaRG cells (13%), and finally the HepG2 cells (6.3%). Indeed, these results contrasted with the clear demonstration of drug metabolism in the HepaRG cells and highlighted the fact that some metabolic capacity in cell lines does not necessarily guarantee a better detection of clinical hepatotoxicants [52].

7.2.3
Differentiated Pluripotent Stem Cells

An alternative to the limitations of the fresh primary hepatocytes and hepatoma cell lines incorporating the advantages of these two models could be provided in the near future by the commercial availability of stem cells. Like the hepatoma lines, stem cells provide a renewable source of human material and if differentiated back into a mature hepatocyte phenotype could provide large numbers of functionally equivalent liver cells unaffected by the genetic changes inherent to carcinogenesis. An *in vitro* model incorporating an infinite supply of human hepatocytes with well-differentiated characteristics would allow for more consistent and relevant results in responses to drug treatment and, since stem cells have been shown to maintain the original liver metabolism of their donor [62], could even incorporate genetic variations of the human population in the screening strategy. Two sources of stem cells are in evaluation today to fulfill these requirements: embryonic and induced pluripotent cells.

7.2.3.1 Embryonic Stem Cells

Human embryonic stem cells (hESCs) are derived from the inner cell mass of *in vitro* fertilization embryos at the blastocyst stage and have demonstrated the ability to differentiate into tissues of all three embryonic germ layers [63]. In addition, these pluripotent progenitors can proliferate indefinitely on a layer of feeder cells in their undifferentiated state.

Although hESCs have the ability to produce teratomas containing several types of differentiated cells in immunodeficient mice and start spontaneously evolving toward an endodermic phenotype in the absence of the feeder layer, homogeneous cellular differentiation to specific tissues has proven challenging. Several laboratories have, with some success, developed differentiation protocols to transform embryonic stem cells into hepatocyte-like cells by replicating the liver maturation process during fetal development [64]. Unfortunately, these differentiation methods produce highly heterogeneous cell populations and investigators were forced to incorporate the expression of fluorescent reporter genes under the control of liver-specific promoters to triage cells with hepatic functionalities. Using this technology and an embryoid body-based differentiation method, Duan *et al.* [65] confirmed the potential of hESCs to differentiate into mature parenchymal cells by demonstrating that purified differentiated hESCs express liver-specific genes at 30–85% of the fresh human hepatocyte values and exhibit liver-specific functions comparable to those of primary liver cells.

In 2008, Hay *et al.* highlighted the importance of the Wnt3a signaling for efficient differentiation to functional hepatic cells [66]. Wnt3a is a member of the Wnt pathway family of secreted glycoproteins thought to coordinate somitogenesis and mesoderm boundary determination during development [67]. They observed that Wnt3a could elicit a rapid and highly efficient cellular progression of the hESC toward hepatic endoderm and in synergy with another protein,

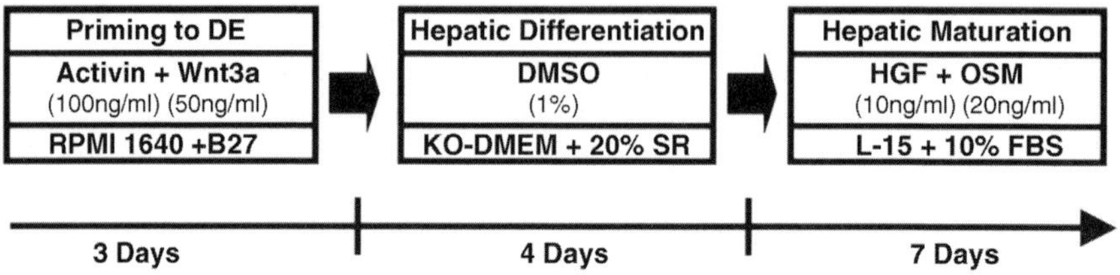

Figure 7.1 hESC differentiation protocol [66]. HGF, hepatocyte growth factor; OSM, oncostatin M.

activin A, produces a viable and predictable model of human hepatic differentiation *in vitro*. Their differentiation protocol is reproduced in Figure 7.1.

H9 embryonic stem cells differentiated using this method into hepatocyte-like cells (HLCs) were characterized for activity and inducibility of CYP3A4 and CYP1A2 and compared with primary hepatocytes for the prediction of hepatotoxicity [68]. The HLCs responded to phenobarbital induction by upregulating four- to fivefold the activity of CYP3A and CYP1A2 after 48 h of incubation. Primary human hepatocytes (*In Vitro* Technologies/BioreclamationIVT, Baltimore, MD) and HLCs were incubated for 1, 4, or 7 days with increasing concentrations of test articles before cell viability and apoptosis were assessed by cellular ATP content and caspase 3/7 activation. All compounds identified as hepatotoxic by the primary human hepatocyte assay were also recognized by the differentiated stem cells, but with a delay in the onset of toxicity. Two different mechanisms of cell death were evident in the study: caspase-dependent apoptosis (nine compounds) and caspase-independent necrosis (six compounds). Overall, the authors reported a sensitivity of 75%, and the drugs that were not predicted by either cell types (dacarbazine, diclofenac, felbamate, isoniazid, and valproic acid) showed either no change or an increase in cellular ATP, suggesting that direct cytotoxicity might not have been an appropriate measure of their cellular effects. Although this study clearly demonstrates the ability of differentiated human embryonic stem cells to perform in toxicology screening assays as well as the traditional primary human hepatocyte monolayer cultures, the application of ESCs in drug discovery is associated with ethical issues. Since the initial preparation requires the destruction of human embryos, hESCs are a controversial source of cells and this perception is not likely to change in the near future. Hence, efforts have been directed toward a different source of stem cells that could eliminate the ethical questions.

7.2.3.2 **Induced Pluripotent Stem Cells**

In 1962, Sir John Gurdon demonstrated in his seminal work on frog embryology that the differentiation of amphibian cells could be reversed to produce a complete clone of the original donor [69]. In showing that the differentiation process was not altering the cellular DNA and that each and every somatic cell in an organism still contained the genetic information sufficient for the formation of all other cell types, he heralded a scientific journey that led to the birth of Dolly the sheep [70] and finally in 2006 the demonstration that a few transcription factors could control the process of dedifferentiation in mammalian cells [71]. A full reprogramming of human somatic cells was achieved in 2007 and the now termed induced pluripotent stem cells (iPSCs) were shown to share the pluripotency and proliferative capabilities of embryonic stem cells. However, since iPSCs do not originate from human embryonic tissues, they are devoid of ethical controversy [72]. As an additional benefit, it appears possible to generate iPSCs from individual with demonstrated clinical phenotypes [62] through the use of non-integrating episomal vectors [73]. Access to such cells could potentially allow the modeling *in vitro* of the genetic diversity encountered in the patient population.

iPSC differentiation toward hepatocyte-like functions has been tried broadly using the methodology developed for embryonic cells. Sullivan *et al.* applied a modified version of the Wnt3a/activin A protocol to the differentiation of iPSCs and reported a differentiation efficiency of 70–90%. The iPSC-derived hepatocytes expressed several liver-specific genes, produced albumin and E-cadherin, and metabolized specific substrates via CYP3A4 and CYP1A2 [74]. Regrettably, expression levels of xenobiotic-metabolizing genes in iPSCs are still not equal to those found in cadaveric liver samples or freshly isolated primary hepatocytes [75] and the cells did not respond to cytochrome P450 induction by phenobarbital [76]. In that study, an attempt to investigate the use of differentiated iPSCs to predict the metabolism-mediated hepatic toxicity of two drug candidates showed that the lower intrinsic CYP450 activity undermined the sensitivity of the assay in comparison with genetically engineered cells (THLE5-B) or differentiated hESCs. At present, differences in the methods and efficiency of differentiation impact gene expression and metabolic activities of the cells. These differences and the absence of optimized culture conditions exclude for now the iPSCs from routine incorporation in toxicology assays for lead optimization [77]. Commercial suppliers have, however, started to address these concerns and recent refinements of the differentiation process have allowed the generation of iPSC-derived hepatocytes with improved cytochrome P450 enzyme activity (Enhanced hiPS-HEP^{TM}, Cellectis, Goteborg, Sweden). In particular, the activity of CYP3A, 1A, 2C9, and 2E1 is now similar to cryopreserved human primary hepatocytes after 20 h in culture. The activity of CYP2C19, 2D6, and 2B6 can be measured as well, although still at lower levels in the hiPSC-derived hepatocytes than the primary cells.[1)] These advances raise the possibility of standardized *in vitro* toxicology assays incorporating human pluripotent stem cells in the near future and support further research toward generating fully mature hepatocytes from individuals with diverse genetic background or DILI patients.

1) J. Edsbagge, Effective tools for the *in vitro* evaluation of chronic hepatotoxicity. Personal communication, 2014. Available at http://www.cellectis-bioresearch.com/cellular-models/admetox/hepatocytes.

7.3 Models to Mitigate Hepatocyte Dedifferentiation

Fresh primary hepatocytes and differentiated stem cells placed in monolayer cultures or suspensions undergo a rapid alteration of gene expression driving them toward a proliferative and apoptosis-resistant phenotype akin to hepatoma cell lines. Essential characteristics of the liver parenchymal cells, such as polarity, bile canalicular transport, and metabolic functions, disappear progressively as a result of profound intracellular signaling changes [78]. Since many of these functions are important contributors to the onset of drug-induced liver damage, models have been developed to correct or overcome these limitations.

7.3.1 Liver Slices

Liver slices have been used for decades to study the hepatic metabolism, toxicity, and efficacy of novel substances. Variability in the thickness of the slices and poor viability of the tissue preparations limited the early use of the technique, but the development of precision slicers in the 1980s enabled the production of reproducible and viable slices [79]. The modern protocol of precision-cut liver slices has been described in detail in a recent review [80]. The preparation and culture of quality liver slices require good technical expertise, but the source of hepatic tissue is of critical importance, as tissue quality directly impacts the viability of the slices during incubation. In animal experiments, the source and time of harvesting can be controlled, but human tissues require careful perfusion with organ preservation solutions and timely processing [81]. This requirement places even greater constraint on the technique than the limitations of primary human hepatocytes, and severely limits the wide application of precision-cut human liver slices in drug discovery.

Hepatic slices conserve the tissue architecture, contain all the cell types found in the liver lobule, show good correlation with *in vivo* metabolism, and maintain zone-specific cytochrome activity [82], allowing the investigation of cellular and zonal mechanisms of toxicity. A toxicogenomics study comparing several hepatic models in rats showed that the gene expression pattern of liver slices was closer to liver samples than cell lines and primary hepatocytes [83]. Various groups have confirmed that albumin production, neoglucogenesis, and phase I and phase II drug metabolism were retained in this model [84]. Drug metabolism and intrinsic clearance appear slower in precision-cut liver slices than in primary hepatocytes and investigators have proposed the existence of a chemical exposure gradient within the slice preventing some hepatocytes at the center from fully participating in the metabolism of compounds [9]. Proper oxygenation of all cells within the slice is critical for the maintenance of viability and metabolic functions [85,86]. Hence, the optimal thickness of a slice appears to be approximately 250 μm or 12–14 cell layers. In tissue slices more than 14 cell layers thick, the innermost cells become hypoxic and die [87]. Even with good oxygenation, necrosis appears after 48–72 h in culture and metabolic enzyme levels decrease over time. Therefore, despite the maintenance of the liver structure and cell–cell interactions, precision-cut liver slices from human tissues are difficult to prepare and use in routine toxicology studies. They remain a better tool for bridging animal and human metabolism and to investigate toxicity mechanisms dependent on the architecture of the liver lobule [88].

7.3.2 Selective Engineering of Metabolism

In the 1980s, carcinogenesis studies uncovered a process creating inside living cells by-products of otherwise harmless chemicals capable of covalently altering nucleic acids [89]. This mechanism called "bioactivation" was linked to the formation of electrophilic and/or free radical metabolites [90] by xenobiotic-metabolizing enzymes. Reactive metabolites cause toxicity by covalently altering important cellular proteins, inactivating critical biological pathways, and ultimately causing the loss of cell membrane integrity. Avoidance of this mechanism is now the norm in drug discovery.

The diverse hepatic enzyme systems involved in the detoxification and clearance of xenobiotics and the high concentration frequently achieved in the hepatic circulation by orally administered chemicals make the liver an important site of bioactivation. In particular, the reactivity of metabolic intermediates generated by the cytochrome P450 (CYP) enzyme superfamily has been associated with the formation of covalent adducts and liver lesions [11,91]. Unfortunately, marked qualitative and/or quantitative interspecies differences have been observed with the CYP450 enzymes, and even within the human population, genetic polymorphisms can affect expression levels or catalytic activity and result in clinically significant differences in drug metabolism [92]. Thus, hepatic toxicity associated with human-specific metabolism or a polymorphic absence of detoxification mechanisms is difficult to observe in preclinical studies.

Recapitulating *in vitro* human CYP450 hepatic metabolism in order to identify reactive or toxic intermediates is an important component of early candidate screening. Unfortunately, primary human hepatocytes in monolayer culture lose CYP450 enzyme activity quickly. Hepatoma cell lines lack most major phase I and phase II metabolizing enzymes [39,93] and are unable to either generate toxic metabolites or accurately reproduce the normal liver detoxification functions. To correct the very low expression of metabolizing enzymes in hepatic cell lines, several investigators have attempted to insert expression vectors containing human CYP450 gene sequences in immortalized hepatocytes [94,95]. Among those, the T-antigen–immortalized human liver epithelial (THLE) cell lines engineered by Dr. A. Pfeifer have been successfully applied to the prediction of metabolism-mediated toxicity in drug discovery [46,96].

The THLE parental cell line (THLE-5B cl5, ATCC CRL-11113) was created by immortalization of healthy adult human hepatocytes using recombinant SV40 T-antigen [97]. The cells were subsequently genetically engineered to express individual cytochrome P450 enzyme in each cell line under the transcriptional control of the cytomegalovirus promoter. This construct produces a high constitutive expression of the enzyme in the absence of induction signals [98]. Cell lines expressing CYP1A2, 2B6, 2C9, 2C19, 2D6, 2E1, and 3A4 are available for licensing from the Office of Technology Transfer at the National Institutes of Health (Rockville, MD). The THLE cell lines were used to develop a high-throughput assay to rapidly detect the hepatic toxicity of drug candidates and their CYP-generated metabolites [46]. This assay relies on differential evaluation of cytotoxicity in four cell lines expressing CYP 3A4, 2C9, 2C19, and 2D6 and the parental nonmetabolizing cell line (THLE-null) to provide an estimation of a compound's toxicity to liver hepatocytes following specific biotransformation pathways. The activity of the four selected CYPs is clinically important because together they account for the majority of small-molecule drug metabolism and patients have significant polymorphisms impacting their enzyme activities [99,100]. The functional expression of the respective P450 enzymes (or lack of in the parental line) has been verified by RT-PCR, Western blotting, and substrate metabolism assays [46,96]. Cells from each THLE line are incubated with serial concentrations of test articles for 24 h using a robotic system and mitochondrial activity is selected for measure of cell viability through the reduction of 3-(4,5-dimethylthiazol-2-yl)-5-(3-carboxymethoxyphenyl)-2-(4-sulfophenyl)-2*H*-tetrazolium (MTS).

Dambach *et al.* evaluated the predictivity of their assay by comparing the IC_{50} values in all five cell lines for 679 marketed pharmaceuticals with the occurrence of DILI in patients. The compounds were classified into "bins" according to clinical literature reports of hepatotoxicity as described in Table 7.3 [41,101]. Using a toxicity threshold of 50 μM, 585/587 nonhepatotoxic drugs (bin 3), 15/21 severely hepatotoxic drugs (bin 1), and 51/71 variably hepatotoxic drugs (bin 2) were appropriately classified, giving the assay a sensitivity of 66% and a specificity of 99%. The dose–response curves for each cell line were compared to identify routes of bioactivation and detoxification, and that information was included in a larger profiling paradigm incorporating results from ADME screens and primary hepatocytes to holistically assess the risk of hepatotoxicity in lead candidates.

Similarly, Gustafsson *et al.* extracted from the scientific literature hepatotoxicity reports for 104 marketed pharmaceuticals with and without liabilities. These compounds were assigned to one of the five categories of concern, with category 1 including drugs ($n = 24$) implicated in fatal liver failures resulting in either withdrawal or black box warnings and category 5 including drugs ($n = 13$) with no report of liver issues in patients [96]. The drugs were assayed using two cell lines, the THLE-null parental line and the THLE-3A4, to facilitate high-throughput screening. Using an IC_{50} of less than 200 μM as threshold of detection, 18 of the compounds in categories 1–3 were reported hepatotoxic, giving the assay a sensitivity of 23%. However, all but two of the drugs that demonstrated toxicity in one or both cell lines had been associated with DILI cases in the clinic, showing that the assay has a high (95%) specificity. Four drugs (cinchophen,

Table 7.3 Classification of validation compounds [101].

Bin 1: "severe hepatotoxic"	Clinical incidence of elevated[a)] liver function tests >1% (correspond to "frequent")	Report of at least two of the following: jaundice in some patients; documented 3+ cases of acute liver failure/fulminant hepatitis; serious hepatic liability reported (e.g., black box warning or withdrawal)
Bin 2: "moderate hepatotoxic"	Clinical incidence between 0.1 and 1% of elevated liver function tests (correspond to "infrequent")	One of the following: jaundice in some patients; anecdotal report (less than 3 cases) of drug-associated hepatitis; moderate hepatic liability reported (e.g., precaution in PDR)
Bin 3: "minimal or not hepatotoxic"	Clinical incidence of elevated liver function tests <0.1% (correspond to "rare")	When elevation of liver function tests is reported, it is not associated with clinical manifestations of liver injury or dysfunctions (e.g., bilirubin changes)

a) More than 3× upper limit of normal (ULN) values.

lumiracoxib, tolcapone, and glibenclamide) caused less toxicity in THLE-3A4 cells than in THLE-null cells, suggesting detoxification by CYP3A4, whereas 11 drugs exhibited bioactivation by CYP3A4. Engineered cells such as the THLE permit the development of assays employing panels of human hepatic cell lines with high levels of specific enzyme activity for the prediction of metabolism-mediated liver injury. Compounds with known DILI liabilities are detected with high specificity, showing that these assays are unlikely to prevent the progression of efficacious candidates by falsely labeling them as hepatotoxicants and can be deployed in early drug discovery. Since the assays only investigate one mechanism of toxicity, and only for the limited number of enzymes expressed in the included cell lines, the sensitivity for clinical DILI remains limited. To improve the representation of human metabolism, it might be tempting to include many more cell lines expressing additional enzymes. However, this extended coverage of human biotransformation routes has to be weighed against the increased technical challenge of maintaining assay performances as well as the increased cost per test article and the reduction in throughput. Recently, adenovirus vectors have been employed to introduce CYP target genes back into HepG2 cells. Since the virus efficiently infects hepatic cell lines and forces expression of the transgene in proportion to the number of infecting viral particles, this technology can be applied to the generation of cells transiently expressing several CYP450 in physiological proportions [102,103]. Such methods would provide a path toward the engineering of fully metabolizing cell lines with a ratio of enzyme activity closely simulating the human liver without the practical difficulties of testing at the same time multiple concentrations of many test articles on several cell lines.

Engineered cell lines produced by transient or stable expression of metabolizing enzymes are an effective and flexible tool to investigate metabolism-mediated toxicity during lead discovery. Within a given chemical series, these cells provide rapid and cost-effective methods to screen for compound bioactivation, investigate detoxification pathways, and model liver metabolism in populations of extensive or poor metabolizers. They only recapitulate one mechanism of toxicity, but as part of a larger optimization strategy can contribute to an early awareness of potential DILI issues and inform subsequent safety studies.

7.4 Understanding Immune-Mediated Hepatotoxicity

iDILI has traditionally been further divided into two categories: metabolic idiosyncrasy and immune idiosyncrasy [3]. In this categorization, metabolic idiosyncrasy refers to a susceptibility to hepatic toxicity based on individual differences in absorption, distribution, metabolism, and elimination (ADME) of the drug. Immune idiosyncrasy implies an active participation of the innate and/or adaptive immune system. At present, this distinction is more clinical than mechanistic. Drugs causing immune-mediated DILI are in general associated with fever, rash, and eosinophilia, and the symptoms of hepatic damage can be detected after a few weeks of dosing. Patients may present with antidrug antibodies or autoantibodies in the serum or demonstrate a proliferative response of blood monocytes to the drug [19]. On rechallenge, the return of liver toxicity is rapid and sometimes dangerous [2]. In contrast, metabolic idiosyncratic reactions can take several months to appear, lack the symptoms of hypersensitivity, and, on rechallenge, may not reproduce the hepatotoxicity at all [104].

There is a considerable amount of overlap between the two categories of idiosyncratic reactions, with drug metabolism suspected of providing the initiating events for an immune reaction, which in turn determine the extent of liver injury [105]. This concept can be summarized in the adaptation of the immunology "danger hypothesis" to idiosyncratic hepatotoxicity presented in Figure 7.2. The core concept is that the immune system is more likely to react against normal or modified liver proteins if it has been primed by some signal of "danger" in the organ. The formation of reactive metabolites and their covalent modification of intracellular macromolecules can in some cases provide both the hapten and the release of danger signals from the stressed cells. By itself, however, modification of intracellular proteins does not always equate to liver injury, as in the case of anesthesiologists exposed to halogenated anesthetics who frequently harbor antibodies directed against trifluoroacetylated liver proteins in the absence of hepatic damages. The "danger" priming the immune system may come from cellular damages caused by the drug or its metabolites, a concomitant infection or inflammatory condition such as viral or bacterial infections, some form of physical injury [106], or the direct activation of antigen-presenting cells (APCs) or T-cells by the drug itself [107]. The presentation of covalently

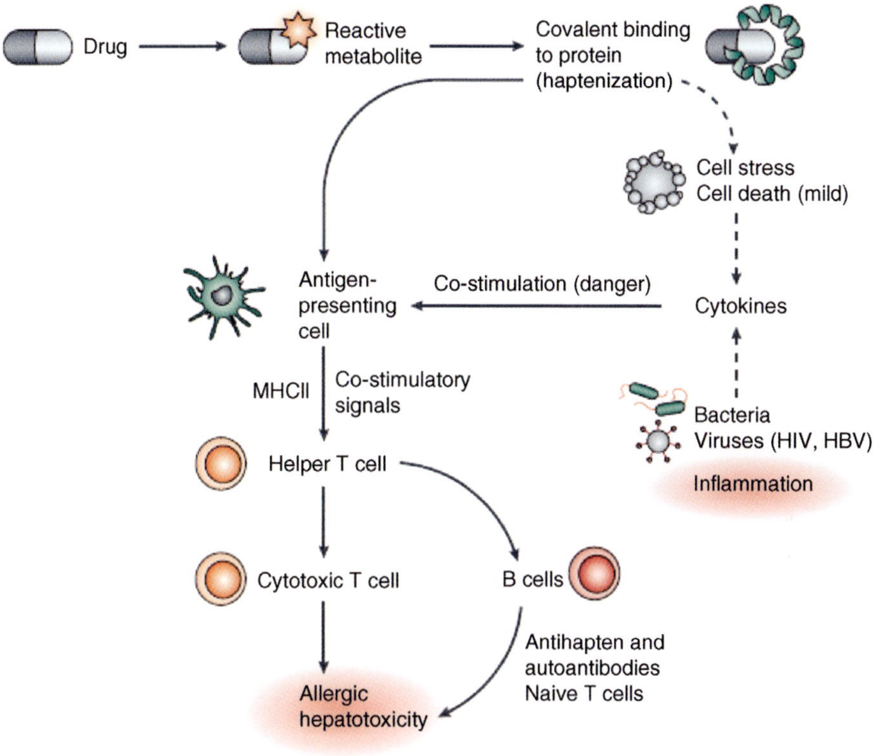

Figure 7.2 The "danger hypothesis" adapted for immune-mediated idiosyncratic hepatotoxicity [104].

altered or native liver proteins by APCs stimulated by the danger signals promotes helper T-cell activation and the targeting of cytotoxic T-cells and B-cell antibodies against the liver.

Accumulating evidence in the literature points toward the role that lymphocytes, macrophages, and neutrophils play in the balance of cell damages and regeneration during idiosyncratic DILI [105]. As our awareness of the importance of inflammation in drug-induced toxicity grew, attempts have been made to incorporate components of the innate and adaptive immune systems into *in vitro* assays for drug-induced liver injury. At this point, however, no extensive validation for liability screening in drug discovery appears to have been published.

7.4.1 Use of Inflammatory Cofactors

The demonstration that drugs associated with human idiosyncratic hepatotoxicity, such as chlorpromazine, ranitidine, diclofenac, or trovafloxacin, could produce liver injury in rodents when administered with an inflammatory stimulant, but not in isolation, focused interest on the role of cytokines in the origin and evolution of DILI [108–111]. These experiments also indicated that the lipopolysaccharide (LPS) treatment was operating in conjunction with some properties of the toxic compounds, as nontoxic drugs from identical therapeutic classes, such as famotidine or levofloxacin, did not produce hepatic injury under the same protocol [109,111]. LPS, a component of the outer membrane of Gram-negative bacteria, activates a variety of intracellular pathways through Toll-like receptors (TLRs) and causes the release of inflammation mediators from nonparenchymal cells [112]. LPS administration has been shown to upregulate plasma concentrations of the proinflammatory cytokines IL-1α, IL-1β, IL-6, INF-γ, and TNF-α, and this effect is specially marked in conjunction with the regeneration signals provided by partial hepatectomy [113].

These observations have been translated into a model of inflammatory cytokine-associated hepatotoxicity using primary hepatocytes or HepG2 cells [114]. By combining rat liver cells with the LPS-regulated cytokines IL-1α, IL-6, INF-γ, and TNF-α, the authors recapitulated the toxicity of ranitidine and trovafloxacin and the lack of toxicity of famotidine and levofloxacin. Combinations of drug/cytokine cocktails identified TNF-α as the most significant contributor to the enhanced toxicity, in agreement with its central role in the LPS-dependent toxicity of trovafloxacin *in vivo* [111,115]. The assay was then applied to the screening of a set of 90 compounds including 53 hepatotoxic drugs. Primary human hepatocytes in Matrigel sandwich culture were exposed to increasing concentrations of the test articles in the presence or absence of a cytokine mix containing IL-1α, IL-6, INF-γ, and TNF-α. Cytotoxicity was measured by lactate dehydrogenase (LDH) release into the culture medium at 24 h posttreatment. The authors observed increased cytotoxicity in the presence of cytokines for 8 of the 43 (19%) idiosyncratic toxicants and only 1 of the 36 (3%) nonhepatotoxic compounds, but only by limiting the dosing concentrations to no more than 100-fold the C_{max} reported in patients. Although they considered these concentration limits a better reflection of clinical exposure, it would be difficult to rely on a similar cutoff in lead optimization since human exposure projections are rarely available at this stage. The experiment was unable to ascertain whether hepatocyte death was initiated by the cytokines in response to drug-induced cellular stress or caused by the drugs themselves following cytokine-mediated sensitization, but it demonstrated that coexposure of idiosyncratic hepatotoxicants and inflammatory cytokines *in vitro* can lead to the synergistic amplification of the mild effects caused by each. This effect appears controlled by four key signaling pathways: Akt, p70 S6 kinase, MEK-ERK, and p38-HSP27, with the MEK-ERK and p38-HSP27 pathways contributing prodeath signaling [116].

This work suggests that proinflammatory conditions could be incorporated into standard hepatotoxicity screening assays with minimum difficulty and that addition may improve the identification of molecules prone to idiosyncratic DILI. It would, however, be important to investigate and validate with a larger set of compounds the specificity of such assay for fear of labeling as toxic and erroneously discarding valuable therapeutic candidates.

7.4.2 Innate Immune System and Inflammasome

The hepatic immune system displays a unique tolerance toward a wide variety of self- and non-self-antigens, likely related to the multiple biotransformation pathways present in the liver and its strong regenerative capacity [117]. In some cases, however, the innate immunity can switch from its normal permissive state toward a proinflammatory one, termed "sterile inflammation" in the absence of foreign pathogens. Sterile inflammation has been linked to a wide variety of hepatic pathologies, among them drug-induced liver injury [21].

In sterile inflammation, the hepatic innate immune system is activated by specific sets of chemical structures recognized as hallmarks of generic pathogen invasions and/or cellular damage. These small molecules, nucleic acids, and proteins are called pathogen-associated molecular patterns (PAMPs) when originating from microbes or viruses, and damage-associated molecular patterns (DAMPs) when released by necrotic cells. Examples of DAMPs are uric acid, high-mobility group protein B1 (HMGB-1), heat shock protein 70 (HSP70), or ATP [118,119]. PAMPs and DAMPs are recognized by an array of surface receptors termed pattern recognition receptors (PRRs) that include the TLRs activated by LPS [120]. Hence, the "danger" signal proposed in the hypothetical mechanism of immune-mediated DILI can now be related to the activation of the pattern recognition receptors. Receptors responsible for sensing DAMPs following tissue injury have been identified on the surface of many cells. Kupffer cells and dendritic cells have received the most attention, but other nonparenchymal cells including the sinusoid endothelium possess surface receptors and signaling pathways capable of initiating inflammation. TLR4 receptors on the surface of hepatocytes have been implicated in the mechanism of sterile liver inflammation following ischemia/reperfusion through production of reactive oxygen species and release of additional danger signals, including HMGB1 [21]. Upon activation, the pattern recognition receptor systems lead to the assembly of multiprotein complexes called inflammasomes [121], which serves as a platform for the activation of the proteolytic enzyme caspase-1. Two broad types of signals are required for full activation of the inflammasomes in most cells: signal 1 is provided by the Toll-like receptors, TLR4 in the case of DILI, and causes transcriptional upregulation of the inflammasome components and substrates such as pro-IL-1β and pro-IL-18. Signal 2 can be provided by a variety of extra- and intracellular sensor molecules such as the Nod-like receptors (NLRs), which trigger upon activation the binding of an adaptor protein called ASC [122]. The complex initiates pro-caspase-1 self-cleavage and the assembly of the active caspase-1. Caspase-1 then cleaves the pro-forms of the cytokines IL-1β and IL-18 to release their active forms, leading to the downstream production of TNF-α and INF-γ [123,124].

The identification of the cytosolic machinery termed the "inflammasome," which converts cellular stress signals (DAMPs) and/or bacterial endotoxin into the production of the proinflammatory cytokine, represents a significant progress in our understanding of the link between inflammation and liver damage. It provides supporting molecular evidence to the "danger hypothesis" model proposed as a mechanism for idiosyncratic DILI. Unfortunately, many elements of the pathophysiology are still poorly understood. The hepatic innate immune functions are performed by a variety of nonparenchymal lymphoid cells including Kupffer cells, natural killer (NK) cells, natural killer T (NKT) cells, and dendritic cells, with cooperation from the endothelium, stellate cells, and hepatocytes themselves. Despite extensive investigations *in vivo* and *in vitro* and clear evidence of innate and adaptive immunity playing a role in acetaminophen-induced hepatic toxicity, the delineation of damaging versus hepatoprotective functions for each of these cells remains controversial [125]. Nonetheless, it is clear that immunity and inflammation do play an important role in both intrinsic and idiosyncratic hepatotoxicity and that our understanding of the mechanisms governing tissue injury and regeneration will require the development of improved *in vitro* models closer to the liver architecture and physiology [28].

7.5 Conclusions

Hepatic toxicity, and in particular idiosyncratic drug-induced liver injury, remains a major concern for the pharmaceutical industry. It is pervasive among small-molecule therapeutics and even reported with some biologics [126]. iDILI detection is difficult in preclinical and clinical studies because of its dependence on rare combinations of drug- and patient-specific conditions to produce the most severe manifestations.

To prevent or minimize hepatotoxicity issues, new chemical entities are studied using *in vitro* models of the human liver in hope of recreating in the laboratory the conditions of clinical toxicity. Primary cultures of hepatocytes are currently the most validated and utilized models to investigate toxicity mechanisms, screen out undesirable compound characteristics, compare human and animal effects, and identify drug–drug interactions. Over the past 10 years, the availability of human tissue and the cryopreservation of hepatocytes have made such progress as to render these studies essentially routine in many pharmaceutical companies. The situation has created an unsustainable demand for human liver tissues, but the development of new methods to differentiate induced pluripotent stem cells into hepatocytes carries the promises of unlimited supply, low cost, reproducibility, and genetic diversity.

The limitation of cytotoxicity endpoints for the prediction of DILI has been demonstrated. DILI can be viewed as the common end result of multiple toxic pathways varying between drugs and patient conditions. Expecting cell cultures to recapitulate all possible routes leading to liver damage into a single common manifestation might be unrealistic. The key cellular mechanisms associated with DILI include CYP-mediated activation of toxicants to reactive metabolites, oxidative stress, mitochondrial injury, membrane transport inhibition, and activation of inflammatory pathways. They should at a minimum be in some way represented in a comprehensive assessment of hepatic toxicity potentials during lead optimization. Until the advance of automated digital microscopy allows the monitoring of all key toxicity mechanisms at the same time, the sequential application of progressively complex *in vitro* models might provide a cost-effective substitute. Using this strategy, an increasingly stringent decision algorithm can be applied to lead selection, with each successive assay providing additional weight of evidence toward the identification of molecules unlikely to cause human DILI. Such "kill-the-loser" approach permits binary decisions on the results of each assay independently and removes undesirable molecules from the candidate pool as early as possible in the optimization process.

Hepatic human cell lines engineered for stable or transient expression of drug-metabolizing enzymes are practical *in vitro* models for routine screening of metabolism-based toxicity in drug discovery. Although cells such as the THLE are designed to permanently overexpress a single enzyme and exhibit a skewed metabolism, they constitute useful tools to maximize toxic metabolite production, emphasize routes of bioactivation, and highlight metabolic "soft spots."

The discovery of damage-associated molecular patterns and inflammasomes began to unravel the molecular pathways linking metabolism and immunology in idiosyncratic DILI. Further progress may require more physiological models of liver lobules bringing together co-cultures of multiple cell types, complex three-dimensional structures, and microfluidics. Several international consortiums are currently working on improving the recognition and prediction of DILI. Among them, the European MIP-DILI [127] aims to further our understanding of the cellular causes of DILI and establish new *in vitro* models more predictive than traditional cell cultures.

References

1 Leise, M.D., Poterucha, J.J., and Talwalkar, J.A. (2014) Drug-induced liver injury. *Mayo Clinic Proceedings*, **89** (1), 95–106.

2 Senior, J.R. (2007) Drug hepatotoxicity from a regulatory perspective. *Clinics in Liver Disease*, **11** (3), 507–524.

3 Zimmerman, H. (1999) *Hepatotoxicity: The Adverse Effects of Drugs and Other Chemicals on the Liver*, 2nd edn, Lippincott Williams & Wilkins, Philadelphia, PA, p. 789.

4 Fontana, R.J. (2013) Pathogenesis of idiosyncratic drug-induced liver injury and clinical perspectives. *Gastroenterology*, **146** (4), 914–928.

5 Agnelli, G., Eriksson, B.I., Cohen, A.T., Bergqvist, D., Dahl, O.E., Lassen, M.R., Mouret, P., Rosencher, N., Andersson, M., Bylock, A., Jensen, E., and Boberg, B. (2009) Safety assessment of new antithrombotic agents: lessons from the EXTEND study on ximelagatran. *Thrombosis Research*, **123** (3), 488–497.

6 Mak, I.W., Evaniew, N., and Ghert, M. (2014) Lost in translation: animal models and clinical trials in cancer treatment. *American Journal of Translational Research*, **6** (2), 114–118.

7 Olson, H., Betton, G., Robinson, D., Thomas, K., Monro, A., Kolaja, G., Lilly, P., Sanders, J., Sipes, G., Bracken, W., Dorato, M., Van Deun, K., Smith, P.,

Berger, B., and Heller, H. (2000) Concordance of the toxicity of pharmaceuticals in humans and in animals. *Regulatory Toxicology and Pharmacology*, **32**, 56–67.

8 Lammert, C., Einarsson, S., Saha, C., Niklasson, A., Bjornsson, E., and Chalasani, N. (2008) Relationship between daily dose of oral medications and idiosyncratic drug-induced liver injury: search for signals. *Hepatology*, **47** (6), 2003–2009.

9 Soldatow, V.Y., Lecluyse, E.L., Griffith, L.G., and Rusyn, I. (2013) *In vitro* models for liver toxicity testing. *Toxicology Research (Cambridge)*, **2** (1), 23–39.

10 Chen, M., Borlak, J., and Tong, W. (2013) High lipophilicity and high daily dose of oral medications are associated with significant risk for drug-induced liver injury. *Hepatology*, **58** (1), 388–396.

11 Park, B.K., Kitteringham, N.R., Maggs, J.L., Pirmohamed, M., and Williams, D.P. (2005) The role of metabolic activation in drug-induced hepatotoxicity. *Annual Review of Pharmacology and Toxicology*, **45** (1), 177–202.

12 Pachkoria, K., Lucena, M.I., Molokhia, M., Cueto, R., Carballo, A.S., Carvajal, A., and Andrade, R.J. (2007) Genetic and molecular factors in drug-induced liver injury: a review. *Current Drug Safety*, **2** (2), 97–112.

13 Lee, W.M. (2003) Drug-induced hepatotoxicity. *The New England Journal of Medicine*, **349** (5), 474–485.

14 Stepan, A.F., Walker, D.P., Bauman, J., Price, D.A., Baillie, T.A., Kalgutkar, A.S., and Aleo, M.D. (2011) Structural alert/reactive metabolite concept as applied in medicinal chemistry to mitigate the risk of idiosyncratic drug toxicity: a perspective based on the critical examination of trends in the top 200 drugs marketed in the United States. *Chemical Research in Toxicology*, **24** (9), 1345–1410.

15 Thompson, R.A., Isin, E.M., Li, Y., Weaver, R., Weidolf, L., Wilson, I., Claesson, A., Page, K., Dolgos, H., and Kenna, J.G. (2011) Risk assessment and mitigation strategies for reactive metabolites in drug discovery and development. *Chemico-Biological Interactions*, **192** (1–2), 65–71.

16 Klaassen, C.D. and Aleksunes, L.M. (2010) Xenobiotic, bile acid, and cholesterol transporters: function and regulation. *Pharmacological Reviews*, **62** (1), 1–96.

17 Pedersen, J.M., Matsson, P., Bergström, C.A.S., Hoogstraate, J., Norén, A., LeCluyse, E.L., and Artursson, P. (2013) Early identification of clinically relevant drug interactions with the human bile salt export pump (BSEP/ABCB11). *Toxicological Sciences*, **136** (2), 328–343.

18 Rodrigues, A.D., Lai, Y., Cvijic, M.E., Elkin, L.L., Zvyaga, T., and Soars, M.G. (2014) Drug-induced perturbations of the bile acid pool, cholestasis, and hepatotoxicity: mechanistic considerations beyond the direct inhibition of the bile salt export pump. *Drug Metabolism and Disposition*, **42** (4), 566–574.

19 Liu, Z.-X. and Kaplowitz, N. (2002) Immune-mediated drug-induced liver disease. *Clinics in Liver Disease*, **6** (3), 755–774.

20 Dykens, J.A. and Will, Y. (2007) The significance of mitochondrial toxicity testing in drug development. *Drug Discovery Today*, **12** (17–18), 777–785.

21 Kubes, P. and Mehal, W.Z. (2012) Sterile inflammation in the liver. *Gastroenterology*, **143** (5), 1158–1172.

22 Friedman, S.L. (2008) Mechanisms of hepatic fibrogenesis. *Gastroenterology*, **134** (6), 1655–1669.

23 Kotecha, R.S., Buckland, A., Phillips, M.B., Cole, C.H., and Gottardo, N.G. (2014) Hepatic sinusoidal obstruction syndrome during chemotherapy for childhood medulloblastoma: report of a case and review of the literature. *Journal of Pediatric Hematology/Oncology*, **36** (1), 76–80.

24 MacGregor, J.T., Collins, J.M., Sugiyama, Y., Tyson, C.A., Dean, J., Smith, L., Andersen, M., Curren, R.D., Houston, J.B., Kadlubar, F.F., Kedderis, G.L., Krishnan, K., Li, A.P., Parchment, R.E., Thummel, K., Tomaszewski, J.E., Ulrich, R., Vickers, A.E., and Wrighton, S.A. (2001) *In vitro* human tissue models in

risk assessment: report of a consensus-building workshop. *Toxicological Sciences*, **59** (1), 17–36.

25 Kmieć, Z. (2001) Cooperation of liver cells in health and disease. *Advances in Anatomy, Embryology and Cell Biology*, **161**, III–XIII, 1–151.

26 Rappaport, A.M. (1977) Microcirculatory units in the mammalian liver. Their arterial and portal components. *Bibliotheca Anatomica*, **16** (Part 2), 116–120.

27 Katz, N.R. (1992) Metabolic heterogeneity of hepatocytes across the liver acinus. *The Journal of Nutrition*, **122** (3 Suppl.), 843–849.

28 LeCluyse, E.L., Witek, R.P., Andersen, M.E., and Powers, M.J. (2012) Organotypic liver culture models: meeting current challenges in toxicity testing. *Critical Reviews in Toxicology*, **42** (6), 501–548.

29 Treyer, A. and Müsch, A. (2013) Hepatocyte polarity. *Comprehensive Physiology*, **3** (1), 243–287.

30 Soars, M.G., McGinnity, D.F., Grime, K., and Riley, R.J. (2007) The pivotal role of hepatocytes in drug discovery. *Chemico-Biological Interactions*, **168** (1), 2–15.

31 Gómez-Lechón, M.J., Donato, M.T., Castell, J.V., and Jover, R. (2004) Human hepatocytes in primary culture: the choice to investigate drug metabolism in man. *Current Drug Metabolism*, **5** (5), 443–462.

32 Blouin, A., Bolender, R.P., and Weibel, E.R. (1977) Distribution of organelles and membranes between hepatocytes and nonhepatocytes in the rat liver parenchyma: a stereological study. *The Journal of Cell Biology*, **72** (2), 441–455.

33 Li, A.P. (2007) Human hepatocytes: isolation, cryopreservation and applications in drug development. *Chemico-Biological Interactions*, **168** (1), 16–29.

34 Loretz, L.J., Li, A.P., Flye, M.W., and Wilson, A.G. (1989) Optimization of cryopreservation procedures for rat and human hepatocytes. *Xenobiotica*, **19** (5), 489–498.

35 Li, A.P. (1999) Overview: hepatocytes and cryopreservation – a personal historical perspective. *Chemico-Biological Interactions*, **121** (1), 1–5.

36 Griffin, S.J. and Houston, J.B. (2005) Prediction of *in vitro* intrinsic clearance from hepatocytes: comparison of suspensions and monolayer cultures. *Drug Metabolism and Disposition*, **33** (1), 115–120.

37 Elaut, G., Henkens, T., Papeleu, P., Snykers, S., Vinken, M., Vanhaecke, T., and Rogiers, V. (2006) Molecular mechanisms underlying the dedifferentiation process of isolated hepatocytes and their cultures. *Current Drug Metabolism*, **7** (6), 629–660.

38 Rowe, C., Goldring, C.E.P., Kitteringham, N.R., Jenkins, R.E., Lane, B.S., Sanderson, C., Elliott, V., Platt, V., Metcalfe, P., and Park, B.K. (2010) Network analysis of primary hepatocyte dedifferentiation using a shotgun proteomics approach. *Journal of Proteome Research*, **9** (5), 2658–2668.

39 Rodríguez-Antona, C., Donato, M.T., Boobis, A., Edwards, R.J., Watts, P.S., Castell, J.V., and Gómez-Lechón, M.-J. (2002) Cytochrome P450 expression in human hepatocytes and hepatoma cell lines: molecular mechanisms that determine lower expression in cultured cells. *Xenobiotica*, **32** (6), 505–520.

40 Godoy, P., Hewitt, N.J., Albrecht, U., Andersen, M.E., Ansari, N., Bhattacharya, S., Bode, J.G., Bolleyn, J., Borner, C., Böttger, J., Braeuning, A., Budinsky, R.A., Burkhardt, B., Cameron, N.R., Camussi, G., Cho, C.-S., Choi, Y.-J., Rowlands, J.C., Dahmen, U., Damm, G., Dirsch, O., Donato, M.T., Dong, J., Dooley, S., Drasdo, D., Eakins, R., Ferreira, K.S., Fonsato, V., Fraczek, J., Gebhardt, R., Gibson, A., Glanemann, M., Goldring, C.E.P., Gómez-Lechón, M.J., Groothuis, G.M.M., Gustavsson, L., Guyot, C., Hallifax, D., Hammad, S., Hayward, A., Häussinger, D., Hellerbrand, C., Hewitt, P., Hoehme, S., Holzhütter, H.-G., Houston, J.B., Hrach, J., Ito, K., Jaeschke, H., Keitel, V., Kelm, J.M., Park, B.K., Kordes, C., Kullak-Ublick, G.A., LeCluyse, E.L., Lu, P., Luebke-Wheeler, J., Lutz, A., Maltman, D.J., Matz-Soja, M., McMullen, P., Merfort, I., Messner, S.,

Meyer, C., Mwinyi, J., Naisbitt, D.J., Nussler, A.K., Olinga, P., Pampaloni, F., Pi, J., Pluta, L., Przyborski, S.A., Ramachandran, A., Rogiers, V., Rowe, C., Schelcher, C., Schmich, K., Schwarz, M., Singh, B., Stelzer, E.H.K., Stieger, B., Stöber, R., Sugiyama, Y., Tetta, C., Thasler, W.E., Vanhaecke, T., Vinken, M., Weiss, T.S., Widera, A., Woods, C.G., Xu, J.J., Yarborough, K.M., and Hengstler, J.G. (2013) Recent advances in 2D and 3D *in vitro* systems using primary hepatocytes, alternative hepatocyte sources and non-parenchymal liver cells and their use in investigating mechanisms of hepatotoxicity, cell signaling and ADME. *Archives of Toxicology*, **87** (8), 1315–1530.

41 Xu, J.J., Diaz, D., and O'Brien, P.J. (2004) Applications of cytotoxicity assays and pre-lethal mechanistic assays for assessment of human hepatotoxicity potential. *Chemico-Biological Interactions*, **150** (1), 115–128.

42 McKim, J.M. (2010) Building a tiered approach to *in vitro* predictive toxicity screening: a focus on assays with *in vivo* relevance. *Combinatorial Chemistry & High Throughput Screening*, **13** (2), 188–206.

43 Greer, M.L., Barber, J., Eakins, J., and Kenna, J.G. (2010) Cell based approaches for evaluation of drug-induced liver injury. *Toxicology*, **268** (3), 125–131.

44 Xu, J.J., Diaz, D., and O'Brien, P.J. (2004) Applications of cytotoxicity assays and pre-lethal mechanistic assays for assessment of human hepatotoxicity potential. *Chemico-Biological Interactions*, **150**, 115–128.

45 O'Brien, P.J., Irwin, W., Diaz, D., Howard-Cofield, E., Krejsa, C.M., Slaughter, M.R., Gao, B., Kaludercic, N., Angeline, A., Bernardi, P., Brain, P., and Hougham, C. (2006) High concordance of drug-induced human hepatotoxicity with *in vitro* cytotoxicity measured in a novel cell-based model using high content screening. *Archives of Toxicology*, **80** (9), 580–604.

46 Dambach, D.M., Andrews, B.A., and Moulin, F. (2005) New technologies and screening strategies for hepatotoxicity: use of *in vitro* models. *Toxicologic Pathology*, **33** (1), 17–26.

47 Thum, T. and Borlak, J. (2008) Detection of early signals of hepatotoxicity by gene expression profiling studies with cultures of metabolically competent human hepatocytes. *Archives of Toxicology*, **82** (2), 89–101.

48 Vass, L., Kelemen, J.Z., Fehér, L.Z., Lorincz, Z., Kulin, S., Cseh, S., Dormán, G., and Puskás, L.G. (2009) Toxicogenomics screening of small molecules using high-density, nanocapillary real-time PCR. *International Journal of Molecular Medicine*, **23** (1), 65–74.

49 Skett, P. (1994) Problems in using isolated and cultured hepatocytes for xenobiotic metabolism/metabolism-based toxicity testing – solutions? *Toxicology In Vitro*, **8** (3), 491–504.

50 Donato, M.T., Lahoz, A., Castell, J.V., and Gómez-Lechón, M.J. (2008) Cell lines: a tool for *in vitro* drug metabolism studies. *Current Drug Metabolism*, **9** (1), 1–11.

51 Kelly, J.H. and Darlington, G.J. (1989) Modulation of the liver specific phenotype in the human hepatoblastoma line Hep G2. *In Vitro Cellular & Developmental Biology*, **25** (2), 217–222.

52 Gerets, H.H.J., Tilmant, K., Gerin, B., Chanteux, H., Depelchin, B.O., Dhalluin, S., and Atienzar, F.A. (2012) Characterization of primary human hepatocytes, HepG2 cells, and HepaRG cells at the mRNA level and CYP activity in response to inducers and their predictivity for the detection of human hepatotoxins. *Cell Biology and Toxicology*, **28** (2), 69–87.

53 Gerets, H.H.J., Hanon, E., Cornet, M., Dhalluin, S., Depelchin, O., Canning, M., and Atienzar, F.A. (2009) Selection of cytotoxicity markers for the screening of new chemical entities in a pharmaceutical context: a preliminary study using a multiplexing approach. *Toxicology In Vitro*, **23** (2), 319–332.

54 Flynn, T.J. and Ferguson, M.S. (2008) Multiendpoint mechanistic profiling of hepatotoxicants in HepG2/C3A human hepatoma cells and novel statistical approaches for development of a

prediction model for acute hepatotoxicity. *Toxicology In Vitro*, **22** (6), 1618–1631.
55 Gripon, P., Rumin, S., Urban, S., Le Seyec, J., Glaise, D., Cannie, I., Guyomard, C., Lucas, J., Trepo, C., and Guguen-Guillouzo, C. (2002) Infection of a human hepatoma cell line by hepatitis B virus. *Proceedings of the National Academy of Sciences of the United States of America*, **99** (24), 15655–15660.
56 Lambert, C.B., Spire, C., Claude, N., and Guillouzo, A. (2009) Dose- and time-dependent effects of phenobarbital on gene expression profiling in human hepatoma HepaRG cells. *Toxicology and Applied Pharmacology*, **234** (3), 345–360.
57 Jossé, R., Aninat, C., Glaise, D., Dumont, J., Fessard, V., Morel, F., Poul, J.-M., Guguen-Guillouzo, C., and Guillouzo, A. (2008) Long-term functional stability of human HepaRG hepatocytes and use for chronic toxicity and genotoxicity studies. *Drug Metabolism and Disposition*, **36** (6), 1111–1118.
58 Guengerich, F.P., Johnson, W.W., Shimada, T., Ueng, Y.F., Yamazaki, H., and Langouët, S. (1998) Activation and detoxication of aflatoxin B1. *Mutation Research*, **402** (1–2), 121–128.
59 Anthérieu, S., Bachour-El Azzi, P., Dumont, J., Abdel-Razzak, Z., Guguen-Guillouzo, C., Fromenty, B., Robin, M.-A., and Guillouzo, A. (2013) Oxidative stress plays a major role in chlorpromazine-induced cholestasis in human HepaRG cells. *Hepatology*, **57** (4), 1518–1529.
60 McGill, M.R., Yan, H.-M., Ramachandran, A., Murray, G.J., Rollins, D.E., and Jaeschke, H. (2011) HepaRG cells: a human model to study mechanisms of acetaminophen hepatotoxicity. *Hepatology*, **53** (3), 974–982.
61 Rogue, A., Lambert, C., Spire, C., Claude, N., and Guillouzo, A. (2012) Interindividual variability in gene expression profiles in human hepatocytes and comparison with HepaRG cells. *Drug Metabolism and Disposition*, **40** (1), 151–158.
62 Rashid, S.T., Corbineau, S., Hannan, N., Marciniak, S.J., Miranda, E., Alexander, G., Huang-Doran, I., Griffin, J., Ahrlund-Richter, L., Skepper, J., Semple, R., Weber, A., Lomas, D.A., and Vallier, L. (2010) Modeling inherited metabolic disorders of the liver using human induced pluripotent stem cells. *The Journal of Clinical Investigation*, **120** (9), 3127–3136.
63 Thomson, J.A. (1998) Embryonic stem cell lines derived from human blastocysts. *Science*, **282** (5391), 1145–1147.
64 Baxter, M.A., Rowe, C., Alder, J., Harrison, S., Hanley, K.P., Park, B.K., Kitteringham, N.R., Goldring, C.E., and Hanley, N.A. (2010) Generating hepatic cell lineages from pluripotent stem cells for drug toxicity screening. *Stem Cell Research*, **5** (1), 4–22.
65 Duan, Y., Catana, A., Meng, Y., Yamamoto, N., He, S., Gupta, S., Gambhir, S.S., and Zern, M.A. (2007) Differentiation and enrichment of hepatocyte-like cells from human embryonic stem cells *in vitro* and *in vivo*. *Stem Cells*, **25** (12), 3058–3068.
66 Hay, D.C., Fletcher, J., Payne, C., Terrace, J.D., Gallagher, R.C.J., Snoeys, J., Black, J.R., Wojtacha, D., Samuel, K., Hannoun, Z., Pryde, A., Filippi, C., Currie, I.S., Forbes, S.J., Ross, J.A., Newsome, P.N., and Iredale, J.P. (2008) Highly efficient differentiation of hESCs to functional hepatic endoderm requires activin A and Wnt3a signaling. *Proceedings of the National Academy of Sciences of the United States of America*, **105** (34), 12301–12306.
67 Saito-Diaz, K., Chen, T.W., Wang, X., Thorne, C.A., Wallace, H.A., Page-McCaw, A., and Lee, E. (2013) The way Wnt works: components and mechanism. *Growth Factors*, **31** (1), 1–31.
68 Szkolnicka, D., Farnworth, S.L., Lucendo-Villarin, B., Storck, C., Zhou, W., Iredale, J.P., Flint, O., and Hay, D.C. (2014) Accurate prediction of drug-induced liver injury using stem cell-derived populations. *Stem Cells Translational Medicine*, **3** (2), 141–148.
69 Gurdon, J.B. (1962) The developmental capacity of nuclei taken from intestinal

epithelium cells of feeding tadpoles. *Journal of Embryology and Experimental Morphology*, **10**, 622–640.

70 Wilmut, I., Schnieke, A.E., McWhir, J., Kind, A.J., and Campbell, K.H. (1997) Viable offspring derived from fetal and adult mammalian cells. *Nature*, **385** (6619), 810–813.

71 Takahashi, K. and Yamanaka, S. (2006) Induction of pluripotent stem cells from mouse embryonic and adult fibroblast cultures by defined factors. *Cell*, **126** (4), 663–676.

72 Zhao, J., Jiang, W., Sun, C., Hou, C., Yang, X.-M., and Gao, J. (2013) Induced pluripotent stem cells: origins, applications, and future perspectives. *Journal of Zhejiang University Science B*, **14** (12), 1059–1069.

73 Chou, B.-K., Mali, P., Huang, X., Ye, Z., Dowey, S.N., Resar, L.M., Zou, C., Zhang, Y.A., Tong, J., and Cheng, L. (2011) Efficient human iPS cell derivation by a non-integrating plasmid from blood cells with unique epigenetic and gene expression signatures. *Cell Research*, **21** (3), 518–529.

74 Sullivan, G.J., Hay, D.C., Park, I.-H., Fletcher, J., Hannoun, Z., Payne, C.M., Dalgetty, D., Black, J.R., Ross, J.A., Samuel, K., Wang, G., Daley, G.Q., Lee, J.-H., Church, G.M., Forbes, S.J., Iredale, J.P., and Wilmut, I. (2010) Generation of functional human hepatic endoderm from human induced pluripotent stem cells. *Hepatology*, **51** (1), 329–335.

75 Si-Tayeb, K., Noto, F.K., Nagaoka, M., Li, J., Battle, M.A., Duris, C., North, P.E., Dalton, S., and Duncan, S.A. (2010) Highly efficient generation of human hepatocyte-like cells from induced pluripotent stem cells. *Hepatology*, **51** (1), 297–305.

76 Medine, C.N., Lucendo-Villarin, B., Storck, C., Wang, F., Szkolnicka, D., Khan, F., Pernagallo, S., Black, J.R., Marriage, H.M., Ross, J.A., Bradley, M., Iredale, J.P., Flint, O., and Hay, D.C. (2013) Developing high-fidelity hepatotoxicity models from pluripotent stem cells. *Stem Cells Translational Medicine*, **2** (7), 505–509.

77 Chen, M., Bisgin, H., Tong, L., Hong, H., Fang, H., Borlak, J., and Tong, W. (2014) Toward predictive models for drug-induced liver injury in humans: are we there yet? *Biomarkers in Medicine*, **8** (2), 201–213.

78 Godoy, P., Hengstler, J.G., Ilkavets, I., Meyer, C., Bachmann, A., Müller, A., Tuschl, G., Mueller, S.O., and Dooley, S. (2009) Extracellular matrix modulates sensitivity of hepatocytes to fibroblastoid dedifferentiation and transforming growth factor beta-induced apoptosis. *Hepatology*, **49** (6), 2031–2043.

79 Smith, P.F., Gandolfi, A.J., Krumdieck, C.L., Putnam, C.W., Zukoski, C.F., Davis, W.M., and Brendel, K. (1985) Dynamic organ culture of precision liver slices for *in vitro* toxicology. *Life Sciences*, **36** (14), 1367–1375.

80 de Graaf, I.A.M., Olinga, P., de Jager, M.H., Merema, M.T., de Kanter, R., van de Kerkhof, E.G., and Groothuis, G.M.M. (2010) Preparation and incubation of precision-cut liver and intestinal slices for application in drug metabolism and toxicity studies. *Nature Protocols*, **5** (9), 1540–1551.

81 Olinga, P., Merema, M., Hof, I.H., de Jong, K.P., Slooff, M.J., Meijer, D.K., and Groothuis, G.M. (1998) Effect of human liver source on the functionality of isolated hepatocytes and liver slices. *Drug Metabolism and Disposition*, **26** (1), 5–11.

82 Heinonen, J.T., Sidhu, J.S., Reilly, M.T., Farin, F.M., Omiecinski, C.J., Eaton, D.L., and Kavanagh, T.J. (1996) Assessment of regional cytochrome P450 activities in rat liver slices using resorufin substrates and fluorescence confocal laser cytometry. *Environmental Health Perspectives*, **104** (5), 536–543.

83 Boess, F., Kamber, M., Romer, S., Gasser, R., Muller, D., Albertini, S., and Suter, L. (2003) Gene expression in two hepatic cell lines, cultured primary hepatocytes, and liver slices compared to the *in vivo* liver gene expression in rats: possible implications for toxicogenomics use of *in vitro* systems. *Toxicological Sciences*, **73** (2), 386–402.

84 Lake, B.G. and Price, R.J. (2013) Evaluation of the metabolism and hepatotoxicity of xenobiotics utilizing precision-cut slices. *Xenobiotica*, **43** (1), 41–53.

85 Drobner, C., Glöckner, R., and Müller, D. (2000) Optimal oxygen tension conditions for viability and functioning of precision-cut liver slices. *Experimental and Toxicologic Pathology*, **52** (4), 335–338.

86 Toutain, H.J., Moronvalle-Halley, V., Sarsat, J.P., Chelin, C., Hoet, D., and Leroy, D. (1998) Morphological and functional integrity of precision-cut rat liver slices in rotating organ culture and multiwell plate culture: effects of oxygen tension. *Cell Biology and Toxicology*, **14** (3), 175–190.

87 Catania, J.M., Pershing, A.M., and Gandolfi, A.J. (2007) Precision-cut tissue chips as an *in vitro* toxicology system. *Toxicology In Vitro*, **21** (5), 956–961.

88 Neyrinck, A.M., Gomez, C., and Delzenne, N.M. (2004) Precision-cut liver slices in culture as a tool to assess the physiological involvement of Kupffer cells in hepatic metabolism. *Comparative Hepatology*, **3** (Suppl. 1), S45.

89 Miller, J.A. and Miller, E.C. (1983) The metabolic activation and nucleic acid adducts of naturally-occurring carcinogens: recent results with ethyl carbamate and the spice flavors safrole and estragole. *British Journal of Cancer*, **48** (1), 1–15.

90 Miller, E.C. and Miller, J.A. (1981) Reactive metabolites as key intermediates in pharmacologic and toxicologic responses: examples from chemical carcinogenesis. *Advances in Experimental Medicine and Biology*, **136** (Part A), 1–21.

91 Ioannides, C. and Lewis, D.F. (2004) Cytochromes P450 in the bioactivation of chemicals. *Current Topics in Medicinal Chemistry*, **4** (16), 1767–1788.

92 Evans, W.E. and Relling, M.V. (1999) Pharmacogenomics: translating functional genomics into rational therapeutics. *Science*, **286** (5439), 487–491.

93 Wilkening, S., Stahl, F., and Bader, A. (2003) Comparison of primary human hepatocytes and hepatoma cell line HepG2 with regard to their biotransformation properties. *Drug Metabolism and Disposition*, **31** (8), 1035–1042.

94 Sawada, M. and Kamataki, T. (1998) Genetically engineered cells stably expressing cytochrome P450 and their application to mutagen assays. *Mutation Research*, **411** (1), 19–43.

95 Crespi, C.L. and Miller, V.P. (1999) The use of heterologously expressed drug metabolizing enzymes – state of the art and prospects for the future. *Pharmacology & Therapeutics*, **84** (2), 121–131.

96 Gustafsson, F., Foster, A.J., Sarda, S., Bridgland-Taylor, M.H., and Kenna, J.G. (2014) A correlation between the *in vitro* drug toxicity of drugs to cell lines that express human P450s and their propensity to cause liver injury in humans. *Toxicological Sciences*, **137** (1), 189–211.

97 Pfeifer, A.M., Cole, K.E., Smoot, D.T., Weston, A., Groopman, J.D., Shields, P.G., Vignaud, J.M., Juillerat, M., Lipsky, M.M., and Trump, B.F. (1993) Simian virus 40 large tumor antigen-immortalized normal human liver epithelial cells express hepatocyte characteristics and metabolize chemical carcinogens. *Proceedings of the National Academy of Sciences of the United States of America*, **90** (11), 5123–5127.

98 Macé, K., Aguilar, F., Wang, J.S., Vautravers, P., Gómez-Lechón, M., Gonzalez, F.J., Groopman, J., Harris, C.C., and Pfeifer, A.M. (1997) Aflatoxin B1-induced DNA adduct formation and p53 mutations in CYP450-expressing human liver cell lines. *Carcinogenesis*, **18** (7), 1291–1297.

99 Rendic, S. and Di Carlo, F.J. (1997) Human cytochrome P450 enzymes: a status report summarizing their reactions, substrates, inducers, and inhibitors. *Drug Metabolism Reviews*, **29** (1–2), 413–580.

100 Watkins, P.B. (1990) Role of cytochromes P450 in drug metabolism and

hepatotoxicity. *Seminars in Liver Disease*, **10** (4), 235–250.

101 Andrews, B.A., Chen, S.-J., Zhu, M., Moulin, F.J.-M., and Flint, O.P. (2003) Evaluation of cytochrome P450-mediated hepatotoxicity using a high throughput robotic system. *Drug Metabolism Reviews*, **35**, 413.

102 Tolosa, L., Donato, M.T., Pérez-Cataldo, G., Castell, J.V., and Gómez-Lechón, M.J. (2012) Upgrading cytochrome P450 activity in HepG2 cells co-transfected with adenoviral vectors for drug hepatotoxicity assessment. *Toxicology In Vitro*, **26** (8), 1272–1277.

103 Tolosa, L., Gómez-Lechón, M.J., Pérez-Cataldo, G., Castell, J.V., and Donato, M.T. (2013) HepG2 cells simultaneously expressing five P450 enzymes for the screening of hepatotoxicity: identification of bioactivable drugs and the potential mechanism of toxicity involved. *Archives of Toxicology*, **87** (6), 1115–1127.

104 Kaplowitz, N. (2005) Idiosyncratic drug hepatotoxicity. *Nature Reviews. Drug Discovery*, **4** (6), 489–499.

105 Adams, D.H., Ju, C., Ramaiah, S.K., Uetrecht, J., and Jaeschke, H. (2010) Mechanisms of immune-mediated liver injury. *Toxicological Sciences*, **115** (2), 307–321.

106 Zhang, X., Zhang, X., Liu, F., Chen, X., Zhu, X., and Uetrecht, J. (2011) Involvement of the immune system in idiosyncratic drug reactions. *Drug Metabolism and Pharmacokinetics*, **26** (1), 47–59.

107 Pichler, W.J., Beeler, A., Keller, M., Lerch, M., Posadas, S., Schmid, D., Spanou, Z., Zawodniak, A., and Gerber, B. (2006) Pharmacological interaction of drugs with immune receptors: the p-i concept. *Allergology International*, **55** (1), 17–25.

108 Buchweitz, J.P., Ganey, P.E., Bursian, S.J., and Roth, R.A. (2002) Underlying endotoxemia augments toxic responses to chlorpromazine: is there a relationship to drug idiosyncrasy? *The Journal of Pharmacology and Experimental Therapeutics*, **300** (2), 460–467.

109 Luyendyk, J.P., Maddox, J.F., Cosma, G.N., Ganey, P.E., Cockerell, G.L., and Roth, R.A. (2003) Ranitidine treatment during a modest inflammatory response precipitates idiosyncrasy-like liver injury in rats. *The Journal of Pharmacology and Experimental Therapeutics*, **307** (1), 9–16.

110 Deng, X., Stachlewitz, R.F., Liguori, M.J., Blomme, E.A.G., Waring, J.F., Luyendyk, J.P., Maddox, J.F., Ganey, P.E., and Roth, R.A. (2006) Modest inflammation enhances diclofenac hepatotoxicity in rats: role of neutrophils and bacterial translocation. *The Journal of Pharmacology and Experimental Therapeutics*, **319** (3), 1191–1199.

111 Shaw, P.J., Hopfensperger, M.J., Ganey, P.E., and Roth, R.A. (2007) Lipopolysaccharide and trovafloxacin coexposure in mice causes idiosyncrasy-like liver injury dependent on tumor necrosis factor-alpha. *Toxicological Sciences*, **100** (1), 259–266.

112 Roth, R.A. and Ganey, P.E. (2010) Intrinsic versus idiosyncratic drug-induced hepatotoxicity – two villains or one? *The Journal of Pharmacology and Experimental Therapeutics*, **332** (3), 692–697.

113 Bergheim, I., Luyendyk, J.P., Steele, C., Russell, G.K., Guo, L., Roth, R.A., and Arteel, G.E. (2006) Metformin prevents endotoxin-induced liver injury after partial hepatectomy. *The Journal of Pharmacology and Experimental Therapeutics*, **316** (3), 1053–1061.

114 Cosgrove, B.D., King, B.M., Hasan, M.A., Alexopoulos, L.G., Farazi, P.A., Hendriks, B.S., Griffith, L.G., Sorger, P.K., Tidor, B., Xu, J.J., and Lauffenburger, D.A. (2009) Synergistic drug–cytokine induction of hepatocellular death as an *in vitro* approach for the study of inflammation-associated idiosyncratic drug hepatotoxicity. *Toxicology and Applied Pharmacology*, **237** (3), 317–330.

115 Liguori, M.J., Ditewig, A.C., Maddox, J.F., Luyendyk, J.P., Lehman-McKeeman, L.D., Nelson, D.M., Bhaskaran, V.M., Waring, J.F., Ganey, P.E., Roth, R.A., and Blomme, E.A.G. (2010) Comparison of TNFα to lipopolysaccharide as an inflammagen to

characterize the idiosyncratic hepatotoxicity potential of drugs: trovafloxacin as an example. *International Journal of Molecular Sciences*, **11** (11), 4697–4714.

116 Cosgrove, B.D., Alexopoulos, L.G., Hang, T., Hendriks, B.S., Sorger, P.K., Griffith, L.G., and Lauffenburger, D.A. (2010) Cytokine-associated drug toxicity in human hepatocytes is associated with signaling network dysregulation. *Molecular BioSystems*, **6** (7), 1195–1206.

117 Tiegs, G. and Lohse, A.W. (2010) Immune tolerance: what is unique about the liver. *Journal of Autoimmunity*, **34** (1), 1–6.

118 Cauwels, A., Rogge, E., Vandendriessche, B., Shiva, S., and Brouckaert, P. (2014) Extracellular ATP drives systemic inflammation, tissue damage and mortality. *Cell Death and Disease*, **5**, e1102.

119 Liao, K.-C. and Mogridge, J. (2013) Activation of the Nlrp1b inflammasome by reduction of cytosolic ATP. *Infection and Immunity*, **81** (2), 570–579.

120 Guicciardi, M.E., Malhi, H., Mott, J.L., and Gores, G.J. (2013) Apoptosis and necrosis in the liver. *Comprehensive Physiology*, **3** (2), 977–1010.

121 Martinon, F., Burns, K., and Tschopp, J. (2002) The inflammasome: a molecular platform triggering activation of inflammatory caspases and processing of proIL-beta. *Molecular Cell*, **10** (2), 417–426.

122 Leemans, J.C., Cassel, S.L., and Sutterwala, F.S. (2011) Sensing damage by the NLRP3 inflammasome. *Immunological Reviews*, **243** (1), 152–162.

123 Latz, E., Xiao, T.S., and Stutz, A. (2013) Activation and regulation of the inflammasomes. *Nature Reviews. Immunology*, **13** (6), 397–411.

124 Hoque, R., Vodovotz, Y., and Mehal, W. (2013) Therapeutic strategies in inflammasome mediated diseases of the liver. *Journal of Hepatology*, **58** (5), 1047–1052.

125 Jaeschke, H., Williams, C.D., Ramachandran, A., and Bajt, M.L. (2012) Acetaminophen hepatotoxicity and repair: the role of sterile inflammation and innate immunity. *Liver International*, **32** (1), 8–20.

126 Ghabril, M., Bonkovsky, H.L., Kum, C., Davern, T., Hayashi, P.H., Kleiner, D.E., Serrano, J., Rochon, J., Fontana, R.J., and Bonacini, M. (2013) Liver injury from tumor necrosis factor-α antagonists: analysis of thirty-four cases. *Clinical Gastroenterology and Hepatology*, **11** (5), 558–564.

127 Opar, A. (2012) Overtaking the DILI Model-T. *Nature Reviews. Drug Discovery*, **11** (8), 585–586.

8
Transporters in the Liver

Bruno Stieger and Gerd A. Kullak-Ublick

8.1
Introduction

The liver is composed of several different cell types, with hepatocytes constituting about 80% of the cells. Hepatocytes are involved in a multitude of physiological processes, the most important being energy homeostasis, synthesis of plasma proteins, detoxification, and bile formation. The latter two processes are highly relevant for drug disposition and thus of great interest during drug development. Bile is continuously produced by hepatocytes and is made up of various components, including bile salts, lipids, and organic anions [1]. Bile salts and lipids together form mixed micelles, which can act as carriers for poorly water-soluble compounds such as cholesterol [2,3]. Bile salts are taken up from portal blood into hepatocytes, where they mix with newly synthesized bile salts and undergo secretion across the canalicular membrane into primary bile. Bile is drained into the intestine, from where bile salts are taken up again in the terminal ileum and transported back to the liver in portal blood. This leads to a cycling of bile salts between the liver and the intestine, which is termed enterohepatic circulation of bile salts. Similarly to many drugs that are handled by the liver, bile salts are amphipathic molecules and as such can be used as model substances for some drugs [4,5]. Hepatocellular handling of bile salts has been reviewed in great depth [6–11] and will therefore not be covered here. The aim of this chapter is to put the role of bile salt and transporters for organic anions into perspective with respect to hepatocellular handling of drugs and the potential pathophysiological consequences of the interaction of drugs with these transporters.

8.2
Role of Organic Anion Transporters for Drug Uptake

Hepatocellular bile salt uptake occurs predominantly in a sodium-dependent manner and is mediated by the sodium taurocholate cotransporting polypeptide (NTCP) [12–14]. In addition, members of the organic anion transporting

Antitargets and Drug Safety, First Edition. Edited by László Urbán, Vinod F. Patel, and Roy J. Vaz.

polypeptide (OATP) superfamily mediate sodium-independent bile salt uptake into hepatocytes [6,15–17].

While NTCP generally is not considered to be a drug transporter, recently evidence has been presented that it can mediate transport of statins [18–21]. OATPs are involved in the transport of a wide variety of (generally large and amphipathic) drugs [15,17,22–27]. Despite the fact that the first OATP was already cloned in 1994 [28], the exact driving force of these transporters is not yet fully understood. Most if not all OATPs have more than one binding site for their substrates [17,26]. It is currently not known whether OATPs can mediate transport of drugs against a concentration gradient. In addition to OATPs, uptake of drugs into the hepatocyte is also mediated by members of the organic anion transporter (OAT) family [29].

Interaction between drugs at the basolateral entry site of endogenous substances into hepatocytes may, at least conceptually, lead to a reduced clearance of such substrates. For example, high-dose intravenous silibinin treatment of patients with a hepatitis C infection may lead to an elevation of serum bilirubin [30,31]. *In vitro* studies with OATP1B1, OATP1B3, and OATP2B1 in a heterologous expression system have demonstrated inhibition of these transporters by silibinin, which in part could explain the observed elevation of serum bilirubin in patients treated with high doses of silibinin [32]. The sodium-dependent bile salt uptake transporter NTCP was recently identified as the protein that mediates the hepatocellular uptake of the hepatitis B and D viruses into hepatocytes [13,33]: NTCP interacts with the myristoylated N-terminal preS1 domain of the large envelope glycoprotein [34], which inhibits the transport function of NTCP [35].

8.3 Drug Interaction with the Bile Salt Export Pump

Bile salts are effluxed from hepatocytes into the canaliculus against a steep concentration gradient by the bile salt export pump (BSEP) [14,36]. There is no backup transporter for the canalicular export of bile salts [36] and an inherited inactivation of this transporter leads to progressive familial intrahepatic cholestasis type 2 [37]. Inhibition of BSEP by drugs [38] or drug metabolites [39] may lead to drug-induced cholestasis [40]. As a consequence of BSEP inhibition, serum bile salt levels may increase, as was shown for bosentan [41]. Bosentan [42] and other drugs known to lead to drug-induced cholestasis [43] are competitive inhibitors of BSEP. These initial observations prompted investigation of the inhibitory potential of a considerable number of drugs with BSEP [44–47].

Inhibition of BSEP leads to an intracellular elevation of bile salts, which may ultimately lead to elevated serum bile salt levels [41]. As bile salts have detergent properties [48], they can damage mitochondria [49,50]. An ongoing intracellular elevation of bile salt concentration will therefore lead to cytotoxicity and, if persistent, to liver injury [51,52]. The antidiabetic drug troglitazone induced severe hepatotoxicity and was withdrawn. The exact mechanism underlying troglitazone-induced liver injury remains somewhat enigmatic; however, mitochondrial toxicity of (a) metabolite(s) appears to be involved [53,54]. Given the potential of troglitazone for inhibiting BSEP, elevation of intracellular bile salts may have aggravated the mitochondrial toxicity of troglitazone metabolites and consequently have led to severe drug-induced liver injury (DILI) in susceptible patients. As troglitazone sulfate also acts as a BSEP inhibitor [55], the transport activity of BSEP may have been considerably impaired. Hence, several mechanisms may be involved in drug-induced liver injury [56].

In addition to a direct interaction of drugs or drug metabolites with BSEP, indirect mechanisms of BSEP inhibition are also of relevance. Bosentan, for example, has a choleretic effect in rats, a process that depends on the function of the multidrug resistance-associated protein 2 (MRP2) [57]. Subsequent *in vitro* experiments showed that bosentan inhibits BSEP, but stimulates MRP2 [58]. Such an indirect inhibition of BSEP has also been reported for a metabolite of the HER1/HER2 inhibitor PKI166 [59]. Furthermore, oral contraceptives as well as pregnancy may also lead to acquired cholestasis. Both estrogen and progesterone metabolites require intact function of MRP2 to inhibit BSEP [38,60,61].

8.4
Susceptibility Factors for Drug–BSEP Interactions

While the consequences of drug-induced cholestasis secondary to BSEP inhibition may be severe, and BSEP inhibition thus represents an important clinical entity, the risk for such events is low [56,62]. This may impede the rapid identification of risk factors for BSEP-mediated liver injury in the context of drug therapy. An analysis of the correlation of $C_{\mathrm{max,unbound}}$ of drugs in plasma did not reveal a clear-cut correlation with drug-induced liver injury and the potential to inhibit BSEP [45]. This is not unexpected, as such a correlation takes neither the transport mechanism for hepatocellular drug uptake nor drug metabolism into account. The genetics of hepatocellular drug uptake systems have been extensively reviewed [5,23,63,64]. To date, the functional characterization of uptake transporter variants has mostly demonstrated a reduced function conferred by the variants, which would protect hepatocytes from drug-induced injury and probably not contribute to an increased risk. In addition to the function of the transport protein, polymorphic variants may lead to altered protein expression levels. Using Western blotting methodology, OATP1B1 and OATP1B3 have been reported to show an up to 70-fold difference of expression in healthy human liver samples [65] and the organic cation transporter 1 (OCT1) up to 80-fold [66]. Using quantitative proteomics, OATPs show an up to 32-fold range of expression [67–69]. NTCP varies eightfold [69] and OCT1, OAT2, and other drug transporters vary up to sixfold [67].

Given that BSEP is a bottleneck for canalicular secretion of bile salts, it is highly probable that BSEP constitutes a susceptibility factor for drug-induced cholestasis. Several studies have been published that highlight the presence of many different allelic variants of the gene coding for BSEP [70–74]. Among the many BSEP variants identified in human genomes, the p.444A variant is the most frequently observed in about 50% of the Caucasian population, albeit with ethnicity-dependent differences in frequency. Studies investigating the role of variants in the promoter of the gene coding for BSEP are only beginning to emerge [75]. Of note, one study reported the association of functional variants of the bile salt sensor FXR with intrahepatic cholestasis of pregnancy, which is an acquired form of liver disease [76]. To the best of our knowledge, no studies associating variants of transcription factors or polymorphisms in the promoter region of the gene coding for BSEP with drug-induced cholestasis have been published so far. Nevertheless, *in vitro* experiments suggest that drugs known to cause liver injury (e.g., troglitazone and benzbromarone) repress BSEP expression [77]. Parenthetically, a variant of PXR has been associated with flucloxacillin-induced liver injury [78]. The expression level of BSEP in healthy human liver correlates with the presence of the p.444A variant, as individuals homozygous for this allele tend to display lower BSEP levels than individuals homozygous for the wild-type allele, with a 20-fold difference in BSEP expression in healthy individuals as assessed by Western blotting [79]. Quantitative proteomics performed on a small number of individuals reported a fourfold variation [67]. In a small cohort of patients, the p.444A variant was found to be associated with drug-induced cholestasis, but not with drug-induced hepatitis [80]. While this variant is also associated with other forms of liver diseases [81,82], studies with larger cohorts of patients suffering from drug-induced cholestasis are needed to understand the contribution of the p.444A variant to drug-induced cholestasis. In addition, given the complex pathogenetic mechanism of drug-induced cholestasis, many additional genes may contribute to the susceptibility for developing drug-induced cholestatic liver injury. A genome-wide association study reported 42 loci to be associated with elevated liver enzymes, among them BSEP [83].

As drug metabolites are substrates of MRP2 [84], this canalicular export system also constitutes a risk factor for drug-induced cholestatic liver disease. Variants of this transporter have been associated with drug-induced liver injury [85,86]. When BSEP function is impaired, basolateral efflux systems (MRP3 and MRP4) are potential salvage systems to lower the burden of bile salts and drug metabolites for hepatocytes [87]. Hence, these two transporters are additional potential susceptibility factors for drug-induced cholestasis [88].

8.5 Role of BSEP in Drug Development

Investigation of the role of specific transporters for new chemical entities is now well established [89]. In 2012, at the second workshop of the International Transporter Consortium, the role of BSEP in the light of drug-induced cholestasis was discussed [90,91]. As there is currently no firm evidence that interaction of a new chemical entity in an *in vitro* assay reliably predicts an increased risk of drug-induced cholestasis, the consortium did not recommend routine testing of BSEP interaction during drug development, a view that is shared by the FDA (http://www.fda.gov/downloads/Drugs/GuidanceComplianceRegulatoryInformation/Guidances/ucm292362.pdf). The European Medicines Agency (EMA) recommends interaction testing of drugs with BSEP during development (http://www.ema.europa.eu/docs/en_GB/document_library/Scientific_guideline/2012/07/WC500129606.pdf). In cases of elevated liver enzymes (alanine aminotransferase or alkaline phosphatase) during clinical trials, testing for inhibition of BSEP by the compound is critical for understanding the mechanism of DILI [92]. The preferred assay for such cases has been defined by the International Transporter Consortium [93]. It has to be emphasized that lack of interaction of the parent drug with BSEP does not rule out the interaction with one or more metabolites. From a bench-side point of view, testing of new chemical entities for their interaction with BSEP is certainly warranted at an early stage of drug development. This may result in an early flag that helps to design the safety plan for clinical trials. However, BSEP inhibition *per se* is not a showstopper since additional factors such as the mode of uptake into hepatocytes, the metabolism of the drug, or the relation of the unbound C_{max} to the inhibitory affinity to BSEP (as expressed by the K_i value or with limited information by the IC_{50} value) are important parameters to be considered. If BSEP interaction has been found during development, determination of serum bile salt levels should certainly complement the clinical parameters needed for the identification of drug-induced liver injury [92]. In case drug metabolites are of concern, a vesicular BSEP assay should be complemented with a system that has the capacity to metabolize drugs, such as sandwich-cultured human hepatocytes [94,95]. Inhibition of BSEP in the absence of clinical data is not an indication for abandoning the development of the new chemical entity in question. For example, cyclosporine A is a potent BSEP inhibitor [38,43–45] and is indeed associated with drug-induced cholestasis in clinical routine [96], but was instrumental for successfully establishing organ transplantation.

As BSEP inhibition is now generally accepted as a mechanism leading to drug-induced cholestatic liver injury, major efforts are currently being undertaken to better understand the complex interplay of additional susceptibility factors and to develop novel models for better prediction and mitigation of the consequences of BSEP inhibition [44,97–102]. Consequently, improved and/or novel algorithms that incorporate data on BSEP interaction of new chemical entities can be expected.

References

1 Esteller, A. (2008) Physiology of bile secretion. *World Journal of Gastroenterology*, **14**, 5641–5649.

2 Hofmann, A.F. (2009) Bile acids: trying to understand their chemistry and biology with the hope of

helping patients. *Hepatology*, **49**, 1403–1418.

3 Hofmann, A.F. and Hagey, L.R. (2008) Bile acids: chemistry, pathochemistry, biology, pathobiology, and therapeutics. *Cellular and Molecular Life Sciences*, **65**, 2461–2483.

4 Hofmann, A.F., Molino, G., Milanese, M., and Belforte, G. (1983) Description and simulation of a physiological pharmacokinetic model for the metabolism and enterohepatic circulation of bile acids in man. Cholic acid in healthy man. *The Journal of Clinical Investigation*, **71**, 1003–1022.

5 Stieger, B. and Meier, P.J. (2011) Pharmacogenetics of drug transporters in the enterohepatic circulation. *Pharmacogenomics*, **12**, 611–631.

6 Meier, P.J. and Stieger, B. (2002) Bile salt transporters. *Annual Review of Physiology*, **64**, 635–661.

7 Alrefai, W.A. and Gill, R.K. (2007) Bile acid transporters: structure, function, regulation and pathophysiological implications. *Pharmaceutical Research*, **24**, 1803–1823.

8 Dawson, P.A., Lan, T., and Rao, A. (2009) Bile acid transporters. *Journal of Lipid Research*, **50**, 2340–2357.

9 Monte, M.J., Marin, J.J., Antelo, A., and Vazquez-Tato, J. (2009) Bile acids: chemistry, physiology, and pathophysiology. *World Journal of Gastroenterology*, **15**, 804–816.

10 Boyer, J.L. (2013) Bile formation and secretion. *Comprehensive Physiology*, **3**, 1035–1078.

11 Zwicker, B.L. and Agellon, L.B. (2013) Transport and biological activities of bile acids. *The International Journal of Biochemistry & Cell Biology*, **45**, 1389–1398.

12 Geyer, J., Wilke, T., and Petzinger, E. (2006) The solute carrier family SLC10: more than a family of bile acid transporters regarding function and phylogenetic relationships. *Naunyn-Schmiedeberg's Archives of Pharmacology*, **372**, 413–431.

13 Anwer, M.S. and Stieger, B. (2014) Sodium-dependent bile salt transporters of the SLC10A transporter family: more than solute transporters. *Pflugers Archiv: European Journal of Physiology*, **466**, 77–89.

14 Stieger, B. (2011) The role of the sodium-taurocholate cotransporting polypeptide (NTCP) and of the bile salt export pump (BSEP) in physiology and pathophysiology of bile formation. *Handbook of Experimental Pharmacology*, **201**, 205–259.

15 Hagenbuch, B. and Gui, C. (2008) Xenobiotic transporters of the human organic anion transporting polypeptides (OATP) family. *Xenobiotica*, **38**, 778–801.

16 Konig, J. (2011) Uptake transporters of the human OATP family. Molecular characteristics, substrates, their role in drug–drug interactions, and functional consequences of polymorphisms. *Handbook of Experimental Pharmacology*, **201**, 1–28.

17 Stieger, B. and Hagenbuch, B. (2014) Organic anion-transporting polypeptides. *Current Topics in Membranes*, **73**, 205–232.

18 Ho, R.H., Tirona, R.G., Leake, B.F., Glaeser, H., Lee, W., Lemke, C.J., Wang, Y., and Kim, R.B. (2006) Drug and bile acid transporters in rosuvastatin hepatic uptake: function, expression, and pharmacogenetics. *Gastroenterology*, **130**, 1793–1806.

19 Choi, M.K., Shin, H.J., Choi, Y.L., Deng, J.W., Shin, J.G., and Song, I.S. (2011) Differential effect of genetic variants of Na^+-taurocholate co-transporting polypeptide (NTCP) and organic anion-transporting polypeptide 1B1 (OATP1B1) on the uptake of HMG-CoA reductase inhibitors. *Xenobiotica*, **41**, 24–34.

20 Greupink, R., Dillen, L., Monshouwer, M., Huisman, M.T., and Russel, F.G. (2011) Interaction of fluvastatin with the liver-specific Na^+-dependent taurocholate cotransporting polypeptide (NTCP). *European Journal of Pharmaceutical Sciences*, **44**, 487–496.

21 Bi, Y.A., Qiu, X., Rotter, C.J., Kimoto, E., Piotrowski, M., Varma, M.V., Ei-Kattan, A.F., and Lai, Y. (2013) Quantitative assessment of the contribution of sodium-dependent taurocholate co-

transporting polypeptide (NTCP) to the hepatic uptake of rosuvastatin, pitavastatin and fluvastatin. *Biopharmaceutics & Drug Disposition*, **34**, 452–461.

22 Kalliokoski, A. and Niemi, M. (2009) Impact of OATP transporters on pharmacokinetics. *British Journal of Pharmacology*, **158**, 693–705.

23 Fahrmayr, C., Fromm, M.F., and Konig, J. (2010) Hepatic OATP and OCT uptake transporters: their role for drug–drug interactions and pharmacogenetic aspects. *Drug Metabolism Reviews*, **42**, 380–401.

24 Fenner, K.S., Jones, H.M., Ullah, M., Kempshall, S., Dickins, M., Lai, Y., Morgan, P., and Barton, H.A. (2012) The evolution of the OATP hepatic uptake transport protein family in DMPK sciences: from obscure liver transporters to key determinants of hepatobiliary clearance. *Xenobiotica*, **42**, 28–45.

25 Obaidat, A., Roth, M., and Hagenbuch, B. (2012) The expression and function of organic anion transporting polypeptides in normal tissues and in cancer. *Annual Review of Pharmacology and Toxicology*, **52**, 135–151.

26 Hagenbuch, B. and Stieger, B. (2013) The SLCO (former SLC21) superfamily of transporters. *Molecular Aspects of Medicine*, **34**, 396–412.

27 Shitara, Y., Maeda, K., Ikejiri, K., Yoshida, K., Horie, T., and Sugiyama, Y. (2013) Clinical significance of organic anion transporting polypeptides (OATPs) in drug disposition: their roles in hepatic clearance and intestinal absorption. *Biopharmaceutics & Drug Disposition*, **34**, 45–78.

28 Jacquemin, E., Hagenbuch, B., Stieger, B., Wolkoff, A.W., and Meier, P.J. (1994) Expression cloning of a rat liver Na^+-independent organic anion transporter. *Proceedings of the National Academy of Sciences of the United States of America*, **91**, 133–137.

29 Burckhardt, G. and Burckhardt, B.C. (2011) *In vitro* and *in vivo* evidence of the importance of organic anion transporters (OATs) in drug therapy. *Handbook of Experimental Pharmacology*, **201**, 29–104.

30 Neumann, U.P., Biermer, M., Eurich, D., Neuhaus, P., and Berg, T. (2010) Successful prevention of hepatitis C virus (HCV) liver graft reinfection by silibinin mono-therapy. *Journal of Hepatology*, **52**, 951–952.

31 Rutter, K., Scherzer, T.M., Beinhardt, S., Kerschner, H., Stattermayer, A.F., Hofer, H., Popow-Kraupp, T., Steindl-Munda, P., and Ferenci, P. (2011) Intravenous silibinin as 'rescue treatment' for on-treatment non-responders to pegylated interferon/ribavirin combination therapy. *Antiviral Therapy*, **16**, 1327–1333.

32 Wlcek, K., Koller, F., Ferenci, P., and Stieger, B. (2013) Hepatocellular organic anion-transporting polypeptides (OATPs) and multidrug resistance-associated protein 2 (MRP2) are inhibited by silibinin. *Drug Metabolism and Disposition*, **41**, 1522–1528.

33 Yan, H., Zhong, G., Xu, G., He, W., Jing, Z., Gao, Z., Huang, Y., Qi, Y., Peng, B., Wang, H., Fu, L., Song, M., Chen, P., Gao, W., Ren, B., Sun, Y., Cai, T., Feng, X., Sui, J., and Li, W. (2012) Sodium taurocholate cotransporting polypeptide is a functional receptor for human hepatitis B and D virus. *eLife*, **1**, e00049.

34 Urban, S., Bartenschlager, R., Kubitz, R., and Zoulim, F. (2014) Strategies to inhibit entry of HBV and HDV into hepatocytes. *Gastroenterology*, **147**, 48–64.

35 Konig, A., Doring, B., Mohr, C., Geipel, A., Geyer, J., and Glebe, D. (2014) Kinetics of the bile acid transporter and hepatitis B virus receptor Na/taurocholate cotransporting polypeptide (NTCP) in hepatocytes. *Journal of Hepatology*, **61**, 867–875.

36 Stieger, B., Meier, Y., and Meier, P.J. (2007) The bile salt export pump. *Pflugers Archiv: European Journal of Physiology*, **453**, 611–620.

37 Jacquemin, E. (2012) Progressive familial intrahepatic cholestasis. *Clinics and Research in Hepatology and Gastroenterology*, **36** (Suppl. 1), S26–35.

38 Stieger, B., Fattinger, K., Madon, J., Kullak-Ublick, G.A., and Meier, P.J.

(2000) Drug- and estrogen-induced cholestasis through inhibition of the hepatocellular bile salt export pump (Bsep) of rat liver. *Gastroenterology*, **118**, 422–430.

39 Funk, C. (2008) The role of hepatic transporters in drug elimination. *Expert Opinion on Drug Metabolism and Toxicology*, **4**, 363–379.

40 Stieger, B. (2010) Role of the bile salt export pump, BSEP, in acquired forms of cholestasis. *Drug Metabolism Reviews*, **42**, 437–445.

41 Fattinger, K., Funk, C., Pantze, M., Weber, C., Reichen, J., Stieger, B., and Meier, P.J. (2001) The endothelin antagonist bosentan inhibits the canalicular bile salt export pump: a potential mechanism for hepatic adverse reactions. *Clinical Pharmacology and Therapeutics*, **69**, 223–231.

42 Noe, J., Stieger, B., and Meier, P.J. (2002) Functional expression of the canalicular bile salt export pump of human liver. *Gastroenterology*, **123**, 1659–1666.

43 Byrne, J.A., Strautnieks, S.S., Mieli-Vergani, G., Higgins, C.F., Linton, K.J., and Thompson, R.J. (2002) The human bile salt export pump: characterization of substrate specificity and identification of inhibitors. *Gastroenterology*, **123**, 1649–1658.

44 Morgan, R.E., Trauner, M., van Staden, C.J., Lee, P.H., Ramachandran, B., Eschenberg, M., Afshari, C., Qualls, C.W., Jr., Lightfoot-Dunn, R., and Hamadeh, H.K. (2010) Interference with bile salt export pump function is a susceptibility factor for human liver injury in drug development. *Toxicological Sciences*, **118**, 485–500.

45 Dawson, S., Stahl, S., Paul, N., Barber, J., and Kenna, J.G. (2012) *In vitro* inhibition of the bile salt export pump correlates with risk of cholestatic drug induced liver injury in man. *Drug Metabolism and Disposition*, **40**, 130–138.

46 Pedersen, J.M., Matsson, P., Bergstrom, C.A., Hoogstraate, J., Noren, A., LeCluyse, E.L., and Artursson, P. (2013) Early identification of clinically relevant drug interactions with the human bile salt export pump (BSEP/ABCB11). *Toxicological Sciences*, **136**, 328–343.

47 Morgan, R.E., van Staden, C.J., Chen, Y., Kalyanaraman, N., Kalanzi, J., Dunn, R.T., 2nd, Afshari, C.A., and Hamadeh, H.K. (2013) A multifactorial approach to hepatobiliary transporter assessment enables improved therapeutic compound development. *Toxicological Sciences*, **136**, 216–241.

48 Hofmann, A.F. and Hagey, L.R. (2014) Bile acid chemistry, biology, and therapeutics during the last 80 years: historical aspects. *Journal of Lipid Research*. doi: 10.1194/jlr.R049437.

49 Krahenbuhl, S., Talos, C., Fischer, S., and Reichen, J. (1994) Toxicity of bile acids on the electron transport chain of isolated rat liver mitochondria. *Hepatology*, **19**, 471–479.

50 Utanohara, S., Tsuji, M., Momma, S., Morio, Y., and Oguchi, K. (2005) The effect of ursodeoxycholic acid on glycochenodeoxycholic acid-induced apoptosis in rat hepatocytes. *Toxicology*, **214**, 77–86.

51 Sokol, R.J., Devereaux, M., Dahl, R., and Gumpricht, E. (2006) "Let there be bile" – understanding hepatic injury in cholestasis. *Journal of Pediatric Gastroenterology and Nutrition*, **43** (Suppl. 1), S4–S9.

52 Tujios, S. and Fontana, R.J. (2011) Mechanisms of drug-induced liver injury: from bedside to bench. *Nature Reviews. Gastroenterology & Hepatology*, **8**, 202–211.

53 Masubuchi, Y. (2006) Metabolic and non-metabolic factors determining troglitazone hepatotoxicity: a review. *Drug Metabolism and Pharmacokinetics*, **21**, 347–356.

54 Julie, N.L., Julie, I.M., Kende, A.I., and Wilson, G.L. (2008) Mitochondrial dysfunction and delayed hepatotoxicity: another lesson from troglitazone. *Diabetologia*, **51**, 2108–2116.

55 Funk, C., Ponelle, C., Scheuermann, G., and Pantze, M. (2001) Cholestatic potential of troglitazone as a possible factor contributing to troglitazone-induced hepatotoxicity: *in vivo* and *in vitro* interaction at the canalicular bile

salt export pump (Bsep) in the rat. *Molecular Pharmacology*, **59**, 627–635.

56 Russmann, S., Kullak-Ublick, G.A., and Grattagliano, I. (2009) Current concepts of mechanisms in drug-induced hepatotoxicity. *Current Medicinal Chemistry*, **16**, 3041–3053.

57 Fouassier, L., Kinnman, N., Lefevre, G., Lasnier, E., Rey, C., Poupon, R., Elferink, R.P., and Housset, C. (2002) Contribution of mrp2 in alterations of canalicular bile formation by the endothelin antagonist bosentan. *Journal of Hepatology*, **37**, 184–191.

58 Mano, Y., Usui, T., and Kamimura, H. (2007) Effects of bosentan, an endothelin receptor antagonist, on bile salt export pump and multidrug resistance-associated protein 2. *Biopharmaceutics & Drug Disposition*, **28**, 13–18.

59 Takada, T., Weiss, H.M., Kretz, O., Gross, G., and Sugiyama, Y. (2004) Hepatic transport of PKI166, an epidermal growth factor receptor kinase inhibitor of the pyrrolo-pyrimidine class, and its main metabolite, ACU154. *Drug Metabolism and Disposition*, **32**, 1272–1278.

60 Akita, H., Suzuki, H., Ito, K., Kinoshita, S., Sato, N., Takikawa, H., and Sugiyama, Y. (2001) Characterization of bile acid transport mediated by multidrug resistance associated protein 2 and bile salt export pump. *Biochimica et Biophysica Acta*, **1511**, 7–16.

61 Vallejo, M., Briz, O., Serrano, M.A., Monte, M.J., and Marin, J.J. (2006) Potential role of trans-inhibition of the bile salt export pump by progesterone metabolites in the etiopathogenesis of intrahepatic cholestasis of pregnancy. *Journal of Hepatology*, **44**, 1150–1157.

62 Russmann, S., Kaye, J.A., Jick, S.S., and Jick, H. (2005) Risk of cholestatic liver disease associated with flucloxacillin and flucloxacillin prescribing habits in the UK: cohort study using data from the UK General Practice Research Database. *British Journal of Clinical Pharmacology*, **60**, 76–82.

63 Zair, Z.M., Eloranta, J.J., Stieger, B., and Kullak-Ublick, G.A. (2008) Pharmacogenetics of OATP (SLC21/SLCO), OAT and OCT (SLC22) and PEPT (SLC15) transporters in the intestine, liver and kidney. *Pharmacogenomics*, **9**, 597–624.

64 Gong, I.Y. and Kim, R.B. (2013) Impact of genetic variation in OATP transporters to drug disposition and response. *Drug Metabolism and Pharmacokinetics*, **28**, 4–18.

65 Nies, A.T., Niemi, M., Burk, O., Winter, S., Zanger, U.M., Stieger, B., Schwab, M., and Schaeffeler, E. (2013) Genetics is a major determinant of expression of the human hepatic uptake transporter OATP1B1, but not of OATP1B3 and OATP2B1. *Genome Medicine*, **5**, 1.

66 Nies, A.T., Koepsell, H., Winter, S., Burk, O., Klein, K., Kerb, R., Zanger, U.M., Keppler, D., Schwab, M., and Schaeffeler, E. (2009) Expression of organic cation transporters OCT1 (SLC22A1) and OCT3 (SLC22A3) is affected by genetic factors and cholestasis in human liver. *Hepatology*, **50**, 1227–1240.

67 Ohtsuki, S., Schaefer, O., Kawakami, H., Inoue, T., Liehner, S., Sato, A., Ishiguro, N., Kishimoto, W., Ludwig-Schwellinger, E., Ebner, T., and Terasaki, T. (2012) Simultaneous absolute protein quantification of transporters, cytochrome P450s and UDP-glucuronosyltransferases as a novel approach for the characterization of individual human liver: comparison with mRNA levels and activities. *Drug Metabolism and Disposition*, **40**, 83–92.

68 Prasad, B., Lai, Y., Lin, Y., and Unadkat, J.D. (2013) Interindividual variability in the hepatic expression of the human breast cancer resistance protein (BCRP/ABCG2): effect of age, sex, and genotype. *Journal of Pharmaceutical Sciences*, **102**, 787–793.

69 Vildhede, A., Karlgren, M., Svedberg, E.K., Wisniewski, J.R., Lai, Y., Noren, A., and Artursson, P. (2014) Hepatic uptake of atorvastatin: influence of variability in transporter expression on uptake clearance and drug–drug interactions. *Drug Metabolism and Disposition*, **42**, 1210–1218.

70 Saito, S., Iida, A., Sekine, A., Miura, Y., Ogawa, C., Kawauchi, S., Higuchi, S., and

Nakamura, Y. (2002) Three hundred twenty-six genetic variations in genes encoding nine members of ATP-binding cassette, subfamily B (ABCB/MDR/TAP), in the Japanese population. *Journal of Human Genetics*, **47**, 38–50.

71 Pauli-Magnus, C., Kerb, R., Fattinger, K., Lang, T., Anwald, B., Kullak-Ublick, G.A., Beuers, U., and Meier, P.J. (2004) BSEP and MDR3 haplotype structure in healthy Caucasians, primary biliary cirrhosis and primary sclerosing cholangitis. *Hepatology*, **39**, 779–791.

72 Lang, T., Haberl, M., Jung, D., Drescher, A., Schlagenhaufer, R., Keil, A., Mornhinweg, E., Stieger, B., Kullak-Ublick, G.A., and Kerb, R. (2006) Genetic variability, haplotype structures, and ethnic diversity of hepatic transporters MDR3 (ABCB4) and bile salt export pump (ABCB11). *Drug Metabolism and Disposition*, **34**, 1582–1599.

73 Kim, S.R., Saito, Y., Itoda, M., Maekawa, K., Kawamoto, M., Kamatani, N., Ozawa, S., and Sawada, J. (2009) Genetic variations of the ABC transporter gene ABCB11 encoding the human bile salt export pump (BSEP) in a Japanese population. *Drug Metabolism and Pharmacokinetics*, **24**, 277–281.

74 Ho, R.H., Leake, B.F., Kilkenny, D.M., Meyer Zu Schwabedissen, H.E., Glaeser, H., Kroetz, D.L., and Kim, R.B. (2010) Polymorphic variants in the human bile salt export pump (BSEP; ABCB11): functional characterization and interindividual variability. *Pharmacogenetics and Genomics*, **20**, 45–57.

75 Kim, M.J., Skewes-Cox, P., Fukushima, H., Hesselson, S., Yee, S.W., Ramsey, L.B., Nguyen, L., Eshragh, J.L., Castro, R.A., Wen, C.C., Stryke, D., Johns, S.J., Ferrin, T.E., Kwok, P.Y., Relling, M.V., Giacomini, K.M., Kroetz, D.L., and Ahituv, N. (2011) Functional characterization of liver enhancers that regulate drug-associated transporters. *Clinical Pharmacology and Therapeutics*, **89**, 571–578.

76 Van Mil, S.W., Milona, A., Dixon, P.H., Mullenbach, R., Geenes, V.L., Chambers, J., Shevchuk, V., Moore, G.E., Lammert, F., Glantz, A.G., Mattsson, L.A., Whittaker, J., Parker, M.G., White, R., and Williamson, C. (2007) Functional variants of the central bile acid sensor FXR identified in intrahepatic cholestasis of pregnancy. *Gastroenterology*, **133**, 507–516.

77 Garzel, B., Yang, H., Zhang, L., Huang, S.M., Polli, J.E., and Wang, H. (2014) The role of bile salt export pump gene repression in drug-induced cholestatic liver toxicity. *Drug Metabolism and Disposition*, **42**, 318–322.

78 Andrews, E., Armstrong, M., Tugwood, J., Swan, D., Glaves, P., Pirmohamed, M., Aithal, G.P., Wright, M.C., Day, C.P., and Daly, A.K. (2010) A role for the pregnane X receptor in flucloxacillin-induced liver injury. *Hepatology*, **51**, 1656–1664.

79 Meier, Y., Pauli-Magnus, C., Zanger, U.M., Klein, K., Schaeffeler, E., Nussler, A.K., Nussler, N., Eichelbaum, M., Meier, P.J., and Stieger, B. (2006) Interindividual variability of canalicular ATP-binding-cassette (ABC)-transporter expression in human liver. *Hepatology*, **44**, 62–74.

80 Lang, C., Meier, Y., Stieger, B., Beuers, U., Lang, T., Kerb, R., Kullak-Ublick, G.A., Meier, P.J., and Pauli-Magnus, C. (2007) Mutations and polymorphisms in the bile salt export pump and the multidrug resistance protein 3 associated with drug-induced liver injury. *Pharmacogenetics and Genomics*, **17**, 47–60.

81 Pauli-Magnus, C., Meier, P.J., and Stieger, B. (2010) Genetic determinants of drug-induced cholestasis and intrahepatic cholestasis of pregnancy. *Seminars in Liver Disease*, **30**, 147–159.

82 Stieger, B. and Geier, A. (2011) Genetic variations of bile salt transporters as predisposing factors for drug-induced cholestasis, intrahepatic cholestasis of pregnancy and therapeutic response of viral hepatitis. *Expert Opinion on Drug Metabolism and Toxicology*, **7**, 411–425.

83 Chambers, J.C., Zhang, W., Sehmi, J., Li, X., Wass, M.N., Van der Harst, P., Holm, H., Sanna, S., Kavousi, M., Baumeister, S.E., Coin, L.J., Deng, G., Gieger, C., Heard-Costa, N.L., Hottenga, J.J., Kuhnel, B., Kumar, V., Lagou, V., Liang, L., Luan, J., Vidal, P.M., Mateo Leach, I., O'Reilly,

P.F., Peden, J.F., Rahmioglu, N., Soininen, P., Speliotes, E.K., Yuan, X., Thorleifsson, G., Alizadeh, B.Z., Atwood, L.D., Borecki, I.B., Brown, M.J., Charoen, P., Cucca, F., Das, D., de Geus, E.J., Dixon, A.L., Doring, A., Ehret, G., Eyjolfsson, G.I., Farrall, M., Forouhi, N.G., Friedrich, N., Goessling, W., Gudbjartsson, D.F., Harris, T.B., Hartikainen, A.L., Heath, S., Hirschfield, G.M., Hofman, A., Homuth, G., Hypponen, E., Janssen, H.L., Johnson, T., Kangas, A.J., Kema, I.P., Kuhn, J.P., Lai, S., Lathrop, M., Lerch, M.M., Li, Y., Liang, T.J., Lin, J.P., Loos, R.J., Martin, N.G., Moffatt, M.F., Montgomery, G.W., Munroe, P.B., Musunuru, K., Nakamura, Y., O'Donnell, C.J., Olafsson, I., Penninx, B.W., Pouta, A., Prins, B.P., Prokopenko, I., Puls, R., Ruokonen, A., Savolainen, M.J., Schlessinger, D., Schouten, J.N., Seedorf, U., Sen-Chowdhry, S., Siminovitch, K.A., Smit, J.H., Spector, T.D., Tan, W., Teslovich, T.M., Tukiainen, T., Uitterlinden, A.G., Van der Klauw, M.M., Vasan, R.S., Wallace, C., Wallaschofski, H., Wichmann, H.E., Willemsen, G., Wurtz, P., Xu, C., Yerges-Armstrong, L.M., Alcohol Genome-wide Association Consortium, Diabetes Genetics Replication and Meta-analyses Study, Genetic Investigation of Anthropometric Traits Consortium, Global Lipids Genetics Consortium, Genetics of Liver Disease Consortium, International Consortium for Blood Pressure, Meta-analyses of Glucose and Insulin-Related Traits Consortium, Abecasis, G.R., Ahmadi, K.R., Boomsma, D.I., Caulfield, M., Cookson, W.O., van Duijn, C.M., Froguel, P., Matsuda, K., McCarthy, M.I., Meisinger, C., Mooser, V., Pietilainen, K.H., Schumann, G., Snieder, H., Sternberg, M.J., Stolk, R.P., Thomas, H.C., Thorsteinsdottir, U., Uda, M., Waeber, G., Wareham, N.J., Waterworth, D.M., Watkins, H., Whitfield, J.B., Witteman, J.C., Wolffenbuttel, B.H., Fox, C.S., Ala-Korpela, M., Stefansson, K., Vollenweider, P., Volzke, H., Schadt, E.E., Scott, J., Jarvelin, M.R., Elliott, P., and Kooner, J.S. (2011) Genome-wide association study identifies loci influencing concentrations of liver enzymes in plasma. *Nature Genetics*, **43**, 1131–1138.

84 Keppler, D. (2011) Multidrug resistance proteins (MRPs, ABCCs): importance for pathophysiology and drug therapy. *Handbook of Experimental Pharmacology*, **201**, 299–323.

85 Choi, J.H., Ahn, B.M., Yi, J., Lee, J.H., Nam, S.W., Chon, C.Y., Han, K.H., Ahn, S.H., Jang, I.J., Cho, J.Y., Suh, Y., Cho, M.O., Lee, J.E., Kim, K.H., and Lee, M.G. (2007) MRP2 haplotypes confer differential susceptibility to toxic liver injury. *Pharmacogenetics and Genomics*, **17**, 403–415.

86 Daly, A.K., Aithal, G.P., Leathart, J.B., Swainsbury, R.A., Dang, T.S., and Day, C.P. (2007) Genetic susceptibility to diclofenac-induced hepatotoxicity: contribution of UGT2B7, CYP2C8, and ABCC2 genotypes. *Gastroenterology*, **132**, 272–281.

87 Geier, A., Wagner, M., Dietrich, C.G., and Trauner, M. (2007) Principles of hepatic organic anion transporter regulation during cholestasis, inflammation and liver regeneration. *Biochimica et Biophysica Acta*, **1773**, 283–308.

88 Kock, K., Ferslew, B.C., Netterberg, I., Yang, K., Urban, T.J., Swaan, P.W., Stewart, P.W., and Brouwer, K.L. (2014) Risk factors for development of cholestatic drug-induced liver injury: inhibition of hepatic basolateral bile acid transporters multidrug resistance-associated proteins 3 and 4. *Drug Metabolism and Disposition*, **42**, 665–674.

89 Giacomini, K.M., Huang, S.M., Tweedie, D.J., Benet, L.Z., Brouwer, K.L., Chu, X., Dahlin, A., Evers, R., Fischer, V., Hillgren, K.M., Hoffmaster, K.A., Ishikawa, T., Keppler, D., Kim, R.B., Lee, C.A., Niemi, M., Polli, J.W., Sugiyama, Y., Swaan, P.W., Ware, J.A., Wright, S.H., Yee, S.W., Zamek-Gliszczynski, M.J., and Zhang, L. (2010) Membrane transporters in drug development. *Nature Reviews. Drug Discovery*, **9**, 215–236.

90 Zamek-Gliszczynski, M.J., Hoffmaster, K.A., Tweedie, D.J., Giacomini, K.M., and

Hillgren, K.M. (2012) Highlights from the International Transporter Consortium second workshop. *Clinical Pharmacology and Therapeutics*, **92**, 553–556.
91 Hillgren, K.M., Keppler, D., Zur, A.A., Giacomini, K.M., Stieger, B., Cass, C.E., and Zhang, L. (International Transporter Consortium) (2013) Emerging transporters of clinical importance: an update from the International Transporter Consortium. *Clinical Pharmacology and Therapeutics*, **94**, 52–63.
92 Aithal, G.P., Watkins, P.B., Andrade, R.J., Larrey, D., Molokhia, M., Takikawa, H., Hunt, C.M., Wilke, R.A., Avigan, M., Kaplowitz, N., Bjornsson, E., and Daly, A.K. (2011) Case definition and phenotype standardization in drug-induced liver injury. *Clinical Pharmacology and Therapeutics*, **89**, 806–815.
93 Brouwer, K.L., Keppler, D., Hoffmaster, K.A., Bow, D.A., Cheng, Y., Lai, Y., Palm, J.E., Stieger, B., and Evers, R. (2013) *In vitro* methods to support transporter evaluation in drug discovery and development. *Clinical Pharmacology and Therapeutics*, **94**, 95–112.
94 Swift, B., Pfeifer, N.D., and Brouwer, K.L. (2010) Sandwich-cultured hepatocytes: an *in vitro* model to evaluate hepatobiliary transporter-based drug interactions and hepatotoxicity. *Drug Metabolism Reviews*, **42**, 446–471.
95 Godoy, P., Hewitt, N.J., Albrecht, U., Andersen, M.E., Ansari, N., Bhattacharya, S., Bode, J.G., Bolleyn, J., Borner, C., Bottger, J., Braeuning, A., Budinsky, R.A., Burkhardt, B., Cameron, N.R., Camussi, G., Cho, C.S., Choi, Y.J., Craig Rowlands, J., Dahmen, U., Damm, G., Dirsch, O., Donato, M.T., Dong, J., Dooley, S., Drasdo, D., Eakins, R., Ferreira, K.S., Fonsato, V., Fraczek, J., Gebhardt, R., Gibson, A., Glanemann, M., Goldring, C.E., Gomez-Lechon, M.J., Groothuis, G.M., Gustavsson, L., Guyot, C., Hallifax, D., Hammad, S., Hayward, A., Haussinger, D., Hellerbrand, C., Hewitt, P., Hoehme, S., Holzhutter, H.G., Houston, J.B., Hrach, J., Ito, K., Jaeschke, H., Keitel, V., Kelm, J.M., Kevin Park, B., Kordes, C., Kullak-Ublick, G.A., Lecluyse, E.L., Lu, P., Luebke-Wheeler, J., Lutz, A., Maltman, D.J., Matz-Soja, M., McMullen, P., Merfort, I., Messner, S., Meyer, C., Mwinyi, J., Naisbitt, D.J., Nussler, A.K., Olinga, P., Pampaloni, F., Pi, J., Pluta, L., Przyborski, S.A., Ramachandran, A., Rogiers, V., Rowe, C., Schelcher, C., Schmich, K., Schwarz, M., Singh, B., Stelzer, E.H., Stieger, B., Stober, R., Sugiyama, Y., Tetta, C., Thasler, W.E., Vanhaecke, T., Vinken, M., Weiss, T.S., Widera, A., Woods, C.G., Xu, J.J., Yarborough, K.M., and Hengstler, J.G. (2013) Recent advances in 2D and 3D *in vitro* systems using primary hepatocytes, alternative hepatocyte sources and non-parenchymal liver cells and their use in investigating mechanisms of hepatotoxicity, cell signaling and ADME. *Archives of Toxicology*, **87**, 1315–1530.
96 Arias, I.M. (1993) Cyclosporin, the biology of the bile canaliculus, and cholestasis. *Gastroenterology*, **104**, 1558–1560.
97 Thompson, R.A., Isin, E.M., Li, Y., Weidolf, L., Page, K., Wilson, I., Swallow, S., Middleton, B., Stahl, S., Foster, A.J., Dolgos, H., Weaver, R., and Kenna, J.G. (2012) *In vitro* approach to assess the potential for risk of idiosyncratic adverse reactions caused by candidate drugs. *Chemical Research in Toxicology*, **25**, 1616–1632.
98 Warner, D.J., Chen, H., Cantin, L.D., Kenna, J.G., Stahl, S., Walker, C.L., and Noeske, T. (2012) Mitigating the inhibition of human bile salt export pump by drugs: opportunities provided by physicochemical property modulation, *in silico* modeling, and structural modification. *Drug Metabolism and Disposition*, **40**, 2332–2341.
99 Chang, J.H., Plise, E., Cheong, J., Ho, Q., and Lin, M. (2013) Evaluating the *in vitro* inhibition of UGT1A1, OATP1B1, OATP1B3, MRP2, and BSEP in predicting drug-induced hyperbilirubinemia. *Molecular Pharmacology*, **10**, 3067–3075.
100 Vinken, M., Landesmann, B., Goumenou, M., Vinken, S., Shah, I., Jaeschke, H.,

Willett, C., Whelan, M., and Rogiers, V. (2013) Development of an adverse outcome pathway from drug-mediated bile salt export pump inhibition to cholestatic liver injury. *Toxicological Sciences*, **136**, 97–106.

101 Ritschel, T., Hermans, S.M., Schreurs, M., van den Heuvel, J.J., Koenderink, J.B., Greupink, R., and Russel, F.G. (2014) *In silico* identification and *in vitro* validation of potential cholestatic compounds through 3D ligand-based pharmacophore modeling of BSEP inhibitors. *Chemical Research in Toxicology*, **27**, 873–881.

102 Rodrigues, A.D., Lai, Y., Cvijic, M.E., Elkin, L.L., Zvyaga, T., and Soars, M.G. (2014) Drug-induced perturbations of the bile acid pool, cholestasis, and hepatotoxicity: mechanistic considerations beyond the direct inhibition of the bile salt export pump. *Drug Metabolism and Disposition*, **42**, 566–574.

9
Mechanistic Modeling of Drug-Induced Liver Injury (DILI)

Kyunghee Yang, Jeffrey L. Woodhead, Lisl K. Shoda, Yuching Yang, Paul B. Watkins, Kim L.R. Brouwer, Brett A. Howell, and Scott Q. Siler

9.1
Introduction

Drug-induced liver injury (DILI) is the most common cause of acute liver failure [1], and is one of the primary reasons for the failure of pharmaceutical agents during drug development. Clinical reports of DILI cases after drug approval may lead to black box warnings, which limit drug use, or withdrawal of drugs from the market. DILI raises significant public health concerns, and also elevates economic burdens on patients by increasing the cost of drug development. Early detection of liver signals during the drug development process will save time and resources and protect patients from potential liver injury. However, the hepatotoxic potential of many chemical entities currently is not well predicted from *in vitro* screening or standard preclinical testing. While multiple experimental systems and approaches are required to accurately predict DILI, systems pharmacology modeling is a useful tool to integrate drug disposition, the underlying biology, and mechanisms of toxicity to predict human DILI.

DILIsym® is a mechanistic, multiscale model of DILI that is implemented in the MATLAB computing platform (The Math Works, Inc., Natick, MA). DILIsym® represents hepatocyte–drug interactions in preclinical species (Sprague-Dawley rats, C57Bl/6 mice, and Beagle dogs) and humans. Mechanistic representation of preclinical species and humans allows the translation of preclinical data to prospective predictions of human hepatotoxicity. DILIsym® includes baseline individuals and virtual populations (SimPops™) for both preclinical and clinical species. Simulations using baseline individuals provide insights into DILI responses in the average individual, whereas DILI responses can be simulated at the population level using SimPops™. DILIsym® spans multiple scales of physiology, from the organ/tissue level to the molecular and cellular levels (Figure 9.1). It consists of multiple drug- and system (biology)-specific submodels. Disposition of drugs/metabolites is described by the physiologically based pharmacokinetic (PBPK) submodel. Examples of system-specific submodels are glutathione (GSH) synthesis and depletion, cellular energy

Antitargets and Drug Safety, First Edition. Edited by László Urbán, Vinod F. Patel, and Roy J. Vaz.

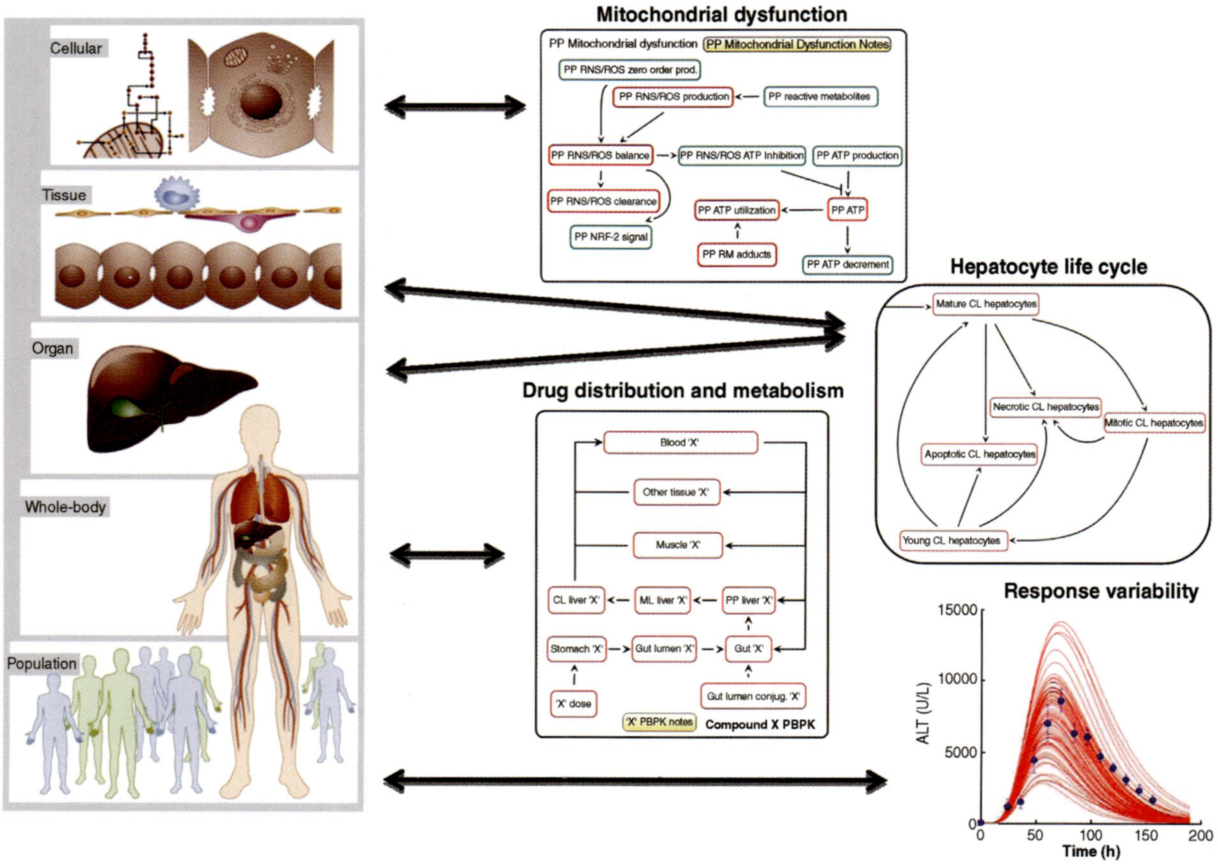

Figure 9.1 Multiscale structure of DILIsym®. (Reprinted with permission from Ref. [2].)

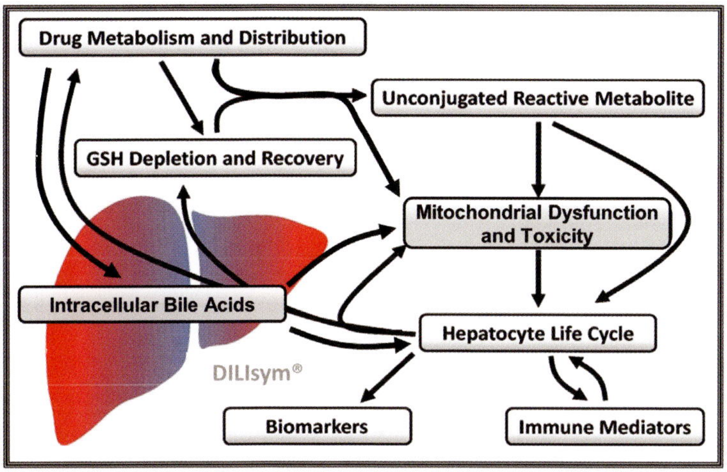

Figure 9.2 Diagram of the overall structure and mechanistic representation of DILIsym®.

balance, hepatocyte life cycle, and biomarkers for liver injury and function (e.g., serum ALT, AST, and total bilirubin). These submodels are integrated mathematically to build a dynamic and quantitative biological network, allowing simulation of time-dependent interactions of drugs/metabolites and a biological system and the resulting changes in hepatic mass, function, and biomarkers.

The current version of DILIsym® (version 3A) represents multiple mechanisms of hepatotoxicity such as oxidative stress, innate immunity, mitochondrial toxicity, and bile acid-mediated toxicity (Figure 9.2). Mechanistic modules and the list of exemplar compounds for each module are listed in Table 9.1. Given the data regarding specific mechanisms underlying DILI, DILIsym® simulates the mechanistic interactions and events from compound administration through the progression of liver injury and regeneration. Each mechanistic module will be discussed in detail in the next section.

9.2 Mechanistic Modules in DILIsym® version 3A

9.2.1 Oxidative Stress-Mediated Toxicity

Reactive metabolites generate reactive nitrogen/oxygen species (RNS/ROS) by various mechanisms such as reduction of cellular antioxidants, protein binding in various locations inside the cell, and direct reactive metabolite–membrane interactions. Depletion of hepatic ATP by RNS/ROS in turn leads to disruptions in other cellular processes, resulting in necrosis [3]. To understand the underlying mechanisms of oxidative stress-mediated DILI processes, acetaminophen

Table 9.1 Mechanistic modules and exemplar compounds within DILIsym® version 3A.

Mechanism of hepatotoxicity	Exemplar compounds	Species
Oxidative stress	Acetaminophen (APAP)	Human, mouse, rat, dog
	3-Hydroxyacetamilide (AMAP)	Mouse
	Methapyrilene (MP)	Human, mouse, rat
	Furosemide	Human, mouse, rat
	Aflatoxin B1	Mouse, rat
Innate immunity	APAP	Human, mouse, rat, dog
	Carbon tetrachloride (CCl4)	Mouse, rat
Mitochondria dysfunction	Etomoxir	Human
	Buprenorphine	Human
	Tolcapone	Human
Bile acid transport inhibition	Glibenclamide	Human, rat
	Troglitazone[a)]	Human, rat
	Pioglitazone[a)]	Human
	Bosentan	Human, rat
	Telmisartan	Human
	CP-724714	Human, rat, dog
	Tolcapone	Human

a) DILIsym® version 3A was used for the troglitazone and pioglitazone simulation, and these compounds are explicitly included in DILIsym® version 3B.

(APAP) was employed as a model hepatotoxic compound. APAP overdose is the predominant cause of clinical DILI cases, including liver failure [4]. APAP presents dose-dependent hepatotoxicity, and numerous studies have shown that hepatic RNS/ROS levels increase following APAP administration [5–12]. APAP generates *N*-acetyl-*p*-benzoquinone imine (NAPQI), a toxic reactive metabolite, by CYP-mediated metabolism. GSH detoxifies NAPQI, but as hepatic GSH is depleted, NAPQI forms protein adducts and induces mitochondrial oxidative stress, leading to cell death.

To simulate oxidative stress-mediated liver injury, submodels representing basic biochemical/physiological processes involved in RNS/ROS production/clearance, GSH dynamics, hepatic ATP dynamics, hepatocyte life cycle, and DILI biomarkers were constructed within DILIsym® using available *in vitro* and *in vivo* data [13]. A PBPK model describing hepatic and systemic disposition of APAP and its metabolites (APAP–sulfate, APAP–glucuronide, and NAPQI) was also constructed. The simulated hepatotoxic responses to APAP (e.g., altered hepatic GSH levels, serum ALT/AST/bilirubin, and prothrombin time) were comparable with measured data from numerous studies in mice, rats, dogs, and humans [13].

N-acetyl cysteine (NAC) is the standard therapy for APAP overdose [14,15], but the optimal treatment protocol (e.g., route of administration and treatment duration) is still in debate. Although it is not feasible to compare different treatment protocols under different clinical scenarios (e.g., length of delay in treatment) in prospective studies with a large number of APAP overdose patients, mechanistic models can be used to do so. Simulations using human SimPops™ within DILIsym® suggested that within 24 h of APAP overdose, standard 72 h oral NAC treatment (loading dose of 140 mg/kg, followed by 70 mg/kg doses every 4 h) is superior to standard 21 h intravenous treatment (loading infusion of 150 mg/kg over 1 h, followed by infusion of 50 mg/kg over 4 h and then infusion of 100 mg/kg over 16 h) [13]. Simulations also provided insights into potential biomarkers that might predict when to terminate NAC treatment safely. It had been suggested that NAC treatment should be stopped when blood APAP drops below detectable levels [16]. Simulations supported the hypothesis that the blood APAP level is predicted to be a reasonable biomarker of hepatic NAPQI when NAC was administered within 24 h of APAP overdose. However, the blood APAP level was predicted to undertreat patients if NAC treatment was started after 24 h of overdose because the elimination of blood APAP was often faster than the elimination of hepatic NAPQI [13]. Investigation of several serum biomarkers using DILIsym® suggested that serum ALT may be a potential biomarker; termination of NAC treatment at the time of peak ALT was predicted to prevent undertreatment of patients [13]. Although it is not recommended to change clinical practice based only on these modeling results, this example illustrates how systems pharmacology models can be used to identify treatment protocols that may require re-examination and help optimize protocols to improve clinical results.

While APAP was selected as a model hepatotoxic compound to investigate oxidative stress-mediated DILI, an analogue of APAP, 3-hydroxyacetamilide (AMAP), was employed as a negative control to validate the model. AMAP initially was patented as a possible alternative to APAP, and has been shown to be less hepatotoxic than APAP in mice. Although various mechanisms for the differential toxicological response between the two isomers have been proposed, the primary mechanism still remains unclear. Thus, DILIsym® was employed to test the plausibility of the proposed mechanistic hypotheses: (a) AMAP generates less reactive metabolites compared with APAP, (b) reactive metabolites of AMAP inhibit AMAP formation by mechanism-based inhibition of CYP2E1, (c) reactive metabolites of AMAP bind to nonspecific cellular proteins at a higher rate than those of APAP, and thus deplete less GSH, and (d) reactive metabolites of AMAP are less potent compared with those of APAP on an equimolar basis. Comparison of simulated results based on each hypothesis with the observed data (e.g., cumulative metabolite accumulation, maximum GSH depletion in the liver, and serum ALT) suggested that hypotheses (a) and (b) are likely to be mechanisms underlying the differences in hepatotoxic potential of APAP and AMAP [17]. These results also indicate that differences in the amount of reactive metabolites generated, rather than differences in processes downstream of reactive metabolite formation, are more likely to be responsible for observed differences in hepatotoxicity. The current DILIsym® model does not have a representation of specific proteins bound to reactive metabolites. Therefore, the alternative hypothesis of selective protein binding (reactive metabolites of APAP selectively bind to critical proteins compared with those of AMAP [18,19]) was not evaluated in this study, which is one of the limitations. Nonetheless, these results demonstrated the utility of systems pharmacology modeling and simulation to investigate the underlying mechanisms of toxicity and differentiate between hepatotoxic and nonhepatotoxic compounds.

Identification of the hepatotoxic potential of compounds early in drug development is desired to save time and resources. Methapyrilene (MP), a hepatotoxic compound that possesses the same mechanism of toxicity as APAP, was selected to evaluate the application of DILIsym® in *in vitro–in vivo* extrapolation. To this end, an MP model was constructed using only *in vitro* data such as log P, pK_a, metabolic partitioning in rat and mouse hepatocytes, and covalent binding in mouse, rat, and human microsomes. Although APAP and MP share the same mechanisms, MP hepatotoxicity has not been reported in mice and humans. Moreover, MP is hepatotoxic in rats, whereas mice and humans are more susceptible to APAP hepatotoxicity. Simulations based only on *in vitro* data correctly predicted species differences in MP hepatotoxicity, supporting the idea that DILIsym® can be used to translate *in vitro* data to predict *in vivo* hepatotoxicity.

9.2.2
Innate Immune Responses

The innate immune system has been shown to participate in the hepatotoxic response to APAP. Necrotic hepatocytes release molecules known as damage-associated molecular patterns (DAMPs), for example, high mobility group box 1 (HMGB1), which can initiate an immune response. Activated innate immune cells release multiple mediators, including tumor necrosis factor (TNF)-α, interleukin (IL)-1β, IL-6, IL-10, and IL-12, transforming growth factor (TGF)-β, acetylated HMGB1, hepatocyte growth factor (HGF), vascular endothelial growth factor (VEGF), monocyte chemoattractant protein (MCP)-1, and macrophage colony-stimulating factor (M-CSF). Many of these mediators are pleiotropic in their activities and could include potentiation of injury, recruitment of additional immune cells, and regulation of both immune cell activity or mediator production and hepatocyte activity or mediator production. Circulating levels of these and other mediators have been measured in preclinical experimental APAP models and sometimes in patients with APAP overdose.

The representation of the innate immune response in DILIsym® version 3A includes two cell populations: macrophages and liver sinusoidal endothelial cells (LSECs). Life cycles of macrophages and LSECs were represented by maturation/differentiation, local proliferation, and apoptosis using available data [20–25]. Activated macrophages produce TNF-α, acetylated HMGB1, and IL-10. TNF-α is represented as a regulatory molecule inducing autocrine TNF-α as well as macrophage IL-10 production. It may also induce cell death via programmed necrosis in energetically compromised hepatocytes. Survival and mitotic activity currently are represented indirectly via stimulation of HGF production. Macrophage-derived acetylated HMGB1 differs from the nonacetylated form released from necrotic or late apoptotic cells [26,27] and is a putative biomarker for immune activation [28]. IL-10 acts as a regulatory molecule, inhibiting the production of TNF-α. Activated LSECs produce TNF-α and HGF. Initial modeling efforts have focused on a select number of cell populations and mediators that have been implicated in APAP hepatotoxicity through preclinical manipulation or clinical measurements. For example, serial measurements from patients with APAP overdose revealed that acetylated HMGB1 was elevated in patients with poor outcomes (death or liver transplant) relative to spontaneous survivors [28]. Other cell types and mediators can be incorporated in future development.

To validate the innate immune response model, multiple immune perturbations combined with APAP administration were simulated. Administration of blocking antibodies to HMBG1 to mice in combination with APAP plays a partially protective role in APAP-induced liver injury based on histology and serum ALT levels [29–31]. Simulations of different APAP doses with anti-HMGB1 in DILIsym® lessened hepatotoxicity in mice, consistent with the observed experimental data. Similarly, simulations using DILIsym® reproduced the alleviation in APAP hepatotoxicity in mice after neutralizing TNF-α as observed *in vivo* in mice [32–35]. These results demonstrated that although the representation of innate immunity in the current version of DILIsym® is relatively simple, it described the innate immune responses after APAP overdose and the resulting enhanced/elevated hepatotoxicity that has been measured experimentally reasonably well.

Carbon tetrachloride (CCl_4) was included in DILIsym® to test the mathematical representation of the innate immune response, following exposure to another compound that generates a reactive metabolite, which is thought to induce oxidative stress and subsequent hepatotoxicity. The innate immune system has been shown to participate in the hepatotoxic response to CCl_4; elevated levels of immune mediators and macrophage accumulation have been reported after administration of a hepatotoxic dose of CCl_4 [36–59]. In DILIsym®, CCl_4-mediated oxidative stress consistent with the measured data was insufficient to recapitulate the observed dose-dependent hepatotoxicity. However, the addition of a second mechanism, mitochondrial dysfunction, which has also been reported in the literature, resulted in the expected hepatotoxicity [50,60]. Simulated liver macrophage accumulation induced by CCl_4 was comparable with observed data in rats and mice [40,56–59]. Furthermore, the range of TNF-α reported in various mouse and rat CCl_4 models was recapitulated across a range of CCl_4 doses. These results ensure that the current innate immune response model within DILIsym® is able to recapitulate the innate immune response observed experimentally.

Similar to APAP, TNF-α neutralization strategies can be protective against CCl_4-mediated hepatotoxicity, although disparate responses have been observed and attributed to the mediator's pleiotropic activities.

9.2.3 Mitochondrial Toxicity

Mitochondria are critical cellular components in DILI, as they are responsible for the vast majority of cellular ATP synthesis. Disruptions in ATP synthesis decrease cellular ATP levels leading to disturbances in other cellular processes and necrotic cell death [3]. Drugs and/or metabolites can disrupt mitochondria ATP production in multiple ways: direct inhibition of ATP synthesis, inhibition of electron transport chain (ETC) flux, or direct reduction of the mitochondria proton gradient via uncoupling. Inhibition of substrate utilization also reduces ATP synthesis. Initiation of the mitochondria permeability transition via changes in reactive nitrogen/oxygen species can also reduce ATP synthesis. Finally, bile acid accumulation by transporter inhibition can also lead to reductions in ATP production by induction of mitochondrial membrane permeabilization [61]. ATP produced from glycolysis can offset disruptions in mitochondria ATP production, particularly if there is ample glycolytic substrate [62].

To construct the mitochondrial toxicity module within DILIsym®, a mathematical model representing *in vitro* studies (MITOsym®) was first developed because most data describing the dynamics associated with mitochondria biochemistry are collected from *in vitro* studies. MITOsym® version 3A includes glucose uptake and glycolysis as well as the dynamic regulation of the mitochondria ETC activity, substrate utilization, and the proton gradient [63]. The cellular biomarkers oxygen consumption rate (OCR) and extracellular acidification rate (ECAR) were used to represent changes in ETC activity and glycolysis, respectively, in HepG2 cells, primary human hepatocytes, and primary rat hepatocytes; experimental data from these cells treated with exemplar mitochondria disruptors, rotenone (ETC complex inhibitor), oligomycin (FoF1 ATPase inhibitor), or FCCP (uncoupling agent) were utilized to optimize MITOsym® [62–65]. Assuming that mitochondrial biochemistry is consistent, the quantitative relationships in these pathways were then translated to DILIsym® from MITOsym®. Substrate provision to mitochondria differs between MITOsym® and DILIsym®; glucose uptake and glycolysis provide the bulk of mitochondria uptake in the cultured cells represented in MITOsym®, whereas the liver takes up only glucose in the postprandial state *in vivo*. Moreover, the liver utilizes fatty acids in both the fed and fasted states [66].

To test the behavior of *in vivo* response to mitochondria disruption in DILIsym®, etomoxir was used as a model hepatotoxic compound. Etomoxir was developed to treat type 2 diabetes and congestive heart failure, but development was stopped due to efficacy and safety issues [67]. Etomoxir inhibits fatty acid beta-oxidation by irreversibly binding to carnitine palmitoyltransferase (CPT)-1 and preventing entry of long-chain fatty acids into the mitochondria matrix [68,69]. Hepatotoxicity was detected during clinical trials; serum ALT elevations were found in a subset of congestive heart failure patients [70]. Thus, etomoxir treatment of heart failure patients was terminated following this clinical trial [67]. A PBPK model of etomoxir was constructed based on a human PK study to simulate the exposure to etomoxir. Inhibition of beta-oxidation by etomoxir was included as the primary mechanism of toxicity, and the quantitative effect was based on *in vitro* fatty acid oxidation inhibition data obtained from human hepatocytes [68]. Simulations suggested that daily dosing of etomoxir was predicted to elicit hepatotoxicity in populations that include variability in drug clearance and meal administration [66,71].

Buprenorphine, a semisynthetic opioid that is used to treat opioid addiction and to control pain, was also employed as an exemplar compound for mitochondria toxicity. Hepatotoxicity has been observed in overdosed patients [72–76]. Buprenorphine has two mechanisms for mitochondria toxicity: direct inhibition of ETC activity and reduction of the mitochondria proton gradients by uncoupling [72]. The simulated hepatotoxic response was comparable with that observed in clinical data using a PBPK model to predict exposure combined with parameters derived from *in vitro* mitochondria toxicity data [72,73,77,78].

9.2.4
Bile Acid-Mediated Toxicity

Bile acids play important roles in the body as lipid emulsifiers and signaling molecules that regulate lipid and glucose homeostasis. However, bile acids can exert toxic effects when present at supraphysiological concentrations in hepatocytes [79]. Bile acid toxicity is, in general, thought to be highly correlated with hydrophobicity; more hydrophobic bile acids are more cytotoxic [80]. Mechanisms of bile acid-induced hepatotoxicity include disruption of cell membranes due to detergent-like properties of the bile acids, disruption of mitochondrial ATP synthesis, and induction of cell necrosis and apoptosis [80]. Therefore, inhibition of hepatic efflux of bile acids by drugs may result in intracellular accumulation of toxic bile acids, leading to hepatotoxicity [81]. *In vitro* vesicular transport studies also suggest that interruption of the bile salt export pump (BSEP)-mediated biliary excretion of bile acids by drugs is a potential risk factor for DILI [82–84].

Bile acids undergo vectorial transport from sinusoidal blood across the basolateral membranes into hepatocytes and across the canalicular membranes into bile. Bile acids exist as anions at physiological pH, and thus are substrates of hepatic transporters. Bile acids are taken up from the sinusoidal blood into hepatocytes primarily by the uptake of transport protein sodium taurocholate cotransporting polypeptide (NTCP); organic anion transporting polypeptides (OATPs) are also capable of transporting bile acids into hepatocytes. Within hepatocytes, bile acids are metabolized and excreted into bile predominantly via BSEP in an ATP-dependent manner [85]. In addition to canalicular excretion, bile acids can also be excreted into sinusoidal blood via multidrug resistance-associated protein (MRP)3, MRP4, and organic solute transporter (OST)-α/β [86–88]. Once excreted into bile, bile acids undergo efficient enterohepatic recirculation; about 90–95% of the bile acids excreted into bile are reabsorbed from the intestinal lumen by apical sodium-dependent bile acid transporter (ASBT) in the terminal ileum or by passive diffusion [89]. Due to the critical physiological and pathophysiological roles of bile acids, homeostasis is tightly regulated through multiple nuclear receptors, including the farnesoid X receptor (FXR), the constitutive androstane receptor (CAR), and the liver X receptor (LXR) [90–92].

The bile acid homeostasis model within DILIsym® represents synthesis, metabolism, transport, and enterohepatic recirculation of lithocholic acid (LCA), chenodeoxycholic acid (CDCA), and their respective conjugates as well as a bulk bile acid that contains the rest of the bile acid species [93]. LCA and CDCA were selected for inclusion in the model because they are known to be hydrophobic, cytotoxic bile acid species [80]. In addition, CDCA is a primary bile acid synthesized from cholesterol in hepatocytes, whereas LCA is a secondary bile acid that is formed by bacterial 7α-dehydroxylation of CDCA in the intestinal lumen. Thus, modeling LCA and CDCA provides the opportunity to explore different behaviors of primary and secondary bile acids in the setting of impaired bile acid transport. Finally, CDCA and CDCA conjugates are reported to be potent activators of FXR [90]; FXR-mediated negative feedback regulation on bile acid synthesis and transport by hepatic accumulation of CDCA species has also been incorporated into the bile acid homeostasis model in DILIsym® [93]. However, mathematical representation of regulation in the current DILIsym® model is empirical due to the lack of understanding of the quantitative effects of hepatic bile acid concentrations on the function of enzymes and transporters involved in bile acid homeostasis. Hepatic bile acid transport processes were represented using saturable Michaelis–Menten kinetics. The K_m values were obtained from available literature, whereas V_{max} values were optimized to a known bile acid profile in humans, dogs, and rats [94,95]. The inhibition of hepatic uptake as well as basolateral and canalicular efflux transporters by drugs can be simulated as competitive or noncompetitive inhibition based on the available data. Hepatic bile acid efflux transporters such as BSEP, MRP3, and MRP4 are ATP-dependent transporters and, thus, depletion of hepatic ATP will result in impaired function of these efflux transporters. The relationship between ATP depletion and impaired transporter function was parameterized using available *in vitro* data [96,97]. In humans and dogs, release of bile acids from the gall bladder into the intestinal lumen is regulated by meals. This aspect was parameterized using *in vivo* bile acid release data in humans [98,99] and dogs [100]. In rats, bile flow and biliary bile acid excretion increase during the dark cycle; this aspect was modeled as increased biliary transport by the meal signal and parameterized using *in vivo* data describing circadian rhythm of bile acid excretion in rats [101].

Available data suggest that serum bile acid profiles in humans and rats show large interindividual variability [94,95]. To account for the population variability, virtual human and rat populations (SimPops™) that include variability in parameters describing bile acid homeostasis were constructed [93]. The bile acid homeostasis model was validated using *in vivo* serum bile acid data from rats administered glibenclamide. Administration of glibenclamide, a potent BSEP and NTCP inhibitor, increased systemic bile acid concentrations in rats; a large variability was observed in rat serum bile acid concentrations after glibenclamide administration [93]. Simulated systemic bile acid concentrations in rat SimPops™ after administration of glibenclamide at different dose levels reasonably described total bile acid concentrations, unconjugated CDCA, conjugated

CDCA (sum of taurine and glycine conjugates), and unconjugated LCA concentrations observed from *in vivo* studies [93]. Results from these *in vivo* rat experiments confirmed the simulated bile acid profile after drug administration and also reemphasize the necessity of population analysis due to the large inter-individual variability in bile acid disposition in the presence of bile acid transport inhibitors.

Construction of a systems pharmacology model revealed that while much is understood qualitatively about bile acid homeostasis, quantitative information essential to the construction of a mechanistic model is still lacking. A sensitivity analysis using human and rat bile acid SimPops™ suggested that the most influential parameters affecting the magnitude of changes in intrahepatic bile acid concentrations after administration of a bile acid transport inhibitor are BSEP expression levels, the rate of intestinal synthesis of LCA, and the magnitude of FXR-mediated regulation on enzymes and transporters [93]. The systems pharmacology modeling revealed important data gaps, facilitated prioritization of knowledge gaps, and thus helped guide experimentation.

One of the important data gaps identified during model construction was the toxicity of bile acids in relation to their hepatic accumulation. It has been widely accepted that intracellular accumulation of BAs results in hepatotoxicity, but, surprisingly, the relationship between hepatocellular BA accumulation and toxicity has not been assessed quantitatively. In order to fill this data gap and link bile acid kinetics to toxicity in DILIsym®, *in vitro* studies were undertaken in sandwich-cultured hepatocytes (SCH) from human, rat, mouse, and dog [102]. SCH were incubated with concentration ranges of LCA or CDCA, and intracellular concentrations of LCA, CDCA, and their conjugates as well as ATP levels were measured at predetermined time points. As described in the previous section, depletion of intracellular ATP results in necrotic cell death [3] and cellular ATP levels are important determinant of necrotic cell death in the current version of DILIsym®. The relationship between intracellular unconjugated LCA or CDCA and ATP levels were parameterized using these *in vitro* data and incorporated into DILIsym®.

The bile acid-mediated hepatotoxicity module consists of submodels representing disposition of drugs and metabolites, physiology and pathophysiology of bile acids, the hepatocyte life cycle, and biomarkers of liver injury (e.g., serum ALT and bilirubin) (Figure 9.3). Hepatic and systemic disposition of drugs/metabolites are simulated using a PBPK model. The bile acid homeostasis model represents hepatobiliary disposition and enterohepatic recirculation of LCA and CDCA species and all other (bulk) bile acids as already described [93]. Using bile acid transport inhibition constants of drugs/metabolites (e.g., K_i and IC_{50}) measured *in vitro*, altered bile acid disposition is simulated. Increased hepatocellular accumulation of bile acids inhibits hepatic ATP synthesis and decreases intracellular ATP concentrations (cellular ATP model), leading to necrotic cell death (hepatocyte life cycle model) and elevations in serum biomarkers of hepatocellular injury and function (e.g., ALT, AST, and bilirubin) (biomarker model). Loss of hepatocytes will subsequently influence drug and bile acid disposition

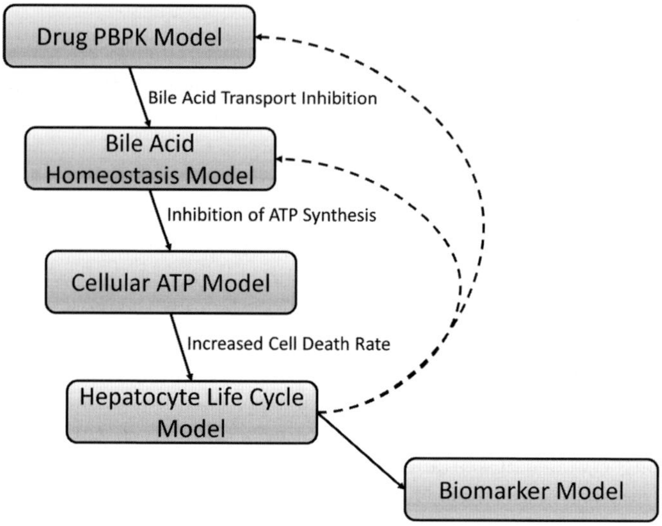

Figure 9.3 Diagram of the bile acid-mediated hepatotoxicity module. (Reprinted with permission from Ref. [103].)

(dashed lines in Figure 9.3), allowing dynamic interaction between kinetics and toxicity mechanisms.

The bile acid-mediated hepatotoxicity module was validated using several exemplar compounds, including troglitazone (TGZ) and bosentan. Pioglitazone and telmisartan, bile acid transport inhibitors that do not induce hepatotoxicity, were employed as negative controls. These exemplar drugs will be discussed in more detail in the following sections.

9.3
Examples of Bile Acid-Mediated Toxicity Module

9.3.1
Troglitazone and Pioglitazone

TGZ was the first thiazolidinedione class drug approved for the treatment of type 2 diabetes. During the clinical trials, serum ALT elevations >3× upper limit of normal (ULN) appeared in about 2% of patients and two cases of jaundice were reported [104], all of which were resolved without serious clinical complications. However, liver failure cases related to TGZ treatment were reported postmarketing, and a black box warning was added to the TGZ label. After the approval of rosiglitazone and pioglitazone, drugs from the same class that exhibited less hepatotoxicity concerns, TGZ was withdrawn from the market. Rosiglitazone was withdrawn due to cardiovascular concerns, but pioglitazone is still used in diabetic patients.

TGZ is known to be one of the most toxic drugs approved, but the mechanisms of hepatotoxicity still remain controversial. One proposed mechanism is inhibition of bile acid transport by TGZ and its major metabolite TGZ sulfate (TS). *In vitro* vesicular transport assays demonstrated that TGZ and TS are potent inhibitors of BSEP, MRP4, and NTCP [83,105,106]. However, the relationship between bile acid transport inhibition and *in vivo* hepatotoxicity has not been evaluated. Thus, DILIsym® was employed to evaluate the hepatotoxic potential of TGZ by bile acid transport inhibition using these *in vitro* data (i.e., inhibition constants of TGZ and TS for bile acid transporters) as model inputs. A PBPK model was developed to describe the disposition of TGZ and TS in humans. The PBPK model of TGZ consisted of a central compartment representing the blood, as well as hepatic and extrahepatic tissues (e.g., muscle and gut) linked to the central compartment by blood flow. Transporter-mediated hepatic uptake and hepatic metabolism (sulfation and glucuronidation) of TGZ were parameterized using available literature data [107,108]. TS disposition was described using a semi-PBPK model that consisted of a central blood compartment, hepatic tissue, and extrahepatic tissues lumped into one compartment. TS was excreted predominantly into bile; TS biliary clearance was parameterized using available *in vitro* data [109].

The low incidence of DILI in TGZ-treated patients indicates that just a subset of treated patients is susceptible to DILI. Consistent with these clinical observations, DILIsym® simulations based on the average baseline human data did not show hepatotoxicity after TGZ administration. Thus, TGZ-mediated hepatotoxicity was simulated in the virtual human population (SimPops™) that included variability in key model parameters describing bile acid and drug disposition [103].

Simulations based on TGZ-mediated bile acid effects adequately predicted the incidence and delayed presentation of TGZ hepatotoxicity in humans (Table 9.2) [103]. In the human SimPops™ orally administered 200–600 mg/day TGZ for 6 months, the incidence of elevated serum ALT >3× ULN was 0.3–5.1%, and the time to peak ALT was 116 ± 60 days [103]. These simulated values were comparable with those observed during the clinical trials: 1.9% and 147 ± 86 days, respectively [104]. Incorporation of population variability into the mechanistic model allowed prediction of rare incidences of hepatotoxicity. Delayed presentation is one of the idiosyncratic characteristics of TGZ-mediated hepatotoxicity, but underlying mechanisms have not been identified. Systems pharmacology modeling suggested that delay in buildup of toxic bile acids in hepatocytes due to FXR-mediated feedback regulation and competitive inhibition of biliary excretion by TGZ and TS might be responsible, in part, for delayed hepatotoxicity. Altogether, these results suggest that bile acid inhibition by TGZ and TS is a plausible mechanism that contributed to TGZ-mediated hepatotoxicity *in vivo* in humans.

Preclinical toxicity testing is a prerequisite to clinical studies. However, animal models (e.g., rats) appear to be less susceptible to bile acid-mediated hepatotoxicity compared with humans, potentially due to species differences in toxic bile acid composition, metabolism, and/or transport of bile acids [110–114].

Table 9.2 Summary of troglitazone (TGZ)-mediated hepatotoxicity in human SimPops™ and clinical trials.

	Simulations[a)]			Clinical trials	
	TGZ 200 mg ($n = 331$)	TGZ 400 mg ($n = 331$)	TGZ 600 mg ($n = 331$)	TGZ 200–600 mg ($n = 2510$)	Placebo ($n = 475$)
ALT > 3× ULN (%)[b)]	0.3	3.0	5.1	1.9	0.6
ALT > 5× ULN (%)[b)]	0.3	1.8	4.2	1.7	N/A
ALT > 8× ULN (%)[b)]	0.3	1.8	3.6	0.9	0
ALT > 30× ULN (%)[b)]	0	0.6	0.9	0.2	0
Time to peak ALT (days)[c)]	180[d)]	118 ± 61	111 ± 61	147 ± 86	N/A
Total bilirubin > 2× (%)[e)]	0.3	1.8	3.6	N/A	N/A
Hy's law cases (%)	0.3	1.8	3.6	N/A	N/A
Jaundice (%)	N/A	N/A	N/A	0.08	0

Reprinted from Ref. [103].
N/A: not available.
a) Each dose level was simulated for 6 months.
b) ULN was 34 U/l in the clinical trials. Baseline serum ALT in human SimPops™ was 30 U/L.
c) Mean ± SD
d) SD was not calculated because only one individual showed ALT elevation > 3× ULN.
e) Baseline serum total bilirubin in human SimPops™ was 0.55 mg/dl.

TGZ-mediated hepatotoxicity was not detected during standard preclinical testing. The bile acid pool in rats consists of more hydrophilic and less toxic trihydroxy bile acids such as cholic acid and muricholic acid [115], whereas more hydrophobic bile acids such as CDCA are abundant in humans. LCA, the most toxic bile acid, is detoxified by 6β-hydroxylation in rats, whereas LCA is predominantly sulfated in humans [114]. To explore species differences in bile acid-mediated TGZ hepatotoxicity, a PBPK model in rats and a rat bile acid homeostasis model were constructed using available rat-specific data, and also a rat SimPops™ was constructed. Simulations demonstrated that no hepatotoxicity was predicted in rat SimPops™ administered with 5 mg/kg (equivalent to the clinical dose) and 25 mg/kg TGZ [103]. Lack of hepatotoxicity in rats was due to lower accumulation of toxic bile acids (CDCA and LCA species in the current version of DILIsym®) in rats compared with humans. These results demonstrated that systems pharmacology modeling incorporating species-specific bile acid and TGZ disposition correctly predicted species differences in TGZ hepatotoxicity.

In contrast to TGZ pioglitazone, another thiazolidinedione class drug, did not increase serum ALT during clinical trials, and clinically apparent liver injury related to pioglitazone treatment is very rare [116]. As a result, pioglitazone is still used in the clinic to treat type 2 diabetes. Interestingly, pioglitazone was also identified as a potent BSEP inhibitor in vesicular transport assays, and has been shown to inhibit the basolateral efflux transporter MRP4 [83]. Steady-state plasma concentrations of TGZ and pioglitazone are comparable (0.939 versus 0.935 μM) [83] and, thus, the hepatotoxic potential of these compounds cannot be differentiated using *in vitro* transporter inhibition and systemic exposure data. In order to translate these data to *in vivo* hepatotoxicity predictions, dynamic changes in the systemic as well as the hepatic exposure of these drugs/metabolites and the complex physiology of bile acid homeostasis (i.e., enterohepatic recirculation and feedback regulation) need to be considered. Therefore, the hepatotoxic potential of pioglitazone due to bile acid transport inhibition was evaluated using DILIsym®. To this end, the pioglitazone PBPK model was constructed, and bile acid inhibition constants obtained from *in vitro* studies were used to simulate altered bile acid disposition and hepatotoxicity after pioglitazone administration. The other submodels (e.g., bile acid homeostasis model, cellular ATP model, hepatocyte life cycle model, and biomarker model) were the same as for the TGZ simulations. Simulations revealed that no hepatotoxicity was predicted in SimPops™ treated with clinical doses of pioglitazone (15, 30, or 45 mg/day) [103]. The lack of hepatotoxicity was explained by the low hepatic exposure of pioglitazone due to extensive hepatic metabolism. In summary, systems pharmacology modeling that integrates physiological information and experimental data was able to predict the differential hepatotoxicity between TGZ and pioglitazone.

9.3.2 Bosentan and Telmisartan

Bosentan is an endothelin receptor agonist that is used for the treatment of pulmonary arterial hypertension. In clinical trials, bosentan caused ALT elevations greater than threefold in 8–18% of patients taking 1000 mg/day, either 500 mg b.i.d. or 1000 mg q.d [117]. Bosentan currently carries a black box warning for hepatotoxicity. Bosentan and its minor metabolite both inhibit BSEP noncompetitively [117]. Furthermore, bosentan inhibits bile acid uptake, although it does so differently in rats and in humans. Researchers have proposed that this difference in bile acid uptake inhibition potency is responsible for the observed species differences in toxicity; bosentan does not cause hepatotoxicity in rats [111,118]. Therefore, bosentan was an ideal test compound for the prediction of species differences in bile acid-mediated hepatotoxicity in DILIsym®.

A bosentan PBPK model was constructed within DILIsym® using available literature data in humans and *in vivo* rat data from the DILI-sim Initiative collaborators [119,120]. Due to the potential contribution of a minor metabolite to BSEP inhibition, both major and minor metabolites of bosentan were included in the PBPK model. Furthermore, bosentan was shown to be a substrate of hepatic uptake transporters [121]; this was included in the PBPK model as well. Simulations were performed on the bile acid human and rat SimPops™ included within DILIsym® version 3A, and toxicity was assessed by the elevation of serum ALT threefold above the model baseline value. The human SimPops™ were given 500 mg b.i.d. bosentan for 30 days; doses for the rat SimPops™ ranged up to 50 mg/kg per day of bosentan for a duration of 30 days.

The results of the bosentan simulations are shown in Table 9.3. After bosentan treatment in the human SimPops™, one individual developed ALT

Table 9.3 SimPops™ simulation results for bosentan and telmisartan.

Drug	Species	Dose (mg/day)	SimPops™	Bile acid transport inhibition	Number of individuals with ALT > 3× baseline	Percentage of individuals with ALT > 3× baseline
Bosentan	Human	1000	Variability in bile acid disposition	Noncompetitive BSEP inhibition	1	0.302%
			Variability in bile acid disposition, bosentan PK, and toxicity	Noncompetitive BSEP inhibition	3	0.906%
			Variability in bile acid disposition 10× lower metabolism	Noncompetitive BSEP inhibition	8	2.42%
			Variability in bile acid disposition	Noncompetitive inhibition of BSEP and basolateral efflux transporters	4	1.21%
	Rat	12.5	Variability in bile acid disposition	Noncompetitive BSEP inhibition	0	0
Telmisartan	Human	50	Variability in bile acid disposition	Competitive BSEP inhibition	0	0
		50	Variability in bile acid disposition	Noncompetitive BSEP inhibition	0	0
		3000	Variability in bile acid disposition	Noncompetitive BSEP inhibition	0	0
		12 000	Variability in bile acid disposition	Noncompetitive BSEP inhibition	1	0.302%

elevations (0.30%). When PK variability was included in the human SimPops™, three individuals developed ALT elevations, and when a genetic polymorphism that impairs bosentan metabolism was modeled, eight individuals developed ALT elevations [120]. While the model successfully predicts that bosentan is a potentially hepatotoxic molecule, the simulated incidence rate of bosentan hepatotoxicity is well below that observed in the clinic.

No individual in the rat SimPops™ developed toxicity, which is consistent with preclinical observations. In order to determine whether the species difference in uptake inhibition was an important factor in the differential toxicity [111], simulations were performed in the rat SimPops™ that removed the bile acid uptake inhibition from the rat model altogether. There was no toxicity predicted by SimPops™ using this model either, suggesting that species difference in the bile acid pool, rather than difference in the uptake inhibition potency, is the dominant factor in explaining the differential toxicity of bosentan in humans and rats.

Telmisartan, an antihypertensive with a low BSEP IC_{50} but with no clinically observed hepatotoxicity liability [83], served as a negative control for our model. The PBPK model for telmisartan was optimized using data available in the literature [122]. The human SimPops™ did not predict toxicity at clinically relevant, once-daily doses (40–80 mg/day), which is in agreement with clinical observations. Increasing doses of telmisartan were also simulated (listed in Table 9.3), and an unrealistically large dose of telmisartan was required to cause toxicity in DILIsym® [120].

A closer look at the mechanistic information available within DILIsym® reveals the true scope of the difference between bosentan and telmisartan. Figure 9.4 shows the minimum average liver ATP of each individual in the human SimPops™ after bosentan (a) and telmisartan (b) dosing. While only one individual in the bosentan-treated SimPops™ lost enough ATP for ALT to rise significantly, many more individuals are suffering some loss in ATP from the baseline value. These individuals might be susceptible to DILI in the presence of additional risk factors (e.g., compromised mitochondrial function due to disease

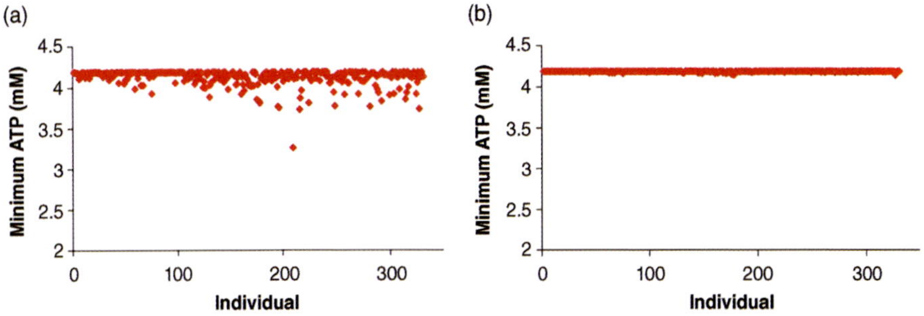

Figure 9.4 Minimum average liver ATP for each individual in the human bile acid SimPops™ after simulated dosing with clinically relevant doses of 1000 mg/day bosentan (a) and 50 mg/day telmisartan (b). (Reprinted with permission from Ref. [120].)

state or coadministered drugs). In contrast, ATP loss in the telmisartan-treated SimPops™ was barely discernable. The difference between the toxic bosentan and the nontoxic telmisartan is clearer here than it would be by simply looking at ALT elevation results. This demonstrates the power of the mechanistic information obtained from DILIsym® simulations that provide context to potentially ambiguous simulation results.

9.4 Conclusions and Future Directions

DILI has a variety of clinical presentations and is mediated by multiple mechanisms. To accurately predict hepatotoxic potential of drugs, perturbation of the biological systems by the drug at multiple sites needs to be understood. Once each perturbation is characterized quantitatively, systems pharmacology modeling can help systematically integrate these data to predict *in vivo* hepatotoxicity. In this chapter, DILIsym®, a systems pharmacology model of DILI, was introduced as an example of a modeling approach. Applications of DILIsym® described in this chapter showed that systems pharmacology modeling can be useful to predict hepatotoxic potential of novel compounds based on *in vitro* and *in vivo* data, which shows how the compound interacts with the relevant biological processes incorporated in the model. As shown in the case of TGZ, systems pharmacology modeling can also illuminate the underlying mechanisms of hepatotoxicity, when unexpected DILI is detected. The TGZ case also demonstrated that rare DILI can be predicted by incorporation of population variability in the mechanistic model. Simulations of hepatotoxic potential of drugs across different species may provide insights into why different species respond differently to the same drug as shown with MP and TGZ. Although it was not discussed in detail in this chapter, systems pharmacology modeling can also be employed in biomarker interpretation. As an example, DILIsym® was used to predict the level of hepatocyte loss after administration of entolimod, a toll-like receptor-5 agonist in development to treat potentially lethal whole-body irradiation, based on the serum ALT time profile data [123].

It is important to point out that construction of systems pharmacology models invariably involves approximation and simplification of the biological system, which may limit accurate predictions of hepatotoxicity. Thus, systems pharmacology models should be considered useful, but not perfect tools to aid in decision-making during drug development. Also, validity of model predictions depends largely on the quality of data used to develop the model. As pointed out multiple times in this chapter, gaps in our knowledge about the biology of DILI may reduce model validity. However, as described in Section 9.2.4, construction of systems pharmacology models facilitates the identification and prioritization of data gaps, which can help guide experimentation. Data generated from these new experiments will, in turn, be employed to refine the model. This iterative process will help expand current knowledge and improve our ability to predict and prevent DILI.

References

1 Lee, W.M. (2003) Drug-induced hepatotoxicity. *The New England Journal of Medicine*, **349**, 474–485.

2 Bhattacharya, S., Shoda, L.K., Zhang, Q., Woods, C.G., Howell, B.A., Siler, S.Q., Woodhead, J.L., Yang, Y., McMullen, P., Watkins, P.B., and Andersen, M.E. (2012) Modeling drug- and chemical-induced hepatotoxicity with systems biology approaches. *Frontiers in Physiology*, **3**, 462.

3 Nieminen, A.L., Saylor, A.K., Herman, B., and Lemasters, J.J. (1994) ATP depletion rather than mitochondrial depolarization mediates hepatocyte killing after metabolic inhibition. *The American Journal of Physiology*, **267**, C67–C74.

4 Lee, W.M. (2008) Acetaminophen-related acute liver failure in the United States. *Hepatology Research*, **38** (Suppl. 1), S3–S8.

5 Burke, A.S., MacMillan-Crow, L.A., and Hinson, J.A. (2010) Reactive nitrogen species in acetaminophen-induced mitochondrial damage and toxicity in mouse hepatocytes. *Chemical Research in Toxicology*, **23**, 1286–1292.

6 Cover, C., Mansouri, A., Knight, T.R., Bajt, M.L., Lemasters, J.J., Pessayre, D., and Jaeschke, H. (2005) Peroxynitrite-induced mitochondrial and endonuclease-mediated nuclear DNA damage in acetaminophen hepatotoxicity. *The Journal of Pharmacology and Experimental Therapeutics*, **315**, 879–887.

7 Knight, T.R., Ho, Y.S., Farhood, A., and Jaeschke, H. (2002) Peroxynitrite is a critical mediator of acetaminophen hepatotoxicity in murine livers: protection by glutathione. *The Journal of Pharmacology and Experimental Therapeutics*, **303**, 468–475.

8 Hinson, J.A., Pike, S.L., Pumford, N.R., and Mayeux, P.R. (1998) Nitrotyrosine–protein adducts in hepatic centrilobular areas following toxic doses of acetaminophen in mice. *Chemical Research in Toxicology*, **11**, 604–607.

9 Bajt, M.L., Knight, T.R., Lemasters, J.J., and Jaeschke, H. (2004) Acetaminophen-induced oxidant stress and cell injury in cultured mouse hepatocytes: protection by *N*-acetyl cysteine. *Toxicological Sciences*, **80**, 343–349.

10 Ghosh, J., Das, J., Manna, P., and Sil, P.C. (2010) Arjunolic acid, a triterpenoid saponin, prevents acetaminophen (APAP)-induced liver and hepatocyte injury via the inhibition of APAP bioactivation and JNK-mediated mitochondrial protection. *Free Radical Biology & Medicine*, **48**, 535–553.

11 Liu, Z.X., Han, D., Gunawan, B., and Kaplowitz, N. (2006) Neutrophil depletion protects against murine acetaminophen hepatotoxicity. *Hepatology*, **43**, 1220–1230.

12 Hanawa, N., Shinohara, M., Saberi, B., Gaarde, W.A., Han, D., and Kaplowitz, N. (2008) Role of JNK translocation to mitochondria leading to inhibition of mitochondria bioenergetics in acetaminophen-induced liver injury. *The Journal of Biological Chemistry*, **283**, 13565–13577.

13 Woodhead, J.L., Howell, B.A., Yang, Y., Harrill, A.H., Clewell, H.J., III, Andersen, M.E., Siler, S.Q., and Watkins, P.B. (2012) An analysis of *N*-acetylcysteine treatment for acetaminophen overdose using a systems model of drug-induced liver injury. *The Journal of Pharmacology and Experimental Therapeutics*, **342**, 529–540.

14 Rumack, B.H., Peterson, R.C., Koch, G.G., and Amara, I.A. (1981) Acetaminophen overdose. 662 cases with evaluation of oral acetylcysteine treatment. *Archives of Internal Medicine*, **141**, 380–385.

15 Heard, K.J. (2008) Acetylcysteine for acetaminophen poisoning. *The New England Journal of Medicine*, **359**, 285–292.

16 Woo, O.F., Mueller, P.D., Olson, K.R., Anderson, I.B., and Kim, S.Y. (2000) Shorter duration of oral *N*-acetylcysteine therapy for acute acetaminophen overdose. *Annals of Emergency Medicine*, **35**, 363–368.

17 Howell, B.A., Siler, S.Q., and Watkins, P.B. (2014) Use of a systems model of drug-induced liver injury (DILIsym(®)) to elucidate the mechanistic differences

between acetaminophen and its less-toxic isomer, AMAP, in mice. *Toxicology Letters*, **226**, 163–172.

18 Streeter, A.J., Bjorge, S.M., Axworthy, D.B., Nelson, S.D., and Baillie, T.A. (1984) The microsomal metabolism and site of covalent binding to protein of 3′-hydroxyacetanilide, a nonhepatotoxic positional isomer of acetaminophen. *Drug Metabolism and Disposition: The Biological Fate of Chemicals*, **12**, 565–576.

19 Rashed, M.S., Myers, T.G., and Nelson, S.D. (1990) Hepatic protein arylation, glutathione depletion, and metabolite profiles of acetaminophen and a non-hepatotoxic regioisomer, 3′-hydroxyacetanilide, in the mouse. *Drug Metabolism and Disposition: The Biological Fate of Chemicals*, **18**, 765–770.

20 Crofton, R.W., Diesselhoff-den Dulk, M.M., and van Furth, R. (1978) The origin, kinetics, and characteristics of the Kupffer cells in the normal steady state. *The Journal of Experimental Medicine*, **148**, 1–17.

21 Bouwens, L., Knook, D.L., and Wisse, E. (1986) Local proliferation and extrahepatic recruitment of liver macrophages (Kupffer cells) in partial-body irradiated rats. *Journal of Leukocyte Biology*, **39**, 687–697.

22 Guilbert, L.J., Winkler-Lowen, B., Smith, A., Branch, D.R., and Garcia-Lloret, M. (1993) Analysis of the synergistic stimulation of mouse macrophage proliferation by macrophage colony-stimulating factor (CSF-1) and tumor necrosis factor alpha (TNF-alpha). *Journal of Leukocyte Biology*, **54**, 65–72.

23 van Furth, R., Elzenga-Claasen, I., van Schadewijk-Nieuwstad, M., Diesselhoff-den Dulk, M.M., Toivonen, H., and Rytomaa, T. (1987) Cell kinetic analysis of a murine macrophage cell line. *European Journal of Cell Biology*, **44**, 93–96.

24 van Furth, R. and Sluiter, W. (1986) Distribution of blood monocytes between a marginating and a circulating pool. *The Journal of Experimental Medicine*, **163**, 474–479.

25 Yamamoto, T., Naito, M., Moriyama, H., Umezu, H., Matsuo, H., Kiwada, H., and Arakawa, M. (1996) Repopulation of murine Kupffer cells after intravenous administration of liposome-encapsulated dichloromethylene diphosphonate. *The American Journal of Pathology*, **149**, 1271–1286.

26 Scaffidi, P., Misteli, T., and Bianchi, M.E. (2002) Release of chromatin protein HMGB1 by necrotic cells triggers inflammation. *Nature*, **418**, 191–195.

27 Bell, C.W., Jiang, W., Reich, C.F., III, and Pisetsky, D.S. (2006) The extracellular release of HMGB1 during apoptotic cell death. *The American Journal of Physiology: Cell Physiology*, **291**, C1318–C1325.

28 Antoine, D.J., Jenkins, R.E., Dear, J.W., Williams, D.P., McGill, M.R., Sharpe, M.R., Craig, D.G., Simpson, K.J., Jaeschke, H., and Park, B.K. (2012) Molecular forms of HMGB1 and keratin-18 as mechanistic biomarkers for mode of cell death and prognosis during clinical acetaminophen hepatotoxicity. *Journal of Hepatology*, **56**, 1070–1079.

29 Yang, R., Zhang, S., Cotoia, A., Oksala, N., Zhu, S., and Tenhunen, J. (2012) High mobility group B1 impairs hepatocyte regeneration in acetaminophen hepatotoxicity. *BMC Gastroenterology*, **12**, 45.

30 Chen, G.Y., Tang, J., Zheng, P., and Liu, Y. (2009) CD24 and Siglec-10 selectively repress tissue damage-induced immune responses. *Science*, **323**, 1722–1725.

31 Antoine, D.J., Williams, D.P., Kipar, A., Laverty, H., and Park, B.K. (2010) Diet restriction inhibits apoptosis and HMGB1 oxidation and promotes inflammatory cell recruitment during acetaminophen hepatotoxicity. *Molecular Medicine (Cambridge, Mass.)*, **16**, 479–490.

32 Blazka, M.E., Elwell, M.R., Holladay, S.D., Wilson, R.E., and Luster, M.I. (1996) Histopathology of acetaminophen-induced liver changes: role of interleukin 1 alpha and tumor necrosis factor alpha. *Toxicologic Pathology*, **24**, 181–189.

33 Blazka, M.E., Wilmer, J.L., Holladay, S.D., Wilson, R.E., and Luster, M.I. (1995)

Role of proinflammatory cytokines in acetaminophen hepatotoxicity. *Toxicology and Applied Pharmacology*, **133**, 43–52.

34 Ishida, Y., Kondo, T., Tsuneyama, K., Lu, P., Takayasu, T., and Mukaida, N. (2004) The pathogenic roles of tumor necrosis factor receptor p55 in acetaminophen-induced liver injury in mice. *Journal of Leukocyte Biology*, **75**, 59–67.

35 Simpson, K.J., Lukacs, N.W., McGregor, A.H., Harrison, D.J., Strieter, R.M., and Kunkel, S.L. (2000) Inhibition of tumour necrosis factor alpha does not prevent experimental paracetamol-induced hepatic necrosis. *The Journal of Pathology*, **190**, 489–494.

36 Chen, Z.Z., Wang, Z.L., Deng, C.Y., Zheng, H., Wang, X.H., Ma, L., Ye, X., Ma, Y.H., Xie, C.F., Chen, L.J., and Wei, Y.Q. (2012) (*Z*)-5-(4-methoxybenzylidene)thiazolidine-2,4-dione protects rats from carbon tetrachloride-induced liver injury and fibrogenesis. *World Journal of Gastroenterology*, **18**, 654–661.

37 Deng, J.S., Chang, Y.C., Wen, C.L., Liao, J.C., Hou, W.C., Amagaya, S., Huang, S.S., and Huang, G.J. (2012) Hepatoprotective effect of the ethanol extract of *Vitis thunbergii* on carbon tetrachloride-induced acute hepatotoxicity in rats through anti-oxidative activities. *Journal of Ethnopharmacology*, **142**, 795–803.

38 Huang, G.J., Deng, J.S., Chiu, C.S., Liao, J.C., Hsieh, W.T., Sheu, M.J., and Wu, C.H. (2012) Hispolon protects against acute liver damage in the rat by inhibiting lipid peroxidation, proinflammatory cytokine, and oxidative stress and downregulating the expressions of iNOS, COX-2, and MMP-9. *Evidence-Based Complementary and Alternative Medicine*, **2012**, 480714.

39 Campo, G.M., Avenoso, A., Campo, S., Ferlazzo, A.M., Micali, C., Zanghi, L., and Calatroni, A. (2004) Hyaluronic acid and chondroitin-4-sulphate treatment reduces damage in carbon tetrachloride-induced acute rat liver injury. *Life Sciences*, **74**, 1289–1305.

40 Lloyd, R.S. and Triger, D.R. (1975) Studies on hepatic uptake of antigen: III. Studies of liver macrophage function in normal rats and following carbon tetrachloride administration. *Immunology*, **29**, 253–263.

41 Wu, Z.M., Wen, T., Tan, Y.F., Liu, Y., Ren, F., and Wu, H. (2007) Effects of salvianolic acid A on oxidative stress and liver injury induced by carbon tetrachloride in rats. *Basic and Clinical Pharmacology and Toxicology*, **100**, 115–120.

42 Quan, J., Piao, L., Wang, X., Li, T., and Yin, X. (2009) Rossicaside B protects against carbon tetrachloride-induced hepatotoxicity in mice. *Basic and Clinical Pharmacology and Toxicology*, **105**, 380–386.

43 Quan, J., Piao, L., Xu, H., Li, T., and Yin, X. (2009) Protective effect of iridoid glucosides from *Boschniakia rossica* on acute liver injury induced by carbon tetrachloride in rats. *Bioscience, Biotechnology, and Biochemistry*, **73**, 849–854.

44 Nakamoto, N., Tada, S., Kameyama, K., Kitamura, K., Kurita, S., Saito, Y., Saito, H., and Ishii, H. (2003) A free radical scavenger, edaravone, attenuates steatosis and cell death via reducing inflammatory cytokine production in rat acute liver injury. *Free Radical Research*, **37**, 849–859.

45 Quan, J., Yin, X., and Xu, H. (2011) *Boschniakia rossica* prevents the carbon tetrachloride-induced hepatotoxicity in rat. *Experimental and Toxicologic Pathology*, **63**, 53–59.

46 Ai, G., Liu, Q., Hua, W., Huang, Z., and Wang, D. (2013) Hepatoprotective evaluation of the total flavonoids extracted from flowers of *Abelmoschus manihot* (L.) Medic: *in vitro* and *in vivo* studies. *Journal of Ethnopharmacology*, **146**, 794–802.

47 Jiang, W., Gao, M., Sun, S., Bi, A., Xin, Y., Han, X., Wang, L., Yin, Z., and Luo, L. (2012) Protective effect of L-theanine on carbon tetrachloride-induced acute liver injury in mice. *Biochemical and Biophysical Research Communications*, **422**, 344–350.

48 Kim, H.Y., Park, J., Lee, K.H., Lee, D.U., Kwak, J.H., Kim, Y.S., and Lee, S.M.

(2011) Ferulic acid protects against carbon tetrachloride-induced liver injury in mice. *Toxicology*, **282**, 104–111.

49 Kiso, K., Ueno, S., Fukuda, M., Ichi, I., Kobayashi, K., Sakai, T., Fukui, K., and Kojo, S. (2012) The role of Kupffer cells in carbon tetrachloride intoxication in mice. *Biological & Pharmaceutical Bulletin*, **35**, 980–983.

50 Knockaert, L., Berson, A., Ribault, C., Prost, P.E., Fautrel, A., Pajaud, J., Lepage, S., Lucas-Clerc, C., Begue, J.M., Fromenty, B., and Robin, M.A. (2012) Carbon tetrachloride-mediated lipid peroxidation induces early mitochondrial alterations in mouse liver. *Laboratory Investigation; A Journal of Technical Methods and Pathology*, **92**, 396–410.

51 Lee, C.H., Park, S.W., Kim, Y.S., Kang, S.S., Kim, J.A., Lee, S.H., and Lee, S.M. (2007) Protective mechanism of glycyrrhizin on acute liver injury induced by carbon tetrachloride in mice. *Biological & Pharmaceutical Bulletin*, **30**, 1898–1904.

52 Louis, H., Van Laethem, J.L., Wu, W., Quertinmont, E., Degraef, C., Van den Berg, K., Demols, A., Goldman, M., Le Moine, O., Geerts, A., and Deviere, J. (1998) Interleukin-10 controls neutrophilic infiltration, hepatocyte proliferation, and liver fibrosis induced by carbon tetrachloride in mice. *Hepatology*, **28**, 1607–1615.

53 Morio, L.A., Chiu, H., Sprowles, K.A., Zhou, P., Heck, D.E., Gordon, M.K., and Laskin, D.L. (2001) Distinct roles of tumor necrosis factor-alpha and nitric oxide in acute liver injury induced by carbon tetrachloride in mice. *Toxicology and Applied Pharmacology*, **172**, 44–51.

54 Yamada, Y. and Fausto, N. (1998) Deficient liver regeneration after carbon tetrachloride injury in mice lacking type 1 but not type 2 tumor necrosis factor receptor. *The American Journal of Pathology*, **152**, 1577–1589.

55 Bruccoleri, A., Gallucci, R., Germolec, D.R., Blackshear, P., Simeonova, P., Thurman, R.G., and Luster, M.I. (1997) Induction of early-immediate genes by tumor necrosis factor alpha contribute to liver repair following chemical-induced hepatotoxicity. *Hepatology*, **25**, 133–141.

56 Minamino, T., Ito, Y., Ohkubo, H., Hosono, K., Suzuki, T., Sato, T., Ae, T., Shibuya, A., Sakagami, H., Narumiya, S., Koizumi, W., and Majima, M. (2012) Thromboxane A(2) receptor signaling promotes liver tissue repair after toxic injury through the enhancement of macrophage recruitment. *Toxicology and Applied Pharmacology*, **259**, 104–114.

57 Karlmark, K.R., Weiskirchen, R., Zimmermann, H.W., Gassler, N., Ginhoux, F., Weber, C., Merad, M., Luedde, T., Trautwein, C., and Tacke, F. (2009) Hepatic recruitment of the inflammatory Gr1+ monocyte subset upon liver injury promotes hepatic fibrosis. *Hepatology*, **50**, 261–274.

58 Matsumoto, A., Kanai, T., Mikami, Y., Chu, P.S., Nakamoto, N., Ebinuma, H., Saito, H., Sato, T., Yagita, H., and Hibi, T. (2013) IL-22-producing RORγt-dependent innate lymphoid cells play a novel protective role in murine acute hepatitis. *PLoS One*, **8**, e62853.

59 Marra, F., DeFranco, R., Grappone, C., Parola, M., Milani, S., Leonarduzzi, G., Pastacaldi, S., Wenzel, U.O., Pinzani, M., Dianzani, M.U., Laffi, G., and Gentilini, P. (1999) Expression of monocyte chemotactic protein-1 precedes monocyte recruitment in a rat model of acute liver injury, and is modulated by vitamin E. *Journal of Investigative Medicine*, **47**, 66–75.

60 Albano, E., Bellomo, G., Carini, R., Biasi, F., Poli, G., and Dianzani, M.U. (1985) Mechanisms responsible for carbon tetrachloride-induced perturbation of mitochondrial calcium homeostasis. *FEBS Letters*, **192**, 184–188.

61 Schulz, S., Schmitt, S., Wimmer, R., Aichler, M., Eisenhofer, S., Lichtmannegger, J., Eberhagen, C., Artmann, R., Tookos, F., Walch, A., Krappmann, D., Brenner, C., Rust, C., and Zischka, H. (2013) Progressive stages of mitochondrial destruction caused by cell toxic bile salts. *Biochimica et Biophysica Acta*, **1828**, 2121–2133.

62 Nadanaciva, S., Rana, P., Beeson, G.C., Chen, D., Ferrick, D.A., Beeson, C.C., and Will, Y. (2012) Assessment of drug-induced mitochondrial dysfunction via altered cellular respiration and acidification measured in a 96-well platform. *Journal of Bioenergetics and Biomembranes*, **44**, 421–427.

63 Yang, Y., Nadanaciva, S., Will, Y., Woodhead, J.L., Howell, B.A., Watkins, P.B., and Siler, S.Q. (2014) MITOsym™: a mechanistic, mathematical model of hepatocellular respiration and bioenergetics. *Pharmaceutical Research*, PMID: 25504454 (Epub Ahead of Print).

64 Mullen, P.J., Zahno, A., Lindinger, P., Maseneni, S., Felser, A., Krahenbuhl, S., and Brecht, K. (2011) Susceptibility to simvastatin-induced toxicity is partly determined by mitochondrial respiration and phosphorylation state of Akt. *Biochimica et Biophysica Acta*, **1813**, 2079–2087.

65 Zahno, A., Brecht, K., Morand, R., Maseneni, S., Torok, M., Lindinger, P.W., and Krahenbuhl, S. (2011) The role of CYP3A4 in amiodarone-associated toxicity on HepG2 cells. *Biochemical Pharmacology*, **81**, 432–441.

66 Shoda, L.K., Woodhead, J.L., Siler, S.Q., Watkins, P.B., and Howell, B.A. (2014) Linking physiology to toxicity using DILIsym®, a mechanistic mathematical model of drug-induced liver injury. *Biopharmaceutics & Drug Disposition*, **35**, 33–49.

67 Lionetti, V., Stanley, W.C., and Recchia, F.A. (2011) Modulating fatty acid oxidation in heart failure. *Cardiovascular Research*, **90**, 202–209.

68 Agius, L., Peak, M., and Sherratt, S.A. (1991) Differences between human, rat and guinea pig hepatocyte cultures: a comparative study of their rates of beta-oxidation and esterification of palmitate and their sensitivity to R-etomoxir. *Biochemical Pharmacology*, **42**, 1711–1715.

69 Bryson, J.M., Cooney, G.J., Wensley, V.R., Phuyal, J.L., and Caterson, I.D. (1996) The effects of the inhibition of fatty acid oxidation on pyruvate dehydrogenase complex activity in tissues of lean and obese mice. *International Journal of Obesity and Related Metabolic Disorders*, **20**, 738–744.

70 Holubarsch, C.J., Rohrbach, M., Karrasch, M., Boehm, E., Polonski, L., Ponikowski, P., and Rhein, S. (2007) A double-blind randomized multicentre clinical trial to evaluate the efficacy and safety of two doses of etomoxir in comparison with placebo in patients with moderate congestive heart failure: the ERGO (etomoxir for the recovery of glucose oxidation) study. *Clinical Science (London, England: 1979)*, **113**, 205–212.

71 Yang, Y., Woodhead, J.L., Howell, B.A., Watkins, P.B., and Siler, S.Q. (2014). Using DILIsym® and MITOsym™ to investigate *in vivo* etomoxir-induced DILI based on *in vitro* data. ASCPT 2014 Annual Meeting, March 18–22, Atlanta, GA.

72 Berson, A., Gervais, A., Cazals, D., Boyer, N., Durand, F., Bernuau, J., Marcellin, P., Degott, C., Valla, D., and Pessayre, D. (2001) Hepatitis after intravenous buprenorphine misuse in heroin addicts. *Journal of Hepatology*, **34**, 346–350.

73 Peyriere, H., Tatem, L., Bories, C., Pageaux, G.P., Blayac, J.P., and Larrey, D. (2009) Hepatitis after intravenous injection of sublingual buprenorphine in acute hepatitis C carriers: report of two cases of disappearance of viral replication after acute hepatitis. *Annals of Pharmacotherapy*, **43**, 973–977.

74 Zuin, M., Giorgini, A., Selmi, C., Battezzati, P.M., Cocchi, C.A., Crosignani, A., Benetti, A., Invernizzi, P., and Podda, M. (2009) Acute liver and renal failure during treatment with buprenorphine at therapeutic dose. *Digestive and Liver Disease*, **41**, e8–e10.

75 Petry, N.M., Bickel, W.K., Piasecki, D., Marsch, L.A., and Badger, G.J. (2000) Elevated liver enzyme levels in opioid-dependent patients with hepatitis treated with buprenorphine. *American Journal on Addictions*, **9**, 265–269.

76 Herve, S., Riachi, G., Noblet, C., Guillement, N., Tanasescu, S., Goria, O., Thuillez, C., Tranvouez, J.L., Ducrotte, P., and Lerebours, E. (2004) Acute hepatitis due to buprenorphine administration.

European Journal of Gastroenterology and Hepatology, **16**, 1033–1037.
77 Saxon, A.J., Ling, W., Hillhouse, M., Thomas, C., Hasson, A., Ang, A., Doraimani, G., Tasissa, G., Lokhnygina, Y., Leimberger, J., Bruce, R.D., McCarthy, J., Wiest, K., McLaughlin, P., Bilangi, R., Cohen, A., Woody, G., and Jacobs, P. (2013) Buprenorphine/Naloxone and methadone effects on laboratory indices of liver health: a randomized trial. *Drug and Alcohol Dependence*, **128**, 71–76.
78 Siler, S.Q. (2013) Using the DILIsym™ and MITOsym™ mathematical models to predict *in vivo* mitochondria-based DILI based on *in vitro* screening data. 246th ACS National Meeting, September 10, Indianapolis, IN.
79 Hofmann, A.F. (1999) Bile acids: the good, the bad, and the ugly. *News in Physiological Sciences*, **14**, 24–29.
80 Perez, M.J. and Briz, O. (2009) Bile-acid-induced cell injury and protection. *World Journal of Gastroenterology*, **15**, 1677–1689.
81 Maillette de Buy Wenniger, L. and Beuers, U. (2010) Bile salts and cholestasis. *Digestive and Liver Disease*, **42**, 409–418.
82 Dawson, S., Stahl, S., Paul, N., Barber, J., and Kenna, J.G. (2012) *In vitro* inhibition of the bile salt export pump correlates with risk of cholestatic drug-induced liver injury in humans. *Drug Metabolism and Disposition: The Biological Fate of Chemicals*, **40**, 130–138.
83 Morgan, R.E., van Staden, C.J., Chen, Y., Kalyanaraman, N., Kalanzi, J., Dunn, R.T., II, Afshari, C.A., and Hamadeh, H.K. (2013) A multifactorial approach to hepatobiliary transporter assessment enables improved therapeutic compound development. *Toxicological Sciences*, **136** (1), 216–241.
84 Pedersen, J.M., Matsson, P., Bergstrom, C.A., Hoogstraate, J., Noren, A., Lecluyse, E.L., and Artursson, P. (2013) Early identification of clinically relevant drug interactions with the human bile salt export pump (BSEP/ABCB11). *Toxicological Sciences*, **136**, 328–343.
85 Meier, P.J. and Stieger, B. (2002) Bile salt transporters. *Annual Review of Physiology*, **64**, 635–661.
86 Akita, H., Suzuki, H., Hirohashi, T., Takikawa, H., and Sugiyama, Y. (2002) Transport activity of human MRP3 expressed in Sf9 cells: comparative studies with rat MRP3. *Pharmaceutical Research*, **19**, 34–41.
87 Rius, M., Hummel-Eisenbeiss, J., Hofmann, A.F., and Keppler, D. (2006) Substrate specificity of human ABCC4 (MRP4)-mediated cotransport of bile acids and reduced glutathione. *The American Journal of Physiology: Gastrointestinal and Liver Physiology*, **290**, G640–G649.
88 Ballatori, N., Li, N., Fang, F., Boyer, J.L., Christian, W.V., and Hammond, C.L. (2009) OST alpha-OST beta: a key membrane transporter of bile acids and conjugated steroids. *Frontiers in Bioscience: a Journal and Virtual Library*, **14**, 2829–2844.
89 Dietschy, J.M. (1968) Mechanisms for the intestinal absorption of bile acids. *Journal of Lipid Research*, **9**, 297–309.
90 Jonker, J.W., Liddle, C., and Downes, M. (2012) FXR and PXR: potential therapeutic targets in cholestasis. *The Journal of Steroid Biochemistry and Molecular Biology*, **130**, 147–158.
91 Beilke, L.D., Aleksunes, L.M., Holland, R.D., Besselsen, D.G., Beger, R.D., Klaassen, C.D., and Cherrington, N.J. (2009) Constitutive androstane receptor-mediated changes in bile acid composition contributes to hepatoprotection from lithocholic acid-induced liver injury in mice. *Drug Metabolism and Disposition: The Biological Fate of Chemicals*, **37**, 1035–1045.
92 Uppal, H., Saini, S.P., Moschetta, A., Mu, Y., Zhou, J., Gong, H., Zhai, Y., Ren, S., Michalopoulos, G.K., Mangelsdorf, D.J., and Xie, W. (2007) Activation of LXRs prevents bile acid toxicity and cholestasis in female mice. *Hepatology*, **45**, 422–432.
93 Woodhead, J.L., Yang, K., Brouwer, K.L.R., Siler, S.Q., Stahl, S.H., Ambroso, J.L., Baker, D., Watkins, P.B., and Howell, B.A. (2014) Mechanistic modeling reveals the critical knowledge gaps in bile acid-mediated DILI. *CPT Pharmacometrics & Systems Pharmacology*, **3**, e123.

94 Trottier, J., Caron, P., Straka, R.J., and Barbier, O. (2011) Profile of serum bile acids in noncholestatic volunteers: gender-related differences in response to fenofibrate. *Clinical Pharmacology and Therapeutics*, **90**, 279–286.

95 Garcia-Canaveras, J.C., Donato, M.T., Castell, J.V., and Lahoz, A. (2012) Targeted profiling of circulating and hepatic bile acids in human, mouse, and rat using a UPLC-MRM-MS-validated method. *Journal of Lipid Research*, **53**, 2231–2241.

96 Hirohashi, T., Suzuki, H., Takikawa, H., and Sugiyama, Y. (2000) ATP-dependent transport of bile salts by rat multidrug resistance-associated protein 3 (Mrp3). *The Journal of Biological Chemistry*, **275**, 2905–2910.

97 Muller, M., Ishikawa, T., Berger, U., Klunemann, C., Lucka, L., Schreyer, A., Kannicht, C., Reutter, W., Kurz, G., and Keppler, D. (1991) ATP-dependent transport of taurocholate across the hepatocyte canalicular membrane mediated by a 110-kDa glycoprotein binding ATP and bile salt. *The Journal of Biological Chemistry*, **266**, 18920–18926.

98 Jazrawi, R.P., Pazzi, P., Petroni, M.L., Prandini, N., Paul, C., Adam, J.A., Gullini, S., and Northfield, T.C. (1995) Postprandial gallbladder motor function: refilling and turnover of bile in health and in cholelithiasis. *Gastroenterology*, **109**, 582–591.

99 Baxter, J.N., Grime, J.S., Critchley, M., and Shields, R. (1985) Relationship between gastric emptying of solids and gall bladder emptying in normal subjects. *Gut*, **26**, 342–351.

100 Jonderko, K. and Bueno, L. (1997) Effect of peripherally and centrally administered calcitonin on gallbladder emptying in dogs. *Journal of Gastroenterology*, **32**, 380–388.

101 Dijkstra, M., Kuipers, F., Smit, E.P., de Vries, J.J., Havinga, R., and Vonk, R.J. (1991) Biliary secretion of trace elements and minerals in the rat: effects of bile flow variation and diurnal rhythms. *Journal of Hepatology*, **13**, 112–119.

102 Yang, K., Woodhead, J.L., St. Claire, R., Watkins, P.B., Siler, S.Q., Howell, B.A., and Brouwer, K.L.R. (2013) The quantitative relationship between intracellular lithocholic acid and hepatotoxicity in rat; incorporation into a mechanistic model of drug-induced liver injury. *The Toxicologist*, **132**, Abstract ID #1059.

103 Yang, K., Woodhead, J.L., Watkins, P.B., Howell, B.A., and Brouwer, K.L.R. (2014) Systems pharmacology modeling predicts delayed presentation and species differences in bile acid-mediated troglitazone hepatotoxicity. *Clinical Pharmacology and Therapeutics*, **96** (5), 589–598.

104 Watkins, P.B. and Whitcomb, R.W. (1998) Hepatic dysfunction associated with troglitazone. *The New England Journal of Medicine*, **338**, 916–917.

105 Funk, C., Ponelle, C., Scheuermann, G., and Pantze, M. (2001) Cholestatic potential of troglitazone as a possible factor contributing to troglitazone-induced hepatotoxicity: *in vivo* and *in vitro* interaction at the canalicular bile salt export pump (Bsep) in the rat. *Molecular Pharmacology*, **59**, 627–635.

106 Yang, K., Yue, W., Koeck, K., Pfeifer, N.D., and Brouwer, K.L.R. (2011) Interaction of troglitazone sulfate with hepatic basolateral and canalicular transport proteins. 2011 AAPS Annual Meeting and Exposition, Washington, DC, p M1301.

107 Izumi, T., Hosiyama, K., Enomoto, S., Sasahara, K., and Sugiyama, Y. (1997) Pharmacokinetics of troglitazone, an antidiabetic agent: prediction of *in vivo* stereoselective sulfation and glucuronidation from *in vitro* data. *The Journal of Pharmacology and Experimental Therapeutics*, **280**, 1392–1400.

108 Chang, C., Pang, K.S., Swaan, P.W., and Ekins, S. (2005) Comparative pharmacophore modeling of organic anion transporting polypeptides: a meta-analysis of rat Oatp1a1 and human OATP1B1. *The Journal of Pharmacology and Experimental Therapeutics*, **314**, 533–541.

109 Lee, J.K., Marion, T.L., Abe, K., Lim, C., Pollock, G.M., and Brouwer, K.L. (2010) Hepatobiliary disposition of troglitazone

and metabolites in rat and human sandwich-cultured hepatocytes: use of Monte Carlo simulations to assess the impact of changes in biliary excretion on troglitazone sulfate accumulation. *The Journal of Pharmacology and Experimental Therapeutics*, **332**, 26–34.

110 Olson, H., Betton, G., Robinson, D., Thomas, K., Monro, A., Kolaja, G., Lilly, P., Sanders, J., Sipes, G., Bracken, W., Dorato, M., Van Deun, K., Smith, P., Berger, B., and Heller, A. (2000) Concordance of the toxicity of pharmaceuticals in humans and in animals. *Regulatory Toxicology and Pharmacology*, **32**, 56–67.

111 Leslie, E.M., Watkins, P.B., Kim, R.B., and Brouwer, K.L. (2007) Differential inhibition of rat and human Na+-dependent taurocholate cotransporting polypeptide (NTCP/SLC10A1)by bosentan: a mechanism for species differences in hepatotoxicity. *The Journal of Pharmacology and Experimental Therapeutics*, **321**, 1170–1178.

112 Herman, J.R., Dethloff, L.A., McGuire, E.J., Parker, R.F., Walsh, K.M., Gough, A.W., Masuda, H., and de la Iglesia, F.A. (2002) Rodent carcinogenicity with the thiazolidinedione antidiabetic agent troglitazone. *Toxicological Sciences*, **68**, 226–236.

113 Chiang, J.Y. (2009) Bile acids: regulation of synthesis. *Journal of Lipid Research*, **50**, 1955–66.

114 Hofmann, A.F. (2004) Detoxification of lithocholic acid, a toxic bile acid: relevance to drug hepatotoxicity. *Drug Metabolism Reviews*, **36**, 703–722.

115 Greim, H., Trulzsch, D., Czygan, P., Rudick, J., Hutterer, F., Schaffner, F., and Popper, H. (1972) Mechanism of cholestasis. 6. Bile acids in human livers with or without biliary obstruction. *Gastroenterology*, **63**, 846–850.

116 Livertox Database (2014) Pioglitazone. Available at http://livertox.nlm.nih.gov/Pioglitazone.htm (last accessed April 9, 2014).

117 Fattinger, K., Funk, C., Pantze, M., Weber, C., Reichen, J., Stieger, B., and Meier, P.J. (2001) The endothelin antagonist bosentan inhibits the canalicular bile salt export pump: a potential mechanism for hepatic adverse reactions. *Clinical Pharmacology and Therapeutics*, **69**, 223–231.

118 Ansede, J.H., Smith, W.R., Perry, C.H., St Claire, R.L., III, and Brouwer, K.R. (2010) An *in vitro* assay to assess transporter-based cholestatic hepatotoxicity using sandwich-cultured rat hepatocytes. *Drug Metabolism and Disposition: The Biological Fate of Chemicals*, **38**, 276–280.

119 Weber, C., Gasser, R., and Hopfgartner, G. (1999) Absorption, excretion, and metabolism of the endothelin receptor antagonist bosentan in healthy male subjects. *Drug Metabolism and Disposition: The Biological Fate of Chemicals*, **27**, 810–815.

120 Woodhead, J.L., Yang, K., Siler, S.Q., Watkins, P.B., Brouwer, K.L., Barton, H.A., Morgan, R.E., Qualls, C., Hamadeh, H., Buntich, S., Kalyanaraman, N., Hickman, D., Mould, A., and Howell, B.A. (2014) Exploring BSEP inhibition-mediated toxicity with a mechanistic model of drug-induced liver injury. *Frontiers in Pharmacology*, **5**, 240.

121 Menochet, K., Kenworthy, K.E., Houston, J.B., and Galetin, A. (2012) Simultaneous assessment of uptake and metabolism in rat hepatocytes: a comprehensive mechanistic model. *The Journal of Pharmacology and Experimental Therapeutics*, **341**, 2–15.

122 Stangier, J., Su, C.A., and Roth, W. (2000) Pharmacokinetics of orally and intravenously administered telmisartan in healthy young and elderly volunteers and in hypertensive patients. *The Journal of International Medical Research*, **28**, 149–167.

123 Howell, B.A., Siler, S.Q., Shoda, L.K., Yang, Y., Woodhead, J.L., and Watkins, P.B. (2014) A mechanistic model of drug-induced liver injury AIDS the interpretation of elevated liver transaminase levels in a phase I clinical trial. *CPT Pharmacometrics & Systems Pharmacology*, **3**, e98.

Section 3
Cardiovascular Side Effects

Antitargets and Drug Safety, First Edition. Edited by László Urbán, Vinod F. Patel, and Roy J. Vaz.

10
Functional Cardiac Safety Evaluation of Novel Therapeutics

Jean-Pierre Valentin, Brian Guth, Robert L. Hamlin, Pierre Lainée, Dusty Sarazan, and Matt Skinner

10.1
Introduction: What Is the Issue?

Over the last two decades, the number of new medicines being launched has fallen sharply despite significant investments in research and development [1–3]. Over the same period, nonclinical and clinical safety has remained a major cause of drug attrition. Such attrition can occur during preclinical or clinical development stages or even postapproval, resulting in withdrawal of marketed products accounting for approximately one-third of all drug discontinuation [4–9]. A recent literature review revealed that cardiovascular toxicity is the main safety reason for drug attrition in nonclinical and clinical development, serious adverse drug reactions (ADRs), and withdrawal from the marketplace [8,10]. The data indicate that phase I clinical trials are very safe, at least from a cardiovascular point of view; this may reflect the effective preclinical testing and elimination of high-risk cardiovascular safety liabilities prior to entering clinical development. However, of more concern is the identification of more subtle, but high-risk, cardiovascular events, either not detected in earlier clinical trials or initially not deemed to be biologically significant or clinically meaningful, but that emerge when drugs are administered for longer periods of time to larger patient populations [8,11–13]. Such high incidence and/or severity of cardiovascular ADRs in late-stage clinical development can lead to prescribing restrictions, additional pre- and/or postapproval monitoring, dose-limiting toxicity, or ultimately drug discontinuation or withdrawal.

Cardiovascular-related drug withdrawal has increased steadily over the last three decades (4, 24, and 44% in the 1980s, 1990s, and 2000s, respectively), and now exceeds hepatotoxicity as a cause for drug withdrawal [14]. The difference in incidence of cardiovascular-related attrition postapproval noted between Fung *et al.* [15] and Stevens and Baker [16] a decade later may reflect the increased cardiovascular attrition related to arrhythmias over the last ~15 years. Out of the 154 drugs discontinued in clinical development for cardiovascular reasons,

Antitargets and Drug Safety, First Edition. Edited by László Urbán, Vinod F. Patel, and Roy J. Vaz.

only 4% were due to QT or torsades de pointes (TdP), 23% due to non-QT type arrhythmia, and 73% due to "other" cardiovascular reasons [14].

Cardiovascular adverse events (AEs) are diverse and can be life threatening; they are observed with both cardiovascular and noncardiovascular pharmaceuticals and affect all components of the cardiovascular system, namely, the heart, blood vessels, and blood constituents. In the context of this chapter, only functional cardiovascular changes (i.e., chronotropy, inotropy, lusitropy, and blood pressure) are considered, with the exclusion of electrocardiographic side effects, and acknowledging that those changes may have structural consequences and vice versa. Cardiovascular side effects can occur after acute (i.e., single-dose administration) or chronic treatment and can be functional and/or structural in nature. Furthermore, the key role of the nervous and renal systems in modulating cardiovascular function should not be neglected.

Although a large number of therapeutic classes are associated with cardiac toxicities, in most cases they are not related to the primary pharmacological target, the therapeutic class, or the chemical class. However, this is not a general rule because (i) cardiotoxicity is a well-established adverse side effect of several drug classes, for example, tyrosine kinase inhibitors as anticancer drugs [17,18], and (ii) some drug physicochemical properties and pharmacophores are associated with a propensity for cardiovascular AEs [19,20]. Based on the 2010 "Drug Information Association Daily Alert," the following cardiovascular AE profile as defined by contribution to product withdrawal from sale and then by attrition during clinical development was obtained: myocardial infarction and heart attack>stroke>QT risk or TdP>thrombotic events or disorder>bleeding> hypertension [14]. The cardiovascular AE profile reported in the United States via the Spontaneous Reporting System and the Adverse Event Reporting System (AERS) of the FDA extracted from PharmaPendium and reported in Laverty *et al.* [10] showed the following ranking order (top 6): arrhythmias>coronary artery disorders>cardiac disorder signs and symptoms>decreased and nonspecific blood pressure effects>heart failures>myo-, epi-, and endocardial disorders. Furthermore, clinical AEs reported with 104 drugs marketed in Japan showed a high incidence of cardiovascular AEs and some significant associations with preclinical changes in cardiovascular parameters (e.g., headache, dizziness, malaise, and hot flushes associated with decreased blood pressure; fever associated with increased blood flow) [21]. Some cardiovascular AEs, such as myocardial ischemia, myocardial necrosis, heart failure, coronary artery disorders, and cardiac valve, pericardial, and endocardial disorders, as well as disorders affecting blood components, do not always appear to be detected during drug development, rather they are reported postapproval suggesting that current preclinical assays and clinical development studies are failing to detect adequately such liabilities. Usually, compounds that cause hypo- or hypertension and tachy- or bradycardia can be detected and this information may be used to manage risk during subsequent development. It is becoming increasingly recognized that small cardiovascular changes may be very relevant to longer term clinical outcomes. For example, it has been suggested that increases in blood pressure as small as 2 mmHg may be associated with increased morbidity and mortality [11], although this view is not shared by all, since convincing clinical studies are not readily available. However, more recent studies suggest that patients experiencing small, chronic drug-induced increases in blood pressure (5 mmHg) or heart rate (5 beats/min) have a 6–23% greater risk of suffering heart failure, cardiac ischemia, or cerebral stroke events [13]. Interestingly, preclinical studies conducted prior to first-in-human trials may be powered to identify only relatively large changes in a given parameter [22]. The true meaning of any observed change is often only understood when a sufficiently large number of patients have been exposed to a given drug for a prolonged period of time. It is possible that even small changes in these parameters result in the impairment of cardiovascular function and/or loss of cardiovascular homeostasis with the potential to damage cardiovascular organ systems as well as other organs (e.g., kidney), precipitating increases in cardiovascular-related mortality and morbidity [11,23,24]. Likewise, vascular inflammation and injury is often reported in preclinical models [25,26], while the clinical relevance and consequence of these observations remains unclear as compounds with a drug-induced vascular injury liability have been successfully developed (e.g., potassium channel openers, phosphodiesterase inhibitors, and endothelin receptor antagonists). Surprisingly, for many vascular disorders reported preclinically (e.g., arteriosclerosis, vascular insufficiency, and vascular necrosis), there remains a lack of data to confidently translate from preclinical observations to humans [23,27]. Because of these unanticipated cardiovascular complications at the level of the patient population, cardiovascular safety is of paramount importance in contemporary drug development, especially in an era marked by increased public scrutiny, escalating industry costs, and limited resources at regulatory agencies.

10.2 Cardiac Function: Definitions and General Principles

10.2.1 Definition and Importance of Inotropy and Difference from Ventricular Function

Inotropy, also called the inotropic state or myocardial contractility, is the force-generating potential of heart muscle and it is easily defined as the velocity of cycling of heavy meromyosin heads (Figure 10.1a). In the context of a contracting muscle, it is the velocity with which the muscle shortens against the imaginary conditions of no hindrance (i.e., no load) to shortening. The units of myocardial contractility are velocity, usually expressed as muscle length/s. Because inotropy is an expression of systolic function and is a prime determinant, along with heart rate and peak tension, of myocardial oxygen consumption, it is extremely important to the clinician, the safety pharmacologist, the toxicologist, the pharmaceutical industry, and the drug regulatory agencies. Although there are no guidances of what decrease in inotropy translates to morbidity

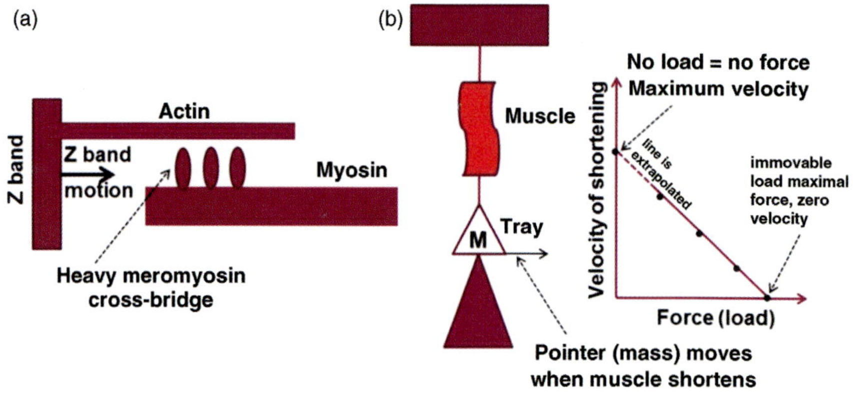

Figure 10.1 (a) Mechanism of myocardial contraction. Contraction of myocardium occurs when heavy meromyosin cross-bridges cycle and pull actin filaments and the Z band to which they are attached. Total force-generating capability depends upon velocity of cycling of a cross-bridge times the number of cross-bridges cycling. (b) Determination of the contractility of a strip of myocardium. As mass in the tray (abscissa) decreases, velocity (ordinate) with which the load moves increases. Maximal velocity is achieved when there is no load.

and/or mortality for a given patient, it is known that diseases and drugs that reduce inotropy are considered risky or at the very least potentially risky [28]. Inotropy is a descriptor of systolic cardiac function, but there is an important distinction between ventricular function, as used in the clinic, and myocardial contractility. Ventricular function refers to the ability of the ventricle to remove blood from a venous reservoir and pump it into and through the arterial tree. In the clinic, function is expressed as cardiac output or ejection fraction. Both indices of function, but not inotropy, are determined also by preload and afterload.

Contractility of a single myocardial fiber can be estimated by placing it in a bath, stimulating it electrically, and measuring, by microphotography, the velocity with which it shortens. Sitting unencumbered in a perfusion bath, the cell appears to be completely unhindered from shortening (i.e., unloaded); however, it is not truly unloaded because it still has to move its own mass. Because that mass is so small and hinders shortening negligibly, the hindrance to shortening can be considered to be nil; therefore, the velocity of shortening can be considered maximal as it is determined solely by the velocity of cycling of heavy meromyosin heads. Since there is, in effect, no hindrance, the maximal velocity is determined by the rate of cycling of only a single cross-bridge; more cross-bridges will produce more force, but since the fiber is considered unloaded and therefore can produce no force, the velocity achieved is the maximal velocity, that is, the definition of contractility.

Contractility of a strip of myocardium may be estimated by suspending one end of the strip to a fixed point and attaching the other end to a (massless) tray loaded with a mass that may be reduced from too heavy to move to masses that are lighter and lighter (Figure 10.1b) and allow faster and faster motion. In the experiment to determine inotropy, the muscle strip is stimulated as lighter and lighter loads are placed on the tray, and the velocity with which the tray moves is measured and graphed against the mass in the tray. Of course, even when there is no mass in the tray and even when the tray is removed, the muscle strip must still shorten against its own mass, so there is never a truly unloaded state. However, the curved line (termed a force–velocity curve, but shown as a straight line in the figure) of velocity of shortening versus load can be extrapolated to intersect the ordinate when the mass would have been nil. Thus, the Y-axis intercept is the maximal velocity, that is, the definition of contractility.

Myocardial contractility may also be approximated, *in situ*, by comparing systolic performance (e.g., cardiac output (CO), stroke volume (SV), developed or peak left ventricular pressure (LVP), maximal rate of rise of LVP ($dLVP/dt_{max}$), and myocardial oxygen consumption (MVO_2)) with the volume (end-diastolic volume (EDV) or preload (PL)) of blood in the ventricle just before it contracts. As mentioned in Section 10.2.2, preload is determined by the forces distending the ventricle (i.e., the end-diastolic pressure (EDP) inside the chamber minus the pleural or pericardial pressure (P_{pl}) outside of the chamber) all divided by the stiffness or elasticity modulus (ε) of the ventricle. Of course, the time for filling is also important, and that time is inversely related to heart rate.

Preload does not alter myocardial contractility (the rate of cycling of any and all heavy meromyosin heads), but it does change the number of heavy meromyosin heads cycling and the avidity with which Ca^{2+} binds to troponin C that permits the cycling. If all else (e.g., hindrance to ejection and myocardial contractility) is constant, the greater the preload (i.e., the greater the stretch on the myocardial fibers just before they contract), the greater will be the force of contraction.

A single curve of systolic function (on the ordinate) versus preload (on the abscissa) was first conceptualized by Elias Cyon, but was popularized almost a decade later by Otto Frank and Ernest Starling. It is called the Frank–Starling curve (Figure 10.2) and represents the "law of the heart," which states that the force of contraction is determined by the degree of stretch on the fibers just before they contract. The more blood in the heart, the more the fibers are stretched, and the more vigorously the heart contracts. Decades later, Wiggers [29] restated and simplified the law of the heart as "the heart pumps out whatever returns to it," and Sarnoff renamed the relationship as heterometric autoregulation, that is, changing (hetero-) fiber length (meters) results in changing force of contraction without other influences (auto-).

Single Frank–Starling curves (Figure 10.2) represent the systolic function for normal inotropy and increased inotropy. Note that, for each curve, as preload increases (i.e., the heart gets larger), the force of contraction also increases. Note also, however, that under a positive inotropic state, for any given preload, the force of contraction is greater for the positive inotropic state than for the normal inotropic state; under a negative inotropic state, the force of contraction is weaker for any given reduction in preload. Thus, the changes in the inotropic

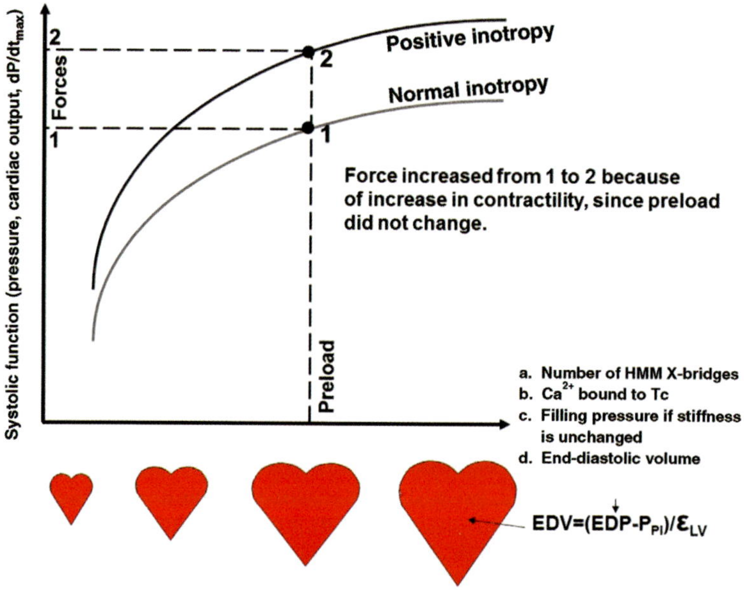

Figure 10.2 Frank–Starling curves showing the "law of the heart" for two inotropic states (see the text for details).

state can be expressed by observing a force of contraction, for any given preload, that is either greater, for a positive inotrope, or lesser, for a negative inotrope, than normal. Finally, note that almost any force of contraction can result from either a change in preload or a change in the inotropic state. Restated, any state of systolic function depends upon both inotropy and preload, and, as will be shown by addressing the pressure–volume loop, systolic function, but not inotropy, may also be changed by altering hindrance to ejection [30].

Measuring contractility from the pressure–volume loop is also discussed in Section 10.2.2 (Figure 10.3). A plot of intraventricular pressure (ordinate) versus ventricular volume (abscissa) during a single cardiac cycle is termed a pressure–volume loop. A family of loops can be generated if individual loops are inscribed as ventricular volume is decreased briefly (for ~8–10 cardiac cycles) by decreasing venous return (usually by occlusion of the caudal vena cava). This maneuver invokes heterometric autoregulation, since as the left ventricle becomes smaller, force of contraction decreases due to fewer heavy meromyosin cross-bridges cycling and decreased avidity with which Ca^{2+} binds to troponin C. The portion of the loop occurring during diastole is discussed under lusitropy. The "gold standard" for expressing myocardial contractility is considered to be the steepness of the slope of the line drawn between points of preload recruitable stroke work obtained during heterometric autoregulation. Discussions by Berghoff, Kass, and Sugawa explain the limits, methods, physiology, and physics behind generation and interpretation of pressure–volume loops. The methodology not

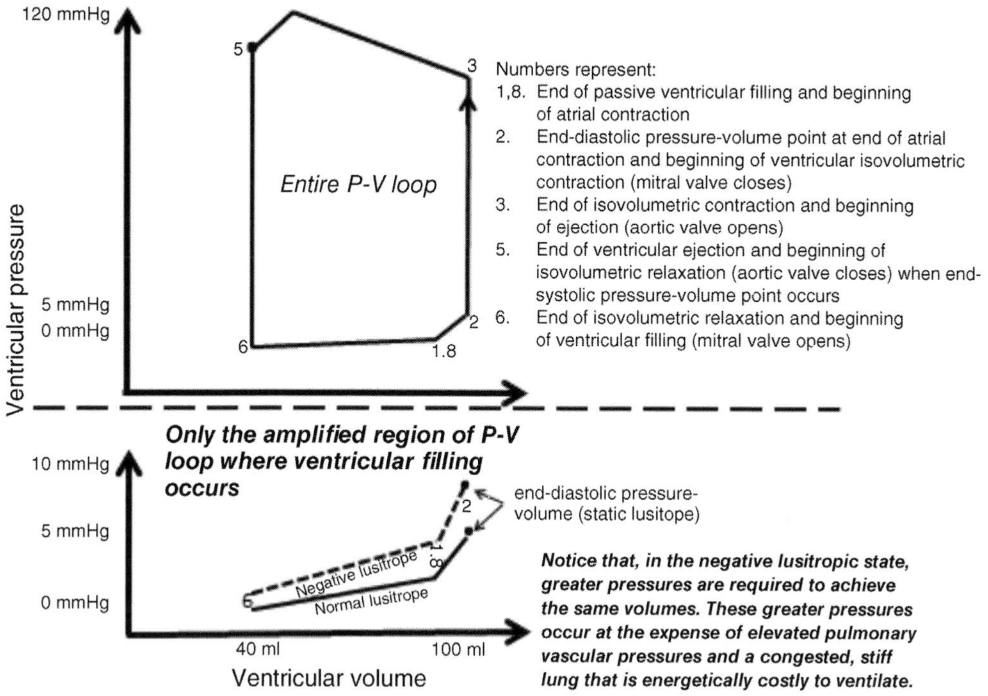

Figure 10.3 Measurement of contractility from the pressure–volume loop (see the text for details).

only produces a load-independent measure of myocardial contractility, but also measures lusitropy, and arterial stiffness, and predicts myocardial oxygen demand. Unfortunately, the pressure–volume loop is relatively difficult to obtain and to interpret, but it becomes essential to identify drug effects on contractility if the drug also alters loading conditions.

10.2.2 Definition and Importance of Lusitropy

Lusitropy is a mechanical property of the heart referring to the ease with which it may be filled. It relates intimately to compliance; therefore, it is the reciprocal of stiffness. In fact, during the contraction and relaxation of the heart, lusitropy is manifested once during isovolumetric relaxation before any ventricular filling occurs, and again during isotonic relaxation when the ventricle actually fills passively and terminally in response to atrial contraction. In clinical cardiology, lusitropy is equally important to inotropy, since equal morbidity and mortality occurs from lusitropic and inotropic incompetence [31,32]. In patients with diabetes, hypertrophic or restrictive cardiomyopathy, many forms of lung disease, or pericardial disease, the vast majority of clinical signs and symptoms (including mortality) stem from lusitropic incompetence. It is highly likely that drugs causing lusitropic incompetence present a high cardiovascular risk. Since it is rarely measured or is measured inadequately or incompletely, this issue still requires confirmation [28,33].

Manifestation(s) of lusitropy may be discussed with reference to the diagram (Figure 10.4), popularized by Carl Wiggers, and modified here to show (a) fluctuations in pressures from within the left atrium, left ventricle, and aorta, (b) fluctuations of volume, wall thickness, and tension of the left ventricle, and (c) fluctuations of blood flow through the coronary arteries nourishing the myocardium. Lusitropy is manifested three times, seen in Figure 10.4 between the vertical lines 5 and 6, 6 and 8, and 1 and 2. Between lines 5 and 6, ventricular pressure and myocardial tension plummet, but neither ventricular volume nor

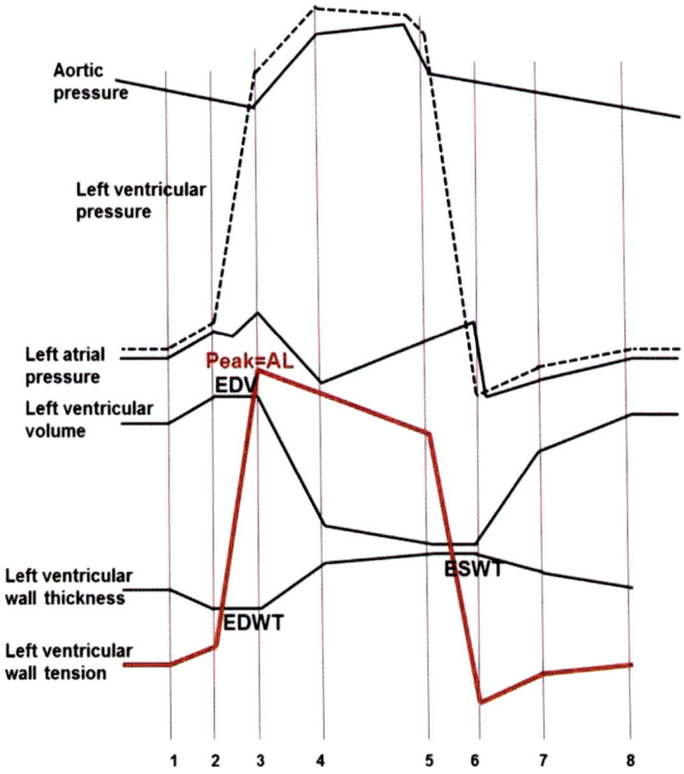

Figure 10.4 A modified Wiggers diagram showing cardiovascular pressures, volumes, wall thickness, and myocardial tension. Left ventricular tension (left ventricular pressure times left ventricular volume (actually radius), all divided by left ventricular wall thickness) is shown in red. Peak tension – the measure of afterload (AL) – occurs at vertical line 3, even though pressure continues to elevate from vertical line 2 to vertical line 3 when tension actually decreases. This occurs because the volume (radius) becomes smaller and the wall thicker as the ventricle ejects. ED, end-diastolic; *V*, volume (or radius); WT, wall thickness.

wall thickness changes. This is termed isovolumetric relaxation because the ventricular myocardium is relaxing, but its volume is not changing (iso). Since both aortic and mitral valves are closed, making the left ventricle a closed chamber, it can neither eject nor be filled. The fall in ventricular pressure occurs because of relaxation of the myocardium, initiated when Ca^{2+} is driven off of troponin C and resequestered into the sarcoplasmic reticulum (SR) through the $SERCa^{2+}$ channel (stabilized by phospholamban) in its membrane. Energy for concentrating or driving Ca^{2+} into the SR comes from hydrolysis of ATP; production of this energy is equally important to that for energy fueling contraction. Thus, with myocardial hypoxia, there will be energy starvation and reduction in both inotropy (making contraction feeble) and lusitropy (making the ventricle stiff). The manifestation of lusitropy that occurs during actual filling of the ventricle occurs at two intervals: (a) between timelines 6 and 8, when there is a relatively rapid rate of filling (6–7) followed by a reduced rate of filling (7–8), and (b) between timelines 1 and 2 when the atrium is contracting.

The force driving the filling of the left ventricle is the pressure gradient between the left atrial pressure (LAP) and the left intraventricular pressure (actually the intraventricular pressure minus the pleural pressure, but pleural pressure is often neglected); the opposition (hindrance) to filling is imposed by the stiffness of the ventricle, properties of the pericardium, the viscosity of blood, physiology of the mitral valve, and, of course, time over which filling forces and opposition to filling are manifested (i.e., the duration of diastole that is inversely related to heart rate). Left atrial pressure (and also left ventricular pressure, when the mitral valve is open) is modulated by a balance between the right ventricle pumping blood through the pulmonary circulation into the left atrium (producing the v-wave of the venous pressure pulse), the left atrial contraction (*vis a tergo*, force from behind), and the left ventricle actually sucking (*vis a fronte*, force from the front) blood out of the atrium, as its relaxation causes a drop in the intraventricular pressure.

The component of lusitropy occurring during isovolumetric relaxation is often estimated by the maximal rate of decrease in LVP with respect to time (dP/dt_{min}) (Figure 10.5). It is also estimated as τ, the time required for LVP to fall approximately 63% from the instant when dP/dt_{min} occurs to the instant when LVP falls below LAP or when LVP falls to between 5 and 10 mmHg. It is important to remember, however, that these events occur before there is any filling of the ventricle, that they depend upon heart rate, and that they represent the rate with which Ca^{2+} is driven off of troponin C and is resequestered into the SR. It is predominantly a physicochemical process, not a mechanical process! Lusitropy may be inferred in the clinic from (a) echocardiograms and/or Doppler signals (e.g., durations of isovolumetric relaxation and estimates of peak filling rates), (b) analysis of left ventricular pressure curves principally of dP/dt_{min}, and (c) auscultation of gallop sounds (S_3 and/or S_4) produced from a relatively stiff heart. However, the "gold standard" to interrogate both inotropy and lusitropy is, no doubt, the pressure–volume loop (Figure 10.3). Highly schematic diagrams of left ventricular pressure versus left ventricular volume during the entire cardiac

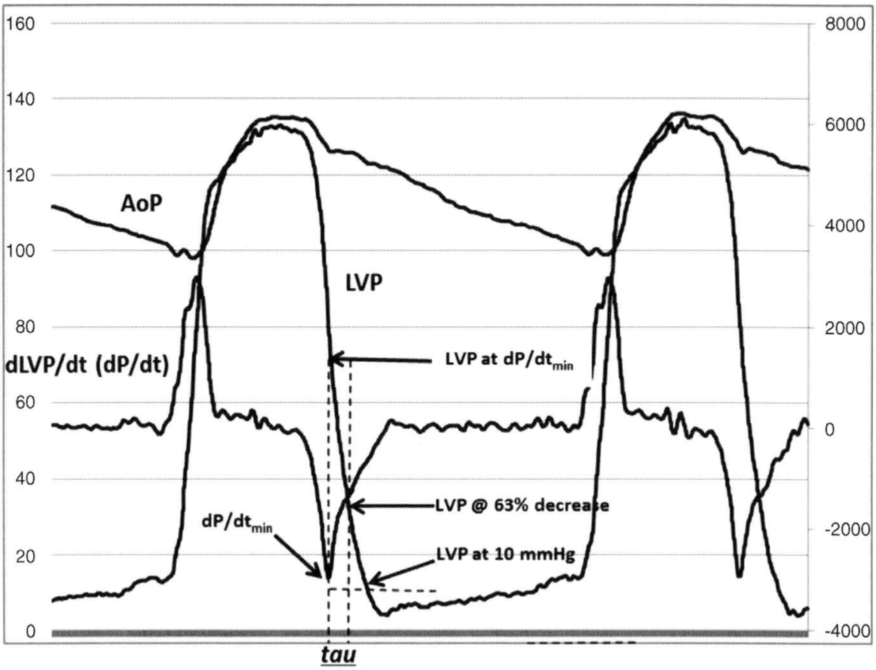

Figure 10.5 Recordings (top to bottom) of aortic pressure (AoP; left axis in mmHg), rate of change of left ventricular pressure (d*P*/d*t* or dLVP/d*t*; right axis in mmHg/s), and left ventricular pressure (LVP; left axis in mmHg).

cycle (Figure 10.3, top) or (amplified) during only ventricular filling (Figure 10.3, bottom) are shown. The slope of the line (6–8) represents the dynamic stiffness (the reciprocal of dynamic lusitropy) of the ventricle indicating the increase in intraventricular pressure as the ventricle fills and volume increases. Because the pressure–volume relationship at end of atrial contraction occurs at a single point representing the end-diastolic pressure–volume relationship (point 2), it may be considered to represent static stiffness (the reciprocal of static lusitropy) and is most often the expression of ventricular stiffness used in the clinic.

A negative lusitropic state is considered undesirable for a number of reasons. First, a stiff ventricle may not achieve an appropriate end-diastolic volume; therefore, according to the Frank–Starling law of the heart, systolic function and cardiac output may be reduced. Second, if cardiac output falls, the reduction in cardiac output translates to reduced emptying of pulmonary venous reservoirs and therefore to pulmonary vascular congestion. Pulmonary venous engorgement elicits a bronchoconstrictory reflex leading to asthma. Furthermore, if a satisfactory end-diastolic volume (i.e., preload) is achieved despite a stiff ventricle, it can occur only if pulmonary vascular pressures are elevated. If pulmonary capillary pressure becomes critically elevated, intravascular volume may transude into the peribronchial spaces, leading to obstructive lung disease, and into other intercellular spaces faster than lymphathics can return it to the vascular compartment, leading to pulmonary edema. Thus, the lung becomes bronchoconstricted, "wet," and stiff, leading to hypoventilation, hypoxia, ventilation–perfusion mismatch, increased energetic costs of ventilation, and fatigue of muscles of ventilation, the causes of morbidity and mortality.

In summary, (1) it must be remembered that, in the clinic, lusitropic incompetence is equally important to inotropic incompetence, (2) lusitropic incompetence may be manifested three times: (a) during isovolumetric relaxation, when the ventricle is not filling, due to a physicochemical process, (b) during passive ventricular filling, and (c) during atrial contraction, (3) it is highly likely that drug- or device-induced negative lusitropy translates to both morbidity and mortality, and (4) lusitropy may be inferred by analysis of the left ventricular pressure pulse or by clinical means, but is best quantified rigorously using P–V loops in both clinical and preclinical studies [34–37].

10.2.3
Components and Importance of the Systemic Arterial Pressure

No characterization of a potential drug is complete without knowledge of the effects on systemic arterial and pulmonary arterial pressures. Small changes may translate to significant morbidity and/or mortality. Valuable information is present in, and there are variable determinants of, each component of the pressure pulse (Figure 10.6): (1) systolic (i.e., highest), (2) diastolic (i.e., lowest), (3) mean

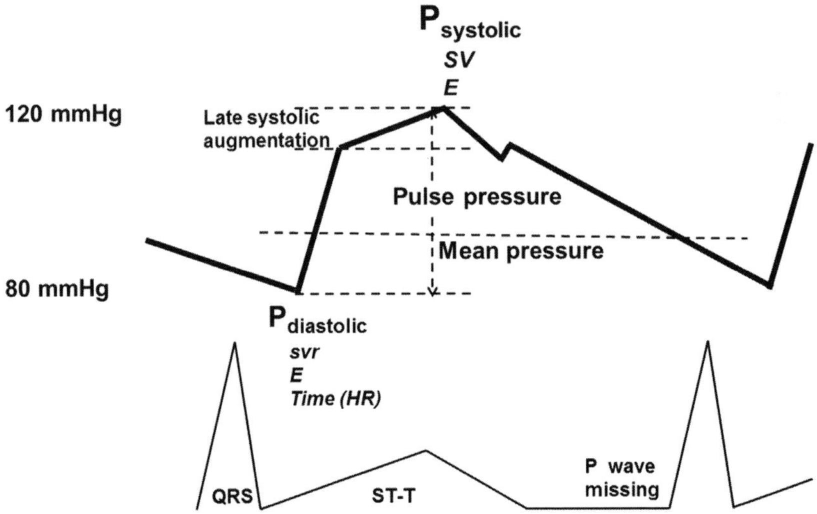

Figure 10.6 Schematic diagram of aortic pressure pulse showing systolic, diastolic, mean, and pulse pressures and late systolic augmentation. The prime determinants of systolic (SV, *E*) and diastolic (svr, *E*, time/HR) pressures appear below each. The electrocardiogram without *P* waves appears below for timing.

(i.e., ~diastolic + one-third of systolic minus diastolic), (4) pulsatile (i.e., systolic minus diastolic), and (5) late systolic augmentation, that is, the pressure difference between peak systolic and when the rising phase of the pressure pulse changes from a rapid to a decreased rate of rise. The systolic pressure is determined by stroke volume and stiffness (ε) of the aorta. The diastolic pressure that is a prime determinant of myocardial oxygen consumption and heart failure is determined by systemic vascular resistance (svr), stiffness of the aorta (ε), and the time between beats, determined by heart rate. Late systolic augmentation, a determinant of arterial physiology, is determined by stiffness (ε) of the aorta. Since the pulse pressure is the difference between systolic and diastolic pressures, it is determined by the determinants of both systolic and diastolic pressures and, when changed, reflects tendencies for consequences of changes of both.

10.2.3.1 Afterload

The role of the left ventricle is to pump blood into and through the systemic arterial tree. The arterioles are so far from the ventricle and the ventricular stroke volume is so modest that the ventricle pumps its stroke volume only into the initial portion of the aorta. The aorta stores energy in its elastic deformation, and when the ventricle is relaxing and filling in preparation for the next ejection, the energy stored in the aorta squeezes the blood within and pumps it through the arterioles. No blood returns to the ventricle because the aortic valve is closed. Therefore, there are two components to the hindrance to ejection from the left ventricle (Figure 10.7): the impedance is the hindrance to moving blood into the initial portion of the aorta resulting from having to overcome the elasticity of the aortic wall, and the systemic vascular resistance is the hindrance to moving blood into capillaries resulting from having to overcome the aperture of the arterioles.

For the clinician, impedance is termed afterload, and it is measured as the peak tension generated by the ventricle necessary to overcome the diastolic pressure in the aorta that keeps closed the aortic valve leaflets and prevents

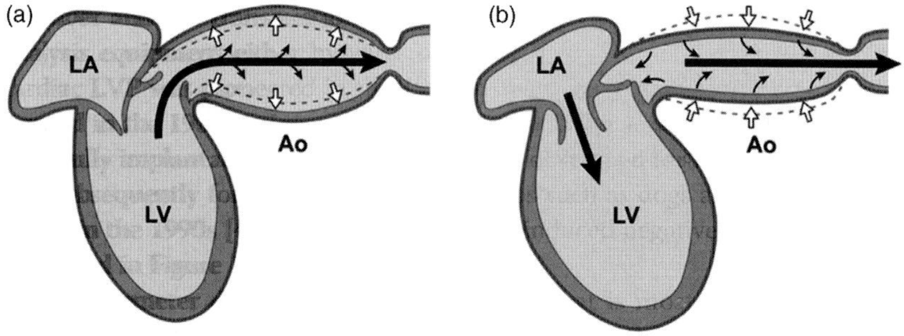

Figure 10.7 Hindrance to flow of blood from the left ventricle (LV) into (a) and through (b) the systemic arterial tree (see the text for details). LA, left atria; Ao, aorta.

ejection. The ventricle is modeled as a thick-walled sphere, and the tension in a thick-walled sphere is roughly equal to the pressure (*P*) inside times the radius (*r*) all divided by the wall thickness (WT). The peak tension is the tension at which *Pr*/WT is maximal. Even though *P* continues to rise after the aortic valve opens, because *r* becomes smaller and WT thicker (as blood is ejected and the ventricle becomes smaller), tension actually decreases during ejection, so afterload (i.e., peak tension) occurs the instant the aortic valve opens at the arterial diastolic pressure.

Afterload is extremely important for two reasons: (1) it is the principal factor that expresses the toll taken on the ventricle to eject and (2) it is a prime determinant of myocardial oxygen consumption/demand. A disease (e.g., dilated cardiomyopathy and aortic stenosis) or drug (e.g., norepinephrine and phenylephrine) that increases afterload increases the effort the ventricle must expend and increases the amount of oxygen consumed to expend that effort. The clinician knows well the importance of increased afterload with heart disease and expends every effort to decrease it.

Afterload can be estimated by measuring end-diastolic (ED) aortic *P*, *r*, and WT. EDP can be measured by sphygmomanometry; EDr and EDWT can be estimated by echocardiography or nuclear magnetic resonance imaging. EDP and EDr, but not EDWT, can be measured using inductance catheters for generating, minimally invasively, pressure–volume loops. All determinants of afterload can be measured from pressure–volume loops generated by more invasive placement of sonomicrometer crystals.

10.3
Methods Available to Assess Cardiac Function

When selecting a method for nonclinical assessment of cardiac function, it is important to consider sensitivity, specificity, translatability to humans, and animal welfare. Each method involves a balance between these attributes, none being the best in all of them. Advantages and disadvantages of various methods have been recently reviewed [38]. Although most of the emphasis in cardiac function assessment is on systolic function (inotropy or contractility), diastolic function (lusitropy or relaxation) is also important, as stated in the previous section.

An important limitation of many indices of cardiac contractility is their dependence on changes in preload, afterload, and heart rate. Preload is the amount of stretch on myocardial fibers at the beginning of systolic contraction (primarily affected by end-diastolic pressure) and afterload is the pressure in the aorta against which the left ventricle must work to eject blood, times preload, all divided by wall thickness. All three factors must be considered, since patients with dilated cardiomyopathy that generate very low arterial pressure but from a dilated, thin-walled ventricle may have enormous afterload. In order to measure contractility, either these three parameters must be kept constant or an index must be used that is independent of changes in any of them, thus only measuring true changes in the intrinsic inotropic state.

At the smallest extreme, myocardial function can be assessed in a laboratory using small samples of cardiac tissue such as papillary muscles, atrial strips, or even individual cardiac myocytes. In addition, a new methodology is under development to measure function in human embryonic or induced pluripotent stem cell-derived cardiomyocytes [39,40].

The only truly preload- and afterload-independent model for assessing cardiac inotropy (and lusitropy) in a whole heart is the time-varying elastance model developed by Suga *et al.* in the 1970s [41]. Using an isolated Langendorff heart preparation with an intraventricular balloon, they were able to demonstrate that the peak elastance, measured at the upper left corner of a family of pressure–volume loops under varying preload or afterload, was a very accurate and load-independent index of the cardiac inotropic state. Unfortunately, this requires sacrificing the animal to extract the heart. Although it can be achieved in nonclinical *in vivo* studies with vascular occluders on the vena cava or aorta (to manipulate loading conditions) and with chamber volume measurements using impedance catheters, it is cumbersome and expensive and is primarily used in basic research or cardiovascular drug discovery studies as opposed to routine drug safety assessment studies.

The most translatable method between nonclinical and human studies is noninvasive echocardiography. Obviously, the method is identical with the exceptions of thoracic anatomical differences and the fact that animals must be physically or chemically restrained during the procedure, whereas human patients will voluntarily comply. Echocardiography is considerably less sensitive as a quantitative measure of systolic and diastolic function than more invasive instrumentation because of its subjective nature and the large amount of technical skill and interoperator variability in the method. Nonetheless, the method is ideal for long-term cardiac assessment, such as in repeat-dose toxicology studies, and it provides structural, in addition to functional, information about the heart.

The most commonly used approach to nonclinical *in vivo* cardiac function assessment is the surgical placement of a pressure sensor in the left ventricular chamber and the transmission of the signal to laboratory data acquisition and analysis equipment either by wires or by telemetry. This method of measuring cardiac LVP was pioneered in the 1950s using wires connected to chart recorders and in the 1960s using externalized wires with backpack telemetry transmitters. Fully implantable pressure telemetry was developed for rodents in the 1980s and subsequently for larger laboratory animals such as dogs and nonhuman primates in the 1990s [42]. An example of drug-induced negative inotropic effect is presented in Figure 10.8.

The parameter derived from an LVP signal that is most commonly used to assess systolic function (inotropy and contractility) is the peak value of the first derivative, or dP/dt_{max}. This event occurs during isovolumic systole and represents the inflection point of the sigmoid ascending pressure waveform, where

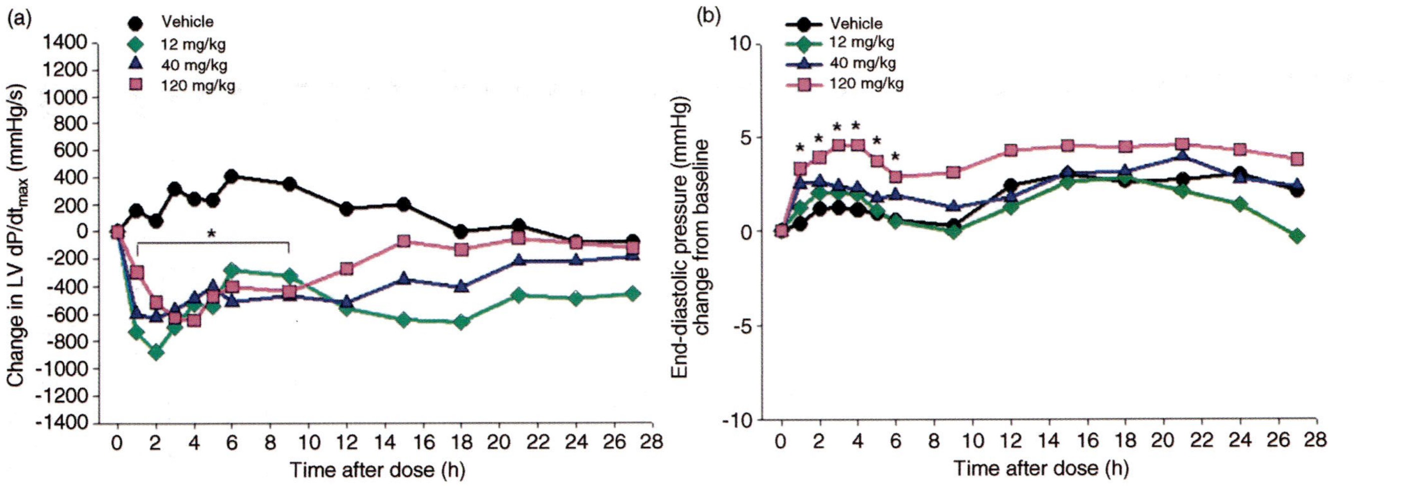

Figure 10.8 Results from administration of a drug that has a negative inotropic effect at all three doses (a). Although the magnitude of the response is similar in the low, mid, and high doses, the duration is clearly dose dependent. (b) LVEDP from the same study. Note that at the high dose, LVEDP is significantly increased, indicating that the heart is failing to adequately eject blood during systole. *$P < 0.05$ versus the vehicle group.

the rate of increase in pressure reaches its peak before the opening of the aortic valve and ejection begins to occur. Although it is preload, afterload, and rate dependent, this parameter is a useful and robust indicator of cardiac contractility when other parameters are measured and controlled [43,44]. Cardiac left ventricular end-diastolic pressure (LVEDP) should also be monitored to allow the correct interpretation of LV dP/dt_{max} results. LVEDP provides a very sensitive measure of short-term changes in preload, which affects the dP/dt_{max} parameter. If a change in dP/dt_{max} is detected, LVEDP should be examined to determine whether a real change in the intrinsic inotropic state occurred or whether it was just a response to a preload change through the Starling mechanism [45]. For example, if dP/dt_{max} increases, but LVEDP also increases, this suggests the possibility of an indirect effect, not a true inotropic change. An increase in LVEDP may provide confirmation of the presence of a strong negative inotropic effect since a weaker contraction will reduce ejection (stroke) volume resulting in incomplete chamber emptying and increased residual blood volume preceding the next contraction. An increase in LVEDP with a concurrent decrease in dP/dt_{max} would obviously not be consistent with a Starling preload-mediated mechanism since the change is in the wrong direction. A potential criticism of relying on LVEDP as an indicator of preload is that it is a pressure measurement and preload is actually a measurement of myocardial fiber length (or ventricular diastolic circumference). End-diastolic ventricular diameter is actually a product of chamber pressure and the compliance of the wall itself (opposite of stiffness). However, for acute pharmacology studies, diastolic compliance can be assumed to be constant since changes are typically a result of structural changes such as fibrosis, which take considerable time to develop. This can become an issue with long-term disease models, where the structure of the ventricular wall does change. As stated earlier, afterload can also affect the dP/dt_{max} parameter, even though the dP/dt_{max} event occurs during isovolumic systole, prior to the opening of the aortic valve and subsequent exposure of the ventricle to the aortic pressure. This too can be related to reduced ejection volume due to the heart pumping against a higher pressure and also through indirect effects on venous return to the heart. Systemic arterial pressure is typically measured with a second pressure sensor whenever LVP is measured, so it is straightforward to determine whether there was a change in afterload that could be indirectly affecting the dP/dt_{max} parameter. An important limitation to relying only on pressure to determine changes in preload or afterload in longer term studies is that the actual structural changes may occur, such as in wall thickness or chamber diameter. If this occurs, changes in wall stress and therefore myocardial fiber length may not correlate directly with pressure changes, as is the case with short-term studies.

Heart rate is a well-known modulator of the cardiac inotropic state, which is reflected in the dP/dt_{max} parameter through the Bowditch staircase (Treppe) effect on myocardial Ca^{2+} [46]. Heart rate should be carefully monitored and if dP/dt_{max} and heart rate both increase or decrease together, it is not possible to determine whether a change in dP/dt_{max} is a direct effect on intrinsic myocardial function or an indirect effect of the concurrent change in heart rate. The impact of a change in heart rate and LV dP/dt_{max} can, however, be estimated if one has determined the relationship between heart rate and LV dP/dt_{max} for the study animals previously [47]. All three of these confounding variables, preload, afterload, and heart rate, can be monitored *in vivo* and should be used to properly interpret left ventricular dP/dt_{max} results, which then provide a convenient and sensitive assessment of cardiac performance.

It is very important for investigators to understand the requirements and limitations of pressure-sensing systems used to measure LVP to avoid the inadvertent collection of inaccurate results and/or artifacts. For an in-depth review of this topic, see Ref. [48]. The most important performance characteristics of a pressure-sensing system for LVP measurement are stability (drift) and frequency response. Depending on the species and heart rate of the experimental animal, a pressure-sensing system with a frequency response of 85–90 Hz is adequate [48–50]. A frequency response lower than that can result in artificially low dP/dt_{max} results and a frequency response much higher is wasteful due to large data storage requirements with higher digital sample rates and can also result in artifacts from nonphysiological high-frequency noise affecting analysis algorithms [48,50].

10.4 What Do We Know About the Translation of the Nonclinical Findings to Humans?

Nonclinical testing of drugs, whether in terms of demonstrating potential clinical efficacy of the drug candidate or establishing drug safety to allow for clinical testing, is based on the assumption that the observation in nonclinical animal models reflects what will be seen later in studies with healthy human volunteers and later in the intended patient population. Despite the critical importance of this basic assumption, together with the fact that most scientists are readily prepared to accept it, there is little data supporting its validity. This situation is also true for studies examining the potential chronotropic, inotropic, lusitropic, or hemodynamic effects of drug candidates in animal models. However, in recent years there has been an increasing effort within the pharmaceutical industry, with the support of drug regulatory agencies, academia, and technologies and service providers, to critically examine the degree of translation between experimental results obtained using nonclinical animal models (with and without disease) of cardiovascular function and results in human trials. The validity of such a translation is the cornerstone of our nonclinical safety testing approach and serves as the justification for the ethical use of animals in the conduct of such studies.

The first regulatory guidance on testing of drugs in models of general or safety pharmacology came from the Japanese Ministry of Health and Welfare. The predictivity of such testing for clinically adverse reactions of drugs was assessed based on drugs registered in Japan, provided data suggesting an important role for such nonclinical studies for predicting clinically relevant effects [21], and also paved the way for the international harmonization of such studies [51]. A similar approach was used to examine the predictive value of data coming from toxicology studies from different pharmaceutical companies on 150 new drugs [52] for anticipating human toxicity. This survey also concluded that *in vivo* toxicology studies were useful in predicting human toxicity. Thus, in general, there is/has been a reason to think that safety pharmacology studies in animal models focusing on cardiovascular effects of new drugs will be useful in predicting cardiovascular effects in humans.

Safety pharmacological studies addressing potential cardiovascular side effects of novel therapeutics are typically performed in both rodent and nonrodent species, including dogs, minipigs, or nonhuman primates. Studies in rodents can be useful to detect potential effects when amounts of a compound are limited and costly, thereby necessitating the need for smaller animals. However, later studies prior to first human studies will use one of the nonrodent species, as recommended in the ICH S7A guidance. Furthermore, in this guidance the use of conscious animals is recommended, although there may be a rationale for the use of an anesthetized animal model, depending on the nature of the test article being evaluated and the particular parameters being explored. In either case, studies should be designed to determine possible dose-dependent effects on parameters, including the heart rate, arterial blood pressure, the contractile state (inotropy), and compliance (lusitropy) of the myocardium. Direct or indirect effects of a test article on any of these properties, as well as on high-pressure baroreceptor function, have been known to translate, in humans, to morbidity and/or mortality.

How well do results obtained from the currently *preferred* nonclinical models of cardiovascular function reflect the results found later in clinical trials? Several recent initiatives, related principally to drug-induced changes in the QT interval duration, have demonstrated that drug-induced alterations in QT of infrahuman mammals translate well to drug-induced alterations of QT in humans [53,54]. Similar datasets for effects on other important parameters of cardiovascular function (e.g., heart rate, systemic arterial blood pressure, and the myocardial contractile state) are emerging. A framework to assess the translation of data obtained during studies of safety pharmacology to humans was suggested [27] and data focusing on the cardiovascular endpoints (heart rate and blood pressure (as well as the QTc interval)) have been reported recently [55]. Cardiovascular data from 113 new drugs (all small molecules) was compiled from seven participating pharmaceutical companies. Data from nonclinical studies were found to predict drug effects on the QT interval, but with poorer predictive ability to detect effects on heart rate and diastolic blood pressure.

Such initiatives have been supported by public–private consortia to bring the involved parties together for prospective study design and data sharing [56]. One such consortium involving the HESI Cardiac Safety Technical Committee [44] addresses myocardial contractility and is based upon a harmonized cardiovascular model using the conscious beagle dog to reflect current common practice [57]. In that initiative, multiple laboratories have performed prospective studies on four compounds (pimobendan, amrinone, atenolol, and itraconazole) chosen for their known inotropic effects in clinical use. The question being addressed is whether or not these inotropic effects would have been detected had studies using the model selected been used. Furthermore, the drug exposures measured in the nonclinical studies are being compared with plasma drug levels known to produce clinically relevant effects in humans. Based on the preliminary data [44], there was good concordance of the data generated across laboratories, with dose-dependent effects on left ventricular dP/dt_{max}, the endpoint used in those studies for assessing LV contractile function, correlating to the drug level achieved. Also, the systemic drug exposures associated with the inotropic effects in the dog model were very similar to those known to cause effects in humans, suggesting good translation between the nonclinical and clinical data, at least for the four drugs tested and with dP/dt_{max} as the primary endpoint.

It is anticipated that with the completion of the ongoing consortium studies, including not only the inotropic state of the heart, but also heart rate and arterial blood pressure, we will have a better understanding of the predictive value of our current nonclinical cardiovascular animal models.

Based on the importance of lusitropy in affecting morbidity and mortality, the incidence of compounds (e.g., endothelins, SERCA and NCX blockers, β-blockers, and inotropes) affecting lusitropy, and the continual search for positive lusitropes, it is clear that exploration of lusitropy should accompany the assessment of chronotropy, dromotropy, and inotropy as preferred targets for potential drugs.

10.5 Risk Assessment

Based on their incidence and impact on drug development, functional cardiovascular adverse effects should, ideally, be investigated all along the drug discovery [58] and development process [10], as presented in Figure 10.9 with activities and objectives aligned to it. Three streams can be separated and are discussed in this section: (i) hazard identification, where unexpected cardiovascular effects linked to the target or the chemical series tested should be detected, (ii) risk assessment, where selected compounds should be profiled to best balance the benefits and the drawbacks of each candidate drug and ensure that clinical trials can take place safely, and (iii) risk management and mitigation, where preclinical studies may be used to help address any remaining safety issues and/or explain any new finding.

10.5.1 Hazard Identification

Once a promising target has been identified during the discovery phase, a review of the potential adverse effects that may be related to the target can also be generated using information gathered from scientific literature, databases, or

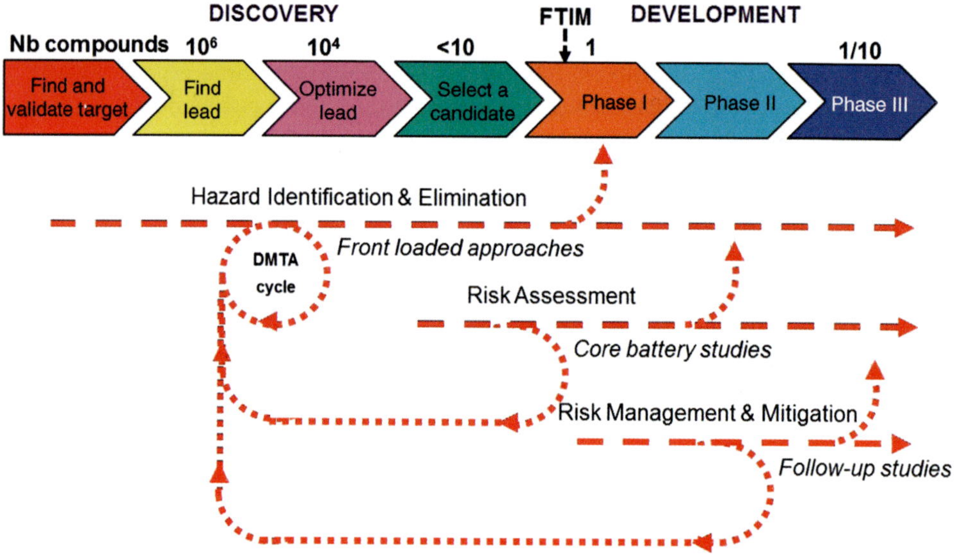

Figure 10.9 Main objectives of the studies intended at assessing cardiac safety liability and their alignment to the drug discovery and development process. Nb compounds, approximate number of compounds synthesized per project; FTIM, first-time-in-man clinical trials; DMTA, design, make, test, and analyze cycle of the drug discovery process. (Modified with permission from Ref. [59].)

bioinformatics tools. This can give a very early identification of potential cardiovascular risks associated with that particular target or pathway and can prompt some early safety investigations using pharmacological approaches with selective compounds or experiments in knock-in/out transgenic mice [60,61]. Although molecular biology has improved significantly over the past few years, the creation of such animals is still time consuming, potentially delaying discovery projects. Surprisingly, while project teams consider the use of these animals for proof-of-concept studies (i.e., target engagement), typically very little is done to identify associated safety concerns [61]. Although thorough cardiovascular assessment in mice is still challenging, simple examinations such as gross necropsy and limited pathology could enable examination of key organs (i.e., heart, kidney, liver, and lungs). This was the case in PAI-1 knockout mice [62] that develop an age-related cardiac fibrosis and were used to explain the exaggerated pharmacology of PAI-1 inhibitors found in late preclinical development [63]. On the other hand, novel technologies such as zinc finger, TALE proteins, and CRISPR are opening new frontiers and promise to speed up the generation of not only transgenic mice but also higher mammals [64,65]. The availability of transgenic rats has already influenced new strategies in early discovery, facilitating functional phenotyping at the very early discovery phases with examples already published on cardiomyopathy pathways [66], and extension of these technologies to rabbits, pigs, and even dogs and primates is expected.

During the search for a lead chemical series, early assessments of cardiovascular and other potential safety issues are performed using *in vitro* pharmacological profiling [67]. Compounds from chemical series of interest are screened *in vitro* against a range of targets, including GPCRs, enzymes (including kinases), ion channels, and transporters, which are distinct from the primary target and usually have known associations with ADRs. Among the hundreds of targets listed in those target profiles, examples of off-target activity of particular concern for cardiovascular safety include α-adrenoceptors (effects on blood pressure), muscarinic M_2 receptor (direct cardiac effects), 5-HT_{2B} (association with valvulopathy), PDE3 (cardiac contractility, blood pressure, and heart rate), VEGFR2 (blood pressure), and multiple kinase inhibitors (cardiac contractility) [67]. These *in vitro* profiling assays can be performed rapidly, require small amounts of compound, and can be used by medicinal chemists to select between chemical series based on promiscuity. Structure–activity relationships can be built at the lead optimization stage with the aim of reducing off-target activity while retaining activity at the primary target. At this stage, there is often no prediction of the human therapeutic plasma concentration and interpretation of the off-target activity is done versus the most appropriate efficacy biomarker. It is therefore very important to characterize well the risk associated with each target, in terms of both potency (IC_{50}, K_i, or other relevant parameters depending on the target) and potential clinical effects, and refer to pharmacology experts to interpret these profiles (i.e., extraction of the most undesirable targets or association of targets). In the best cases, a prediction of the expected human exposures is available and can complete or replace the use of efficacy target values. Such a case is presented for a kinase inhibitor in Figure 10.10, where the pharmacological profile was used to quantify safety margins and give a first estimation of the potential risk of eliciting ADRs in humans. By repeating this profiling with the most relevant lead compounds synthesized, chemical series and compounds can be compared and those with the best safety margins selected for progression to the next stage of drug discovery.

Alongside pharmacological profiling, *in vitro* functional tests have been developed using rat primary cardiomyocytes [68] or more recently myocytes obtained from human induced pluripotent stem cells with tests amenable to middle- and sometimes high-throughput screening [69]. These tests can supplement the identification of cardiovascular hazards by measuring simple parameters such as beating rate or cell contraction strength and help define an optimized risk assessment strategy.

10.5.2
Risk Assessment

The early identification of hazards impacts the next phases of drug development and may trigger bespoke safety assessments to complement the standard early safety models each company has defined. This strategy is usually a combination

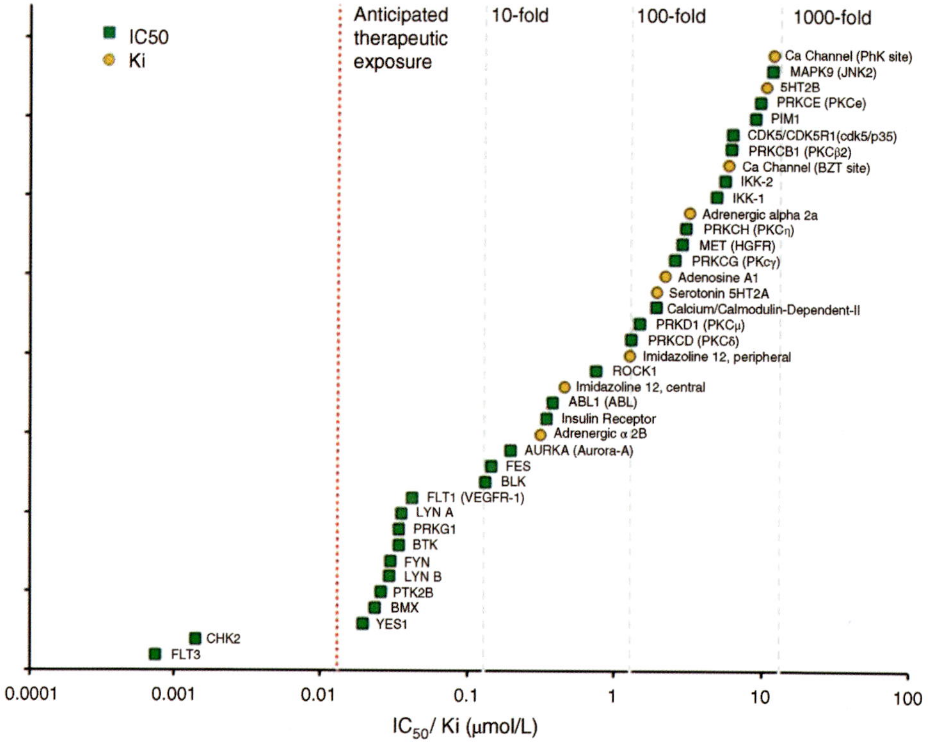

Figure 10.10 Hazard identification of a kinase inhibitor using *in vitro* pharmacological profiling. The candidate compound was screened against a broad range of targets including GPCRs, enzymes (including kinases), ion channels, and transporters to identify interactions that may cause adverse effects in humans. Affinity at the targets was quantified by calculating IC_{50} or K_i. The anticipated human therapeutic exposure and margins from this are indicated with the vertical lines.

of *in vitro* or *ex vivo* models such as isolated vessels or isolated heart, anesthetized animals such as the guinea pig that enable the combined assessment of *in vivo* electrophysiology and hemodynamics [70–72], and also conscious animal models such as rat or nonrodent telemetry, depending on how critical is the information for decision making in a project context. Once a drug candidate is selected and progressed into preclinical development, standard *in vivo* GLP core battery assessments must be performed to assess cardiovascular safety. At a minimum, these must include assessments of blood pressure, heart rate, and ECG [51]. The cardiovascular risk assessment is often supplemented with follow-up studies, or measurements of additional parameters, for example, LV dP/dt_{max}, that may provide a greater depth of understanding of physiological effects than that provided by the core battery. The core battery cardiovascular assessment should be well standardized following published best practices to ensure that conclusions are aligned to clinical thresholds of concern with

		Maximum acceptability of the safety studies								
		Minor			Moderate			Major		
Therapeutic indication	Existing therapy	100	10	1	100	10	1	100	10	1
Minor disease	Good	X								
	Partially effective / side effects		X							
	Poor / none			X						
Debilitating disease	Good				X					
	Partially effective / side effects					X				
	Poor / none						X			
Life-threatening disease	Good							X		
	Partially effective / side effects								X	
	Poor / none									X

Figure 10.11 Risk assessment matrix. Outcomes to the left of the line (within the green zone) are acceptable, whereas those lying to the right of the line of identity (within the red zone) demonstrate a clear unacceptable risk. Those lying near the line (crosses) require close examination before a decision of progression is made. The values 1, 10, and 100 indicate a multiple of the anticipated, predicted, or measured therapeutic exposure, respectively. (Adapted with permission from Ref. [73].)

sufficient sensitivity for all parameters [57]. Pharmacodynamic and pharmacokinetic data from all the relevant studies are combined, along with the human predicted therapeutic concentration, and the resulting dataset forms the basis of the integrated risk assessment used to assess the risk of progressing further into first-in-human studies.

By grading (i) the outcome of any safety finding (e.g., minor, moderate, or major), (ii) the intended disease indication (e.g., minor, debilitating, or life threatening), and (iii) the existing therapies available (e.g., good, partially effective, or none), a risk/benefit profile can be generated as shown in Figure 10.11. Outcomes far to the left of the line (within the green zone) have favorable risk/benefit ratio that would support progression into humans, whereas those lying to the right of the line of identity (within the red zone) demonstrate a clear unacceptable risk. Those lying near the line require close examination before a decision of progression is made [73].

Figure 10.12 shows an integrated risk assessment used to assess the potential for a compound to affect cardiac contractility in humans. The compound caused dose-dependent decreases in left ventricular $\mathrm{d}P/\mathrm{d}t_{\max}$ in both anesthetized and conscious dogs. Additional investigations *in vitro* in isolated myocytes and a rat Langendorff preparation demonstrated a direct effect on contractility at similar

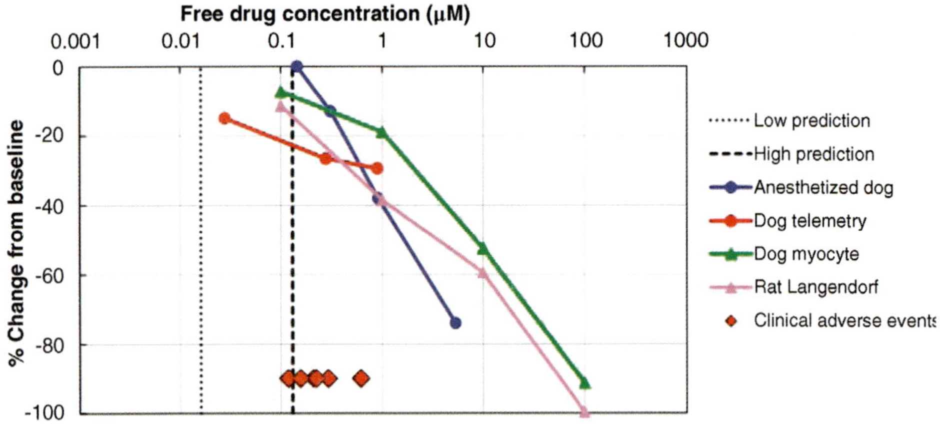

Figure 10.12 Integrated risk assessment to evaluate the potential of a candidate compound to affect cardiac contractility in humans. Data show the mean effects on left ventricular dP/dt_{max} in anesthetized and conscious dogs and isolated rat heart and the effects on sarcomere shortening in isolated dog myocytes all plotted against free drug concentration. The free plasma concentrations at which clinical adverse effects were subsequently observed are also indicated.

concentrations. This profile was considered a major risk given the small safety margins, but since reversibility of effect was shown in the dog telemetry study and since the compound was intended for a life-threatening indication with poor existing treatments, it progressed into FTIM trials. The preclinical risk assessment provided valuable information to determine human starting doses, identification of relevant biomarkers for measurement in the clinic (troponins and ejection fraction by echocardiography), and guidance for the patient risk management plan that included strict inclusion and exclusion criteria relating to a preexisting cardiac disease [74]. Cardiotoxicity, detected as changes in plasma troponin levels and reduction in ejection fraction, ultimately proved to be the dose-limiting toxicity in the clinical trials and was the main reason for discontinuation of the compound.

10.5.3
Risk Management

If the risk/benefit ratio favors progression of a compound into clinical development despite the compound carrying some cardiovascular safety concerns, additional preclinical safety studies may be beneficial. These studies should provide more information about the mechanism of the adverse cardiovascular effect that will hopefully provide more reassurance to the clinical team that the compound can progress safely to large-scale clinical trials. Demonstrating an understanding of the mechanism of an adverse cardiovascular effect can also improve the chances of regulatory approval. As an example, hypertension was shown to be a side-effect of potential concern during phase II clinical trials for fostamatinib, a small-molecule kinase inhibitor developed in the indication of rheumatoid arthritis. Elevations in arterial blood pressure of 2–5 mmHg were observed in patients after 1 month of treatment [75,76]. Preclinical investigations were initiated to investigate the potential mechanism of this blood pressure elevation [77]. Fostamatinib was shown to increase arterial blood pressure in telemetered and anesthetized rats. An increase in cardiac output was ruled out since the anesthetized preparation and an isolated rat heart assay revealed no positive inotropic or chronotropic effects. The effects were shown to be due to an increased vascular resistance and, using isolated vessels and *in vivo* assays, to be an indirect effect related to inhibition of VEGF-mediated nitric oxide release. Indeed, *in vitro* receptor profiling had previously revealed that fostamatinib inhibited several other kinases in addition to its primary target including VEGFR2 activity. Knowledge of the molecular mechanism allowed for a better clinical risk management strategy based on the preexisting clinical experience with VEGF inhibitors used for targeting tumors for which an association with hypertension had been previously demonstrated [78].

10.5.4
Risk Mitigation

Preclinical cardiovascular studies have also been utilized to provide risk mitigation strategies following identification of adverse cardiovascular events during clinic trials. It may therefore be acceptable for a compound to progress although adverse effects have been identified if the benefit/risk ratio is still acceptable. At this stage of clinical development, no further adjustments can be made to the compound properties and it is important to provide a mitigation plan to offer as many options as possible to the supporting clinical experts. As such, ensuring that adverse effects are reversible and that clinical antidotes have been identified is of critical importance. An example is the vascular disrupting agent ZD6126 developed as a chemotherapy for solid tumors. A small proportion of the patients in the phase I study experienced adverse cardiovascular effects indicative of myocardial ischemia including reduced left ventricular ejection fraction and increased plasma troponin concentration [79]. A rat telemetry model was used to investigate the underlying mechanism and ZD6126 was shown to cause increased blood pressure and tachycardia and increases in plasma troponin I after a single dose [80]. Histopathological assessment of the animals also revealed necrosis, hemorrhage, and inflammatory cell infiltration within the left and right ventricles. When the animals were pretreated with a combination of a β-blocker and a calcium channel antagonist, the cardiovascular effects were abolished, as were the increases in plasma troponin and histopathological changes (Figure 10.13). Pretreatment also had no impact on the antitumor effect of ZD6126 in preclinical models. These data had important implications suggesting that the cardiac adverse effects could be mitigated with antihypertensive therapy, thus facilitating continuation of the clinical trials.

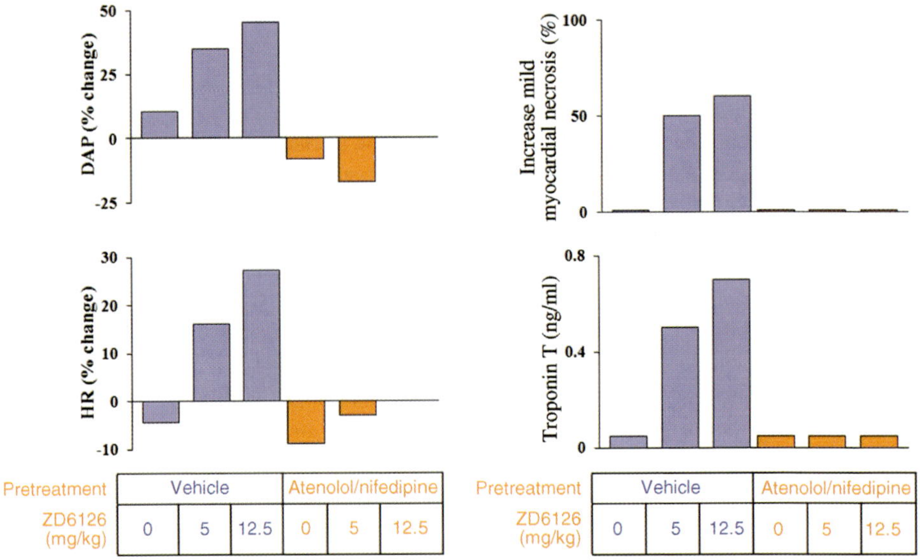

Figure 10.13 Effect of ZD6126 alone following pretreatment with the β-adrenoceptor antagonist, atenolol, and the calcium channel blocker, nifedipine, on heart rate (HR), diastolic arterial pressure (DAP), plasma troponin levels, and myocardial necrosis. When the animals were pretreated with a combination of a β-blocker and a calcium channel antagonist, the cardiovascular effects were abolished, as were the increases in plasma troponin and histopathological changes.

Although the development cycle and examples provided in this chapter deal with small molecules, the situation is not significantly different for biologics and has been recently addressed in a workshop summarized by Baumann *et al.* [63]. For those compounds, the risk of off-target effects is reduced due to high specificity for their pharmacological target. However, adverse effects can be the consequence of exaggerated pharmacology and less frequently expected toxicity. Very little safety testing is performed during the discovery phase, rather taking place during preclinical toxicity studies with dedicated functional assessments, tissue distribution for PK/PD relationship, and a larger use of nonhuman primates or minipigs as nonrodent species. New challenges will probably arise with less conventional entities than peptides or large molecules such as bispecific antibodies, silent RNAs, and nanobodies.

The risk of causing cardiovascular adverse events is assessed throughout the drug development process encompassing identification of hazards during early discovery, assessment of risk before the FTIM trials, and management and mitigation of risk during clinical development. Given that, for novel therapeutics, cardiovascular safety remains a major cause of drug attrition, adverse drug reactions, and drug withdrawals, it is clear that significant challenges remain. Identification of the most appropriate strategies to assess the cardiovascular risk of more novel therapeutic products will also be an area of focus over the coming years.

10.6 Summary, Recommendations, and Conclusions

Drug-induced functional cardiovascular changes (i.e., chronotropy, inotropy, lusitropy, and hypo/hypertension) and associated sequelae account for a significant proportion of adverse events. This is not surprising knowing the complex cardiac physiology and associated pharmacology controlling the inotropic and lusitropic status of the myocardium, and associated regulation of heart rate (chronotropy) and arterial blood pressure. When selecting a method for nonclinical assessment of cardiac function, it is important to consider sensitivity, specificity, translatability to humans, and animal welfare aspects. Methods include, but are not limited to, *in vitro* approaches (e.g., isolated Langendorff heart, isolated vessels, and isolated cells) and anesthetized and conscious *in vivo* animal models in small and large animal species using invasive and noninvasive approaches. In recent years, there has been an increasing effort within the pharmaceutical industry, with the support of drug regulatory agencies, academia, and technologies and service providers, to critically examine the degree of translation between experimental results obtained using nonclinical, healthy and diseased animal models of cardiovascular function and results in human trials. The validity of such a translation is the cornerstone of the nonclinical safety testing approach. In drug discovery and development, the nonclinical data are used in three ways for hazard identification, risk assessment, risk management and mitigation. Ultimately, it is of paramount importance to develop novel therapeutics that have an acceptable cardiovascular safety profile in order to benefit the majority of patients.

List of Abbreviations

ADRs	adverse drug reactions
AERS	Adverse Event Reporting System
AEs	adverse events
dP/dt_{max}	maximum value of the first derivative of pressure (peak positive rate of change)
FDA	Food and Drug Administration
FTIM	first time in man
GLP	Good Laboratory Practice
HESI	Health and Environmental Sciences Institute
ICH	International Conference on Harmonisation
LVEDP	left ventricular end-diastolic pressure
LVP	left ventricular pressure

References

1 Munos, B. (2009) Lessons from 60 years of pharmaceutical innovation. *Nature Reviews. Drug Discovery*, **8**, 959–968.

2 Holdren, J.P., Lander, E., Press, W., Savitz, M., Blerbaum, R., Gates, J.S., Jr., Cassel, C., Gorenberg, M., Jackson, S.A., Chyba, C., Levin, R.C., Mirkin, C., Schaal, B., Schmidt, E., Molina, M., Schrag, D., Shaw, D.E., Moniz, E.J., Zewall, A., Mundle, C., and Penhoet, E. (2012) Report to the President on "propelling innovation in drug discovery, development and evaluation". US President's Council of Advisors on Science and Technology (PCAST), September 25, 2012. Available at http://www.whitehouse.gov/sites/default/files/microsites/ostp/pcast-fda-final.pdf. (accessed December 13, 2014).

3 Hay, M., Thomas, D.W., Craighead, J.L., Economides, C., and Rosenthal, J. (2014) Clinical development success rates for investigational drugs. *Nature Biotechnology*, **32**, 40–51.

4 Kennedy, T. (1997) Managing the drug discovery/development interface. *Drug Discovery and Development*, **2**, 436–444.

5 Lasser, K.E., Allen, P.D., Woolhandler, S.J., Himmelstein, D.U., Wolfe, S.M., and Bor, D.H. (2002) Timing of new black box warnings and withdrawals for prescription medications. *The Journal of the American Medical Association*, **287**, 2215–2220.

6 Kola, I. and Landis, J. (2004) Can the pharmaceutical industry reduce attrition rates? *Nature Reviews. Drug Discovery*, **3**, 711–715.

7 Shah, R.R. (2006) Can pharmacogenetics help rescue drugs withdrawn from the market? *Pharmacogenomics*, **7**, 889–908.

8 Redfern, W.S., Ewart, L., Hammond, T.G., Bialecki, R., Kinter, L., Lindgren, S., Pollard, C.E., Roberts, R., Rolf, M.G., and Valentin, J.-P. (2010) Impact and frequency of different toxicities throughout the pharmaceutical life cycle. *The Toxicologist*, **114**, 1081.

9 Cook, D., Brown, D., Alexander, R., March, R., Morgan, P., Satterthwaite, G., and Pangalos, M.N. (2014) Lessons learned from the fate of AstraZeneca's drug pipeline: a five-dimensional framework. *Nature Reviews. Drug Discovery*. doi: 10.1038/nrd4309.

10 Laverty, H., Benson, C., Cartwright, E., Cross, M., Garland, C., Hammond, T., Holloway, C., McMahon, N., Milligan, J., Park, B., Pirmohamed, M., Pollard, C., Radford, J., Roome, N., Sager, P., Singh, S., Suter, T., Suter, W., Trafford, A., Volders, P., Wallis, R., Weaver, R., York, M., and Valentin, J. (2011) How can we improve our understanding of cardiovascular safety liabilities to develop safer medicines? *British Journal of Pharmacology*, **163** (4), 675–693.

11 Lewington, S., Clarke, R., Qizilbash, N., Peto, R., and Collins, R. (Prospective Studies Collaboration) (2002) Age-specific relevance of usual blood pressure to vascular mortality: a meta-analysis of individual data for one million adults in 61 prospective studies. *Lancet*, **360**, 1903–1913.

12 Joy, T.R. and Hegele, R.A. (2008) The failure of torcetrapib: what have we learned? *British Journal of Pharmacology*, **154**, 1379–1381.

13 Paul, L., Hastie, C.E., Li, W.S., Harrow, C., Muir, S., Connell, J.M., Dominiczak, A.F., McInnes, G.T., and Padmanabhan, S. (2010) Resting heart rate pattern during follow-up and mortality in hypertensive patients. *Hypertension*, **55**, 567–574.

14 Valentin, J.-P., Kenna, J.G., Lainée, P., Redfern, W.S., Roberts, S., and Hammond, T.G. (2012) A literature-based analysis of cardiovascular adverse events impacting on drug development. *Journal of Pharmacological and Toxicological Methods*, **66** (2), 173.

15 Fung, M., Thornton, A., Mybeck, K., Wu, J.H., Hornbuckle, K., and Muniz, E. (2001) Evaluation of the characteristics of safety withdrawal of prescription drugs from worldwide pharmaceuticals markets – 1960 to 1999. *Drug Information Journal*, **35**, 293–317.

16 Stevens, J.L. and Baker, T.K. (2009) The future of drug safety testing: expanding the view and narrowing the focus. *Drug Discovery Today*, **14**, 162–167.

17 Mellor, H.R., Bell, A.R., Valentin, J.P., and Robert, R.R. (2011) Cardiotoxicity associated with targeting kinase pathways in cancer. *Toxicological Sciences*, **120** (1), 14–32.
18 Shah, R.R., Morganroth, J., and Shah, D.R. (2013) Cardiovascular safety of tyrosine kinase inhibitors: with a special focus on cardiac repolarisation (QT interval). *Drug Safety*, **36**, 295–316.
19 Leeson, P.D. and Springthorpe, B. (2007) The influence of drug-like concepts on decision-making in medicinal chemistry. *Nature Reviews. Drug Discovery*, **6**, 881–890.
20 Gavaghan, C.L., Arnby, C.H., Blomberg, N., Strandlund, G., and Boyer, S. (2007) Development, interpretation and temporal evaluation of a global QSAR of hERG electrophysiology screening data. *Journal of Computer-Aided Molecular Design*, **21** (4), 189–206.
21 Igarashi, T., Nakane, S., and Kitagawa, T. (1995) Predictability of clinical adverse reactions of drugs by general pharmacology studies. *The Journal of Toxicological Sciences*, **20**, 77–92.
22 Guth, B.D., Bass, A.S., Briscoe, R., Chivers, S., Markert, M., Siegl, P.K., and Valentin, J.P. (2009) Comparison of electrocardiographic analysis for risk of QT interval prolongation using safety pharmacology and toxicological studies. *Journal of Pharmacological and Toxicological Methods*, **60**, 107–116.
23 Valentin, J.P., Keisu, M., and Hammond, T.G. (2009) Predicting human adverse drug reactions from non-clinical safety studies, in *Clinical Trials Handbook* (ed. S.C. Gad), John Wiley & Sons, Inc., Hoboken, NJ, pp. 87–113.
24 Chalmers, J. and Arima, H. (2010) Importance of blood pressure lowering in type 2 diabetes: focus on ADVANCE. *Journal of Cardiovascular Pharmacology*, **55**, 340–347.
25 Brott, D., Jones, H., Gould, S., Valentin, J.P., Evans, G., Richardson, R.J., and Louden, C. (2005) Current status and future directions for diagnostic markers of drug-induced vascular injury. *Cancer Biomarkers*, **1**, 15–28.
26 Louden, C., Brott, D., Katein, A., Kelly, T., Gould, S., Jones, H., Betton, G., Valentin, J.P., and Richardson, R.J. (2006) Biomarkers and mechanisms of drug-induced vascular injury in non-rodents. *Toxicologic Pathology*, **34**, 19–26.
27 Valentin, J.-P., Bialecki, R., Ewart, L., Hammond, T., Leischmann, D., Lindgren, S., Martinez, V., Pollard, C., Redfern, W., and Wallis, R. (2009) A framework to assess the translation of safety pharmacology data to humans. *Journal of Pharmacological and Toxicological Methods*, **60**, 152–158.
28 Owan, T.E., Hodge, D.O., Herges, R.M., Jacobsen, S.J., Roger, V.L., and Redfield, M.M. (2006) Trends in prevalence and outcome of heart failure with preserved ejection fraction. *The New England Journal of Medicine*, **355** (3), 251–259.
29 Wiggers, C.J. (1957) Cardiac physiology of fifty years ago. *Circulation Research*, **5** (2), 121–124.
30 Katz, L.N. (1921) Factors modifying the duration of ventricular systole. *The Journal of Laboratory and Clinical Medicine*, **6**, 291–311.
31 Nagayama, T., Takimoto, E., Sadayappan, S., Mudd, J.O., Seidman, J.G., Robbins, J., and Kass, D.A. (2007) Control of *in vivo* left ventricular contraction/relaxation kinetics by myosin binding protein C: protein kinase A phosphorylation dependent and independent regulation. *Circulation*, **116**, 2399–2408.
32 Liu, C.P., Ting, C.T., Lawrence, W., Maughan, W.L., Chang, M.S., and Kass, D.A. (1993) Diminished contractile response to increased heart rate in intact human left ventricular hypertrophy: systolic versus diastolic determinants. *Circulation*, **88**, 1893–1906.
33 Leite-Moreira, A.F. (2006) Current perspectives in diastolic dysfunction and diastolic heart failure. *Heart*, **92**, 712–718.
34 Westermann, D., Kasner, M., Steendijk, P., Spillmann, F., Riad, A., Weitmann, K., Hoffmann, W., Poller, W., Pauschinger, M., Schultheiss, H.P., and Tschöpe, C. (2008) Role of left ventricular stiffness in heart failure with normal ejection fraction. *Circulation*, **117**, 2051–2060.

35 Uesugi, M., Ojima, A., Taniguchi, T., Miyamoto, N., and Sawada, K. (2014) Low-density plating is sufficient to induce cardiac hypertrophy and electrical remodeling in highly purified human iPS cell-derived cardiomyocytes. *Journal of Pharmacological and Toxicological Methods*, **69**, 177–188.

36 Troughton, R.W., Prior, D.L., Frampton, C.M., Nash, P.J., Pereira, J.J., Martin, M., Fogarty, A., Morehead, A.J., Starling, R.C., Young, J.B., Thomas, J.D., Lauer, M.S., and Klein, A.L. (2005) Usefulness of tissue Doppler and color M-mode indexes of left ventricular diastolic function in predicting outcomes in systolic left ventricular heart failure (from the ADEPT study). *The American Journal of Cardiology*, **96**, 257–262.

37 Paulus, W.J., Tschope, C., Sanderson, J.E., Rusconi, C., Flachskampf, F.A., Rademakers, F.E., Marino, P., Smiseth, O.A., De Keulenaer, G., Leite-Moreira, A.F., Borbély, A., Edes, I., Handoko, M.L., Heymans, S., Pezzali, N., Pieske, B., Dickstein, K., Fraser, A.G., and Brutsaert, D.L. (2007) How to diagnose diastolic heart failure: a consensus statement on the diagnosis of heart failure with normal left ventricular ejection fraction by the Heart Failure and Echocardiography Associations of the European Society of Cardiology. *European Heart Journal*, **28**, 2539–2550.

38 Sarazan, R.D., Mittelstadt, S., Guth, B., Koerner, J., Zhang, J., and Pettit, S. (2011) Cardiovascular function in nonclinical drug safety assessment: current issues & opportunities. Perspectives from the Health & Environmental Sciences Institute (HESI). *International Journal of Toxicology*, **30** (3), 272–286.

39 Scott, C.W., Peters, M.F., and Dragan, Y.P. (2013) Human induced pluripotent stem cells and their use in drug discovery for toxicity testing. *Toxicology Letters*, **219** (1), 49–58.

40 Liu, W., Deng, Y., Liu, Y., Gong, W., and Deng, W. (2013) Stem cell models for drug discovery and toxicology studies. *Journal of Biochemical and Molecular Toxicology*, **27** (1), 17–27.

41 Suga, H., Sagawa, K., and Shoukas, A.A. (1973) Load independence of the instantaneous pressure–volume ratio of the canine left ventricle and effects of epinephrine and heart rate on the ratio. *Circulation Research*, **32**, 314–322.

42 Sarazan, R.D. and Schweitz, K.T.R. (2009) Standing on the shoulders of giants: Dean Franklin and his remarkable contributions to physiological measurements in animals. *Advances in Physiology Education*, **33**, 144–156.

43 Markert, M., Klummp, A., Trautmann, T., Mayer, K., Stubhan, M., and Guth, B. (2007) The value added by measuring myocardial contractility "*in vivo*" in safety pharmacology profiling of drug candidates. *Journal of Pharmacological and Toxicological Methods*, **56**, 213–211.

44 Engwall, M.J., Walisser, J.A., Saul, J., Sarazan, R.D., Guth, B., Markert, M., Skinner, M., Guillon, J.-M., Ottinger, S., Heyen, J.R., Cools, F., Hoffmann, P.K., Rossmann, E.I., and Pierson, J.B. (Health and Environmental Sciences Institute Integrated Strategies Working Group) (2013) Update on the evaluation of drug-induced changes in the cardiac inotropy in dogs. Safety Pharmacology Society Annual Meeting, Rotterdam (Abstract).

45 Patterson, S.W., Piper, H., and Starling, E.H. (1914) The regulation of the heart beat. *The Journal of Physiology*, **48**, 465–513.

46 Katz, A.M. (1977) *Physiology of the Heart*, Raven Press, New York.

47 Markert, M., Trautmann, T., Gross, M., Ege, A., Mayer, K., and Guth, B. (2012) Evaluation of a method to correct the contractility index LV$dP/dt_{max}$ for changes in heart rate. *Journal of Pharmacological and Toxicological Methods*, **66** (2), 98–105.

48 Sarazan, R.D., Kroehle, J.P., and Main, B.W. (2012) Left ventricular pressure, contractility and dP/dt_{max} in nonclinical drug safety assessment studies. *Journal of Pharmacological and Toxicological Methods*, **66**, 71–78.

49 Barry, W.H., Marlon, A.M., Adams, M., and Harrison, D.C. (1975) Effect of varying differentiator frequency response on

recorded peak d*P*/d*t*. *Cardiovascular Research*, **9**, 433–439.

50 Anonymous (2000) ICHS7A: Safety Pharmacology Studies for Human Pharmaceutical. CPMP/ICH/539/00, London. Available at http://www.ema.europa.eu/docs/en_GB/document_library/Scientific_guideline/2009/09/WC500002831.pdf. (accessed December 13, 2014).

51 Sarazan, R.D. (2014) Cardiovascular pressure measurement in safety assessment studies: technology requirements and potential errors. *Journal of Pharmacological and Toxicological Methods*. doi: 10.1016/j.vascn.2014.06.003.

52 Olson, H., Betton, G., Robinson, D., Thomas, K., Monro, A., Kalaja, G., Lilly, P., Sanders, J., Sipes, G., Bracken, W., Dorato, M., Van Deun, K., Smith, P., Berger, B., and Heller, A. (2000) Concordance of the toxicity of pharmaceuticals in humans and in animals. *Regulatory Toxicology and Pharmacology*, **32**, 56–67.

53 Parkinson, J., Visser, S.A.G., Jarvis, P., Pollard, C., Valentin, J.-P., Yates, J.W.T., and Ewart, L. (2013) Translational pharmacokinetic–pharmacodynamic modeling of QTc effects in dog and human. *Journal of Pharmacological and Toxicological Methods*, **68**, 357–366.

54 Koerner, J., Valentin, J.P., Willard, J., Park, E.J., Bi, D., Link, W.T., Fiszman, M., Kozeli, D., Skinner, M., Vargas, H.M., Cantilena, L., Gintant, G., Wisialowski, T., and Pettit, S. (2013) Predictivity of non-clinical repolarization assay data for clinical TQT data in FDA database. Proceedings of the 33rd Annual Meeting of the American College of Toxicology (ACT 2012), Orlando, FL.

55 Ewart, L., Aylott, M., Deurinck, M., Engwall, M., Gallacher, D.J., Geys, H., Jarvis, P., Ju, H., Leischman, D., Leong, L., McMahon, N., Mead, A., Millikin, P., Suter, W., Teisman, A., Van Ammel, K., Vargas, H.M., Wallis, R., and Valentin, J.-P. (2014) The concordance between preclinical and phase I cardiovascular assessment from a cross-company data sharing initiative. *Toxicological Sciences*, **142** (2), 427–435.

56 Pierson, J., Berridge, B.R., Brooks, M.B., Dreher, K., Koerner, J., Schultze, A.E., Sarazan, R.D., Valentin, J.-P., Vargas, H.M., and Pettit, S.D. (2013) A public–private consortium advances cardiac safety evaluation: achievements of the HESI cardiac safety technical committee. *Journal of Pharmacological and Toxicological Methods*, **68**, 7–12.

57 Leishman, D.J., Beck, T.W., Dybdal, N., Gallacher, D.J., Guth, B.D., Holbrook, M., Roche, B., and Wallis, R. (2012) Best practice in the conduct of key nonclinical cardiovascular assessments in drug development: current recommendations from the Safety Pharmacology Society. *Journal of Pharmacological and Toxicological Methods*, **65**, 93–101.

58 Hughes, J.P., Rees, S., Kalindjian, S.B., and Philpott, K.L. (2010) Principles of early drug discovery. *British Journal of Physiological Optics*, **162**, 1239–1249.

59 Valentin, J.-P., Pollard, C., Lainée, P., and Hammond, T. (2010) Value of non-clinical cardiac repolarization assays in supporting the discovery and development of safer medicines. *British Journal of Pharmacology*, **159** (1), 25–33.

60 Hornberg, J.J., Laursen, M., Brenden, N., Persson, M., Thougaard, A.V., Toft, D.B., and Mow, T. (2014) Exploratory toxicology as an integrated part of drug discovery. Part I: why and how. *Drug Discovery Today*, **13**, S1359–6446.

61 Redfern, W.S. and Valentin, J.-P. (2013) Transgenic animals in safety pharmacology, in *Drug Discovery and Evaluation: Safety and Pharmacokinetic Assays* (eds H.G. Vogel, F.J. Hock, J. Maas, and J. Mayer), Springer, Berlin.

62 Xu, Z., Castellino, F.J., and Ploplis, V.A. (2010) Plasminogen activator inhibitor-1 (PAI-1) is cardioprotective in mice by maintaining microvascular integrity and cardiac architecture. *Blood*, **115** (10), 2038–2047.

63 Baumann, A., Flagella, K., Forster, R., de Haan, L., Kronenberg, S., Locher, M., Richter, W.F., Theil, F., and Todd, M. (2014) New challenges and opportunities in nonclinical safety testing of biologics. *Regulatory Toxicology and Pharmacology*, **69** (2), 226–233.

64 Mali, P., Esvelt, K.M., and Church, G.M. (2013) Cas9 as a versatile tool for engineering biology. *Nature Methods*, **10** (10), 957–963.
65 Krasteva, P.V. (2014) CRISPR snapshots of a gene-editing tool. *Nature Methods*, **11** (4), 365.
66 Luedde, M., Flögel, U., Knorr, M., Grundt, C., Hippe, H.J., Brors, B., Frank, D., Haselmann, U., Antony, C., Voelkers, M., Schrader, J., Most, P., Lemmer, B., Katus, H.A., and Frey, N. (2009) Decreased contractility due to energy deprivation in a transgenic rat model of hypertrophic cardiomyopathy. *Journal of Molecular Medicine*, **87** (4), 411–422.
67 Bowes, J., Brown, A.J., Hamon, J., Jarolimek, W., Sridhar, A., Waldron, G., and Whitebread, S. (2012) Reducing safety-related drug attrition: the use of *in vitro* pharmacological profiling. *Nature Reviews. Drug Discovery*, **11** (12), 909–922.
68 Nguyen, P.D., Hsiao, S.T., Sivakumaran, P., Lim, S.Y., and Dilley, R.J. (2012) Enrichment of neonatal rat cardiomyocytes in primary culture facilitates long-term maintenance of contractility *in vitro*. *American Journal of Physiology. Cell Physiology*, **303**, C1220–C1228.
69 Carlson, C., Koonce, C., Aoyama, N., Einhorn, S., Fiene, S., Thompson, A., Swanson, B., Anson, B., and Kattman, S. (2013) Phenotypic screening with human iPS cell-derived cardiomyocytes: HTS-compatible assays for interrogating cardiac hypertrophy. *Journal of Biomolecular Screening*, **18** (10), 1203–1211.
70 Johnson, D.M., Geys, R., Lissens, J., and Guns, P.J. (2012) Drug-induced effects on cardiovascular function in pentobarbital anesthetized guinea-pigs: invasive LVP measurements versus the QA interval. *Journal of Pharmacological and Toxicological Methods*, **66** (2), 152–159.
71 Marks, L., Borland, S., Philp, K., Ewart, L., Lainée, P., Skinner, M., Kirk, D., and Valentin, J.-P. (2012) The role of the anaesthetised guinea-pig in the preclinical cardiac safety evaluation of drug candidate compounds. *Toxicology and Applied Pharmacology*, **263** (2), 171–183.
72 Morissette, P., Nishida, M., Trepakova, E., Imredy, J., Lagrutta, A., Chaves, A., Hoagland, K., Hoe, C.M., Zrada, M.M., Travis, J.J., Zingaro, G.J., Gerenser, P., Friedrichs, G., and Salata, J.J. (2013) The anesthetized guinea pig: an effective early cardiovascular derisking and lead optimization model. *Journal of Pharmacological and Toxicological Methods*, **68** (1), 137–49.
73 Redfern, W.S., Wakefield, I.D., Prior, H., Pollard, C.E., Hammond, T.G., and Valentin, J.-P. (2002) Safety pharmacology – a progressive approach. *Fundamental and Clinical Pharmacology*, **16** (3), 161–73.
74 Lainée, P., Philp, K., Harmer, A., Bridgland-Taylor, M., Moors, J., Knight, R., and Valentin, J.-P. (2012) Cardiac contractility assessment: a case study with clear impact and relevance of preclinical data. *Journal of Pharmacological and Toxicological Methods*, **66** (2), 174.
75 Weinblatt, M.E., Kavanaugh, A., Genovese, M.C., Musser, T.K., Grossbard, E.B., and Magilavy, D.B. (2010) An oral spleen tyrosine kinase (Syk) inhibitor for rheumatoid arthritis. *The New England Journal of Medicine*, **363**, 1303–1312.
76 Genovese, M.C., Kavanaugh, A., Weinblatt, M.E., Peterfy, C., DiCarlo, J., White, M.L., O'Brien, M., Grossbard, E.B., and Magilavy, D.B. (2011) An oral Syk kinase inhibitor in the treatment of rheumatoid arthritis: a three-month randomized, placebo-controlled, phase II study in patients with active rheumatoid arthritis that did not respond to biologic agents. *Arthritis and Rheumatism*, **63**, 337–345.
77 Skinner, M., Philp, K., Lengel, D., Coverley, L., Lamm Bergström, E., Glaves, P., Musgrove, H., Prior, H., Jefferies, G., Braddock, M., Valentin, J.-P., Huby, R., Curwen, J., Duffy, P., and Harmer, A. (2014) The contribution of VEGF signalling to fostamatinib-induced blood pressure elevation. *British Journal of Pharmacology*, **171** (9), 2308–2320.
78 Small, H.Y., Montezano, A.C., Rios, F.J., Savoia, C., and Touyz, R.M. (2014) Hypertension due to antiangiogenic cancer therapy with vascular endothelial

growth factor inhibitors: understanding and managing a new syndrome. *The Canadian Journal of Cardiology*, **30** (5), 534–543.

79 LoRusso, P.M., Gadgeel, S.M., Wozniak, A., Barge, A.J., Jones, H.K., DelProposto, Z.S., DeLuca, P.A., Evelhoch, J.L., Boerner, S.A., and Wheeler, C. (2008) Phase I clinical evaluation of ZD6126, a novel vascular-targeting agent, in patients with solid tumors. *Investigational New Drugs*, **26** (2), 159–167.

80 Gould, S., Westwood, F.R., Curwen, J.O., Ashton, S.E., Roberts, D.W., Lovick, S.C., and Ryan, A.J. (2007) Nifedipine on ZD6126-induced cardiac toxicity in rats. *Journal of the National Cancer Institute*, **99** (22), 1724–1728.

11
Safety Aspects of the $Ca_v1.2$ Channel

Berengere Dumotier and Martin Traebert

11.1
Introduction

The $Ca_v1.2$ calcium channels, referred to as L-type voltage-dependent calcium channels, play a vital role in cardiac cells. They are involved in all steps constituting a cardiac cycle. Together with other depolarizing currents, they transform an initial electrical stimulus into a mechanical action. The calcium channels are responsible for the cellular depolarization and the pacemaker activity in the sinoatrial (SA) node; they conduct the influx through the atrioventricular (AV) node, initiate the contraction–relaxation cycle (CICR: calcium-induced calcium release), and maintain the plateau phase of the ventricular action potentials (APs) until calcium ions are extruded from the cytosol. $Ca_v1.2$ channels generate long-lasting currents with minor voltage-dependent inactivation. In cardiac cells, $Ca_v1.2$ inactivation by calcium itself is occurring slowly in parallel to the AP plateau phase, subsequently controlling downstream signal transduction and coordinating contraction and relaxation cycles. $Ca_v1.2$ channels are regulated by the sympathetic nervous system and they are linked to G-protein-coupled receptors. It is essential to keep in mind that the $Ca_v1.2$ channels are macromolecular complexes associated with other proteins such as β-adrenergic receptors (β-ADRs), G proteins, cyclases, phosphodiesterases (PDEs), kinases, protein phosphatases, and anchoring proteins taking part in numerous pathways interfering with the function of the $Ca_v1.2$ channels. This chapter summarizes the principal $Ca_v1.2$ channel functions and regulation in the heart and describes how new molecular entities can modulate the function of $Ca_v1.2$ channels *in vivo* and how the latter represents a potential safety risk.

11.2
Structure of $Ca_v1.2$ Channels

$Ca_v1.2$ channels belong to a family of high-voltage activated calcium channels, $Ca_v1.1$, $Ca_v1.2$, $Ca_v1.3$, and $Ca_v1.4$, also referred to as L-type calcium channels

Antitargets and Drug Safety, First Edition. Edited by László Urbán, Vinod F. Patel, and Roy J. Vaz.

for the long-lasting current they generate when they are activated. The $Ca_v1.2$ α1C (1,4-dihydropyridine (DHP)-sensitive) subunit (SU) is highly expressed in cardiac muscle, importantly located in ventricles. In nodal cells and atrial myocytes, $Ca_v1.3$ α1D (encoded by CACNA1D gene) is present [1]. In excitable tissues, calcium channels are constituted by a minimum of four SUs: the α1 pore-forming SU and the auxiliary (regulatory) SUs also involved in anchorage and trafficking (α2/δ and β). Molecules interfering with $Ca_v1.2$ channels rarely affect the regulatory proteins but rather interact with the α1 pore-forming SU. This chapter will, therefore, essentially focus on α1 SU and regulatory β SU.

11.2.1
α-Subunit of $Ca_v1.2$ Channel

The α1C SU is the pore-forming protein of the $Ca_v1.2$ channel in an adult healthy cardiac myocyte and is encoded by the CACNA1C gene [2]. It is a 190–250 kDa protein containing four homologous repeats (I–IV) connected through cytoplasmic loops. Each repeat has six predicted transmembrane segments (S1–S6) and a reentrant pore-forming loop (P-loop) between S5 and S6. The S6 segments build the inner pore [3], and the positively charged amino acids of the S4 segment form part of the voltage sensor. The movement of this sensor in response to voltage changes results in channel opening and closing. At resting membrane potential, $Ca_v1.2$ channels are in a closed state. From a drug development point of view, it is important to know that the majority of drug- and toxin-binding sites are located on $Ca_v\alpha1$ [4,5]. $Ca_v1.2$ channels are strongly regulated by another type of inactivation that depends on Ca^{2+} influx, namely, Ca^{2+}-dependent inactivation (CDI), which serves as a negative-feedback mechanism. CDI is mediated by the ubiquitous Ca^{2+}-sensing protein calmodulin (CaM), which is constitutively bound to the $Ca_v\alpha1$ COOH terminus (see Section 11.2.2) [6]. In addition, glutamates of the P-loop play a role in the reaction to extracellular acidification that can occur during episodes of ischemia. Hence, the $Ca_v\alpha1$ subunit possesses all of the significant key characteristics that define a $Ca_v1.2$ channel, including pharmacological and biophysical properties such as gating, ion selectivity, and permeation.

11.2.2
β-Subunit of $Ca_v1.2$ Channel

Purified $Ca_v1.2$ channels contain a tightly bound cytosolic $Ca_v\beta$ protein. There are four subfamilies of $Ca_v\beta$s (β1–β4), each with splice variants, encoded by four distinct genes. All four $Ca_v\beta$s can dramatically enhance Ca^{2+} channel currents when they are coexpressed in heterologous expression systems along with a Ca_v1 or Ca_v2 α1 subunit [7–9]. $Ca_v\beta$s also change the voltage dependence and kinetics of activation and inactivation [10,11]; however, they do not affect ion permeation [12,13]. In addition, $Ca_v\beta$ is required for the modulation of

Ca_v1 channels by protein kinases, G proteins, and small RGK (Rem, Rem2, Rad, and Gem/Kir) proteins (for review, see Ref. [14]).

The α1 subunit of Ca_v1 channels cannot reach the membrane by itself; it shows no surface expression and produces very small or no currents when expressed without auxiliary subunits. Coexpression of $Ca_v\beta$ with $Ca_v\alpha1$ increases currents by orders of magnitude. The current increase reflects enhanced channel expression on the plasma membrane and also an increase in channel open probability [15,16]. Once the Ca^{2+} channel complex reaches the plasma membrane, $Ca_v\beta$ significantly modulates the gating behavior of the channel complex.

The main features of gating modulation are the enhancement of voltage-dependent activation (VDA) and voltage-dependent inactivation (VDI) as well as voltage-dependent facilitation (VDF) All $Ca_v\beta$s shift the voltage dependence of activation to more hyperpolarized voltages and increase the speed of activation. β2a is unique in that it inhibits VDI. VDI reduces the amount of Ca^{2+} entering the cell following depolarization and decreases the number of channels responsive to subsequent depolarizations. VDI is observed as a gradual increase in L-type current during high-frequency action potentials [14]. The exact molecular mechanism of CDI is still an area of extensive research, as is the relationship between CDI and VDI, but a recent study shows that two of the elements critical for VDI, $Ca_v\beta$ and a rigid IS6-AID linker, are also essential for CDI [6].

11.3
Function of $Ca_v1.2$ Channels in Cardiac Tissue

$Ca_v1.2$ channels play a vital role in cardiac cells. They are involved in all steps constituting a cardiac cycle. Together with other depolarizing currents, they transform an initial electrical stimulus into a mechanical action. The calcium channels are responsible for initiating the pacemaker activity in the SA node; they conduct the influx through the AV node, initiate the contraction–relaxation cycle (CICR; initially proposed by Fabiato and Fabiato [17), and maintain the plateau phase of the ventricular APs until calcium ions are extruded from the cytosol, mainly through the Na/Ca exchanger (NCX) and the sarcoplasmic reticulum (SR) calcium ATPase, SERCA2, allowing low diastolic calcium concentrations and myocardial relaxation (Figure 11.1). Altered SERCA2 functions will reduce the removal of calcium from the cytosol (diastolic calcium accumulation), lead to intracellular calcium overload, enhance the extrusion of calcium through NCX, and finally deplete the SR calcium load at rest. In proportion, at the next beat, the quantity of released calcium from the SR will decrease and diminish the myocardial contractility (negative inotropy). These pathological changes are observed in the context of heart failure together with additional RyR2 (type 2 ryanodine receptor) dysfunctions promoting intracellular calcium overload (for review, see Ref. [18]). $Ca_v1.2$ are also involved in controlling gene transcription in cardiomyocytes. Dysregulation of their kinetics, of inactivation process, of expression levels, or of external pathways directly influencing $Ca_v1.2$ channels

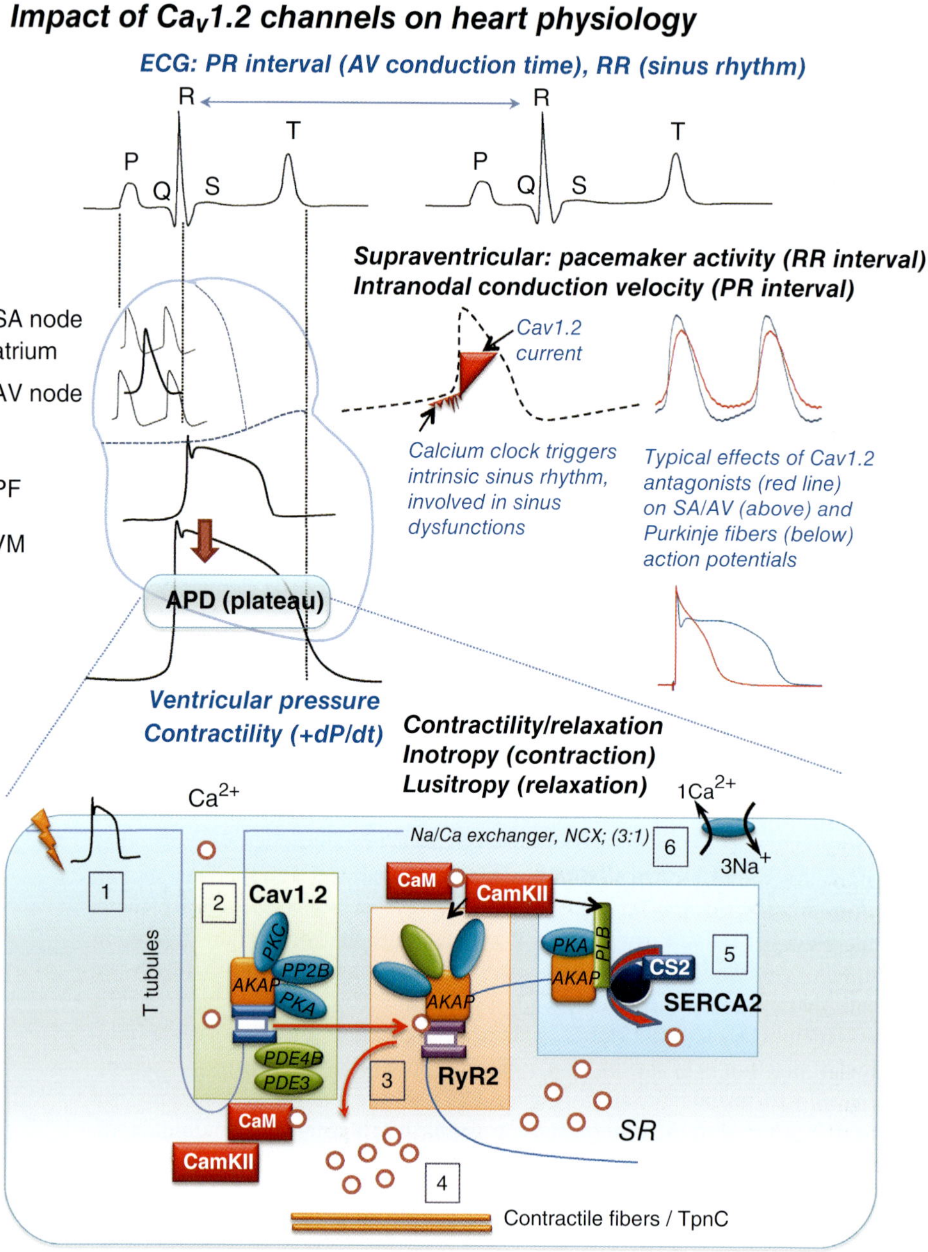

Figure 11.1 Schematic overview of the implication of $Ca_v1.2$ channels on heart physiology. (Top) $Ca_v1.2$ channels are responsible for initiating the pacemaker activity in the SA node; they conduct the influx through the AV node, maintain the plateau phase of the APs, and initiate the contraction–relaxation cycle. (Bottom) Upon membrane depolarization (1), $Ca_v1.2$ channels are activated (2) and serve as an amplification mechanism via calcium

can lead to cardiac arrhythmias or disability of the myocardium to respond to its primary vital function, that is, contract in a synchronized manner and distribute the blood in the whole body according to physical needs.

11.3.1
Role in Conduction and Contractility

$Ca_v1.2$ channels are strongly involved in the myocardial contractility properties through the excitation–contraction process. Before the influx goes through the entire myocardium, $Ca_v1.2$ channels are responsible for generating and conducting this influx from the sinoatrial node to the auriculoventricular (AV) node where the conduction speed will increase along the His bundle due to an increased proportion of fast inward sodium channels. $Ca_v1.2$ channels, therefore, constitute an important piece of the heart rhythm control. The β-adrenergic stimulation (see Section 11.3.2), by increasing the $Ca_v1.2$ current (e.g., the funny current (I_f) [19]), exerts a direct control of the rate of diastolic depolarization, which while increasing augments heart rhythm. $Ca_v1.2$ channels in the pacemaker nodal cells are under the strong influence of PDE3 and PDE4 regulating intracellular cAMP levels in their close vicinity. They constitute an important mediation pathway involved in the cardiostimulant effect of serotonin in human heart [20]. Currently in the clinic, PDE3 inhibitors (i.e., milrinone and enoximone) are used to improve cardiac performance through positive inotropic, lusitropic, and vasodilatory actions [21]. However, several clinical trials showed that long-term use of PDE3 inhibitors (i.e., milrinone) increased the mortality of patients (i.e., sudden death) suffering from congestive heart failure (CHF) [22].

PDE4 enzymes have been described to influence the RyR2 complex in its function to release calcium from the SR. In theory, PDE4D deficiency could therefore be responsible for the observed "leaky" RyR2, contributing to heart failure and arrhythmias. In the clinic, PDE4 inhibitors are developed for the treatment of chronic obstructive pulmonary disease/asthma. However, some of them were withdrawn from clinical development due to emesis and vasculitis. This apparent discrepancy between the PDE4 potential to affect myocardial contractility based on structural biology and the clinical evidence of side effects of different nature is highlighting the need for additional investigative work to better characterize the significance and role of PDE4 enzymes in human heart (for review, see Ref. [23]). $Ca_v1.2$ currents are responsible for upstroke of the action potential in the SA node (primary pacemaker center of the heart) and in the AV node. In these tissues, the diastolic potential is relatively low (between −60 and −40 mV)

release from the sarcoplasmic reticulum through RyR2 (3) for triggering myocardial contraction (4). Calcium ions are extruded from the cell by SERCA2 (5) and the Na/Ca exchanger (6). Constitutive proteins and modulators of $Ca_v1.2$ and of the main contributors to the cardiac contraction and relaxation cycle are shown. For details, please refer to the text. APD: action potential duration; AV: atrioventricular; CS2: calstabin 2 (FKPB12.6); ECG: electrocardiogram; PF: Purkinje fiber; SA: sinoatrial; VM: ventricular myocyte.

resulting in complete inactivation of the fast sodium channels. The conduction of the SA influx to the AV node is therefore characterized by a low conduction velocity compared with that observed in ventricular myocytes (where fast sodium channels are responsible for the conduction speed). $Ca_v1.2$ channel antagonists (i.e., dihydropyridines; see Section 11.4.1) not only are known to affect the peripheral vascular resistance but can also slow intracardiac conduction, this being usually observed with non-DHP compounds such as diltiazem or verapamil overdosage. On the electrocardiogram (Figure 11.1), $Ca_v1.2$ blockade can be seen as important bradycardia (slow rate), a prolongation of the PR interval (intranodal conduction delay, decreased conduction speed between the atrial and the ventricular myocardium), atrioventricular block (stop of influx propagation between atria and ventricles), and left bundle branch block (stop of propagation in the left ventricle). These rhythm disturbances are characteristic of strong depression of the $Ca_v1.2$ channels, depressing then automatism from the SA node and conduction of cardiac electrical stimulus. The predominant role of $Ca_v1.2$ channels in initiating the influx from the nodal cells that will further propagate through the atrium forms the basis of the therapeutic use of calcium channel antagonists to control supraventricular arrhythmias such as atrial fibrillation (AF) or flutter and paroxysmal supraventricular tachycardia [24].

In cardiomyocytes, $Ca_v1.2$ channels are present in the sarcolemma; however, a majority of $Ca_v1.2$ channels are localized in the T-tubules (forming dyadic clefts) where they are tightly connected to the sarcoplasmic reticulum to trigger the CICR through RyR2 receptors. However, it became more and more evident in the recent years that microdomains exist in the control of the intracellular calcium concentration ([25]; for review, see Ref. [26]) through clusters of $Ca_v1.2$ associated with clusters of RyR2 receptors, leading to a variety of cluster population, even outside the dyads [27]. T-tubules are also the sites of biological changes in structure/function of $Ca_v1.2$/RyR2 clusters as observed in chronic diseases such as heart failure or ventricular hypertrophy observed in animal models and human tissues.

11.3.2 Modulation of $Ca_v1.2$ Channels

$Ca_v1.2$ channels undergo negative and positive feedbacks modulating their functions. Pathways controlling the calcium-dependent inactivation process (e.g., calmodulin/CamKII interaction) will therefore affect $Ca_v1.2$ channels.

$Ca_v1.2$ channels are voltage-dependent channels activated at membrane potential above −40 mV. These are characterized by a long-lasting inward calcium current entering the cell. They exhibit three modes of gating: in mode 0, the channel is closed (open-channel probability is zero); in mode 1, the channel exhibits successive brief openings (open-channel probability increases); and in mode 2, the channel exhibits very long openings. The β-adrenergic stimulation of $Ca_v1.2$ channels shifts the channels from mode 0 to mode 1 [28]. Dihydropyridine agonists or β-adrenergic stimulation shifts $Ca_v1.2$ to mode 2.

11.3.2.1 Voltage- and Calcium-Dependent Facilitation

Voltage-dependent facilitation represents an increase in current amplitude after repetitive stimulation, the phenomenon being, by nature, frequency-dependent. Repetitive depolarizations (increased rate) slow the $Ca_v1.2$ decay kinetics [29], augmenting the calcium current in a graded manner with increasing frequencies. The *positive staircase*, that is, *increase in the peak calcium current*, is a mechanism developing slowly, involving a calcium-dependent phosphorylation step induced by an increased calcium entry through the channels. In contrast, the fast facilitation of $Ca_v1.2$ current is thought to result from an attenuation of CDI (see Section 11.3.2.3) because of decreased release of calcium from the SR.

11.3.2.2 Sympathetic Stimulation and Kinase Regulation

$Ca_v1.2$ channels mediate the sympathetic stimulation of the heart mainly through β-ADR. During sympathetic stimulation, catecholamines bind to β-ADR (mainly types 1 and 2 in cardiomyocytes, activate the G protein Gαs by inducing the exchange of GDP for GTP on Gαs). Gαs dissociates from the Gβγ complex and stimulates production of cAMP by the adenylyl cyclase (AC) [30], which in turn activates the cAMP-dependent protein kinase A (PKA) [31,32], which phosphorylates and activates, among other target proteins (i.e., troponin I and phospholamban (PLN)), the βSU of the $Ca_v1.2$ channels (for review, see Refs [33,34]). This, basically, constitutes the main pathway for the positive inotropic effects of the cardiac adrenergic stimulation. Importantly, the β2-ADR can inhibit AC through its ability to activate G_i, thus limiting cAMP production. These parallel mechanisms are essential in restricting the impact of PKA-dependent regulation of $Ca_v1.2$ in cardiac myocytes. Altering one step will have an impact on the other. The β-adrenergic pathway is involved in normal and pathological modifications of the $Ca_v1.2$ functions [35–37]. This can be observed in chronic diseases where the contractile capacity of the myocardium is diminished (i.e., heart failure and left ventricular hypertrophy). In addition, PKCα activation participates in the regulation of the myocardial contractility [32] through a decrease in the SERCA2 activity and subsequently a reduced calcium release during the systole, hence affecting the contractility process [38]. However, mechanism of PKCα and $Ca_v1.2$ channel α SU interaction in normal and diseased hearts is still a matter of ongoing investigations.

Different $Ca_v1.2$ subpopulations coexist in a cardiomyocyte. Functions and regulation of these subpopulations of $Ca_v1.2$ channels depend on their localization (for review, see Ref. [39]). Indeed, the cAMP/PKA signaling pathways on $Ca_v1.2$ channels are not homogeneously distributed throughout the cardiomyocyte. Caveolae (plasma membrane invaginations) mainly contain β1- and β2-ADRs → AC → PKA cascade. Associated with $Ca_v1.2$ and caveolin-3 (CAV-3) in caveolae, β-ADRs can stimulate cAMP production that regulates channel activity. In contrast, in dyadic junctions, where caveolae are absent, β-ADRs associated with $Ca_v1.2$ and caveolin-3 can, in addition, control the activity of RyR2 and PLN. A-kinase anchoring proteins (AKAPs) are closely involved in the functions of the $Ca_v1.2$ channels. They are responsible for the tight anchoring of

PKA [40] and guarantee an efficient communication with other signaling proteins, recruiting phosphodiesterases and protein phosphatases [41]. Different AKAPs have also been found to regulate β1- or β2-ADRs depending on their localization. The production of cAMP induced by β2-ADR is specifically observed in T-tubules of normal adult cardiac myocytes; the β1-ADR-induced cAMP production is distributed in the whole plasma membrane, that is, more globally (for details, see Refs [39,42,43]).

11.3.2.3 Inactivation

The inactivation of $Ca_v1.2$ channels prevents intracellular calcium overload. The VDI of $Ca_v1.2$ channels plays a minor role in this respect compared with other mechanisms. The CDI of $Ca_v1.2$ channels, in contrast to VDI, is a key factor [44]. CDI is a major determinant of the duration of the cardiac action potential. A slowed inactivation of $Ca_v1.2$ channels can disturb the balance between inward (sodium/calcium) and outward currents (mainly potassium) and delay the repolarization phase. CDI can be regarded as a safety mechanism ensuring the end of calcium entry into the cell following reactivation of $Ca_v1.2$ channels, preventing then the development of abnormalities in the repolarization phase [45].

Abnormal inactivation of $Ca_v1.2$ has been demonstrated to be responsible for a genetic disorder of mutated channels causing both cardiac dysfunction and autism (Timothy syndrome [46]). Abnormal $Ca_v1.2$ channel inactivation leads to a prolonged inward $Ca_v1.2$ current during the systole, delays the cardiac refractoriness, and predisposes one to life-threatening arrhythmia [46]. The mechanism underlying the Timothy syndrome primarily affects VDI, and not the CDI. CDI-related congenital diseases are involved in the generation of catecholamine-induced polymorphic ventricular tachycardia (CPVT) and arrhythmogenic right ventricular dysplasia/cardiomyopathy type 2 (ARVD2), following RyR2 dysfunction [47,48].

11.3.2.4 Regulation by Calmodulin

In parallel, the $Ca_v1.2$ channels are controlled by an intracellular calcium-dependent protein CaM. It interferes with $Ca_v1.2$ channels as a constitutive calcium sensor. Calcium entering through the cell binds to calmodulin, changing the conformation of the $Ca_v1.2$ channel, and then promoting the VDI of the channel [49]. Calmodulin is in fact a central regulator of $Ca_v1.2$. However, calmodulin acts as a calcium sensor for both positive and negative modulation [6].

When bound to calcium ions, CaM participates in the "calcium-dependent facilitation" of the $Ca_v1.2$ channels, a concept describing the increase in the inward calcium current as the intracellular calcium concentration augments [50]. This activity of the calcium-binding protein CaM is mediated through modulation of $Ca_v1.2$ channels by the calmodulin-dependent protein kinase II (CaMKII), which is highly sensitive to intracellular calcium increase. This intracellular protein has been initially proposed as a modulator of the CaM protein, impacting the kinetic of effects of CaM on $Ca_v1.2$ channels [51] and central in the control of intracellular calcium homeostasis (for review, see Ref. [52]).

CaMKII triggers the phosphorylation of $Ca_v1.2$ channels and their activation and catalyzes the phosphorylation of PLN that results in the alleviation of the SERCA2 inhibition, both processes running in parallel to facilitate the myocardial inotropy and lusitropy, respectively [53]. Because the quantity of calcium going through the $Ca_v1.2$ channels is small compared with the calcium released from the RyR2 receptors (a ratio of approximately 20/80), it is easy to understand that RyR2 receptors play a crucial role in the inactivation mechanism of $Ca_v1.2$ channels [54]. Hyperphosphorylation of RyR2 by CaMKII can increase SR calcium leak during the diastole [55] promoting arrhythmia through delayed afterdepolarization (DAD)-related abnormalities [45]. Conversely, CaMKII inhibition could prevent arrhythmias [53]. Specific blockers are being developed to treat catecholamine-dependent polymorphic ventricular tachycardia [47].

Calcineurin (also called protein phosphatase 2B (PP2B)) is a phosphatase activated by calcium–calmodulin complex, and hence is primarily affected by calcium entry through $Ca_v1.2$ channels [56]. Calcineurin is able to dephosphorylate the α1 SU of $Ca_v1.2$ [57] and therefore to modulate its activity. Role and function of calcineurin differ in normal and diseased hearts. Expression and function of this phosphatase has been found to be dramatically increased in patients with myocardial hypertrophy and heart failure, that is, conditions accompanied by diastolic calcium overload. Failing cardiomyocytes are exposed to structural remodeling involving proteins deeply involved in the contractility apparatus. Cardiac remodeling characterizing heart failure results from the activation of the calcineurin–nuclear factor of activated T cells (NFAT) signaling pathway, which initiates the expression of genes specific to hypertrophy or heart failure (for review, see Ref. [58]).

11.3.2.5 Indirect Regulation of $Ca_v1.2$ Channels

Various cyclic nucleotide PDEs regulate intracellular cAMP concentration in cardiomyocytes and therefore cardiac inotropy. PDEs are also often observed in complexes with AKAPs, scaffolding proteins that set together PKA and other enzymes involved in the cAMP signaling regulation. PDEs and AKAPs are known to build signaling complexes with β-ADRs (see Section 11.3.2.2). Molecules that inhibit PDE are potent cardiotonic agents used for their ability to support myocardial inotropy in the context of heart failure [59]. Contractile effects of these medications result from inhibition of cAMP degradation and a subsequent increase in cytosolic cAMP inevitably stimulating cAMP-dependent protein kinase A, which finally results in an opening of the $Ca_v1.2$ channel and an increased cytosolic calcium released from SR. At least four different PDE families exist in mammalian cardiac tissue, PDE1, PDE2, PDE3, and PDE4. PDE1 is activated by calcium–calmodulin complex, PDE2 is activated by cGMP, PDE3 preferentially hydrolyzes cAMP, and PDE4 is specific for cAMP.

Several PDE4 subtypes coexist in the myocardium (A, B, C, and D); however, only A, B, and D subtypes exist in cardiomyocytes. PDE4B and PDE4D have been described in the $Ca_v1.2$ complex as being a critical regulator of the $Ca_v1.2$ channel activity during β-ADR stimulation in cardiac cells [60]. Specifically,

PDE4B mediates the β1-ADR stimulation of $Ca_v1.2$ channels [61], limiting calcium entry and calcium overload-related arrhythmias. PDE4D subtype also plays an important role in the regulation of CICR in cardiomyocytes in association with the SERCA2 complex [62]. It is important to note that PDE subtype profile in animals dramatically differs from that observed in humans, and in the same species across tissues [63]. PDE3 and PDE4 regulating intracellular cAMP levels in the close vicinity of $Ca_v1.2$ channels constitute an important mediation pathway involved in the cardiostimulant effect of serotonin in human heart [20].

Currently in the clinic, PDE3 inhibitors (i.e., milrinone and enoximone) are used to improve cardiac performance. The positive inotropic (improved contraction), lusitropic (improved relaxation), and vasodilatory actions of PDE3 inhibitors resulting in improved cardiac output justify the use of these molecules as a therapy for the acute treatment of CHF when administrated acutely [21]. However, several clinical trials showed that long-term use of PDE3 inhibitors (i.e., milrinone) increased the mortality of patients (i.e., sudden death) suffering from CHF, thus abolishing the hopes of using this class of compounds to augment cardiac output chronically [22]. The adverse effects of PDE3 after chronic treatment could result from pathological remodeling (i.e., calcium overload-induced apoptosis) leading to cardiac dysfunctions not compatible with survival [64].

11.3.3
$Ca_v1.2$ and Cardiac Diseases

Cardiac $Ca_v1.2$ channels are deeply involved in the excitation–contraction coupling [65]. Dysregulation of these channels is, therefore, responsible for numerous mechanical and/or electrical pathologies. Heart diseases including $Ca_v1.2$ dysfunctions include long QT syndrome and sudden death [66], chronic atrial fibrillation, ischemic heart diseases, or heart failure [39,53].

In heart failure, the myocardial contractile force is diminished, partially following elevated diastolic calcium levels, depleted SR, and then excitation–contraction coupling. Heart failure is characterized by structural remodeling affecting $Ca_v1.2$ channels and many regulatory proteins modulating these channels. T-tubule architecture also shows dramatic decrease in functional $Ca_v1.2$ channels together with disruption of macromolecular signaling pathways (density, localization, and kinetics) involved in direct or indirect $Ca_v1.2$ modulation such as β-ADR regulation [53]. For instance, PDE3A expression has been found to be dramatically reduced in human failing heart with dilated and ischemic cardiomyopathy. Loss of PDE4D from the macromolecular complex of the RyR2 receptors is also involved, causing the calcium leak from the SR and intracellular calcium overload [67,68]. Because PKCα is taking part in the contractility process of the myocardium, it was thought that targeting this kinase could have a protective effect against calcium overload in the context of heart failure. However, the clinical studies published have not revealed a therapeutic benefit to date [69].

11.4 Pharmacology of $Ca_v1.2$ Channels: Translation to the Clinic

11.4.1 $Ca_v1.2$ Antagonists: Impact on Electromechanical Functions

$Ca_v1.2$ channels can be referred to as DHP-sensitive channels because of the high affinity and selectivity of the 1,4-DHP to this channel. However, there are two different classes of $Ca_v1.2$ channel antagonists: dihydropyridine and non-dihydropyridine depending on their respective binding sites to the channel. An excellent review focusing on the cardiovascular pharmacotherapy of calcium channel blockers has recently been published [24].

The therapeutic use of $Ca_v1.2$ blockers results from their selectivity to cardiac versus vascular $Ca_v1.2$ channels. For example, DHPs are vascular selective and are used in the clinic to treat high blood pressure (for review, see Ref. [70]). Among these compounds is the prototype nifedipine, and related members, amlodipine, felodipine, nicardipine, nimodipine, nisoldipine, nitrendipine, lacidipine, and lercanidipine. DHP antagonists preferentially bind to $Ca_v1.2$ channels in their active conformation, leading to a more potent inhibition at depolarized potentials (so-called use dependency). Importantly, alternative splicing of $Ca_v1.2$ has been described to impact the DHP sensitivity to $Ca_v1.2$ channels in cardiac and smooth muscles [71]. Non-dihydropyridines, in addition to the same indications, also display antiarrhythmic properties in supraventricular arrhythmias, that is, atrial fibrillation or flutter. Phenylalkylamines, such as verapamil, are indeed more selective for myocardium. These molecules reduce myocardial oxygen demand by reversing coronary vasospasm, and are therefore often used to treat angina. Benzothiazepine (BTZ) calcium channel blockers show both cardiac depressant and vasodilator actions [72].

Because they are deeply involved in the CICR process, the rationale for using calcium channel blockers is that their inhibition could protect the myocardium against calcium overload. Indeed, structural damages associated with prolonged intracellular calcium overload play a central role in activating calcium-dependent pathways involved in hypertrophy and cardiac dysfunction such as heart failure. The number of $Ca_v1.2$ channels has been shown to differ between hypertrophied and normal hearts. However, several clinical trials were unable to reveal a clear therapeutic benefit in the treatment of hypertrophy or heart failure (for review, see Refs [73,74]). In consideration of treating cardiac arrhythmias, non-DHPs can be used for acute conversion of reentrant supraventricular tachycardia and to regulate ventricular rhythm in the case of atrial fibrillation [75].

Adverse side effects commonly observed with calcium channel blockers are (i) drug interaction due to inhibition of drug metabolism (drug-specific, unrelated to $Ca_v1.2$ inhibition), (ii) atrioventricular block and bradycardia (mainly with non-DHPs), (iii) hypotension and headache due to peripheral vasodilation (mainly with DHPs), (iv) tachycardia and palpitations (as well with BTZ [76]). Finally, pedal edema is one of the most common adverse effects of the calcium channel antagonists (DHPs and non-DHPs), and its incidence reaches 80% at very high dosages [24]. The mechanism responsible for pedal edema is unclear.

11.5 Prediction of $Ca_v1.2$ Off-Target Liability

11.5.1 $Ca_v1.2$ in Cardiomyocytes Derived from iPS Cells

Cardiomyocytes derived from human induced pluripotent stem (iPS) cells offer a great potential tool for drug discovery and development. Many activities are ongoing to create and validate iPS cardiomyocytes but also other cell types for pharmacological and off-target screening assays. Expression profiling and similar investigation showed that iPS cardiomyocytes exhibit a gene transcription profile for the main proteins involved in the intracellular calcium cycling as well as the contractility process (e.g., SERCA2, $Ca_v1.2$, and RyR2) that is quite similar to adult human and nonhuman primate heart tissues. The gene encoding the L-type Ca^{2+} channel (CACNA1C/$Ca_v1.2$) and its regulatory subunit (CACNA2D2/$\alpha 2\delta 2$) can be detected in those iPS cardiomyocytes [77] and $Ca_v1.2$ is involved as in native human cardiomyocytes in the plateau phase of the cardiac action potential as well as in the intracellular Ca^{2+} homeostasis and contractility. Despite the relatively brief maturation period, *in vitro* iPS-derived cardiomyocytes (iPS-CMs), or cardiomyocytes from embryonic stem cells, express functional intracellular calcium handling components comparable to native cardiomyocytes, albeit in a somewhat immature state [78].

In hiPSC/hESC-CMs, the mechanism of excitation–contraction coupling remains contentious. Some reports support classical model of excitation–contraction coupling [79,80]. Alternatively, it was suggested that Ca^{2+} used by the contractile machinery was provided by transsarcolemmal influx and not by SR Ca^{2+} release [81]. Potential differences could be explained by differences in the T-tubule organization.

However, the measurements on intracellular Ca^{2+} transients are still an important tool to capture indirect effects on $Ca_v1.2$ channels but more importantly to identify potential effects on cardiac cellular contractility. In fact, it has been demonstrated that inhibition of $Ca_v1.2$ channels by nifedipine leads to a decreased Ca^{2+} transient in iPS cardiomyocytes. This shows that $Ca_v1.2$ is functionally expressed in these cells and that it contributes to the intracellular calcium cycling [77,80].

There are a couple of different assays and technologies available but the underlying principle is in most cases comparable and requires the loading of the iPS cardiomyocytes with calcium-sensitive dyes for up to 15 min before Ca^{2+} transients can be visualized by specific excitation light.

Because of the functional presence of $Ca_v1.2$ in iPS cardiomyocytes, these cells were recently used to investigate the cellular mechanism behind the cardiac arrhythmia of patients suffering from Timothy syndrome. As described above, the basis for this syndrome originates from a mutation of $Ca_v1.2$, which is characterized by QT prolongation, ventricular tachycardia, and autism. The Timothy syndrome ventricular-like cardiomyocytes exhibit deficits in contraction, electrical signaling, and calcium handling, as revealed by live cell imaging and electrophysiological studies [82].

References

1 Lipscombe, D. (2002) L-type calcium channels: highs and new lows. *Circulation Research*, **90**, 933–935.

2 Venetucci, L., Denegri, M., Napolitano, C., and Priori, S.G. (2012) Inherited calcium channelopathies in the pathophysiology of arrhythmias. *Nature Reviews Cardiology*, **9**, 561–575.

3 Zhen, X.G., Xie, C., Fitzmaurice, A., Schoonover, C.E., Orenstein, E.T., and Yang, J. (2005) Functional architecture of the inner pore of a voltage-gated Ca^{2+} channel. *The Journal of General Physiology*, **126**, 193–204.

4 Catterall, W.A. (2000) Structure and regulation of voltage-gated Ca^{2+} channels. *Annual Review of Cell and Developmental Biology*, **16**, 521–555.

5 Catterall, W.A. (2005) International Union of Pharmacology. XLVIII. Nomenclature and structure–function relationships of voltage-gated calcium channels. *Pharmacological Reviews*, **57**, 411–425.

6 Zuhlke, R.D., Pitt, G.S., Deisseroth, K., Tsien, R.W., and Reuter, H. (1999) Calmodulin supports both inactivation and facilitation of L-type calcium channels. *Nature*, **399**, 159–162.

7 Mikami, A., Imoto, K., Tanabe, T., Niidome, T., Mori, Y., Takeshima, H., Narumiya, S., and Numa, S. (1989) Primary structure and functional expression of the cardiac dihydropyridine-sensitive calcium channel. *Nature*, **340**, 230–233.

8 Pragnell, M., De Waard, M., Mori, Y., Tanabe, T., Snutch, T.P., and Campbell, K.P. (1994) Calcium channel β-subunit binds to a conserved motif in the I–II cytoplasmic linker of the α1-subunit. *Nature*, **368**, 67–70.

9 Shistik, E., Ivanina, T., Puri, T., Hosey, M., and Dascal, N. (1995) Ca^{2+} current enhancement by α2/δ and β subunits in *Xenopus* oocytes: contribution of changes in channel gating and α1 protein level. *The Journal of Physiology*, **489**, 55–62.

10 Josephson, I.R. and Varadi, G. (1996) The β subunit increases Ca^{2+} currents and gating charge movements of human cardiac L-type Ca^{2+} channels. *Biophysical Journal*, **70**, 1285–1293.

11 Singer, D., Biel, M., Lotan, I., Flockerzi, V., Hofmann, F., and Dascal, N. (1991) The roles of the subunits in the function of the calcium channel. *Science*, **253**, 1553–1557.

12 Gollasch, M., Ried, C., Liebold, M., Haller, H., Hofmann, F., and Luft, F.C. (1996) High permeation of L-type Ca^{2+} channels at physiological [Ca^{2+}]: homogeneity and dependence on the α1-subunit. *American Journal of Physiology. Cell Physiology*, **271**, C842–C850.

13 Wakamori, M., Mikala, G., Schwartz, A., and Yatani, A. (1993) Single-channel analysis of a cloned human heart L-type Ca^{2+} channel α1 subunit and the effects of a cardiac β subunit. *Biochemical and Biophysical Research Communications*, **196**, 1170–1176.

14 Buraei, Z. and Yang, J. (2010) The β subunit of voltage-gated Ca^{2+} channels. *Physiological Reviews*, **90**, 1461–1506.

15 Dolphin, A.C. (2003) β Subunits of voltage-gated calcium channels. *Journal of Bioenergetics and Biomembranes*, **35**, 599–620.

16 Birnbaumer, L., Qin, N., Olcese, R., Tareilus, E., Platano, D., Costantin, J., and Stefani, E. (1998) Structures and functions of calcium channel β subunits. *Journal of*

Bioenergetics and Biomembranes, **30**, 357–375.

17 Fabiato, A. and Fabiato, F. (1979) Calcium and cardiac excitation–contraction coupling. *Annual Review of Physiology*, **41**, 473–484.

18 Goldhaber, J. and Philipson, K. (2013) Cardiac sodium–calcium exchange and efficient excitation–contraction coupling: implications for heart disease. *Advances in Experimental Medicine and Biology*, **961**, 355–364.

19 DiFrancesco, D. (1995) The pacemaker current (I_f) plays an important role in regulating SA node pacemaker activity. *Cardiovascular Research*, **30**, 307–308.

20 Weninger, S., Van Craenenbroeck, K., Cameron, R.T., Vandeput, F., Movsesian, M.A., Baillie, G.S., and Lefebvre, R.A. (2014) Phosphodiesterase 4 interacts with the 5-HT4(b) receptor to regulate cAMP signaling. *Cellular Signalling*, **26**, 2573–2582.

21 Jaski, B.E., Fifer, M.A., Wright, R.F., Braunwald, E., and Colucci, W.S. (1985) Positive inotropic and vasodilator actions of milrinone in patients with severe congestive heart failure. Dose–response relationships and comparison to nitroprusside. *The Journal of Clinical Investigation*, **75**, 643–649.

22 Amsallem, E., Kasparian, C., Haddour, G., Boissel, J.P., and Nony, P. (2005) Phosphodiesterase III inhibitors for heart failure. *Cochrane Database of Systematic Reviews*, **1** (Art. No.: CD002230). doi: 10.1002/14651858.CD002230.pub2.

23 Houslay, M.D., Baillie, G.S., and Maurice, D.H. (2007) cAMP-specific phosphodiesterase-4 enzymes in the cardiovascular system. A molecular toolbox for generating compartmentalized cAMP signaling. *Circulation Research*, **100**, 950–966.

24 Godfraind, T. (2014) Calcium channel blockers in cardiovascular pharmacotherapy. *Journal of Cardiovascular Pharmacology and Therapeutics*, **19**, 501–515.

25 Soeller, C. and Baddeley, D. (2012) Super-resolution imaging of EC coupling protein distribution in the heart. *Journal of Molecular and Cellular Cardiology*, **58**, 32–40.

26 Sipido, K.R. and Cheng, H. (2013) T-tubules and ryanodine receptor microdomains: on the road to translation. *Cardiovascular Research*, **98**, 159–161.

27 Shaw, R.M. and Colecraft, H.M. (2013) L-type calcium channel targeting and local signalling in cardiac myocytes. *Cardiovascular Research*, **98**, 177–186.

28 Yue, D.T., Herzig, S., and Marban, E. (1990) β-Adrenergic stimulation of calcium channels occurs by potentiation of high-activity gating modes. *Proceedings of the National Academy of Sciences of the United States of America*, **87**, 753–757.

29 Barrere-Lemaire, S., Piot, C., Leclercq, F., Nargeot, J., and Richard, S. (2000) Facilitation of L-type calcium currents by diastolic depolarization in cardiac cells: impairment in heart failure. *Cardiovascular Research*, **47**, 336–349.

30 Hardman, J.G., Robison, G.A., and Sutherland, E.W. (1971) Cyclic nucleotides. *Annual Review of Physiology*, **33**, 311–336.

31 Kemp, B.E., Bylund, D.B., Huang, T.S., and Krebs, E.G. (1975) Substrate specificity of the cyclic AMP-dependent protein kinase. *Proceedings of the National Academy of Sciences of the United States of America*, **72**, 3448–3452.

32 Kamp, T.J. and Hell, J.W. (2000) Regulation of cardiac L-type calcium channels by protein kinase A and protein kinase C. *Circulation Research*, **87**, 1095–1102.

33 Haase, H., Bartel, S., Karczewski, P., Morano, I., and Krause, E.G. (1996) *In-vivo* phosphorylation of the cardiac L-type calcium channel beta-subunit in response to catecholamines. *Molecular and Cellular Biochemistry*, **163–164**, 99–106.

34 Weiss, S., Oz, S., Benmocha, A., and Dascal, N. (2013) Regulation of cardiac L-type Ca^{2+} channel $Ca_V1.2$ via the β-adrenergic–cAMP–protein kinase A pathway: old dogmas, advances, and new uncertainties. *Circulation Research*, **113**, 617–631.

35 Brodde, O.E., Bruck, H., and Leineweber, K. (2006) Cardiac adrenoceptors: physiological and pathophysiological

relevance. *Journal of Pharmacological Sciences*, **100**, 323–337.

36 Gorelik, J., Wright, P.T., Lyon, A.R., and Harding, S.E. (2013) Spatial control of the βAR system in heart failure: the transverse tubule and beyond. *Cardiovascular Research*, **98**, 216–224.

37 Lymperopoulos, A., Rengo, G., and Koch, W.J. (2013) Adrenergic nervous system in heart failure: pathophysiology and therapy. *Circulation Research*, **113**, 739–753.

38 Braz, J.C., Gregory, K., Pathak, A., Zhao, W., Sahin, B., Klevitsky, R., Kimball, T.F., Lorenz, J.N., Nairn, A.C. *et al.* (2004) PKC-alpha regulates cardiac contractility and propensity toward heart failure. *Nature Medicine*, **10**, 248–254.

39 Best, J.M. and Kamp, T.J. (2012) Different subcellular populations of L-type Ca^{2+} channels exhibit unique regulation and functional roles in cardiomyocytes. *Journal of Molecular and Cellular Cardiology*, **52**, 376–387.

40 Dessauer, C.W. (2009) Adenylyl cyclase–a-kinase anchoring protein complexes: the next dimension in cAMP signaling. *Molecular Pharmacology*, **76**, 935–941.

41 Skroblin, P., Grossmann, S., Schäfer, G., Rosenthal, W., and Klussmann, E. (2010) Mechanisms of protein kinase A anchoring. *International Review of Cell and Molecular Biology*, **283**, 235–330.

42 Harvey, R.D. and Hell, J.W. (2013) $Ca_V1.2$ signaling complexes in the heart. *Journal of Molecular and Cellular Cardiology*, **58**, 143–152.

43 Flynn, R. and Altier, C. (2013) A macromolecular trafficking complex composed of β-adrenergic receptors, A-kinase anchoring proteins and L-type calcium channels. *Journal of Receptor and Signal Transduction Research*, **33**, 172–176.

44 Haack, J.A., Rosenberg, R.L., Hardman, J.G., Robison, G.A., and Sutherland, E.W. (1994) Calcium-dependent inactivation of L-type calcium channels in planar lipid bilayers. *Biophysical Journal*, **66**, 1051–1060.

45 Dumotier, B.M. (2014) A straightforward guide to the basic science behind arrhythmogenesis. *Heart*. doi: 10.1136/heartjnl-2014-305647.

46 Splawski, I., Timothy, K.W., Sharpe, L.M. *et al.* (2004) $Ca_V1.2$ calcium channel dysfunction causes a multisystem disorder including arrhythmia and autism. *Cell*, **119**, 19–31.

47 Priori, S.G. and Chen, S.R. (2011) Inherited dysfunction of sarcoplasmic reticulum Ca^{2+} handling and arrhythmogenesis. *Circulation Research*, **108**, 871–883.

48 Gomez, A.M. and Richard, S. (2004) Mutant cardiac ryanodine receptors and ventricular arrhythmias: is 'gain-of-function' obligatory? *Cardiovascular Research*, **64**, 3–5.

49 Dzhura, I., Wu, Y., Colbran, R.J., Balser, J.R., and Anderson, M.E. (2000) Calmodulin kinase determines calcium-dependent facilitation of L-type calcium channels. *Nature Cell Biology*, **2**, 173–177.

50 Halling, D.B., Aracena-Parks, P., and Hamilton, S.L. (2005) Regulation of voltage-gated Ca^{2+} channels by calmodulin. *Science's STKE: Signal Transduction Knowledge Environment*. doi: 10.1126/stke. 3152005re15.

51 Nie, H.G., Hao, L.Y., Xu, J.J., Minobe, E., Kameyama, A., and Kameyama, M. (2007) Distinct roles of CaM and Ca^{2+}/CaM-dependent protein kinase II in Ca^{2+}-dependent facilitation and inactivation of cardiac L-type Ca^{2+} channels. *The Journal of Physiological Sciences*, **57**, 167–173.

52 Neely, A. and Hidalgo, P. (2014) Structure–function of proteins interacting with the α1 pore-forming subunit of high-voltage-activated calcium channels. *Frontiers in Physiology*, **5**, 1–19.

53 Luo, M. and Anderson, M. (2013) Mechanisms of altered Ca^{2+} handling in heart failure. *Circulation Research*, **113**, 690–708.

54 Kabulova, Z. (2003) Inactivation of L-type calcium channels in cardiomyocytes. Experimental and theoretical approaches. *General Physiology and Biophysics*, **22**, 441–454.

55 Fischer, T.H., Herting, J., Tirilomis, T., Renner, A., Neef, S., Toischer, K., Ellenberger, D., Förster, A., Schmitto, J.D., Gummert, J., Schöndube, F.A., Hasenfuss, G., Maier, L.S., and Sossalla, S. (2013) Ca^{2+}/calmodulin-dependent protein

kinase II and protein kinase A differentially regulate sarcoplasmic reticulum Ca^{2+} leak in human cardiac pathology. *Circulation*, **128**, 970–981.

56 Gao, H., Wang, F., Wang, W., Makarewich, C.A., Zhang, H., Kubo, H., Berretta, R.M., Barr, L.A., Molkentin, J.D., and Houser, S.R. (2012) Ca^{2+} influx through L-type Ca^{2+} channels and transient receptor potential channels activates pathological hypertrophy signaling. *Journal of Molecular and Cellular Cardiology*, **53**, 657–667.

57 Tandan, S., Wang, Y., Wang, T.T. *et al.* (2009) Physical and functional interaction between calcineurin and the cardiac L-type Ca^{2+} channel. *Circulation Research*, **105**, 51–60.

58 Wang, Y., Tandan, S., and Hill, J.A. (2014) Calcineurin-dependent ion channel regulation in heart. *Trends in Cardiovascular Medicine*, **24**, 14–22.

59 Feneck, R. (2007) Phosphodiesterase inhibitors and the cardiovascular system. *Critical Care & Pain*, **7**, 203–207.

60 Leroy, J., Richter, W., Mika, D., Castro, L.R., Abi-Gerges, A., Xie, M., Scheitrum, C., Lefebvre, F., Schittl, J. *et al.* (2011) Phosphodiesterase 4B in the cardiac L-type Ca^{2+} channel complex regulates Ca^{2+} current and protects against ventricular arrhythmias in mice. *The Journal of Clinical Investigation*, **121**, 2651–2661.

61 Mika, D., Richter, W., Westenbroek, R.E., Catterall, W.A., and Conti, M. (2014) PDE4B mediates local feedback regulation of β_1-adrenergic cAMP signaling in a sarcolemmal compartment of cardiac myocytes. *Journal of Cell Science*, **127**, 1033–1042.

62 Beca, S., Helli, P.B., Simpson, J.A., Zhao, D., Farman, G.P., Jones, P.P., Tian, X., Wilson, L.S., Ahmad, F., Chen, S.R., Movsesian, M.A., Manganiello, V., Maurice, D.H., Conti, M., and Backx, P.H. (2011) Phosphodiesterase 4D regulates baseline sarcoplasmic reticulum Ca^{2+} release and cardiac contractility, independently of L-type Ca^{2+} current. *Circulation Research*, **109**, 1024–1030.

63 Richter, W., Xie, M., Scheitrum, C., Krall, J., Movsesian, M.A., and Conti, M. (2011) Conserved expression and functions of PDE4 in rodent and human heart. *Basic Research in Cardiology*, **106**, 249–262.

64 Movsesian, M., Wever-Pinzon, O., and Vandeput, F. (2011) PDE3 inhibition in dilated cardiomyopathy. *Current Opinion in Pharmacology*, **11**, 707–713.

65 Beers, D.M. (2002) Cardiac excitation–contraction coupling. *Nature*, **415**, 198–205.

66 Hennessey, J.A., Boczek, N.J., Jiang, Y.H., Miller, J.D., Patrick, W., Pfeiffer, R., Sutphin, B.S., Tester, D.J., Barajas-Martinez, H., Ackerman, M.J., Antzelevitch, C., Kanter, R., and Pitt, G.S. (2014) A CACNA1C variant associated with reduced voltage-dependent inactivation, increased $Ca_V1.2$ channel window current, and arrhythmogenesis. *PLoS One*, **9**, e106982.

67 Marks, A.R. (2013) Calcium cycling proteins and heart failure: mechanisms and therapeutics. *The Journal of Clinical Investigation*, **123**, 46–52.

68 Marx, S.O. and Marks, A.R. (2013) Dysfunctional ryanodine receptors in the heart: new insights into complex cardiovascular diseases. *Journal of Molecular and Cellular Cardiology*, **58**, 225–231.

69 Lincoff, A.M., Roe, M., Aylward, P., Galla, J., Rynkiewicz, A., Guetta, V., Zelizko, M., Kleiman, N., White, H., McErlean, E. *et al.* (PROTECTION AMI Investigators) (2014) Inhibition of delta-protein kinase C by delcasertib as an adjunct to primary percutaneous coronary intervention for acute anterior ST-segment elevation myocardial infarction: results of the PROTECTION AMI randomized controlled trial. *European Heart Journal*, **35**, 2516–2523.

70 Cataldi, M. and Bruno, F. (2012) 1,4-Dihydropyridines: the multiple personalities of a blockbuster drug family. *Translational Medicine*, **4**, 12–26.

71 Welling, A., Ludwig, A., Zimmer, S., Klugbauer, N., Flockerzi, V., and Hofmann, F. (1997) Alternatively spliced IS6 segments of the alpha 1C gene determine the tissue-specific dihydropyridine sensitivity of cardiac and vascular smooth muscle L-type

Ca^{2+} channels. *Circulation Research*, **81**, 526–532.

72 O'Connor, S.E., Grosset, A., and Janiak, P. (1999) The pharmacological basis and pathophysiological significance of the heart rate-lowering property of diltiazem. *Fundamental & Clinical Pharmacology*, **13**, 145–153.

73 Bodi, I., Mikala, G., Koch, S., Akhter, S.A., and Schwartz, A. (2005) The L-type calcium channel in the heart: the beat goes on. *The Journal of Clinical Investigation*, **115**, 3306–3317.

74 Packer, M. *et al.* (1996) Effect of amlodipine on morbidity and mortality in severe chronic heart failure. Prospective Randomized Amlodipine Survival Evaluation Study Group. *The New England Journal of Medicine*, **335**, 1107–1114.

75 Camm, A.J., Kirchhof, P., Lip, G.Y., Schotten, U., Savelieva, I., Ernst, S., Van Gelder, I.C., Al-Attar, N., Hindricks, G. *et al.* (2010) Guidelines for the management of atrial fibrillation: the task force for the management of atrial fibrillation of the European Society of Cardiology (ESC). *European Heart Journal*, **31**, 2369–2429.

76 Mason, R.P. (2008) Scientific rationale for combination of a calcium channel antagonist and an HMG-CoA reductase inhibitor: a new approach to risk factor management. *Drugs*, **68**, 885–900.

77 Puppala, D., Collis, L.P., Sun, S.Z., Bonato, V., Chen, X., Anson, B., Pletcher, M., Fermini, B., and Engle, S.J. (2013) Comparative gene expression profiling in human-induced pluripotent stem cell-derived cardiocytes and human and cynomolgus heart tissue. *The Journal of Toxicological Sciences*, **131**, 292–301.

78 Satin, J., Itzhaki, I., Rapoport, S., Schroder, E.A., Izu, L., Arbel, G., Beyar, R., Balke, C.W., Schiller, J., and Gepstein, L. (2008) Calcium handling in human embryonic stem cell-derived cardiomyocyte. *Stem Cells*, **26**, 1961–1972.

79 Zhu, W.Z., Santana, L.F., and Laflamme, M.A. (2009) Local control of excitation–contraction coupling in human embryonic stem cell-derived cardiomyocytes. *PLoS One*, **4**, e5407.

80 Itzhaki, I., Rapoport, S., Huber, I., Mizrahi, I., Zwi-Dantsis, L. *et al.* (2011) Calcium handling in human induced pluripotent stem cell derived cardiomyocytes. *PLoS One*, **6**, e18037.

81 Dolnikov, K., Shilkrut, M., Zeevi-Levin, N., Gerecht-Nir, S., Amit, M. *et al.* (2006) Functional properties of human embryonic stem cell-derived cardiomyocytes: intracellular Ca^{2+} handling and the role of sarcoplasmic reticulum in the contraction. *Stem Cells*, **24**, 236–245.

82 Yazawa, M. and Dolmetsch, R.E. (2013) Modeling Timothy syndrome with iPS cells. *Journal of Cardiovascular Translational Research*, **6**, 1–9.

12
Cardiac Sodium Current ($Na_v1.5$)

Gary Gintant

12.1
Background and Scope

A fast inward sodium current (I_{NaF}) flowing through the voltage-gated cardiac sodium channel assemblages (consisting of the pore-forming $Na_v1.5$ and associated β-subunits and accessory proteins) is responsible for the upstroke of fast response-type action potentials in working atrial and ventricular myocardium. Besides ensuring nondecremental propagation essential for the orderly sequence of atrial and ventricular electrical activation, this current also defines refractoriness (and hence the ability to generate and propagate premature responses involved in proarrhythmia). By affecting intracellular sodium activity, this current can affect cardiac contractility and longer term cellular signaling.

Intraventricular conduction is manifest as the QRS interval on the surface ECG, and reduction of I_{NaF} leads to QRS interval prolongation resulting from decreased conduction velocity. Decreases in I_{NaF} increase the risk for conduction block, especially in diseased or injured hearts. Concerns regarding potential proarrhythmic effects of drugs blocking I_{NaF} remain, at least in part, from the Cardiac Arrhythmia Suppression Trials (also known as CAST) published some 25 years ago [1–3]. CAST was a placebo-controlled, double-blinded, multicenter trial designed to evaluate the effect of three antiarrhythmic drugs that affected I_{NaF} (encainide, flecainide, and moricizine) in postmyocardial infarction patients with ventricular arrhythmias. Mechanistically, the intent was to block cardiac sodium current sufficiently to prolong refractoriness and prevent the initiation and conduction of premature impulses that give rise to reentrant proarrhythmia. Despite early studies demonstrating the ability of encainide and flecainide to suppress frequent premature ventricular contractions, studies with these two drugs were prematurely stopped because of excessive mortality in patients. However, additional studies with flecainide for the treatment of atrial proarrhythmia support its present-day use (despite its ability to block I_{NaF}) in appropriate patients without significant cardiac disease [4]. It should be noted that different drugs vary in their potency to block and demonstrate very different characteristics for block of I_{NaF}, and that additional electrophysiological effects

Antitargets and Drug Safety, First Edition. Edited by László Urbán, Vinod F. Patel, and Roy J. Vaz.

(including those affecting repolarization) may play an important contributory role in defining overall proarrhythmic liabilities with sodium channel blocking drugs.

A recent study linked the use of noncardiac drugs that reduce cardiac excitability (a parameter intricately linked to I_{NaF}) with sudden cardiac arrest (SCA). The ARREST study is an ongoing, prospective, community-based initiative designed to establish the genetic and clinical determinants of SCA in the general population with an emphasis on drug effects [5]. This study concluded that nortriptyline, a drug that blocks I_{NaF}, increased the risk of sudden cardiac arrest in the general population, particularly in the presence of genetic and/or nongenetic factors (including polypharmacology) that affect cardiac excitability by reducing I_{NaF}. This conclusion mirrors the experience with drugs that block the repolarizing hERG/I_{Kr} current to elicit proarrhythmia affected by delayed repolarization, in that either exaggerated effects (high exposures) or concomitant factors (multiple-hit hypothesis) are typically necessary to elicit proarrhythmia for drugs that may affect minimal to moderate QT prolongation.

While the CAST trial results did provide reason for concern for drugs shown to affect I_{NaF} in diseased myocardium, it also left many unanswered questions [6,7]. For example, the relationship between QRS prolongation and proarrhythmic risk in patients without overt cardiac pathology is unknown. A recent prospective study demonstrated that each 10 ms increase in QRS duration was associated with a 27% higher risk for sudden cardiac death in a population-based sample of 2049 men aged 42–60 years (adjusted for clinically relevant risk factors, mean follow-up period of 19.1 years) [8]. It should be recognized that this individual study result does not necessarily apply to expectations with drug-induced QRS prolongation. On a practical note, as the QRS interval represents the first component of the QT interval, it is necessary to separate the contribution from QRS prolongation in evaluating delayed repolarization based on QT interval prolongation when assessing this much-watched surrogate marker of proarrhythmia; in such cases, the JT interval may be a more accurate marker for changes in ventricular repolarization. Finally, concerns related to block of I_{NaF} include the potential for negative inotropic effects that result from reduced intracellular calcium concentrations affected by reduced sodium influx to modulate the activity of the cardiac Na^+/Ca^{2+} exchange pump [9], although this relationship is complex [10,11].

The propensity to pharmacologically reduce I_{NaF} stretches across multiple therapeutic areas. A recent study by Lounkine and coworkers [12] described a computational approach to predict unintended "off-target"-based adverse drug reactions. Of the 656 marketed drugs tested on the 73 "side effect" targets, each drug modulated an average of 7 safety targets, with more than 10% acting on approximately half of the targets. Based on the drug set tested, the most promiscuous target identified was $Na_v1.5$, followed by 5-HT_{2B} serotonin receptor, 5-HT_{2A} serotonin receptor, and α2a adrenergic receptor. Another recent pharma-based *in vitro* study describing the effects of 355 compounds on cardiac conduction reported that approximately one-third of compounds affected conduction (32% of compounds slowed conduction and 3% accelerated conduction [13]). Finally, a functional screening study demonstrated that approximately 25% of the 400 drugs were shown to block activity of human $Na_v1.3$, consistent with concerns regarding early screening for activity against sodium channels [14]. For a clinical perspective on characterizing drugs modulating I_{NaF} during drug development, the reader is referred to a recent overview of drug effects on cardiac conduction [15].

More recently, an appreciation of the role of a late sodium current (I_{NaL}) flowing during the action potential plateau has re-emerged (see below). This current (which is much smaller (but more sustained) than I_{NaF} and harder to measure) may play a prominent role in proarrhythmic activity linked to early and delayed afterdepolarizations as well as contractile dysfunction related to alterations in sodium homeostasis. Although substantial evidence suggests that I_{NaL} contributes to abnormal electrophysiological characteristics of pathological and diseased myocardium, the role of I_{NaL} in modulating repolarization and contractility in normal working myocardium is more controversial at present.

This chapter will briefly highlight some basic aspects of cardiac sodium channel structure, function, and electrophysiological effects in relation to the evaluation of potential off-target actions of novel pharmacological agents that may affect cardiac sodium currents, ventricular conduction, and ventricular proarrhythmia. Evolving gaps and controversies are highlighted, including discussion of the present use and future potential of stem cell-derived cardiomyocytes for evaluating drug effects on human cardiac sodium current.

12.2 Structure and Function

12.2.1 Molecular Biology

Sodium channels are members of a superfamily of voltage-dependent ion channels that include potassium and calcium channels. The pore-forming α-subunit of the voltage-dependent cardiac sodium channel (recognized as $Na_v1.5$, and encoded by SCN5A gene) is an integral transmembrane protein that is part of a complex structure consisting of a large (260 kDa) pore-forming α-subunit, associated β-subunits, and partner proteins (including channel interactive proteins (ChiPs)). The pore structure consists of four homologous membrane domains (termed DI–DIV), each comprised of seven transmembrane spanning helices (termed S1–S6). Although the pore-forming α-subunit provides for functional current, the kinetics and voltage dependence of gating are modified by the β-subunits and other accessory proteins [16]. At present, there are 11 genes known to code for voltage-gated sodium channels and 9 functionally expressed channels ($Na_v1.1$–1.9, with $Na_v1.1$–1.3 and $Na_v1.6$–1.9 termed "neuronal type," $Na_v1.4$ expressed in skeletal muscle, and $Na_v1.5$ the cardiac-specific isoform), sharing 50% amino acid sequence homology (see Ref. [17] for a review). The nine mammalian sodium channel isoforms that have been identified and functionally expressed are all greater than 50% identical in amino acid sequence in transmembrane and extracellular domains [18]. These structural similarities play a role in defining off-target effects of drugs targeting neuronal sodium channel targets related to pain, CNS, and muscular disorders. An excellent review of progress made in understanding voltage-gated sodium channels over the last 60 years has recently been published [16].

It is now appreciated that the mechanisms responsible for congenital sodium channel-dependent cardiac arrhythmias extend beyond those affecting the channel's biophysical properties and must include consideration of components of the $Na_v1.5$ macromolecular complex. Indeed, these proteins modulate channel expression, localization, modulation, and function, and may support (or target) specific subcellular sites for channel isoforms within the myocyte, providing a heterogeneous population of $Na_v1.5$. Proteins shown to associate with $Na_v1.5$ may be classified as (1) anchoring/adaptor proteins, (2) enzymes interacting with and modifying the channel, and (3) proteins modulating the biophysical properties of $Na_v1.5$ upon binding. For example, the $Na_v1.5$ complex located at intercalated disk regions includes the adaptor protein ankyrin-G and calcium/calmodulin-dependent protein kinase II (CaMKII) that depends on the interaction with the cytoskeletal actin-associated protein β-IV-spectrin [19]. A point to consider here is the potential for novel therapeutics to interact with various structures within the sodium channel macromolecular complex to affect functional sodium current with chronic drug exposures. These effects will likely not be detected with acute studies measuring sodium currents flowing through α-subunits expressed in heterologous expression systems. An analogous argument was recently presented in regard to phenotypic variability not ascribed to mutation-dependent changes in channel function that arise from additional modifiers of channel behavior arising from alterations in transcription, RNA processing, translation, posttranslational modifications, and protein degradation [20]. The reader is referred to recent reviews detailing the complex interactions of SCN5A and components in cardiac electrophysiology and general physiology [21–23].

12.2.2 SCN5A Mutations Related to Congenital Long QT Syndromes

Much knowledge of the structure and functional characteristics of $Na_v1.5$ has been gleaned from studies of congenital cardiac arrhythmias linked to sodium channelopathies. Long QT syndromes (LQTS) are characterized by prolonged QT intervals and increased risk of sudden cardiac death due to a particular ventricular tachyarrhythmia known as torsades de pointes occurring in the setting of slow heart rates [24]. At least eleven types of LQTS have been recognized, each type linked to mutations in genes encoding an ion channel or subunits/regulatory proteins. Gain-of-function mutations in SCN5A that affect sodium channel inactivation (and enhance depolarizing inward current) are linked to LQT3, an LQT type that encompasses approximately 15% of LQTS. To delay repolarization (a surrogate marker for proarrhythmia), a mutation must enhance net inward current. Mutations from LQT3 patients often elicit gain of functions leading to enhanced residual, sustained, or persistent non-inactivating sodium current (often loosely termed late sodium current, I_{NaL}). Functional effects of discovered mutations are typically studied in heterologous expression systems (see Ref. [25]), although future studies will likely rely more on patient-specific induced pluripotent stem cell-derived cardiomyocytes [26].

I_{NaL} represents a small amplitude current (~1% of the peak I_{NaF}) that flows during the higher resistance plateau phase of the ventricular action potential. The role of this small (and difficult to measure in its native form without toxins to enhance function) current in prolonging repolarization and generating cardiac arrhythmias has been validated in quantitative models of the ventricular action potential, and is currently the target of novel pharmacological antiarrhythmic therapeutics. Anemone toxin II (ATXII) is a well-known peptide that enhances I_{NaL} that has proven useful in identifying novel therapeutics that block this exaggerated current [27].

12.2.3
Evidence for Multiple Functional Types of Cardiac Sodium Channels and Heterogeneous Distribution

Controversy exists regarding the presence and functional role of sodium channel subtypes in ventricular myocytes. A recent immunohistochemical study evaluated the level of expression and subcellular localization of sodium channel α- and β-subunits in human atrial myocytes [28]. They reported $Na_v1.1$–1.6 isoforms in different locations within myocytes, with $Na_v1.5$ (located in a striated pattern on the cell surface at the z-lines together with β2 subunits) accounting for approximately 88% of total sodium channel staining. Functional studies combining patch clamp recordings and contractility measures show that tetrodotoxin (TTX)-sensitive (non-$Na_v1.5$) isoforms accounted for up to 27% of the total sodium current in human atria and were required for maximal contractility. These findings are generally consistent with studies demonstrating TTX-sensitive sodium current responsible for 10 and 22% of peak sodium current in canine ventricle and Purkinje fibers, respectively [29], 20% of peak sodium current in rat ventricular myocytes [30], and 8% of peak sodium current in mouse ventricular myocytes [31]. A comparable study evaluating localization of sodium channel subtypes in mouse ventricular myocytes also showed TTX-sensitive channels to account for approximately 23% of sodium channels, with TTX-resistant sodium channels representing 77% of total channel staining [32]. The functional roles of multiple sodium channel isoforms in human heart remain to be fully defined.

It has been proposed that multiple pools of $Na_v1.5$ are located on lateral membranes, intercalated disks, and T-tubules within a myocyte (see Ref. [33] for a review). More recently, clustering of functional $Na_v1.5$ channels (defined using scanning ion conductance microscopy and patch clamp techniques) on the sarcolemmal membrane has been described, with clusters of various densities, most crowded in the crest region (around T-tubules) and surrounded by areas lacking functional sodium channels [34].

12.3 Physiological Role and Drug Actions

12.3.1 Fast Sodium Current (I_{NaF}): Conduction and Refractoriness

The upstroke of the action potential of working atrial and ventricular myocardium (as well as specialized conducting system comprised of Purkinje fibers) is initiated by a rapid depolarization of the membrane potential (beyond the threshold potential) to elicit a regenerative influx of sodium ions (I_{NaF}) resulting from the rapid activation and inactivation of voltage-dependent sodium channels. This rapid (lasting only a few ms) and large (up to 400 pA/pF) inward transient (with upstroke velocities ranging from 200 to 300 V/s for ventricular myocardium and up to 1000 V/s for Purkinje fibers) ensures rapid, nondecremental propagation of working myocardium and triggers the complex sequence of events responsible for cardiac contraction. Block of I_{NaF} results in slowed intraventricular conduction, manifest as prolongation of the QRS duration (a measure of ventricular conduction) and prolongation of the PR interval (reflecting the combined effects on atrial and nodal conduction and conduction through specialized ventricular conduction pathways (Purkinje fibers) leading to working myocardium).

For an isolated myocyte, the peak inward sodium current is proportional to the maximum rate of rise of the upstroke (V_{max}) when a comparable configuration is maintained [35]. For a propagating action potential, changes in peak sodium conductance during the upstroke are proportional to fractional changes in V_{max} (provided that membrane capacitance does not change and the background currents are small at the time of V_{max} [36,37]). Although such measures have been largely eclipsed by voltage clamp-based approaches, it should be appreciated that they reflect the response of intact, native currents and integrated systems (subunits and associated proteins) measured at physiological temperatures that are responsive to posttranslational modification that could include metabolic influences, channel trafficking into and out of the membrane, and potential redistribution of channels with electrophysiological remodeling. It should also be recognized that I_{NaF} is only one of the active generator properties of cardiac membranes that, when combined with passive properties, defines cardiac excitability and influences propagation [38,39].

In the simpler functional models describing their behavior, sodium channels are said to cycle through three functional states with each cardiac action potential. Specifically, channels are said to reside in a resting (nonconducted) state in fully polarized cardiac fibers and transition to an open, conducting state upon depolarization. In general, most drugs block sodium channels by binding to the activated (open) or inactivated (rather than resting) state of the channel. This open state is short-lived, as channels rapidly undergo inactivation, resulting in channel closure and termination of the fast inward sodium current transient. Channels are said to remain in the inactivated state until the membrane potential repolarizes, during which time voltage- and time-dependent recovery from inactivation ensues, enabling subsequent channel activation upon depolarization and defining refractoriness. One can easily measure drug-induced changes in refractoriness using standard voltage clamp techniques using two-pulse clamp protocols, with the second pulse progressively moving toward the end of the first pulse. In myocytes, tissues, or whole hearts, one can assess drug effects on refractoriness based on responses to premature stimuli applied during later stages of repolarization. Refractoriness measured with premature stimuli will be influenced by the time- and voltage-dependent recovery from inactivation as well as the configuration of repolarization.

12.3.2
Late (or Residual or Slow) Sodium Current (I_{NaL})

In contrast to the larger transient peak I_{NaF} responsible for the action potential upstroke, a small fraction of sodium channels may conduct inward depolarizing current later during the plateau of the action potential. This current, termed I_{NaL}, has been implicated in sustaining the action potential plateau, defining the action potential duration, and modulates intracellular sodium (and hence contractility). At least three mechanisms may underlie gain-of-function mutations of cardiac Na channels, namely transient failure of channel inactivation (burst gating), steady-state channel reopening ("window current" [40]), and channel reopening resulting from faster recovery from inactivation and membrane potentials that facilitate the activation transition during repolarization (nonequilibrium gating [41]). All these mechanisms may conceivably represent potential effects of novel pharmacological therapeutics. The definition (or possible multiple identities) of I_{NaL} requires further resolution, possibly with specific I_{NaL} blocking agents as they are discovered.

It should be recognized that recent interest in I_{NaL} represents a "rediscovery" of sodium plateau currents. Earlier demonstrations that low concentrations of the specific sodium channel blocker tetrodotoxin shortened repolarization and reduced inward current in the plateau range of potentials (without affecting upstroke velocity, and hence I_{NaF}) were interpreted as evidence of a sodium "window" current, a "persistent" sodium current, multiple states of inactivation, or a slowly inactivating sodium current [40,42–44], mainly on the basis of effects of the neurotoxin tetrodotoxin. Also of note were initial studies demonstrating that the polypeptide ATXII elicited a sustained sodium current in cardiac fibers that was blocked by low concentrations of local anesthetic-type agents [27,45].

Subsequent interest in sodium plateau current was fueled by the demonstration that gain-of-function mutations affecting cardiac sodium channel inactivation were linked to a congenital long QT syndrome (LQT3) that encompasses approximately 15% of congenital long QT syndromes (see Refs [21,46] for reviews). *In vitro* models of LQT3 using induced pluripotent stem cell-derived cardiomyocytes have also aided our understanding of this aberrant form of inactivation [47]. The readers are referred to Refs [48–50] for more recent reviews of I_{NaL}, its potential role in proarrhythmia, regulation of intracellular sodium and cardiac contractility [51], and its potential as a therapeutic drug target.

Regarding off-target effects of evolving drugs, Lacerda *et al.* [52] postulated that alfuzosin (a non-antiarrhythmic drug) acted to delay ventricular repolarization not by blocking a repolarizing potassium current, but by increasing the probability of late sodium channel openings, significantly shortening the slow time constant for recovery from inactivation, and increasing burst duration (between two- and threefold) and the number of openings per burst. These depolarizing effects (which occurred at concentrations consistent with supratherapeutic clinical exposures) raise the possibility that other QT prolonging drugs may also act by increasing I_{NaL} (compared with, for example, "classic" block of i_{Kr}/hERG current). It is currently uncertain whether the potential liability for torsades de pointes proarrhythmia for acquired QT prolongation differs from that related to block of hERG potassium current based on this alternative I_{NaL}-dependent mechanism.

The physiological role of I_{NaL} is still under study and not clearly defined. (Indeed, one can argue that I_{NaL} should be further defined or classified based on the need for toxins or pathological conditions to enhance the current.) Under normal conditions, some studies suggest that I_{NaL} acts to maintain the action potential plateau of guinea pig ventricular myocytes [53,54] and may contribute to transmural heterogeneity of repolarization in guinea pigs and dogs [55,56]. However, experiments with a recent potent and selective inhibitor GS967 (shown to block ATXII-stimulated I_{NaL} with an IC_{50} of 0.13 μM and shown to mitigate or reverse experimentally induced arrhythmias in rabbit myocytes and hearts) caused minimal shortening of the action potential duration of isolated rabbit ventricular myocytes at 0.1 μM, and only 6% shortening at 1 μM concentration [57]. It should be noted that I_{NaL} can be recorded from human $Na_v1.5$ channels in heterologous expression systems [58] and human ventricular myocytes [59]. It has also been suggested that one component of I_{NaL} may be due to noncardiac-type sodium channels [60]. What is certain is that I_{NaL} is increased with some congenital long QT3 syndromes, as well as some pathological or stressed conditions such as myocardial ischemia, heart failure, and oxidative stress [49,61].

Pharmacological studies of I_{NaL} have been hampered by lack of selectivity of agents for I_{NaL} versus I_{NaF}. For example, flecainide (class 1C) elicits use-dependent block of peak I_{NaF} and I_{NaL}, with a somewhat higher selectivity for I_{NaL} (2.9–5-fold [61]). While ranolazine is a drug widely cited as a blocker of I_{NaL}, it also inhibits multiple other cardiac currents, including hERG/i_{Kr}, at somewhat comparable concentrations [62], which will affect its overall electrophysiological profile [63]. Clearly, the identity (or identities) and functional role (or roles) of I_{NaL} in ventricular repolarization of normal hearts will be better defined with more selective (and specific) I_{NaL} blocking agents.

Finally, one must consider that multiple sodium channel isoforms may exist in the heart in different locations and under different experimental and pathological conditions. For example, Yang *et al.* recently reported that a selective blocker of $Na_v1.8$ (the gene product of SCN10A) shortened the action potential in mouse and rabbit myocytes and reversed ATXII-induced early afterdepolarizations [64]. Neuronal-type sodium channels residing within couplons (the functional units consisting of sarcolemmal L-type calcium channels with the dyadic cleft responsible for Ca^{2+} sparks) may activate sufficient reverse Na^+/Ca^{2+} exchanger (NCX) to prime the junctional cleft with Ca^{2+} to modulate contractility in rabbit myocytes [65]. In addition, $Na_v1.8$ functionally present in intracardiac neurons (and able to regulate neuronal action potential firing frequency) may affect cardiac conduction through neural activity by mechanisms not fully understood [66]. These results may help explain genome-wide association studies linking SCN10A expression to PR and QRS intervals. Such results highlight the need for integrated subcellular, cellular, and whole-organ responses in understanding the role of sodium channel isoforms and I_{NaL} in cardiac electrophysiology and potential off-target effects of evolving pharmacological therapeutics.

12.3.3
Drug Effects on I_{NaF}

In general, small molecule/local anesthetic-type drugs block cardiac fast inward sodium current by interacting with a generalized receptor site located in the channel pore (see Ref. [67] for a review). This is in contrast to toxins that bind to at least seven different sites, five of which are located or accessed from the extracellular side of the membrane (see reviews in Refs [68,69]). $Na_v1.5$ is one of three voltage-gated sodium channels that are described as tetrodotoxin-resistant (the others being $Na_v1.8$ and $Na_v1.9$). Block of cardiac sodium current by small molecules is complex, as drug binding (and hence channel block) is modulated by the state of the channel (e.g., in the simplest models, resting, open, or inactivated states). This effect has been termed "state-dependent block." Thus, the extent of channel block is dependent on the rate of stimulation or electrical activity (use-dependent block) and the voltage prior to initiation of the upstroke (voltage-dependent block). Underlying these effects is time- and voltage-dependent modulation of the rates of drug association and dissociation. In general, the time course of block of I_{NaF} during a single depolarizing pulse is not as prominent an issue for I_{NaF} compared with other (slower) cardiac currents (e.g., i_{Kr}/hERG current) due to the rapid activation and inactivation of the sodium transient. Block of I_{NaF} by drugs is recognized as a dynamic process, with drug binding (block) and dissociating (unblock) from channels as they cycle through various resting, open, and inactivated states prior to reopen with the next stimulus or heartbeat. Recovery from block (unblock, representing dissociation of drug from the channel) is an important consideration for defining drug effects, as slow recovery from block enables "accumulation of block" and use-dependent effects (see below). Drugs with slow recovery from block relative to the time course of terminal cardiac repolarization (ranging approximately 100 ms) may demonstrate slowed recovery from inactivation and prolongation of refractoriness (the ability to generate a premature action potential), thus limiting frequency of firing and affecting initiation and propagation of premature impulses. Whether this effect is pro- or antiarrhythmic depends on the kinetics of drug block and unblock, the electrophysiological substrate (including heterogeneity of refractoriness [70]), and cardiac rhythm [71–73] and is beyond the scope of this chapter.

12.3.3.1 **Voltage-Dependent Block**

It is well known that most drugs that block $Na_v1.5$ demonstrate a greater effect at less polarized membrane potentials. This effect, termed "voltage-dependent block," was first characterized based on studies characterizing drug effects on maximum upstroke velocities of normally versus partially depolarized ventricular fibers. One of the first demonstrations of voltage-dependent block of $Na_v1.5$ using voltage clamp techniques was shown by Bean *et al.* [74] who demonstrated that potency of block from depolarized holding potentials (−65 mV, approximately 10 μM) was 40 times less than that observed at hyperpolarized potentials (−120 mV, approximately 400 μM). Voltage-dependent block can cause preferential impairment and block of conduction in partially depolarized, ischemic, and infarcted regions of the myocardium (without affecting normally polarized fibers), and may be responsible for augmenting impaired conduction in diseased myocardium that may lead to reentrant proarrhythmia. Thus, the evaluation of a drug's local anesthetic effects based solely on responses (upstrokes or ionic current measures) measured from normally polarized (or hyperpolarized) cells or tissues is not sufficient to assess local anesthetic effects of drugs on I_{NaF}.

12.3.3.2 **Use-Dependent Block (and Tonic Block)**

Use-dependent block refers to the greater block that accumulates with repeated electrical activity (and cycling of channels through conducting and non-conducting states) as, for example, with more rapid rhythms. Use-dependent block in cardiac tissues was first demonstrated with the reversible exaggeration of effects of quinidine on the V_{max} of action potential upstrokes of guinea pig papillary muscles at faster stimulation rates [75] and subsequently demonstrated by numerous voltage clamp experiments [76]. Use-dependent block can also be studied noninvasively clinically based on QRS prolongation with different levels of electrical activity or rates [77]. In contrast, tonic block refers to residual block that occurs at hyperpolarized potentials during periods of slow and infrequent activity. Clearly, use-dependent block will influence the evaluation of block potency in voltage clamp experiments and may modulate a drug's effect on cardiac conduction; evaluation of drug effects on QRS duration at slow stimulation rates of rhythms may not be sufficient to assess potential local anesthetic effects of drugs on I_{NaF}. An instructive example of a thorough study assessing use-dependent block of I_{NaF} using automated patch clamp techniques (and comparing results with other methods) was published by Penniman *et al.* [78]. Block that is evident with slow stimulation (in fully repolarized fibers) may represent slow recovery from block (if due to prior activity) or block of channels in the resting state, depending on the kinetics of block recovery relative to the voltage clamp pulses used to evaluate recovery.

12.3.3.3 Models of Block and Classification Schemes Based on Antiarrhythmic Drug Effects

Two earlier simpler schemes have been postulated to explain the molecular mechanisms responsible for use-dependent block. The modulated receptor hypothesis, proposed by Hille [79] and Hondeghem and Katzung [80] presumes a single receptor site that changes affinity for a drug based on the functional state of the channel (resting, open, and inactivated states), with drug association blocking current flow. Specifically, this model postulates shifts in equilibrium resulting from a variable affinity receptor and modified inactivation gate kinetics of drug-complexed channels. As the affinity of either the open or the inactivated state is greater than that of the resting state, the number of blocked channels increases with increased cycling of the channel with repetitive activity. Further, drugs may gain access to the receptor site via hydrophilic and hydrophobic pathways, allowing state-independent interactions with the receptor. Starmer *et al.* proposed a second scheme (the guarded receptor hypothesis [81]) that suggests the receptor affinity remains constant and inactivation gate kinetics remain unmodified, but that drug access to the receptor site varies with the functional state of the channel ("guarded" channel gating, with access varying during the course of an action potential). Both models provide a basic framework for appreciating the dynamic aspects of sodium current block, although more sophisticated models may provide for more detailed granularity when describing the kinetics of block onset and recovery. The reader is referred to Ref. [82] for a recent review of state-dependent modulation of sodium channel block.

The full biophysical characterization of I_{NaF} block by a drug can be arduous, and could include measures of block to resting channels (resting state affinity, K_r), affinity to depolarized state (K_i, inactivation state affinity), kinetics of onset and recovery from block (onset and offset of block with change in pulse rate/stimulation frequency), and changes in voltage dependence of steady-state inactivation at multiple test concentrations (see Ref. [83] for an example with $Na_v1.2$). Characterizing and comparing multiple biophysical effects and chemical properties with therapeutic activities and profiles (besides single IC_{50} potency values) provides a more comprehensive view of potential functional effects to assess and confirm in subsequent *in vitro* studies targeting safety margins for conduction. Such early detailed characterizations are made feasible with the advent of automated patch platforms, each with unique advantages (see, for example, Refs [78,84,85]; see Ref. [86] for a detailed description of one approach). However, variability of such data (e.g., in the evaluation of IC_{50} values and Hill coefficients) is a concern that should be considered [87].

It is informative to consider categories of drugs that block I_{NaF} based on a framework proposed by Vaughan Williams [88] that classifies antiarrhythmic drug effects based on the extent of block of sodium current and cardiac conduction. In general, this model considers differences based on the kinetics of recovery of block (that define use-dependency [89]). Specifically, drugs demonstrating prominent local anesthetic effects (class I drugs) are subdivided on the basis of differences in use-dependent block of normally polarized ventricular tissues at physiological stimulation rates: class IA agents cause moderate use-dependent block due to intermediate use-dependent block kinetics (quinidine, procainamide, and disopyramide), class IB agents cause minimal use-dependent block due to rapid use-dependent block kinetics (lidocaine, tocainide, and mexiletine), and class IC agents cause profound reduction of the action potential upstroke and conduction velocity due to slow use-dependent block kinetics (flecainide, encainide, and lorcainide). Differences in the kinetics of use-dependent block are also evident in rate-dependent differences in conduction velocity *in vitro*. For example, lidocaine typically minimally affects QRS duration (little block accumulation due to rapid unblock kinetics), while procainamide causes a measurable increase due to a moderate amount of block accumulation (21% increase [90]) and the slower class IC agent flecainide causes prominent QRS prolongation at physiological heart rates due to greater accumulation of blocked channels [91].

12.3.4
Indirect Modulation of I_{NaF}

Until recently, I_{NaF}, along with the sodium–calcium exchanger and sodium–hydrogen exchanger, was considered the main contributor to sodium entry in cardiac myocytes. Balanced by an electrogenic Na–K ATPase, these primary systems maintain low intracellular sodium levels (Na_i) that modulate calcium cycling, contractility, metabolism, and longer term expression of cardiac proteins. The extent to which I_{NaL} may modulate cardiac contractility remains to be fully elucidated. Cardiac sodium channels are modulated by various factors. One system that has received great attention recently is Ca^{2+}/CaMKII, a serine/threonine kinase capable of phosphorylating various effectors, including sites affecting gating of $Na_v1.5$. CaMKII phosphorylation of multiple phosphorylation sites of the DI–DII cytoplasmic linker of $Na_v1.5$ shifts the voltage dependence of inactivation toward more negative potentials, slows recovery from inactivation, and increases I_{NaL} [51,92]. Similar loss-of-function inactivation gating effects are also associated with PKA-dependent phosphorylation of this cytoplasmic linker. The hyperpolarizing shift in the voltage dependence of inactivation as well as enhanced inactivation could lead to slowed conduction and contribute to reentrant arrhythmias. Finally, enhancement of I_{NaL} by CaMKII can also lead to arrhythmia arising from delayed repolarization. Additional studies have demonstrated that PKA- and PKC-dependent mechanisms can acutely regulate the intracellular distribution and molecular mobility of cardiac sodium channels in HEK cells stably expressing SCN5A [93], and the current may be metabolically modulated by activation of sigma receptors [94] and oxidative stress with proarrhythmic consequences [95].

12.4 Methodology

In silico/Binding	Ionic currents	Cellular- and tissue-based	Organ-based	Animal-based
Approaches	*Approaches*	*Approaches*	*Approaches*	*Approaches*
QSAR/ Displacement of ligands from binding sites	Manual patch – whole-cell, cell-attached patch	Action potential recordings	Ventricular wedge preparations	Small, large animals
	Automated patch – giga-seal or population patch	Upstroke, refractoriness	Langendorff – whole heart	Anesthetized versus telemeterized
				Paced versus nonpaced
	Preparations	*Preparations*	*Experimental parameters*	
	Heterologous expression	Myocytes (nonhuman, human)	Extracellular field potentials	*Experimental parameters*
	Myocytes (nonhuman, human)	Stem cell-derived cardiomyocytes	QRS interval	QRS duration
	Stem cell cardiomyocytes	Tissues – papillary muscles, Purkinje fibers, trabeculae	Conduction velocity	Conduction velocity
			Refractoriness	Neurohumoral, autonomic
	Experimental parameters	*Experimental parameters*	Torsades de pointes proarrhythmia	Hemodynamic modulation
	Block potency (IC_{50} values)	Block potency	Contractility	Contractility
	Kinetics, voltage dependence	Rate dependence		
		Voltage dependence		
		Metabolic modulation		
		Conduction velocity		
		Refractoriness		
		Contractility		

The multiple approaches available to interrogate effects of emerging compounds on $Na_v1.5$ reflect the rich history of studies of pharmacological effects on sodium currents, conduction, and proarrhythmia in heart and other excitable tissues. In general, the appropriateness and utility of various methodologies will depend on the intent of the assay (hazard identification versus risk assessment) and purpose of assay (prioritize and rank order larger number of compounds for further characterization or assess risk of a few later stage candidates) at different stages of drug discovery. Earlier studies (presented at leftward side of the table) are typically simpler, faster, and less expensive, and are more focused on informing of potential hazards, while later studies (rightward side of the table) involve more integrated systems, are slower, but may be easier to translate to clinical observations. For example, binding studies to unique sites in the inner cavity of the pore may be useful in early compound selection, but are difficult to translate regarding effects on QRS that can be monitored in (early) clinical studies. It should be recognized that one can always move toward less integrated systems (leftward direction in the table) to understand an effect on cardiac conduction or refractoriness if one is detected at later stages of drug discovery or clinical development. However, it would make little sense to study binding of a drug candidate near final selection if *in vitro* (ionic current) and *in vivo* (QRS prolongation) measures all showed minimal effects.

An integrated assessment of drug effects on cardiac sodium currents would ideally employ multiple approaches that provide *in vitro* and *in vivo* levels of confidence regarding translation of early preclinical findings. A recent study demonstrated the ability to differentiate between "good" (lidocaine-like) and "bad" (flecainide-like (strong use-dependent block)) sodium channel blocking activities using multiple *in vitro* approaches (block of human cardiac I_{Na} in transfected CHO cells), rabbit Purkinje fibers (measuring upstroke characteristics), arterially perfused left ventricular wedge preparations (measuring QRS/conduction velocity), and rabbit Langendorff hearts [13]. Another recent study illustrated an integrated approach for the preclinical evaluation of evolving drug candidates on cardiac conduction (with experimental elements including patch clamp studies, QRS interval measures in isolated Langendorff preparations, and PR and QRS measures in dogs or nonhuman primates; see Ref. [96]). The *in vitro* studies by Lu *et al.* also demonstrated the enhanced effects of flecainide with myocardial ischemia [13], confirming prior findings that flecainide results in more marked depression of conduction in ischemia/reperfused myocardium in a conscious canine model of sudden cardiac death [97]. This confirmation highlights the utility of benchmarking and mechanistic studies when assessing proarrhythmic risk of $Na_v1.5$ channel block.

12.4.1 Use of Human Stem Cell-Derived Cardiomyocytes

Human stem cell-derived cardiomyocytes represent the newest emerging preparation for evaluating drug effects on cardiac electrophysiology, including functional studies of drug effects on $Na_v1.5$. Recordings of I_{NaF} and I_{NaL} from stem cell-derived myocyte preparations have been published [98–100], and most studies demonstrate effects on various sodium current measures with known sodium channel blocking agents. In one of the first electrophysiological reports describing drug effects on human embryonic stem cell-derived cardiomyocytes, Peng *et al.* [101] demonstrated sensitivity of action potential upstrokes to block by lidocaine and quinidine. Sheng *et al.* [102] reported substantial differences in action potential and sodium currents at late-stage (day 0) *in vitro* differentiation, with higher sodium current density with human induced pluripotent stem cell-derived cardiomyocytes compared with human embryonic stem cell-derived cardiomyocytes. Also in this study, sensitivity to lidocaine was considerably reduced in embryonic versus induced cardiomyocyte preparations, while sensitivity to TTX was higher in embryonically derived preparations. Qu *et al.* [103] reported that drug-induced reduction of the action potential upstroke of embryonic stem cell-derived cardiomyocytes was less sensitive compared with increased QRS interval changes in the isolated rabbit heart.

As one might expect for an evolving use of a new preparation, the interpretation of sodium current studies should, at present, be considered with caution. First, it is likely that genuine differences in the electrophysiological characteristics of stem cell-derived cardiomyocytes are present between vendors, with time in culture, and, in general, stability of preparations. Often, these preparations are described as being electrophysiologically "immature," with less i_{K1} density (responsible for setting the partially depolarized resting membrane potential compared with native ventricular myocardium) and more i_F current (contributing to diastole and pacemaker activity; see Ref. [100]). These deficiencies are consistent with the hallmark spontaneous beating activity reported of most human stem cell-derived cardiac preparations (hSC-CMs). The enhanced automaticity and partially depolarized membrane potentials of hSC-CMs would be expected to modulate $Na_v1.5$ block based on voltage-dependent inactivation as well as rate- and voltage-dependent modulation of block. However, it is also possible that more fundamental differences may exist between various hSC-CM preparations and human adult ventricular myocytes. For example, Jonsson reported that the addition of ATXII elicited an increase in late I_{Na} in only 3 of the 13 embryonic-derived SC-CMs [100]. Additional factors worth considering when using stem cell-derived cardiomyocytes include differences in vendors/preparations, heterogeneous electrophysiological phenotypes, experimental conditions, lack of standards, and differences in levels of maturation of cardiomyocytes. Such differences should matter less when using voltage clamp protocols compared with action potential studies (due to the more controlled nature of the former studies). Future advances in stem cell maturation/differentiation should provide more robust human preparations for *in vitro* studies of all cardiac ionic currents. Such advances, coupled with "patterned growth" of myocytes, should provide for evaluation of drug effects on cardiac conduction under normal and pathological disease states/simulated conditions to better translate proarrhythmic risk of drug candidates (see Ref. [104] for a recent review).

12.5 Translation of Effects on I_{NaF}: Relation to Conduction Velocity and Proarrhythmia

It is often difficult to translate *in vitro* or *in vivo* preclinical findings to clinical effects that can be reproducibly, reliably, and simply measured in subjects or patients; in most cases, we must rely on measures of QRS prolongation from ECGs recorded under stable, controlled clinical conditions. As such, prolongation of QRS duration can be considered as a rough surrogate marker for conduction-based (reentrant) proarrhythmia (and in a manner analogous to the role of QT prolongation as a surrogate marker for torsades de pointes proarrhythmia).

A recent study by Harmer *et al.* [105] explored the relationship between drug-induced block of I_{NaF} with effects on QRS duration: block was assessed using an automated electrophysiology-based approach (IonWorks assay), and QRS prolongation was evaluated based on the published literature. To assess risk, IC_{50} values for block were compared with published reports of the corresponding unbound ("f" for free) plasma concentrations attained during clinical use, providing an IC_{50}/fC_{max} ratio. They reported that 67% of QRS prolonging drugs had IC_{50}/fC_{max} ratios less than 30, while 55 non-QRS prolonging drugs had ratios greater than 100. Further, they reported that for 37 drugs QRS prolongation was observed at free plasma concentrations that were about 15-fold lower than the corresponding IC_{50} values for block. These authors concluded that a margin of 30–100-fold between hNa_v IC_{50} and fC_{max} appears to confer an acceptable degree of safety from QRS prolongation, with QRS prolongation occurring on average at free plasma concentrations below IC_{50} values for block. Similarly, (1) a recent study by Heath *et al.* [106] demonstrated that free plasma concentrations of flecainide and mexiletine 6–30-fold below IC_{50} values for block of $hNa_v1.5$ were sufficient to prolong the QRS interval/duration by 10–20% in preclinical and clinical studies, and (2) an abstract by Cordes *et al.* [107] concluded that free plasma concentrations approximately 3–11-fold below the IC_{50} values for sodium current block were sufficient to produce QRS widening.

The above translational studies are somewhat surprising, considering the high current density of $hNa_v1.5$ in ventricular myocytes (and presumably high "depolarization reserve" [108]). Computer simulations of cardiac propagation describe a nonlinear relationship between conduction and reduced maximal sodium conductance, with a 50% decrease in conductance resulting in only modest reduction of conduction velocity from 55 to 32 cm/s [109]. This study also suggested that extreme QRS prolongation is necessary for intraventricular conduction failure in normal hearts. The sensitivity of ventricular conduction effects from sodium current block may be related to the platforms and experimental conditions used to determine block potency (simply characterized using IC_{50} values) that may include potential difference in properties of overexpressed sodium channels in HEK/CHO cells versus native myocytes, experimental conditions (room temperature, low extracellular sodium conditions), voltage protocols used (often no consideration of voltage or rate dependence), and bath concentrations (possible differences between achieved versus nominal exposures). It is also likely that the retrospective analysis of clinical responses is biased toward lower drug exposures. Despite these concerns, minimal sodium current block appears to be sufficient to slow cardiac conduction in normal myocardium based on limited present practices for evaluating sodium current block.

Advances in cardiac monitoring in early clinical trials and automated ECG analysis have made it easier to interrogate effects of drugs on ventricular conduction (QRS duration) in early clinical studies. Given that preclinical data suggest a potential clinical liability for QRS prolongation with a promising clinical candidate, it should be possible to derisk candidates by directly evaluating clinical responses early in clinical development (as in early clinical dose-ascending phase I tolerability studies). Ideally, this test would be conducted with normal subjects. Such efforts require consideration of the statistical power of clinical studies to reliably detect small changes in the QRS duration.

12.6 Conclusions

Although many questions remain, our knowledge of cardiac sodium channels and functional currents (both I_{NaF} and I_{NaL}) is clearly advancing. We have a clear understanding of how drugs may directly modulate I_{NaF}, a renewed appreciation of the potential role of I_{NaL} in cardiac repolarization and contractility, and are gaining a better appreciation of other mechanisms for modulation of cardiac sodium current realized through subunit interactions and accessory proteins. Furthermore, the use of automated patch techniques has revolutionized the early characterization of drug effects on I_{NaF} expressed in heterologous expression systems, and the further refinement of human stem cell-derived cardiomyocytes holds much promise for evaluation of short-term and longer term effects of drugs on cardiac sodium current (as well as effects on cardiac conduction for syncytial monolayer preparations and those subject to patterned growth). A remaining challenge is to translate effects observed in preclinical studies to clinical effects on conduction and proarrhythmic liability.

Arguably, there is no consensus as to the lowest magnitude of I_{NaF} block that is considered detrimental, or the amount of QRS prolongation observed clinically that is associated with meaningful risk. A challenge that remains for preclinical studies of drug effects on sodium current(s) is how to calibrate risk when a small preclinical signal is consistently found in more than one preclinical assay (at concentrations appropriate to therapeutic exposures) that may or may not be reflected in measures of intraventricular conduction in normal hearts. Although one might consider the use of preclinical disease models to evaluate potential risks, such models are complex, often difficult to replicate, and require greater numbers to calibrate regarding assay sensitivity compared with perceived human risk. The vision for the future could perhaps include the use of bioengineered human stem cell preparations or "hearts on chips" to provide a better risk assessment across normal versus diseased cardiac preparations to better understand conduction and proarrhythmic liabilities. Such an approach would prevent the rejection of novel therapeutics from all patients on the basis of potential safety liabilities relegated to selected patient populations.

References

1 Anonymous (1989) Preliminary report: effect of encainide and flecainide on mortality in a randomized trial of arrhythmia suppression after myocardial infarction. The Cardiac Arrhythmia Suppression Trial (CAST) Investigators. *The New England Journal of Medicine*, **321** (6), 406–412.

2 Pratt, C.M. and Moye, L.A. (1900) The Cardiac Arrhythmia Suppression Trial: background, interim results and implications. *The American Journal of Cardiology*, **65** (4), 20B–29B.

3 Echt, D.S., Liebson, P.R., Mitchell, L.B., Peters, R.W., Obias-Manno, D., Barker, A.H., Arensberg, D., Baker, A., Friedman, L., Greene, H.L. *et al.* (1991) Mortality and morbidity in patients receiving encainide, flecainide, or placebo. The Cardiac Arrhythmia Suppression Trial. *The New England Journal of Medicine*, **324** (12), 781–788.

4 Apostolakis, S., Oeff, M., Tebbe, U., Fabritz, L., Breithardt, G., and Kirchhof, P. (2013) Flecainide acetate for the treatment of atrial and ventricular arrhythmias. *Expert Opinion on Pharmacotherapy*, **14** (3), 347–357.

5 Bardai, A., Amin, A.S., Blom, M.T., Bezzina, C.R., Berdowski, J., Langendijk, P.N., Beekman, L., Klemens, C.A., Souverein, P.C., Koster, R.W., de Boer, A., and Tan, H.L. (2013) Sudden cardiac arrest associated with use of a non-cardiac drug that reduces cardiac excitability: evidence from bench, bedside, and community. *European Heart Journal*, **34** (20), 1506–1516.

6 Akhtar, M., Breithardt, G., Camm, A.J., Coumel, P., Janse, M.J., Lazzara, R., Myerburg, R.J., Schwartz, P.J., Waldo, A.L., Wellens, H.J. *et al.* (1990) CAST and beyond. Implications of the Cardiac Arrhythmia Suppression Trial. Task Force of the Working Group on Arrhythmias of the European Society of Cardiology. *Circulation*, **81** (3), 1123–1127.

7 Nattel, S. (1998) Experimental evidence for proarrhythmic mechanisms of antiarrhythmic drugs. *Cardiovascular Research*, **37** (3), 567–577.

8 Kurl, S., Mäkikallio, T.H., Rautaharju, P., Kiviniemi, V., and Laukkanen, J.A. (2012) Duration of QRS complex in resting electrocardiogram is a predictor of sudden cardiac death in men. *Circulation*, **125** (21), 2588–2594.

9 Ito, K., Nagafuchi, K., Taga, A., Yorikane, R., and Koike, H. (1996) Possible involvement of altered Na^+–Ca^{2+} exchange in negative inotropic effects of class I antiarrhythmic drugs on rabbit and rat ventricles. *Journal of*

Cardiovascular Pharmacology, **27** (3), 355–361.

10 Aronsen, J.M., Swift, F., and Sejersted, O.M. (2013) Cardiac sodium transport and excitation–contraction coupling. *Journal of Molecular and Cellular Cardiology*, **61**, 11–19.

11 Despa, S. and Bers, D.M. (2013) Na^+ transport in the normal and failing heart – remember the balance. *Journal of Molecular and Cellular Cardiology*, **61**, 2–10.

12 Nigsch, F., Lounkine, E., McCarren, P., Cornett, B., Glick, M., Azzaoui, K., Urban, L., Marc, P., Müller, A., Hahne, F., Heard, D.J., and Jenkins, J.L. (2011) Computational methods for early predictive safety assessment from biological and chemical data. *Expert Opinion on Drug Metabolism and Toxicology*, **7** (12), 1497–1511.

13 Lu, H.R., Rohrbacher, J., Vlaminckx, E., Van Ammel, K., Yan, G.X., and Gallacher, D.J. (2010) Predicting drug-induced slowing of conduction and pro-arrhythmia: identifying the 'bad' sodium current blockers. *British Journal of Pharmacology*, **160** (1), 60–76.

14 Huang, C.J., Harootunian, A., Maher, M.P., Quan, C., Raj, C.D., McCormack, K., Numann, R., Negulescu, P.A., and González, J.E. (2006) Characterization of voltage-gated sodium-channel blockers by electrical stimulation and fluorescence detection of membrane potential. *Nature Biotechnology*, **24** (4), 439–446.

15 Nada, A., Gintant, G.A., Kleiman, R., Gutstein, D.E., Gottfridsson, C., Michelson, E.L., Strnadova, C., Killeen, M., Geiger, M.J., Fiszman, M.L., Koplowitz, L.P., Carlson, G.F., Rodriguez, I., and Sager, P.T. (2013) The evaluation and management of drug effects on cardiac conduction (PR and QRS intervals) in clinical development. *American Heart Journal*, **165** (4), 489–500.

16 Catterall, W.A. (2012) Voltage-gated sodium channels at 60: structure, function and pathophysiology. *The Journal of Physiology*, **590** (Part 11), 2577–2589.

17 Savio-Galimberti, E., Gollob, M.H., and Darbar, D. (2012) Voltage-gated sodium channels: biophysics, pharmacology, and related channelopathies. *Frontiers in Pharmacology*, **11** (3), 124.

18 Catterall, W.A., Perez-Reyes, E., Snutch, T.P., and Striessnig, J. (2005) International Union of Pharmacology. XLVIII. Nomenclature and structure–function relationships of voltage-gated calcium channels. *Pharmacological Reviews*, **57** (4), 411–425.

19 Hund, T.J., Koval, O.M., Li, J., Wright, P.J., Qian, L., Snyder, J.S., Gudmundsson, H., Kline, C.F., Davidson, N.P., Cardona, N., Rasband, M.N., Anderson, M.E., and Mohler, P.J. (2010) A β(IV)-spectrin/CaMKII signaling complex is essential for membrane excitability in mice. *The Journal of Clinical Investigation*, **120** (10), 3508–3519.

20 Liu, M., Yang, K.C., and Dudley, S.C., Jr. (2014) Cardiac sodium channel mutations: why so many phenotypes? *Nature Reviews Cardiology*. doi: 10.1038/nrcardio.2014.85.

21 Adsit, G.S., Vaidyanathan, R., Galler, C.M., Kyle, J.W., and Makielski, J.C. (2013) Channelopathies from mutations in the cardiac sodium channel protein complex. *Journal of Molecular and Cellular Cardiology*, **61**, 34–43.

22 Song, W. and Shou, W. (2012) Cardiac sodium channel $Na_v1.5$ mutations and cardiac arrhythmia. *Pediatric Cardiology*, **33** (6), 943–949.

23 Rook, M.B., Evers, M.M., Vos, M.A., and Bierhuizen, M.F. (2012) Biology of cardiac sodium channel $Na_v1.5$ expression. *Cardiovascular Research*, **93** (1), 12–23.

24 Kannankeril, P., Roden, D.M., and Darbar, D. (2010) Drug-induced long QT syndrome. *Pharmacological Reviews*, **62** (4), 760–781.

25 Calloe, K., Refaat, M.M., Grubb, S., Wojciak, J., Campagna, J., Thomsen, N.M., Nussbaum, R.L., Scheinman, M.M., and Schmitt, N. (2013) Characterization and mechanisms of action of novel $Na_V1.5$ channel mutations associated with Brugada syndrome. *Circulation:*

Arrhythmia and Electrophysiology, **6** (1), 177–184.
26 Davis, R.P., Casini, S., van den Berg, C.W., Hoekstra, M., Remme, C.A., Dambrot, C., Salvatori, D., Oostwaard, D.W., Wilde, A.A., Bezzina, C.R., Verkerk, A.O., Freund, C., and Mummery, C.L. (2012) Cardiomyocytes derived from pluripotent stem cells recapitulate electrophysiological characteristics of an overlap syndrome of cardiac sodium channel disease. *Circulation*, **125** (25), 3079–3091.
27 Isenberg, G. and Ravens, U. (1984) The effects of the *Anemonia sulcata* toxin (ATX II) on membrane currents of isolated mammalian myocytes. *The Journal of Physiology*, **357**, 127–149.
28 Kaufmann, S.G., Westenbroek, R.E., Maass, A.H., Lange, V., Renner, A., Wischmeyer, E., Bonz, A., Muck, J., Ertl, G., Catterall, W.A., Scheuer, T., and Maier, S.K. (2013) Distribution and function of sodium channel subtypes in human atrial myocardium. *Journal of Molecular and Cellular Cardiology*, **61**, 133–141.
29 Haufe, V., Cordeiro, J.M., Zimmer, T., Wu, Y.S., Schiccitano, S., Benndorf, K., and Dumaine, R. (2005) Contribution of neuronal sodium channels to the cardiac fast sodium current I_{Na} is greater in dog heart Purkinje fibers than in ventricles. *Cardiovascular Research*, **65** (1), 117–127.
30 Duclohier, H. (2005) Neuronal sodium channels in ventricular heart cells are localized near T-tubules openings. *Biochemical and Biophysical Research Communications*, **334** (4), 1135–1140.
31 Haufe, V., Camacho, J.A., Dumaine, R., Günther, B., Bollensdorff, C., von Banchet, G.S., Benndorf, K., and Zimmer, T. (2005) Expression pattern of neuronal and skeletal muscle voltage-gated Na^+ channels in the developing mouse heart. *The Journal of Physiology*, **564** (Pt 3), 683–696.
32 Westenbroek, R.E., Bischoff, S., Fu, Y., Maier, S.K., Catterall, W.A., and Scheuer, T. (2013) Localization of sodium channel subtypes in mouse ventricular myocytes using quantitative immunocytochemistry. *Journal of Molecular and Cellular Cardiology*, **64**, 69–78.
33 Shy, D., Gillet, L., and Abriel, H. (2013) Cardiac sodium channel $Na_V1.5$ distribution in myocytes via interacting proteins: the multiple pool model. *Biochimica et Biophysica Acta*, **1833** (4), 886–894.
34 Bhargava, A., Lin, X., Novak, P., Mehta, K., Korchev, Y., Delmar, M., and Gorelik, J. (2013) Super-resolution scanning patch clamp reveals clustering of functional ion channels in adult ventricular myocyte. *Circulation Research*, **112** (8), 1112–1120.
35 Cohen, I., Attwell, D., and Strichartz, G. (1981) The dependence of the maximum rate of rise of the action potential upstroke on membrane properties. *Proceedings of the Royal Society of London. Series B, Biological Sciences*, **214** (1194), 85–98.
36 Roberge, F.A. and Boucher, L. (1990) Estimation of fractional changes in peak g_{Na}, $-g_{Na}$, E_{Na}, and h infinity (V) of cardiac cells from V_{max} of the propagating action potential. *IEEE Transactions on Bio-Medical Engineering*, **37** (5), 489–499.
37 King, J.H., Huang, C.L., and Fraser, J.A. (2013) Determinants of myocardial conduction velocity: implications for arrhythmogenesis. *Frontiers in Physiology*, **28** (4), 154.
38 Arnsdorf, M.F. and Bigger, J.T., Jr. (1976) The effect of procaine amide on components of excitability in long mammalian cardiac Purkinje fibers. *Circulation Research*, **38** (2), 115–122.
39 Jack, J.J.B., Noble, D., and Tsien, R.W. (1975) *Electric Current Flow in Excitable Cells*, Clarendon Press, Oxford.
40 Attwell, D., Cohen, I., Eisner, D., Ohba, M., and Ojeda, C. (1979) The steady state TTX-sensitive ("window") sodium current in cardiac Purkinje fibres. *Pflugers Archiv: European Journal of Physiology*, **379** (2), 137–142.
41 Clancy, C.E., Tateyama, M., Liu, H., Wehrens, X.H., and Kass, R.S. (2003) Non-equilibrium gating in cardiac Na^+ channels: an original mechanism of

arrhythmia. *Circulation*, **107** (17), 2233–2237.

42 Coraboeuf, E., Deroubaix, E., and Coulombe, A. (1979) Effect of tetrodotoxin on action potentials of the conducting system in the dog heart. *The American Journal of Physiology*, **236** (4), H561–H567.

43 Carmeliet, E. (1987) Slow inactivation of the sodium current in rabbit cardiac Purkinje fibres. *Pflugers Archiv: European Journal of Physiology*, **408** (1), 18–26.

44 Gintant, G.A., Datyner, N.B., and Cohen, I.S. (1984) Slow inactivation of a tetrodotoxin-sensitive current in canine cardiac Purkinje fibers. *Biophysical Journal*, **45** (3), 509–512.

45 Nishio, M., Ohmura, T., Kigoshi, S., and Muramatsu, I. (1991) Supersensitivity to tetrodotoxin and lignocaine of sea anemone toxin II-treated sodium channel in guinea-pig ventricular muscle. *British Journal of Pharmacology*, **104** (2), 504–508.

46 Amin, A.S., Asghari-Roodsari, A., and Tan, H.L. (2010) Cardiac sodium channelopathies. *Pflugers Archiv: European Journal of Physiology*, **460** (2), 223–237.

47 Ma, D., Wei, H., Zhao, Y., Lu, J., Li, G., Sahib, N.B., Tan, T.H., Wong, K.Y., Shim, W., Wong, P., Cook, S.A., and Liew, R. (2013) Modeling type 3 long QT syndrome with cardiomyocytes derived from patient-specific induced pluripotent stem cells. *International Journal of Cardiology*, **168** (6), 5277–5286.

48 Moreno, J.D. and Clancy, C.E. (2012) Pathophysiology of the cardiac late Na current and its potential as a drug target. *Journal of Molecular and Cellular Cardiology*, **52** (3), 608–619.

49 Remme, C.A. and Bezzina, C.R. (2010) Sodium channel (dys)function and cardiac arrhythmias. *Cardiovascular Therapy*, **28** (5), 287–294.

50 Zaza, A. and Rocchetti, M. (2013) The late Na^+ current – origin and pathophysiological relevance. *Cardiovascular Drugs and Therapy*, **27**, 61–68.

51 Grandi, E. and Herren, A.W. (2014) CaMKII-dependent regulation of cardiac Na^+ homeostasis. *Frontiers in Pharmacology*, **10** (5), 41.

52 Lacerda, A.E., Kuryshev, Y.A., Chen, Y., Renganathan, M., Eng, H., Danthi, S.J., Kramer, J.W., Yang, T., and Brown, A.M. (2008) Alfuzosin delays cardiac repolarization by a novel mechanism. *The Journal of Pharmacology and Experimental Therapeutics*, **324** (2), 427–433.

53 Kiyosue, T. and Arita, M. (1989) Late sodium current and its contribution to action potential configuration in guinea pig ventricular myocytes. *Circulation Research*, **64** (2), 389–397.

54 Horvath, B., Banyasz, T., Jian, Z., Hegyi, B., Kistamas, K., Nanasi, P.P., Izu, L.T., and Chen-Izu, Y. (2013) Dynamics of the late Na^+ current during cardiac action potential and its contribution to afterdepolarizations. *Journal of Molecular and Cellular Cardiology*, **64**, 59–68.

55 Main, M.C., Bryant, S.M., and Hart, G. (1998) Regional differences in action potential characteristics and membrane currents of guinea-pig left ventricular myocytes. *Experimental Physiology*, **83** (6), 747–761.

56 Zygmunt, A.C., Eddlestone, G.T., Thomas, G.P., Nesterenko, V.V., and Antzelevitch, C. (2001) Larger late sodium conductance in M cells contributes to electrical heterogeneity in canine ventricle. *American Journal of Physiology. Heart and Circulatory Physiology*, **281** (2), H689–H697.

57 Belardinelli, L., Liu, G., Smith-Maxwell, C., Wang, W.Q., El-Bizri, N., Hirakawa, R., Karpinski, S., Li, C.H., Hu, L., Li, X.J., Crumb, W., Wu, L., Koltun, D., Zablocki, J., Yao, L., Dhalla, A.K., Rajamani, S., and Shryock, J.C. (2013) A novel, potent, and selective inhibitor of cardiac late sodium current suppresses experimental arrhythmias. *The Journal of Pharmacology and Experimental Therapeutics*, **344** (1), 23–32.

58 Marangoni, S., Di Resta, C., Rocchetti, M., Barile, L., Rizzetto, R., Summa, A., Severi, S., Sommariva, E., Pappone, C., Ferrari, M., Benedetti, S., and Zaza, A.

(2011) A Brugada syndrome mutation (p. S216L) and its modulation by p. H558R polymorphism: standard and dynamic characterization. *Cardiovascular Research*, **91** (4), 606–616.
59 Maltsev, V.A. and Undrovinas, A.I. (2006) A multi-modal composition of the late Na^+ current in human ventricular cardiomyocytes. *Cardiovascular Research*, **69** (1), 116–127.
60 Biet, M., Barajas-Martínez, H., Ton, A.T., Delabre, J.F., Morin, N., and Dumaine, R. (2012) About half of the late sodium current in cardiac myocytes from dog ventricle is due to non-cardiac-type Na^+ channels. *Journal of Molecular and Cellular Cardiology*, **53** (5), 593–598.
61 Zaza, A., Belardinelli, L., and Shryock, J.C. (2008) Pathophysiology and pharmacology of the cardiac "late sodium current". *Pharmacology & Therapeutics*, **119** (3), 326–339.
62 Antzelevitch, C., Belardinelli, L., Zygmunt, A.C., Burashnikov, A., Di Diego, J.M., Fish, J.M., Cordeiro, J.M., and Thomas, G. (2004) Electrophysiological effects of ranolazine, a novel antianginal agent with antiarrhythmic properties. *Circulation*, **110** (8), 904–910.
63 Trenor, B., Gomis-Tena, J., Cardona, K., Romero, L., Rajamani, S., Belardinelli, L., Giles, W.R., and Saiz, J. (2013) *In silico* assessment of drug safety in human heart applied to late sodium current blockers. *Channels (Austin, TX)*, **7** (5), 249–262.
64 Yang, T., Atack, T.C., Stroud, D.M., Zhang, W., Hall, L., and Roden, D.M. (2012) Blocking *SCN10A* channels in heart reduces late sodium current and is antiarrhythmic. *Circulation Research*, **111** (3), 322–332.
65 Torres, N.S., Larbig, R., Rock, A., Goldhaber, J.I., and Bridge, J.H. (2011) Na^+ currents are required for efficient excitation–contraction coupling in rabbit ventricular myocytes: a possible contribution of neuronal Na^+ channels. *The Journal of Physiology*, **588** (Pt 21), 4249–4260.
66 Verkerk, A.O., Remme, C.A., Schumacher, C.A., Scicluna, B.P., Wolswinkel, R., de Jonge, B., Bezzina, C.R., and Veldkamp, M.W. (2012) Functional $Na_v1.8$ channels in intracardiac neurons: the link between SCN10A and cardiac electrophysiology. *Circulation Research*, **111** (3), 333–343.
67 Fozzard, H.A., Sheets, M.F., and Hanck, D.A. (2011) The sodium channel as a target for local anesthetic drugs. *Frontiers in Pharmacology*, **2**, 68.
68 Stevens, M., Peigneur, S., and Tytgat, J. (2011) Neurotoxins and their binding areas on voltage-gated sodium channels. *Frontiers in Pharmacology*, **2**, 71.
69 Chen, R. and Chung, S.H. (2014) Mechanism of tetrodotoxin block and resistance in sodium channels. *Biochemical and Biophysical Research Communications*, **446** (1), 370–374.
70 Han, J. and Moe, G.K. (1964) Nonuniform recovery of excitability in ventricular muscle. *Circulation Research*, **14**, 44–60.
71 Hoffman, B.F. and Rosen, M.R. (1981) Cellular mechanisms for cardiac arrhythmias. *Circulation Research*, **49** (1), 1–15.
72 Zipes, D.P. (2003) Mechanisms of clinical arrhythmias. *Journal of Cardiovascular Electrophysiology*, **14** (8), 902–912.
73 Coronel, R., Wilms-Schopman, F.J., and Janse, M.J. (2010) Anti- or profibrillatory effects of Na^+ channel blockade depend on the site of application relative to gradients in repolarization. *Frontiers in Physiology*, **1**, 10.
74 Bean, B.P., Cohen, C.J., and Tsien, R.W. (1983) Lidocaine block of cardiac sodium channels. *The Journal of General Physiology*, **81** (5), 613–642.
75 Johnson, E.A. and McKinnon, M.G. (1957) The differential effect of quinidine and pyrilamine on the myocardial action potential at various rates of stimulation. *The Journal of Pharmacology and Experimental Therapeutics*, **120** (4), 460–468.
76 Makielski, J.C., Undrovinas, A.I., Hanck, D.A., Sheets, M.F., Nesterenko, V.V., Alpert, L.A., Rosenshtraukh, L.V., and Fozzard, H.A. (1988) Use-dependent block of sodium current by ethmozin in voltage-clamped internally perfused canine cardiac Purkinje cells. *Journal of*

Molecular and Cellular Cardiology, **20** (3), 255–265.

77 Sadanaga, T., Ogawa, S., Okada, Y., Tsutsumi, N., Iwanaga, S., Yoshikawa, T., Akaishi, M., and Handa, S. (1993) Clinical evaluation of the use-dependent QRS prolongation and the reverse use-dependent QT prolongation of class I and class III antiarrhythmic agents and their value in predicting efficacy. *American Heart Journal*, **126** (1), 114–121.

78 Penniman, J.R., Kim, D.C., Salata, J.J., and Imredy, J.P. (2010) Assessing use-dependent inhibition of the cardiac Na^+ current (I_{Na}) in the PatchXpress automated patch clamp. *Journal of Pharmacological and Toxicological Methods*, **62** (2), 107–118.

79 Hille, B. (1977) Local anesthetics: hydrophilic and hydrophobic pathways for the drug–receptor reaction. *The Journal of General Physiology*, **69** (4), 497–515.

80 Hondeghem, L.M. and Katzung, B.G. (1977) Time- and voltage-dependent interactions of antiarrhythmic drugs with cardiac sodium channels. *Biochimica et Biophysica Acta*, **472** (3–4), 373–398.

81 Starmer, C.F., Grant, A.O., and Strauss, H.C. (1984) Mechanisms of use-dependent block of sodium channels in excitable membranes by local anesthetics. *Biophysical Journal*, **46** (1), 15–27.

82 Wang, G.K. and Strichartz, G.R. (2012) State-dependent inhibition of sodium channels by local anesthetics: a 40-year evolution. *Biochemistry (Moscow) Supplement Series A: Membrane and Cell Biology*, **6** (2), 120–127.

83 Lenkey, N., Karoly, R., Lukacs, P., Vizi, E.S., Sunesen, M., Fodor, L., and Mike, A. (2010) Classification of drugs based on properties of sodium channel inhibition: a comparative automated patch-clamp study. *PLoS One*, **5** (12), e15568.

84 Castle, N., Printzenhoff, D., Zellmer, S., Antonio, B., Wickenden, A., and Silvia, C. (2009) Sodium channel inhibitor drug discovery using automated high throughput electrophysiology platforms. *Combinatorial Chemistry & High Throughput Screening*, **12** (1), 107–122.

85 Kirsch, G.E. (2010) Mechanistic ion channel screening for drug discovery. DDD.

86 Liu, Y. (2014) Electrophysiological studies of voltage-gated sodium channels using QPatch HT, an automated patch-clamp system. *Current Protocols in Pharmacology*, **65**, 11.14.1–11.14.45.

87 Elkins, R.C., Davies, M.R., Brough, S.J., Gavaghan, D.J., Cui, Y., Abi-Gerges, N., and Mirams, G.R. (2013) Variability in high-throughput ion-channel screening data and consequences for cardiac safety assessment. *Journal of Pharmacological and Toxicological Methods*, **68** (1), 112–122.

88 Vaughan Williams, E.M. (1984) A classification of antiarrhythmic actions reassessed after a decade of new drugs. *Journal of Clinical Pharmacology*, **24** (4), 129–147.

89 Campbell, T.J. (1983) Kinetics of onset of rate-dependent effects of class I antiarrhythmic drugs are important in determining their effects on refractoriness in guinea-pig ventricle, and provide a theoretical basis for their subclassification. *Cardiovascular Research*, **17** (6), 344–352.

90 Morady, F., DiCarlo, L.A., Jr., Baerman, J.M., and Krol, R.B. (1985) Rate-dependent effects of intravenous lidocaine, procainamide, and amiodarone on intraventricular conduction. *Journal of the American College of Cardiology*, **6** (1), 179–185.

91 Ranger, S., Talajic, M., Lemery, R., Roy, D., and Nattel, S. (1989) Amplification of flecainide-induced ventricular conduction slowing by exercise. A potentially significant clinical consequence of use-dependent sodium channel blockade. *Circulation*, **79** (5), 1000–1006.

92 Wagner, S., Dybkova, N., Rasenack, E.C., Jacobshagen, C., Fabritz, L., Kirchhof, P., Maier, S.K., Zhang, T., Hasenfuss, G., Brown, J.H., Bers, D.M., and Maier, L.S. (2006) Ca^{2+}/calmodulin-dependent protein kinase II regulates cardiac Na^+ channels. *The Journal of Clinical Investigation*, **116** (12), 3127–3138.

93 Hallaq, H., Wang, D.W., Kunic, J.D., George, A.L., Jr., Wells, K.S., and Murray, K.T. (2012) Activation of protein kinase C alters the intracellular distribution and mobility of cardiac Na^+ channels. *American Journal of Physiology. Heart and Circulatory Physiology*, **302** (3), H782–H789.

94 Johannessen, M., Ramachandran, S., Riemer, L., Ramos-Serrano, A., Ruoho, A.E., and Jackson, M.B. (2009) Voltage-gated sodium channel modulation by sigma-receptors in cardiac myocytes and heterologous systems. *American Journal of Physiology. Cell Physiology*, **296** (5), C1049–C1057.

95 Pezhouman, A., Madahian, S., Stepanyan, H., Ghukasyan, H., Qu, Z., Belardinelli, L., and Karagueuzian, H.S. (2014) Selective inhibition of late sodium current suppresses ventricular tachycardia and fibrillation in intact rat hearts. *Heart Rhythms*, **11** (3), 492–501.

96 Erdemli, G.1., Kim, A.M., Ju, H., Springer, C., Penland, R.C., and Hoffmann, P.K. (2012) Cardiac safety implications of $hNa_v1.5$ blockade and a framework for pre-clinical evaluation. *Frontiers in Pharmacology*, **3**, 6.

97 Kou, W.H., Nelson, S.D., Lynch, J.J., Montgomery, D.G., DiCarlo, L., and Lucchesi, B.R. (1987) Effect of flecainide acetate on prevention of electrical induction of ventricular tachycardia and occurrence of ischemic ventricular fibrillation during the early postmyocardial infarction period: evaluation in a conscious canine model of sudden death. *Journal of the American College of Cardiology*, **9** (2), 359–365.

98 Ma, J., Guo, L., Fiene, S.J., Anson, B.D., Thomson, J.A., Kamp, T.J., Kolaja, K.L., Swanson, B.J., and January, C.T. (2011) High purity human-induced pluripotent stem cell-derived cardiomyocytes: electrophysiological properties of action potentials and ionic currents. *American Journal of Physiology. Heart and Circulatory Physiology*, **301** (5), H2006–H2017.

99 Honda, M., Kiyokawa, J., Tabo, M., and Inoue, T. (2011) Electrophysiological characterization of cardiomyocytes derived from human induced pluripotent stem cells. *Journal of Pharmacological Sciences*, **117** (3), 149–159.

100 Jonsson, M.K., Vos, M.A., Mirams, G.R., Duker, G., Sartipy, P., de Boer, T.P., and van Veen, T.A. (2012) Application of human stem cell-derived cardiomyocytes in safety pharmacology requires caution beyond hERG. *Journal of Molecular and Cellular Cardiology*, **52** (5), 998–1008.

101 Peng, S., Lacerda, A.E., Kirsch, G.E., Brown, A.M., and Bruening-Wright, A. (2010) The action potential and comparative pharmacology of stem cell-derived human cardiomyocytes. *Journal of Pharmacological and Toxicological Methods*, **61** (3), 277–286.

102 Sheng, X., Reppel, M., Nguemo, F., Mohammad, F.I., Kuzmenkin, A., Hescheler, J., and Pfannkuche, K. (2012) Human pluripotent stem cell-derived cardiomyocytes: response to TTX and lidocaine reveals strong cell to cell variability. *PLoS One*, **7** (9), 45963.

103 Qu, Y., Gao, B., Fang, M., and Vargas, H.M. (2013) Human embryonic stem cell derived cardiac myocytes detect hERG-mediated repolarization effects, but not $Na_v1.5$ induced depolarization delay. *Journal of Pharmacological and Toxicological Methods*, **68** (1), 74–81.

104 Blazeski, A., Zhu, R., Hunter, D.W., Weinberg, S.H., Zambidis, E.T., and Tung, L. (2012) Cardiomyocytes derived from human induced pluripotent stem cells as models for normal and diseased cardiac electrophysiology and contractility. *Progress in Biophysics and Molecular Biology*, **110** (2–3), 166–177.

105 Harmer, A.R., Valentin, J.P., and Pollard, C.E. (2011) On the relationship between block of the cardiac Na^+ channel and drug-induced prolongation of the QRS complex. *British Journal of Pharmacology*, **164** (2), 260.

106 Heath, B.M., Cui, Y., Worton, S., Lawton, B., Ward, G., Ballini, E., Doe, C.P., Ellis, C., Patel, B.A., and McMahon, N.C. (2011) Translation of flecainide- and mexiletine-induced cardiac sodium

channel inhibition and ventricular conduction slowing from nonclinical models to clinical. *Journal of Pharmacological and Toxicological Methods*, **63** (3), 258–268.

107 Cordes, J., Li, C., Dugas, J., Austin-LaFrance, R., Lightbown, I., Engwall, M., Sutton, M., and Steidl-Nichols, J. (2009) Translation between *in vitro* inhibition of the cardiac $Na_v1.5$ channel and preclinical and clinical QRS widening. Meeting of the Safety Pharmacology Society (Abstract).

108 Gintant, G.A., Gallacher, D.J., and Pugsley, M.K. (2011) The 'overly-sensitive' heart: sodium channel block and QRS interval prolongation. *British Journal of Pharmacology*, **164** (2), 254–259.

109 Shaw, R.M. and Rudy, Y. (1997) Ionic mechanisms of propagation in cardiac tissue. Roles of the sodium and L-type calcium currents during reduced excitability and decreased gap junction coupling. *Circulation Research*, **81** (5), 727–741.

13
Circulating Biomarkers for Drug-Induced Cardiotoxicity: Reverse Translation from Patients to Nonclinical Species

Gül Erdemli, Haisong Ju, and Sarita Pereira

13.1
Introduction

Drug-induced cardiovascular effects, such as arrhythmias and alteration of cardiac contractility and blood pressure, can be adverse and life threatening. Predictably, cardiovascular safety is the leading cause of drug discontinuation in all phases of drug discovery and development as well as the post-approval stage in the United States [1–3]. Following the withdrawal of terfenadine (Seldane) from the US market due to serious cardiac events (torsade de pointes, ventricular fibrillation, and sudden death) and deaths associated with the drug, a series of regulations and guidelines were put in place by the Health Authorities to help protect the public from potential adverse cardiac events [4,5]. As a result, it is now standard practice in the pharmaceutical industry to profile drug candidates routinely for potential effects on the cardiovascular system by *in vitro* and *in vivo* assays [6,7].

Drug candidates that are shown to be safe in nonclinical studies and in healthy volunteers, however, may still cause serious cardiovascular adverse reactions when administrated in larger groups of patients for longer periods of time [2]. This indicates that routine nonclinical methods may not be effective in identifying all adverse effects, particularly those associated with chronic treatments or that emerge in high-risk patient groups. This is an important aspect in late-stage clinical development as new or unexpected adverse reactions may result in a delay in regulatory approvals that could potentially prevent or delay patients' access to new medicines and have significant financial consequences for industry. This emphasizes the importance of the development of additional predictive and specific biomarkers for comprehensive nonclinical cardiovascular safety assessment to minimize the overall attrition rate and to improve the cardiovascular safety of future medicines.

In this chapter, we review the circulating biomarkers for the evaluation of the cardiovascular risk of new drug candidates and their utilization in the integrated risk assessment. We focus on clinically validated biomarkers with emphasis on reverse translation from human to nonclinical species. However, there may be

Antitargets and Drug Safety, First Edition. Edited by László Urbán, Vinod F. Patel, and Roy J. Vaz.

Table 13.1 Overview of cardiac biomarkers.

Cardiac phenotype	Cardiac biomarker
Cardiomyocyte damage	cTns, H-FABP, myosin light chain, CK-MB, Myb, glycogen phosphorylase BB, miRNA (miR-208 and miR-133), and serum amyloid A (SAA)
Myocardial dysfunction	B-type natriuretic peptide, N-terminal fragment proBNP, endothelin, miRNA, and mid-regional pro-adrenomedullin (MR-proADM)
Myocardial ischemia	Ischemia-modified albumin, unbound free fatty acids, and growth differentiation factor (GDF)-15
Inflammation	White blood cell count, myeloperoxidase, soluble CD40 ligand, monocyte chemoattractant protein; C-reactive protein, TNF-α, and interleukins
Hypertrophy/fibrosis	Matrix metalloproteinases, collagen propeptides, galectin-3, and soluble ST2

novel biomarkers for which translational information is not readily available (Table 13.1). Comprehensive coverage of such markers is not within the scope of this chapter and readers are referred to recent reviews [8–11].

13.2 Cardiac Troponins

There are three isoforms of cardiac troponins (cTns), including troponin I (cTnI, 24 kDa), troponin T (cTnT, 37 kDa), and troponin C (cTnC, 20 kDa) [12]. The troponins form a complex in the thin filament of contractile apparatus and play an important role in regulating cardiac contraction. cTnC is identical to troponin C in skeletal muscle and therefore is not useful for diagnosis of myocardial infarction/injury. The structure of cTnT and cTnI is unique and differs from that of skeletal muscle. Although the majority of cTns are regulatory contractile proteins and bound in the contractile apparatus in cardiomyocytes, a very small fraction of cTnT (6%) and cTnI (3%) exists as free form in the cytosol of cardiac myocytes [13]. These free-form cTns can be released into blood at early stage of insult to the heart even without irreversible myocyte injury. cTnI and cTnT are well-established biomarkers for the diagnosis and prognosis of acute myocardial infarction in clinical medicine [14–16]. It has been shown that cTns provide distinct advantages over conventional creatine kinase isoenzymes (such as CK-MB) for diagnosing acute myocardial infarction due to high specificity and wider window of detection [14]. In 2000, a joint committee of the European Society of Cardiology and the American College of Cardiology issued new criteria for the diagnosis of acute myocardial infarction by emphasizing the importance of cTn changes [17]. cTns have supplanted CK-MB as the biomarker of choice for the detection of myocardial injury since 2000 and now cTns are the preferred biomarkers in the universal definition of myocardial infarction [18]. In addition to diagnosing myocardial infarction, the elevation of cTns has also been associated with high mortality in patients with acute coronary syndrome and in the general population [15,19,20].

Based on the high sensitivity and specificity in diagnosing myocardial infarction in clinical practice, cTns have been reverse translated into nonclinical applications for detecting myocardial injury. In fact, cTnI and cTnT were considered specific, sensitive, and robust biomarkers of myocardial damage by an Expert Working Group in 2004 [21]. Both cTnI and cTnT are good examples of how this reverse translation has effectively been done, which led to relatively rapid acceptance of these biomarkers in nonclinical research for detecting drug-induced cardiac injury in toxicity testing.

Since the epitopes of troponins are highly conserved across species, immunoassays for human cTns can also be applied to animal studies. In a paper published in 2008, O'Brien summarized at least 68 nonclinical toxicology studies that validated cTns as effective biomarkers of drug-induced cardiac injury [22,23]. Nonclinical validation studies have shown that elevation of blood cTn levels is dose-dependent and associated with morphological changes in the heart. Further, the duration and amplitude of the increase in blood cTn levels are correlated with the severity of drug-induced histopathological changes.

Immunoassays of cTns have been improved and optimized over the last 15 years or so. In 2006, O'Brien evaluated six immunoassays for cTnI and cTnT to assess the cross-species reactivity and to detect drug-induced myocardial injury [24]. Drug-induced myocardial injury in humans and toxicological observations in animals may be subtle and the amount of cTns released into the blood may be much less than that released after myocardial infarction. Drugs (dobutamine, isoproterenol, and phosphodiesterase-4 inhibitors) that are known to cause myocardial injury were tested in rats or dogs. As expected, all these drugs caused significant increases in serum cTns. Further, cTnI values obtained from animals immediately before necropsy correlated closely with the histopathological findings. Over the years, the sensitivity of the modern cTn assays has also improved significantly. For example, the detection range of cTnT was 100–15 000 ng/l in the early assays, while the sensitivity of the fourth-generation immunoassays is 10 ng/l [25]. Some recent assays (also called ultra- or high-sensitivity assays) have even higher sensitivity (0.09–5 ng/ml) [25].

The biological half-life of human cTns is relatively short (90 min for cTnI and 120 min for cTnT) [22]. The half-lives of cTnI and cTnT in rat hearts are estimated to be 3.2 and 3.5 days, respectively [26]. The diagnostic window of cTns extends from a few hours to 14 days after myocardial infarction. It is conceivable that the detection window will be highly variable in drug-induced myocardial injury depending on the severity of myocardial damage and the frequency of dosing. cTns can be released from the myocardium through various mechanisms, including myocyte injury/necrosis, normal turnover of cardiac myocytes, apoptosis, increased sarcolemmal permeability, and the formation and release of membrane blebs. In addition, some clinical conditions such as heart failure, cardiomyopathy, arrhythmias, pulmonary artery embolism, or hypertension could also lead to elevated Tns in blood by unknown mechanisms. Thus, nonclinical evaluation of Tns should take the above disease conditions into consideration.

Once released into bloodstream, cTns circulate in various forms, TnI–TnC binary and TnT–TnI–TnC ternary complexes. cTns are degraded by proteases (calpain I, caspases, and matrix metalloproteinase 2) [25]. Proteolytic degradation around the epitope region severely compromised the detection of proteolytic fragment forms of cTnI by the monoclonal antibody. In contrast, the phosphorylation status near the epitope region did not significantly affect the antibody recognition of cTnI [27]. Ideal cTn assays should be able to measure total cTn and all relevant degradation products to achieve optimum sensitivity. Although the exact mechanisms of cTn elimination are not fully understood, they are likely cleared via the reticuloendothelial system due to their relatively large molecular size. However, recent evidence suggested that cTnT may be fragmented into molecules small enough for excretion from urine. Thus, impaired renal function and/or alteration of urine volume could also change circulating levels of cTnT.

It has been reported that stress induced by handling or restraint or cardiac injury associated with blood collection by cardiac puncture can also cause a cTn increase in animals. There are gender- and age-dependent changes in cTn in rats. Six-to-eight-month-old male rats have 10-fold greater serum cTnI than age-matched females and 3-month-old rats. It is now known that cTns are only stable below −70 °C for storage [23]. Multiple freeze–thaw cycles can cause significant loss of activity and should be avoided. Rare false positives have occurred with circulating heterophilic antibodies or autoantibodies, fibrin clots, and incomplete serum separation. Hemolysis has negligible contribution to cTn increase. Whole blood or plasma is preferred for cTn assessment since both ethylenediaminetetraacetic acid (EDTA) and heparin can interfere with the cTn assay [16].

In clinical medicine, an increased cTn concentration is defined as the value exceeding the 99th percentile of the normal reference population (upper reference limit, or URL). However, the normal range of cTn in species such as rats and dogs has not yet been established.

13.3 Natriuretic Peptides

The natriuretic peptide (NP) family includes five structurally similar but genetically distinct peptides: atrial natriuretic peptide (ANP), urodilatin, B-type natriuretic peptide (BNP), C-type natriuretic peptide, and D-type natriuretic peptide [28,29]. Of these, ANP and BNP are transcribed and primarily produced in the myocytes of the atria and ventricles, respectively [28–30]. BNP is synthesized as a 134-amino acid preprohormone that is cleaved to prohormone (proBNP), a 108-amino acid precursor. The biologically active 32-amino acid C-terminal and biologically inactive 76-amino acid N-terminal BNP

(NT-proBNP) are released into plasma via cleavage of proBNP in response to myocardial stretch or strain due to pressure or volume overload and/or inflammation [29,31,32]. ANP and BNP play a key role in the cardiac pressure and volume homeostasis by promoting systemic arterial dilation, natriuresis, and diuresis [28,29].

ANP and BNP have similar physiological effects: inhibition of sympathetic activity and the renin–angiotensin–aldosterone system, vascular and pulmonary smooth muscle relaxation, and increase in endothelial permeability [29]. As a result, they decrease systemic vascular resistance and blood pressure in addition to increasing glomerular filtration rate and urine output. BNP also has antimitogenic, anti-ischemic, and positive lusitropic effects and is believed to mitigate adverse cardiovascular remodeling [32]. It is proposed that these two natriuretic peptides work as an integrated system responding to volume overload and myocardial wall tension. ANP may be the first responder to these stimuli, while BNP acts as a backup in prolonged myocardial overload [29,33,34]. Circulating levels of BNP correlate with the magnitude and pattern of ventricular hypertrophy and the severity of left ventricular dysfunction. Therefore, BNP has been proposed to be a more specific marker of left ventricular hypertrophy and overload than ANP that is released mainly in response to atrial overload.

Natriuretic peptides exert their effects via three membrane receptors: NPR-A, NPR-B, and NPR-C. NPR-A and NPR-B are the guanylyl cyclase-coupled receptors expressed in various tissues, including adrenal glands, brain, and vascular and pulmonary smooth muscles, and are responsible for most of their physiological effects. BNP is believed to exert its effects mainly via activation of NPR-A [29].

BNP is also expressed in noncardiac tissues, such as brain and adrenal glands. However, BNP expression in the heart increases in cardiac diseases with pressure or volume overload. Thus, it is believed that the ventricular tissue is the main source of circulating BNP in pathophysiological conditions [29,30]. BNP does not bind to plasma proteins and is quickly cleared from the plasma by ectoenzyme neutral endopetidase and by NPR-C mainly via kidneys with a half-life of around 20 min. NT-proBNP is biologically inactive and generally believed to have longer half-life than BNP [28]. However, a recent study by Kroll *et al.* has shown that NT-proBNP is cleared from the circulation with a similar half-life (~20 min) in humans [35].

Because there is no significant BNP stored in the heart, increased BNP levels require increased synthesis [29,36]. proBNP is present in secretory granules in cardiomyocytes and upon secretion it is cleaved into BNP1–32 and NT-proBNP1–76. In circulation, a small amount of proBNP can also be detected in addition to BNP and NT-proBNP in heart failure patients and healthy subjects [29]. How the disease state might affect the metabolism of proBNP-derived peptides, their individual circulating levels, or their relative ratios is yet not fully understood [37,38]. Several routine laboratory tests approved by Heath Authorities are commercially available. These assays are designed to detect the total amount of analyte. BNP and NT-proBNP assays do not display significant cross-reactivity for each other, but they cross-react with proBNP in various degrees [29,39].

Despite their well-established role in the diagnosis and prognosis of heart failure, there is no consensus on the diagnostic utility of natriuretic peptides in drug-induced cardiotoxicity. Urbanova *et al.* investigated the changes in natriuretic peptide levels in patients treated with anthracyclines [40]. Despite some promising results, the analysis failed to show a clear relationship between the anthracycline cardiac toxicity and natriuretic peptide levels. High variability in natriuretic peptide levels, interactions with various bioactive agents and differences in analytical methods are some of the factors limiting the interpretation of these studies [40]. In addition, the incidence and severity of the anthracycline-induced cardiotoxicity can be influenced by several factors, including pre-existing heart disease, genetic background, age, gender, exposure to radiotherapy, and other cardiotoxic chemotherapy. Therefore, better controlled, long-term studies are required to clarify the role of natriuretic peptides in anthracycline-induced cardiotoxicity and drug-induced cardiotoxicity in general.

Given the established value in the clinical practice, natriuretic peptides are prospective candidates for translational biomarkers for cardiac pathophysiologies such as mechanical stress and heart failure remodeling in animal models. Rat has been the preferred species to assess natriuretic peptide levels due to the ability to use commercially available antibodies for detection [41]. Rat-specific assays have also been described to measure NT-proBNP in rat serum [42,43]. Using an immunoaffinity-based liquid chromatography–mass spectrometry assay, Berna *et al.* showed that NT-proBNP levels increased significantly in cardiac hypertrophy in rats [43]. They also reported that increases in NT-proBNP levels were corroborated with the heart weight and magnetic resonance imaging of left ventricle. However, in this study a detailed analysis of the relationship between the biomarker levels and the measures of cardiac hypertrophy confirming the causal relationship was not presented [43]. Langenickel *et al.* analyzed cardiac natriuretic peptide mRNA expression at a different stage of heart failure and showed that in compensated heart failure models ANP and BNP plasma concentrations were elevated and ANP mRNA expression was induced in both ventricles, while ventricular BNP mRNA expression was unchanged [34]. BNP mRNA expression was upregulated only in overt heart failure when cardiac hypertrophy was further increased and pulmonary congestion, elevated end-diastolic pressures, and decreased cardiac contractility were present, indicating a possible role of BNP as a marker of the transition from compensated to overt heart failure [34]. Using a deconvolution analysis in an acute volume overload sheep model, Pemberton *et al.* showed that plasma NT-proBNP measurements could be a stable and sensitive marker of cardiac function, including early cardiac decompensation [28].

A body of evidence supporting the role of natriuretic peptides in the diagnosis and monitoring of drug-induced cardiotoxicity is also emerging. Bharti *et al.* have studied the antihypertrophic effect of SB-204,741, a 5-hydroxytryptamine receptor 2B (5-HT_{2B}) receptor blocker, and SB-216,763, a glycogen synthase kinase 3β (GSK-3β) inhibitor, in isoproterenol-induced cardiac hypertrophy rat model and showed that both compounds improved BNP levels in isoproterenol-challenged myocardium [44]. Casopitant, a potent and selective neurokinin 1 (NK1) receptor antagonist, was developed for depression and anxiety. The cardiac toxicity, including increased heart weight and myocardial degeneration/necrosis, was observed after 39-week oral administration of casopitant in dogs [45]. To investigate the onset, progression, and reversibility of the cardiac changes, several circulating biomarkers and echocardiography imaging were studied and compared with heart weight at different time points of postmortem examination. The NT-proBNP was the first biomarker to show an increase at 2 weeks onward preceding the anatomical and functional changes. Furthermore, while cardiovascular observations such as left ventricular mass increases recovered after treatment withdrawal, NT-proBNP levels were maintained indicating the sensitivity of NT-proBNP as an early biomarker of functional cardiac impairment [45].

13.4 Novel/Exploratory Biomarkers: H-FABP, miRNA, and Genomic Biomarkers

In addition to cTns, ANP, and BNP, some new biomarkers also show promise in detecting drug-induced cardiotoxicity. Heart fatty acid-binding protein (H-FABP) is a low molecular weight protein (15 kDa) abundant in cardiac muscle and rapidly released following the onset of cardiomyocyte injury [46]. H-FABP has been evaluated as an early marker for cardiomyocyte and other tissue injury [47,48]. The time courses of H-FABP and cTns were compared in isoproterenol-induced myocardial injury in rats in a recent study [49]. The results from this study indicated that H-FABP could be an early marker for myocardial injury but considered to be less sensitive and nonspecific. The lack of specificity is a concern for applying H-FABP in the drug-induced myocardial injury since drugs often cause multiple tissue injuries in addition to the myocardium.

Recently, it has been reported that microRNAs (miRNAs) may be useful as biomarkers of acute myocardial infarction and other cardiovascular diseases. miRNAs are endogenous small noncoding RNAs, 21–25 nucleotides in length. Wang *et al.* showed that the muscle-enriched miRNAs such as miR-133a and cardiac-specific miR-208 are elevated in human plasma after myocardial infarction [50]. Further studies revealed that the levels of circulating miR-133a were positively correlated with the severity of coronary artery stenosis. Receiver operating characteristic (ROC) analysis showed that miR-133a had considerable diagnostic accuracy for coronary heart disease [51]. However, the feasibility of using miRNA to detect drug-induced myocardial injury needs to be further investigated.

A recent study using cardiac toxic compounds and noncardiac toxic compounds evaluated the utility of genomic biomarkers and compared them with established cTnI in rats [52]. In this study, several new genomic biomarkers (*Spp1* and *Timp1*) exhibited much higher diagnostic accuracy than that observed for plasma cTnI. Furthermore, the multiple-genomic biomarker model could predict potential drug-induced cardiotoxicity in rats in the absence of any cardiac histopathological lesions or elevation of cTnI. It is conceivable that further evaluation of novel genomic biomarkers may help identify new circulating biomarkers for cardiotoxicity. In addition, genomic biomarkers can facilitate mechanistic understanding of drug-induced cardiotoxicity.

13.5 Regulatory Perspective

While regulatory authorities typically require all drugs and biologics to undergo an evaluation of cardiovascular toxicity as outlined in International Conference on Harmonisation (ICH) S6 [53] and ICH S7A [54], no specific guidance was available for conducting the testing. There is an increased regulatory emphasis on the development of reliable biomarkers for cardiac toxicity that has prompted the formation of Health and Environmental Sciences Institute (HESI) and the Cardiac Safety Research Consortium (CSRC). The Food and Drug Administration (FDA)'s Critical Path Initiative in 2004 highlighted the urgency for accelerating nonclinical and clinical research on these markers, in addition to developing evidentiary standards for their use. The Cardiac Troponin Biomarker Safety Working Group was formed in 2008 within HESI to discuss and assess the application of cTns in nonclinical, clinical, and regulatory settings, and to address their translation from nonclinical applications to clinical studies. A consensus statement and recommendations are published by Berridge *et al.* and summarized in Table 13.2 [55].

The Biomarker Qualification Review Team (BQRT) at FDA has qualified serum/plasma cTnI and cTnT in nonclinical drug development studies in rats and dogs in 2012 in the following context of use:

a) Drugs with previous indication of cardiac structural damage: cTn testing can be estimated at the lowest toxic dose or at the highest nontoxic dose for the selection of doses for human testing. Specifically, cTns may serve as clinical chemistry correlate to histology; for example, lower doses without increases in cTn can support no observable effect level (NOEL) identified by histology.
b) Pharmacological class of drugs with known cardiac structural damage and histopathology does not reveal structural damage: cTns can support or refute inference of low cardiotoxic potential.
c) Evidence of unexpected cardiac structural toxicity in nonclinical study: retroactive examination of serum/plasma for cTns can determine no observed adverse effect level (NOAEL) or lowest observed adverse effect level (LOAEL) to support inclusion of cTn testing in subsequent safety assessment studies.

Table 13.2 Nonclinical use of cardiac troponins.

Points of consensus	Considerations and recommendations for nonclinical monitoring
• Sensitive and specific biomarkers of active cardiomyocellular injury in nonclinical species (rodents, rabbits, dogs, and nonhuman primates) but not of myocardial fibrosis, cardiomyocyte hypertrophy, and arrhythmias	• Measurement of cTns is not standard: a. Broad or routine monitoring of *in vivo* studies together with clinical chemistry (aspartate aminotransferase (AST), alanine aminotransferase (ALT), blood urea nitrogen (BUN), and creatinine) b. Directed monitoring where cardiotoxicity is identified or suspected
• Real-time assessment of cardiac injury and morphological assessment of preclinical models in repeat-dose studies preferably over varying time for rodents and limited to clinical observations (hematology of whole blood, serum chemistry) in nonrodents	• Selection of cTn assay: importance of relative sensitivity and specificity in relation to test species. New assays require appropriate analytical validation and biologic qualification prior to use
• Choice of commercial assay for species with demonstrated cross-species immune reactivity and precision	• Appropriate cTn reference intervals: established in each preclinical laboratory together with relevant population cTn reference intervals for species, strain, sex, and age
• New ultrasensitive assays with the ability to detect smaller changes in cTns and physiological levels can influence interpretation of clinically meaningful cardiac injury	• Data interpretation similar to routine clinical chemistry/hematology tests considers individual animal variability, change over time, differences in group means, dose response, and so on
• Correlation of temporal kinetics and magnitude of increases in cTns to myocardial injury (progression, mechanism, and pathological insult)	• Inconsistencies between changes in cTn concentrations and corresponding cardiac histopathology
• Assessment of cTn in animal models of cardiac injury can reveal concentrations outside of the expected biological variation for which microscopic lesions are not noted	• Extrapolation of preclinical cTns to clinical data
• Ultrasensitive analytical assay has potential to detect cardiac injury in short-duration studies prior to onset of morphological injury as "predictive biomarker"	
• Long-term implications of increases in cTns and cardiac injury can be assessed with drug-free periods in *in vivo* studies	

Because of limited published data and inconsistent results, the BQRT has not qualified cTns in monkey yet; however, FDA highly encourages collecting cTn data in monkey. Sufficient knowledge of the time course of damage by drug can allow for sampling that will help accurately capture cTn elevation.

However, FDA and the BQRT emphasized that effective implementation of cTns into nonclinical drug development studies still requires demonstration of three conditions in order to conclude that absence of an increase in cTnT and/or cTnI values demonstrates absence of cardiac structural damage. These conditions are (1) validation of assay for the species and laboratory conditions of use; (2) sufficient knowledge of time course of damage by drug in order to accurately capture troponin elevation resulting from ongoing or active damage; and (3) understanding of relevance of nonclinical metabolite profile to humans [56].

13.6 Conclusions and Future Perspectives

Cardiac toxicity is an important issue in the development of new drugs. In order to minimize late-stage attrition, it is essential to identify the risk as early as possible and implement effective follow-up strategies. Therefore, there is an urgent need to identify reliable, noninvasive, and translational biomarkers of drug-induced cardiotoxicity. The integration of translational biomarkers is expected to increase the diagnostic and prognostic power of the cardiac toxicity assessment in nonclinical and clinical development of new drugs. Although still exploratory, some of these nonstandard biomarkers can provide a signal of potential undesired effects in the heart, offering early evidence of treatment-related cardiac changes and accurately characterizing the onset and progression of cardiac lesions.

Due to the long history of using biomarkers, such as cTns and natriuretic peptides, as noninvasive methods of diagnosing and treating cardiovascular diseases in the clinic, it is quite attractive to consider their reverse translation to nonclinical toxicology assessment for early detection of drug-induced cardiotoxicity. As described above in detail, the measurement of cTns in blood is used in the clinic extensively as a noninvasive, reliable diagnostic and prognostic tool for acute myocardial infarction and is considered the gold standard for biomarkers in myocardial injury [14,16]. Their usage also extended to nonclinical studies for drug-induced cardiotoxicity where they could be used when the test article being evaluated is from a class of compound that has previously been shown to induce myocardial injury. When there is an indication of cardiac structural damage with a particular drug, cTn testing can help estimate the lowest toxic dose or the highest nontoxic dose to help choose doses for human testing. Further optimizing cTn assays and establishing normal value range especially the 99th percentile cutoff for species (rat, dog, monkey, and minipig) commonly used in nonclinical studies, however, are required prior to routine implementation in nonclinical research. Similarly, BNP and NT-proBNP have been used extensively in clinical practice as biomarkers for diagnostic, prognostic, and therapeutic monitoring of heart failure [28,32,57]. Even though their role in the clinical and nonclinical assessment of drug-induced cardiac toxicity is not fully ascertained, they appear as promising candidates to increase the power of the standard cardiac toxicity assessments. However, more studies are warranted prior to routine application in nonclinical safety assessment to establish the confidence in the role of natriuretic peptides in toxicological assessment of drug-induced cardiac hypertrophy in nonclinical species.

Drug-induced cardiotoxicity may not be effectively identified due to the gaps in our knowledge concerning biology and pathophysiology during nonclinical toxicity testing, which is a challenge to toxicologists, physicians, and regulators. Using biomarkers of cardiac structure and/or functional changes in nonclinical and clinical drug development continues to be challenging because of the uncertainty around data interpretation. If results are interpreted incorrectly, further development of a potentially useful drug may be abandoned. The validation of predictive and specific biomarkers for monitoring drug-induced cardiotoxicity noninvasively both in nonclinical species and in the clinic is a pressing need for the development of safe medicines. With increased clinical experience in biomarkers for cardiac injury and heart failure, qualifying these biomarkers for nonclinical use in drug discovery and early development is likely to decrease late-stage attrition and facilitate the delivery of safe medicines to patients. The coordinated efforts with regulators, industry, and academia to facilitate the validation and qualification of promising biomarkers would be the key to success.

References

1 Piccini, J.P., Whellan, D.J., Berridge, B.R., Finkle, J.K., Pettit, S.D., Stockbridge, N., Valentin, J.P., Vargas, H.M., and Krucoff, M.W. (2009) Current challenges in the evaluation of cardiac safety during drug development: translational medicine meets the Critical Path Initiative. *American Heart Journal*, **158**, 317–326.

2 Laverty, H., Benson, C., Cartwright, E., Cross, M., Garland, C., Hammond, T., Holloway, C., McMahon, N., Milligan, J., Park, B., Pirmohamed, M., Pollard, C., Radford, J., Roome, N., Sager, P., Singh, S., Suter, T., Suter, W., Trafford, A., Volders, P., Wallis, R., Weaver, R., York, M., and Valentin, J. (2011) How can we improve our understanding of cardiovascular safety liabilities to develop safer medicines? *British Journal of Pharmacology*, **163**, 675–693.

3 Sarazan, R.D., Mittelstadt, S., Guth, B., Koerner, J., Zhang, J., and Pettit, S. (2011) Cardiovascular function in nonclinical drug safety assessment: current issues and opportunities. *International Journal of Toxicology*, **30**, 272–286.

4 Josefson, D. (1997) Hay fever drug to be banned by the FDA. *BMJ*, **314**, 248.

5 Erdemli, G. and Martin, L.R. (2014) Integrated risk assessment of cardiac safety in drug discovery and development, in *Predictive ADMET: Integrated Approaches in Drug Discovery and Development* (eds L. Urban and J. Wang), John Wiley & Sons, Inc., Hoboken, NJ.

6 Hanton, G. (2007) Preclinical cardiac safety assessment of drugs. *Drugs R&D*, **8**, 213–228.

7 Picard, S., Goineau, S., Guillaume, P., Henry, J., Hanouz, J.L., and Rouet, R. (2011) Supplemental studies for

cardiovascular risk assessment in safety pharmacology: a critical overview. *Cardiovascular Toxicology*, **11**, 285–307.

8 Marrer, E. and Dieterle, F. (2010) Impact of biomarker development on drug safety assessment. *Toxicology and Applied Pharmacology*, **243**, 167–179.

9 Gaggin, H.K. and Januzzi, J.L., Jr. (2013) Biomarkers and diagnostics in heart failure. *Biochimica et Biophysica Acta*, **1832**, 2442–2450

10 Sheikh, A., Xia, K., Salma, U., Yang, T., and Peng, J. (2014) Diagnosis, prognosis and therapeutic role of circulating miRNAs in cardiovascular diseases. *Heart, Lung and Circulation*, **23**, 503–510

11 Liu, Y., Parman, T., Schneider, B., Song, B., Galande, A.K., Anderson, D., and Mirsalis, J. (2013) Serum biomarkers reveal long-term cardiac injury in isoproterenol-treated African green monkeys. *Journal of Proteome Research*, **12**, 1830–1837

12 Greaser, M.L. and Gergely, J. (1973) Purification and properties of the components from troponin. *The Journal of Biological Chemistry*, **248**, 2125–2133

13 Babuin, L. and Jaffe, A.S. (2005) Troponin: the biomarker of choice for the detection of cardiac injury. *Canadian Medical Association Journal*, **173**, 1191–1202.

14 Katus, H.A., Remppis, A., Neumann, F.J., Scheffold, T., Diederich, K.W., Vinar, G., Noe, A., Matern, G., and Kuebler, W. (1991) Diagnostic efficiency of troponin T measurements in acute myocardial infarction. *Circulation*, **83**, 902–912

15 Mueller, M., Vafaie, M., Biener, M., Giannitsis, E., and Katus, H.A. (2013) Cardiac troponin T: from diagnosis of myocardial infarction to cardiovascular risk prediction. *Circulation Journal*, **77**, 1653–1661

16 Thygesen, K., Mair, J., Katus, H., Plebani, M., Venge, P., Collinson, P., Lindahl, B., Giannitsis, E., Hasin, Y., Galvani, M., Tubaro, M., Alpert, J.S., Biasucci, L.M., Koenig, W., Mueller, C., Huber, K., Hamm, C., and Jaffe, A.S. (2010) Recommendations for the use of cardiac troponin measurement in acute cardiac care. *European Heart Journal*, **31**, 2197–2204

17 Alpert, J.S., Thygesen, K., Antman, E., and Bassand, J.P. (2000) Myocardial infarction redefined: a consensus document of the joint European Society of Cardiology/American College of Cardiology Committee for the redefinition of myocardial infarction. *Journal of the American College of Cardiology*, **36**, 959–969

18 Jaffe, A.S., Ravkilde, J., Roberts, R., Naslund, U., Apple, F.S., Galvani, M., and Katus, H. (2000) It's time for a change to a troponin standard. *Circulation*, **102**, 1216–1220

19 Mueller, M., Vafaie, M., Biener, M., Giannitsis, E., and Katus, H.A. (2013) Cardiac troponin T. *Circulation Journal*, 77 (7), 1653–1661.

20 Saunders, J.T., Nambi, V., de Lemos, J.A., Chambless, L.E., Virani, S.S., Boerwinkle, E., Hoogeveen, R.C., Liu, X., Astor, B.C., Mosley, T.H., Folsom, A.R., Heiss, G., Coresh, J., and Ballantyne, C.M. (2011) Cardiac troponin T measured by a highly sensitive assay predicts coronary heart disease, heart failure, and mortality in the atherosclerosis risk in communities study. *Circulation*, **123**, 1367–1376.

21 Wallace, K.B., Hausner, E., Herman, E., Holt, G.D., MacGregor, J.T., Metz, A.L., Murphy, E., Rosenblum, I.Y., Sistare, F.D., and York, M.J. (2004) Serum troponins as biomarkers of drug-induced cardiac toxicity. *Toxicologic Pathology*, **32**, 106–121

22 Adamcova, M., Sterba, M., Simunek, T., Potacova, A., Popelova, O., Mazurova, Y., and Gersl, V. (2005) Troponin as a marker of myocardiac damage in drug-induced cardiotoxicity. *Expert Opinion on Drug Safety*, **4**, 457–472

23 O'Brien, P.J. (2008) Cardiac troponin is the most effective translational safety biomarker for myocardial injury in cardiotoxicity. *Toxicology*, **245**, 206–218

24 O'Brien, P.J., Smith, D.E., Knechtel, T.J., Marchak, M.A., Pruimboom-Brees, I., Brees, D.J., Spratt, D.P., Archer, F.J., Butler, P., Potter, A.N., Provost, J.P., Richard, J., Snyder, P.A., and Reagan, W.J. (2006) Cardiac troponin I is a sensitive, specific biomarker of cardiac injury in

laboratory animals. *Laboratory Animals*, **40**, 153–171

25 Vasatova, M., Pudil, R., Horacek, J.M., and Buchler, T. (2013) Current applications of cardiac troponin T for the diagnosis of myocardial damage. *Advances in Clinical Chemistry*, **61**, 33–65.

26 Martin, A.F. (1981) Turnover of cardiac troponin subunits. Kinetic evidence for a precursor pool of troponin-I. *The Journal of Biological Chemistry*, **256**, 964–968

27 Guy, M.J., Chen, Y.C., Clinton, L., Zhang, H., Zhang, J., Dong, X., Xu, Q., Ayaz-Guner, S., and Ge, Y. (2013) The impact of antibody selection on the detection of cardiac troponin I. *Clinica Chimica Acta: International Journal of Clinical Chemistry*, **420**, 82–88

28 Pemberton, C.J., Johnson, M.L., Yandle, T.G., and Espiner, E.A. (2000) Deconvolution analysis of cardiac natriuretic peptides during acute volume overload. *Hypertension*, **36**, 355–359

29 Mair, J. (2008) Biochemistry of B-type natriuretic peptide: where are we now? *Clinical Chemistry and Laboratory Medicine: CCLM/FESCC*, **46**, 1507–1514

30 Hasegawa, K., Fujiwara, H., Doyama, K., Mukoyama, M., Nakao, K., Fujiwara, T., Imura, H., and Kawai, C. (1993) Ventricular expression of atrial and brain natriuretic peptides in dilated cardiomyopathy. An immunohistocytochemical study of the endomyocardial biopsy specimens using specific monoclonal antibodies. *The American Journal of Pathology*, **142**, 107–116

31 Schwab, T.R., Edwards, B.S., Heublein, D.M., and Burnett, J.C., Jr. (1986) Role of atrial natriuretic peptide in volume-expansion natriuresis. *The American Journal of Physiology*, **251**, R310–R313

32 Mahadavan, G., Nguyen, T.H., and Horowitz, J.D. (2014) Brain natriuretic peptide: a biomarker for all cardiac disease? *Current Opinion in Cardiology*, **29**, 160–166

33 Grantham, J.A., Borgeson, D.D., and Burnett, J.C., Jr. (1997) BNP: pathophysiological and potential therapeutic roles in acute congestive heart failure. *The American Journal of Physiology*, **272**, R1077–R1083

34 Langenickel, T., Pagel, I., Hohnel, K., Dietz, R., and Willenbrock, R. (2000) Differential regulation of cardiac ANP and BNP mRNA in different stages of experimental heart failure. *American Journal of Physiology. Heart and Circulatory Physiology*, **278**, H1500–H1506

35 Kroll, M.H., Twomey, P.J., and Srisawasdi, P. (2007) Using the single-compartment ratio model to calculate half-life. NT-proBNP as an example. *Clinica Chimica Acta: International Journal of Clinical Chemistry*, **380**, 197–202.

36 Yoshimura, M., Yasue, H., Okumura, K., Ogawa, H., Jougasaki, M., Mukoyama, M., Nakao, K., and Imura, H. (1993) Different secretion patterns of atrial natriuretic peptide and brain natriuretic peptide in patients with congestive heart failure. *Circulation*, **87**, 464–469

37 Seferian, K.R., Tamm, N.N., Semenov, A.G., Mukharyamova, K.S., Tolstaya, A.A., Koshkina, E.V., Kara, A.N., Krasnoselsky, M.I., Apple, F.S., Esakova, T.V., Filatov, V.L., and Katrukha, A.G. (2007) The brain natriuretic peptide (BNP) precursor is the major immunoreactive form of BNP in patients with heart failure. *Clinical Chemistry*, **53**, 866–873

38 Semenov, A.G., Seferian, K.R., Tamm, N.N., Artem'eva, M.M., Postnikov, A.B., Bereznikova, A.V., Kara, A.N., Medvedeva, N.A., and Katrukha, A.G. (2011) Human pro-B-type natriuretic peptide is processed in the circulation in a rat model. *Clinical Chemistry*, **57**, 883–890

39 Mesmin, C., Renvoise, M., Becher, F., Ezan, E., and Fenaille, F. (2012) MS-based approaches to unravel the molecular complexity of proprotein-derived biomarkers and support their quantification: the examples of B-type natriuretic peptide and apelin peptides. *Bioanalysis*, **4**, 2851–2863

40 Urbanova, D., Urban, L., Danova, K., and Simkova, I. (2008) Natriuretic peptides: biochemical markers of anthracycline cardiac toxicity? *Oncology Research*, **17**, 51–58

41 Henderson, K.A., Borders, R.B., Ross, J.B., Huwar, T.B., Travis, C.O., Wood, B.J., Ma, Z.J., Hong, S.P., Vinci, T.M.,

and Roche, B.M. (2013) Effects of tyrosine kinase inhibitors on rat isolated heart function and protein biomarkers indicative of toxicity. *Journal of Pharmacological and Toxicological Methods*, **68**, 150–159

42 Colton, H.M., Stokes, A.H., Yoon, L.W., Quaile, M.P., Novak, P.J., Falls, J.G., Kimbrough, C.L., Cariello, N.F., Jordan, H.L., and Berridge, B.R. (2011) An initial characterization of N-terminal-proatrial natriuretic peptide in serum of Sprague Dawley rats. *Toxicological Sciences*, **120**, 262–268

43 Berna, M., Ott, L., Engle, S., Watson, D., Solter, P., and Ackermann, B. (2008) Quantification of NTproBNP in rat serum using immunoprecipitation and LC/MS/MS: a biomarker of drug-induced cardiac hypertrophy. *Analytical Chemistry*, **80**, 561–566

44 Bharti, S., Singh, R., Chauhan, S.S., Hussain, T., Al-Attas, O.S., and Arya, D.S. (2012) Phosphorylation of Akt/GSK-3beta/eNOS amplifies 5-HT2B receptor blockade mediated anti-hypertrophic effect in rats. *FEBS Letters*, **586**, 180–185

45 Casartelli, A., Lanzoni, A., Comelli, R., Crivellente, F., Defazio, R., Dorigatti, R., Fasdelli, N., Faustinelli, I., Pagliarusco, S., Tontodonati, M., and Cristofori, P. (2011) A novel and integrated approach for the identification and characterization of drug-induced cardiac toxicity in the dog. *Toxicologic Pathology*, **39**, 361–371

46 Glatz, J.F., van der Vusse, G.J., Simoons, M.L., Kragten, J.A., van Dieijen-Visser, M.P., and Hermens, W.T. (1998) Fatty acid-binding protein and the early detection of acute myocardial infarction. *Clinica Chimica Acta: International Journal of Clinical Chemistry*, **272**, 87–92.

47 Uitterdijk, A., Sneep, S., van Duin, R.W., Krabbendam-Peters, I., Gorsse-Bakker, C., Duncker, D.J., van der Giessen, W.J., and van Beusekom, H.M. (2013) Serial measurement of hFABP and high-sensitivity troponin I post-PCI in STEMI: how fast and accurate can myocardial infarct size and no-reflow be predicted? *American Journal of Physiology. Heart and Circulatory Physiology*, **305**, H1104–H1110

48 Pelsers, M.M., Hermens, W.T., and Glatz, J.F. (2005) Fatty acid-binding proteins as plasma markers of tissue injury. *Clinica Chimica Acta: International Journal of Clinical Chemistry*, **352**, 15–35.

49 Clements, P., Brady, S., York, M., Berridge, B., Mikaelian, I., Nicklaus, R., Gandhi, M., Roman, I., Stamp, C., Davies, D., McGill, P., Williams, T., Pettit, S., Walker, D., and Turton, J. (2010) Time course characterization of serum cardiac troponins, heart fatty acid-binding protein, and morphologic findings with isoproterenol-induced myocardial injury in the rat. *Toxicologic Pathology*, **38**, 703–714

50 Wang, G.K., Zhu, J.Q., Zhang, J.T., Li, Q., Li, Y., He, J., Qin, Y.W., and Jing, Q. (2010) Circulating microRNA: a novel potential biomarker for early diagnosis of acute myocardial infarction in humans. *European Heart Journal*, **31**, 659–666

51 Wang, F., Long, G., Zhao, C., Li, H., Chaugai, S., Wang, Y., Chen, C., and Wang, D.W. (2013) Plasma microRNA-133a is a new marker for both acute myocardial infarction and underlying coronary artery stenosis. *Journal of Translational Medicine*, **11**, 222.

52 Nishimura, Y., Morikawa, Y., Kondo, C., Tonomura, Y., Fukushima, R., Torii, M., and Uehara, T. (2013) Genomic biomarkers for cardiotoxicity in rats as a sensitive tool in preclinical studies. *Journal of Applied Toxicology*, **33**, 1120–1130

53 ICH (1997) Guidance for Industry: S6 Preclinical Safety Evaluation of Biotechnology-Derived Pharmaceuticals. Available at http://www.fda.gov/downloads/Drugs/GuidanceComplianceRegulatoryInformation/Guidances/UCM074957.pdf (accessed May 26, 2014).

54 ICH (2001) Guidance for Industry: S7A Safety Pharmacology Studies for Human Pharmaceuticals. Available at http://www.fda.gov/downloads/Drugs/GuidanceComplianceRegulatoryInformation/Guidances/UCM074959.pdf (accessed May 26, 2014).

55 Berridge, B.R., Pettit, S., Walker, D.B., Jaffe, A.S., Schultze, A.E., Herman, E., Reagan, W.J., Lipshultz, S.E., Apple, F.S., and York, M.J. (2009) A translational approach to detecting drug-induced cardiac injury with cardiac troponins: consensus and recommendations from the Cardiac Troponins Biomarker Working Group of the Health and Environmental Sciences Institute. *American Heart Journal*, **158**, 21–29

56 CDER (2012) Biomarker Qualification Decision Letter on Circulating Cardiac Troponins. Available at http://www.fda.gov/downloads/Drugs/DevelopmentApprovalProcess/DrugDevelopmentTools-QualificationProgram/UCM294644.pdf (accessed May 31, 2014).

57 Cowie, M.R., Jourdain, P., Maisel, A., Dahlstrom, U., Follath, F., Isnard, R., Luchner, A., McDonagh, T., Mair, J., Nieminen, M., and Francis, G. (2003) Clinical applications of B-type natriuretic peptide (BNP) testing. *European Heart Journal*, **24**, 1710–1718

14
The Mechanistic Basis of hERG Blockade and the Proarrhythmic Effects Thereof

Robert A. Pearlstein, K. Andrew MacCannell, Qi-Ying Hu, Ramy Farid, and José S. Duca

14.1
Introduction

The pioneering efforts of many laboratories (notably those of Sanguinetti [1–3], Keating [1], Mitcheson [4,5], Brown [6–8], Rampe [8,9], and Hondeghem [10–12]) ultimately led to the discovery of a clear cause–effect relationship between Ether-à-go-go-related gene (hERG) dysfunction/blockade and torsade de pointes arrhythmia (TdP) [3,13,14]. As a result, several marketed drugs were withdrawn [3], and *in vitro* hERG safety profiling, mitigation, and *in vivo* risk assessment practices were, introduced [3,15]. Awareness of hERG safety has helped to greatly diminish blockade-related mortality and morbidity. However, such gains were arguably achieved more from attrition of offending compounds (often late in preclinical development) than successful mitigation. As such, risk from hERG blockade has not truly diminished, but has instead shifted from the clinic to preclinical discovery. Limitations of hERG mitigation/circumvention continue to hamper afflicted drug discovery projects to varying degrees [15,16]. Key limitations include the following:

1) High susceptibility of hERG to inadvertent blockade by drug-like molecules.
2) Poorly understood nature of hERG structure–activity relationships, which typically involve robust and persistent activity within entire chemical series [17].
3) Lack of clear guidance for proarrhythmic risk assessment of early preclinical candidates due to
   a) uncertainty in *in vitro* assay data caused by poor solubility and/or poor permeability and other limitations (see below),
   b) uncertainty/controversy concerning the true relationship between *in vitro* potency and proarrhythmic endpoints, compounded by the lack of *in vivo* exposure data for early-stage compounds, and
   c) lack of clear priorities in the lead optimization workflow (what to fix first?).

Antitargets and Drug Safety, First Edition. Edited by László Urbán, Vinod F. Patel, and Roy J. Vaz.

Building on the work of others [18–24], we offer novel insights about the fundamental relationship between hERG dysfunction and proarrhythmia, based on simulations of the human cardiac action potential (AP) [23] under increasing levels of hERG blockade. We report a newly identified chemical substructure present in a large fraction of known hERG blockers that, together with our proposed binding mechanism, may assist in consolidating seemingly diverse, local blocker structure–activity relationships into a global paradigm. We demonstrate that *in vitro* electrophysiology-based methods used to measure blocker potency on the subphysiological timescale do not unambiguously recapitulate hERG binding under *in vivo* conditions. Finally, we propose knowledge-based hERG safety assessment and mitigation strategies informed by improved understanding of the dynamic relationship between blocker binding kinetics, hERG channel occupancy, and the proarrhythmic effects thereof.

14.1.1
The Role of hERG Dysfunction/Blockade in Promoting Early After Depolarizations

The ion currents of both nonvoltage- and voltage-gated ion channels drive the time-dependent membrane potential ($V_m(t)$) comprising the cardiac AP [3,25]. All voltage-gated ion channels switch between nonconducting (closed/deactivated, open/inactivated) and conducting (open/activated) states at channel-specific rates and $V_m(t)$ [3,25]. Reduction in the baseline potassium currents of hERG (referred to as I_{Kr}) or KCNQ1-minK (referred to as I_{Ks}) due to inherited or acquired dysfunction [3,25] results in graded alteration of the instantaneous slope and morphology of the AP waveform (which we refer to as $dV_m(t)/dt$) (Figure 14.1). Such alterations are mirrored in the electrocardiogram as lengthening of the QT interval (abbreviated as LQT) [25,26]. Hondeghem was among the first to associate particular changes in $dV_m(t)/dt$ over time with TdP arrhythmia (see below) [18,26–28]. The signature tail current of hERG, which dominates $dV_m(t)/dt$ late in the AP cycle, plays a key role in the innate suppression of abnormal calcium-driven early after depolarizations (EADs) (see below). We begin with an overview of the molecular mechanisms underlying the normal AP and proarrhythmic abnormalities thereof:

1) *State transitions of hERG determine instantaneous* I_{Kr} *current and* $-dV_m(t)/dt$ *during the AP*

   We estimated hERG gating kinetics based on AP simulations using the O'Hara–Rudy model [23]. Depolarization triggers rapid opening (magenta curve in Figure 14.2) and synchronous inactivation (cyan curve in Figure 14.2) of the hERG channel population over the first ~25 ms of the cardiac AP (phase 0). The population is fully open by ~40 ms, but only ~8% activated. Slow recovery from inactivation ensues during AP phase 2 until ~200 ms (orange curve in Figure 14.2), which transitions to rapid acceleration at phase 3 (~260 ms and $V_m \approx -40$ mV). Slow deactivation occurs between ~125 and 225 ms (brown curve in Figure 14.2),

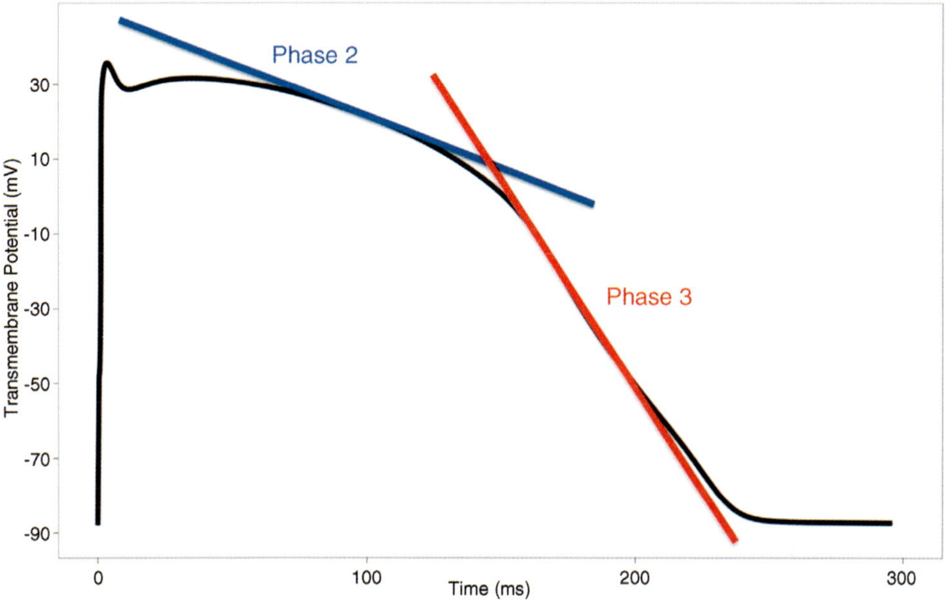

Figure 14.1 Simulated cardiac AP in M cells. The rate of change of $V_m(t)$ (i.e., $-dV_m(t)/dt$) during AP phases 2 and 3 is denoted by the teal and red tangent lines, respectively.

followed by rapid acceleration during phase 3. The rates of deactivation and recovery converge at ~260 ms, at which point the net activated channel population reaches ~55% of the total, and I_K ($=I_{Kr}+I_{Ks}$) reaches $I_{K(peak)}$ ($=I_{Kr(peak)}+I_{Ks}$). AP termination at ~350–400 ms is driven by hERG, KCNQ1, and Kir2.1 (I_{K1}). These timings agree favorably with experimental measurements performed by Zhou *et al.* using an AP-like command voltage protocol [29]. HERG opening and inactivation occurred within the first ~21 ms postdepolarization, followed by recovery from inactivation at ~340 ms and deactivation between ~340 and 574 ms.

2) *Voltage-gated ion channel state transitions are signaled by* $-dV_m(t)/dt$

The instantaneous slope of the AP waveform is determined by the relative balance of total outward (I_K) and inward currents (I_{Na} and I_{Ca}) [3,25]. The shallow nature of $-dV_m(t)/dt$ during AP phase 2 is conveyed by the slight predominance of outward I_K current (teal tangent line in Figure 14.1). The slope of $V_m(t)$ steepens as the I_K/I_{Ca} ratio becomes proportionately larger, undergoing $I_{K(peak)}$-driven maximal steepening during AP phase 3 (red tangent line in Figure 14.1). $I_{K(peak)}$ current is normally dominated by $I_{Kr(peak)}$, but shifts toward the more slowly activating I_{Ks} current under conditions of hERG dysfunction (extra capacity of I_K has been referred to as the "repolarization reserve" [30]). Slowing of $-dV_m(t)/dt$ during AP phase

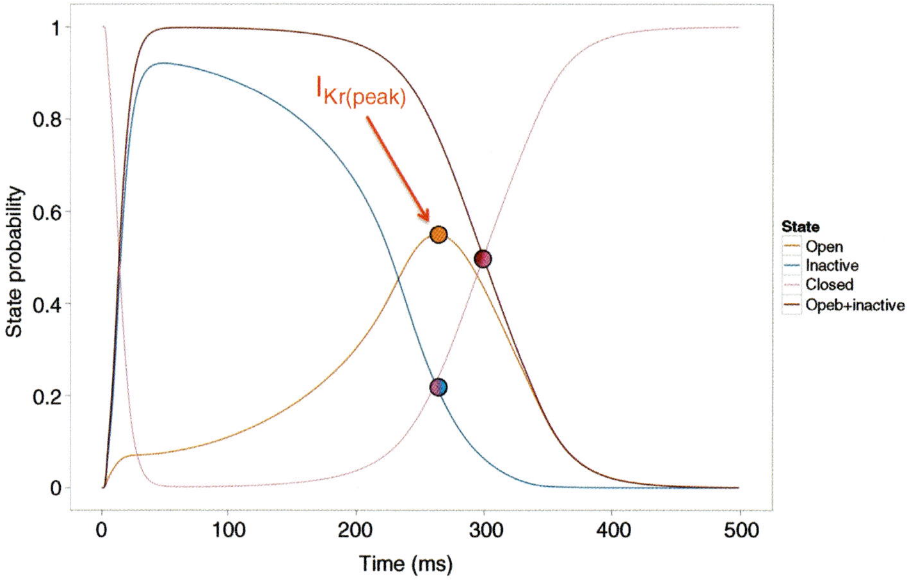

Figure 14.2 Simulated time-dependent state transitions in hERG triggered by changes in $V_m(t)$. The channel population is initially closed (deactivated). Upon depolarization, the population rapidly accelerates toward the fully open/inactivated state (brown curve). The population then transitions from the inactivated (cyan curve) to the activated (orange curve) and deactivated (magenta curve) states, reaching the maximal current ($I_{Kr(peak)}$) at ~275 ms (orange circle), corresponding to ~22% inactivated, 22% deactivated, and 55% activated channels (magenta/cyan circle).

2 due to hERG or KCNQ1 dysfunction/blockade manifest as *isomorphic* AP prolongation (occurring at ~10% or greater loss of I_{Kr} current in our simulations). Slowing of $-dV_m(t)/dt$ during AP phase 3 at higher levels of hERG or KCNQ1 dysfunction/blockade and concomitant $I_{K(peak)}$ reduction manifest as *nonisomorphic* AP prolongation (referred to as "triangulation" by Hondeghem *et al.* [11,12]).

3) *Mistimed calcium channel reopening triggers abnormal depolarizations*

Ca$_v$1.2 calcium channels (which conduct $I_{Ca\text{-}L}$ current) normally activate during the AP *upstroke* (phase 0) between $V_m = -40$ and $+10$ mV (reaching $I_{Ca\text{-}L(peak)}$ at ~0 mV), followed by voltage- and calcium-dependent deactivation between $V_m = +10$ and -40 mV on the *downstroke* [25]. Abnormal slowing of $-dV_m(t)/dt$ during AP phase 2 (Figure 14.3), wherein V_m dwells above the Ca$_v$1.2 activation voltage, prolongs the open time of Ca$_v$1.2 channels (manifesting as isomorphic AP lengthening and LQT). However, abnormal slowing of $-dV_m(t)/dt$ below the rate of Ca$_v$1.2 activation, late in phase 2 or phase 3 (causing $V_m(t)$ to dwell below 0 mV), triggers graded opening of closed Ca$_v$1.2 channels and aberrant $I_{Ca\text{-}L}$ current [31] (appearing as a shoulder in the AP waveform) (Figure 14.4).

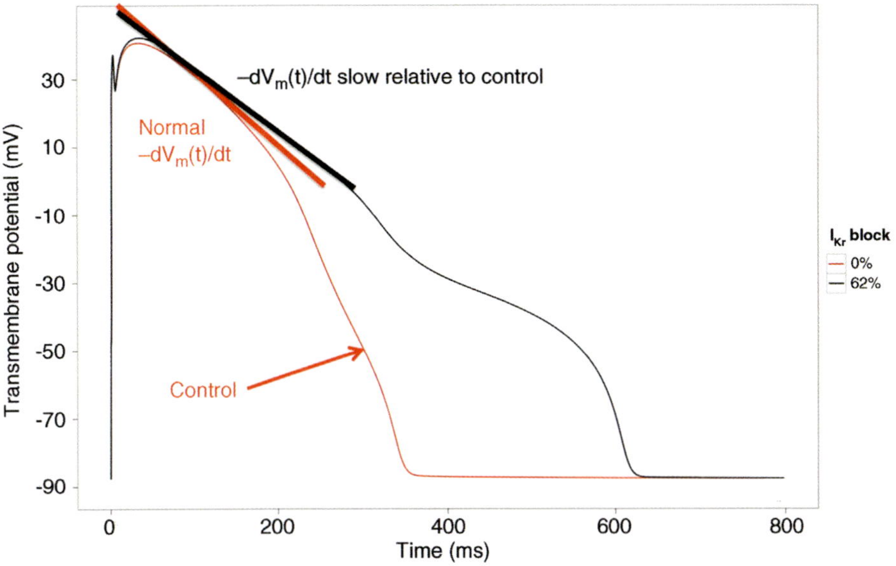

Figure 14.3 Simulated cardiac AP in M cells. Subcritical knockdown of normal baseline I_{Kr} (red tangent line) caused by hERG dysfunction slows deactivation of $Ca_v1.2$ channels and $-dV_m(t)/dt$ during phase 2 (black tangent line), manifesting as prolongation of the AP.

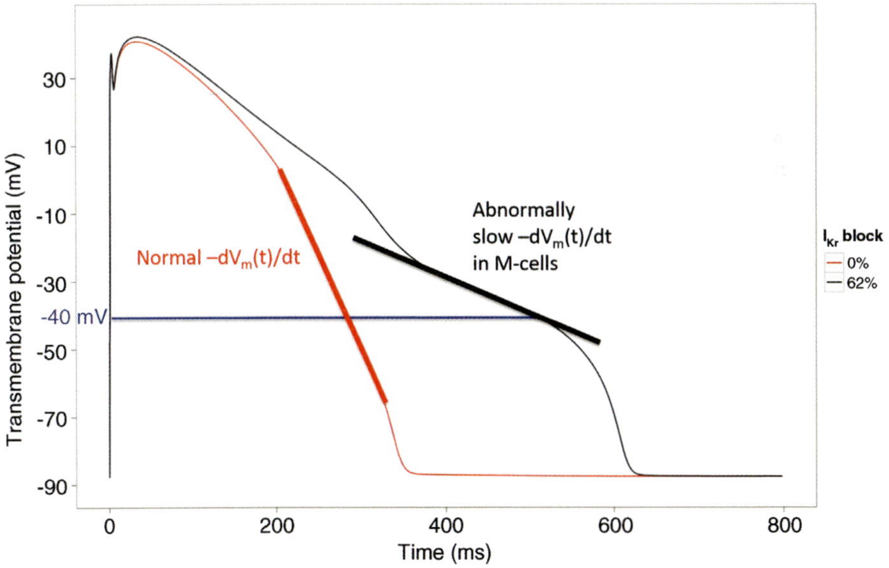

Figure 14.4 Simulated cardiac AP in M cells. Critical knockdown of normal baseline I_{Kr} (red tangent line) caused by hERG dysfunction promotes abnormal reopening of $Ca_v1.2$ channels at about −40 mV (blue line), and slows $-dV_m(t)/dt$ during phase 3 (black tangent line). The resulting graded I_{Ca-L} current manifests as an abnormal shoulder in phase 3.

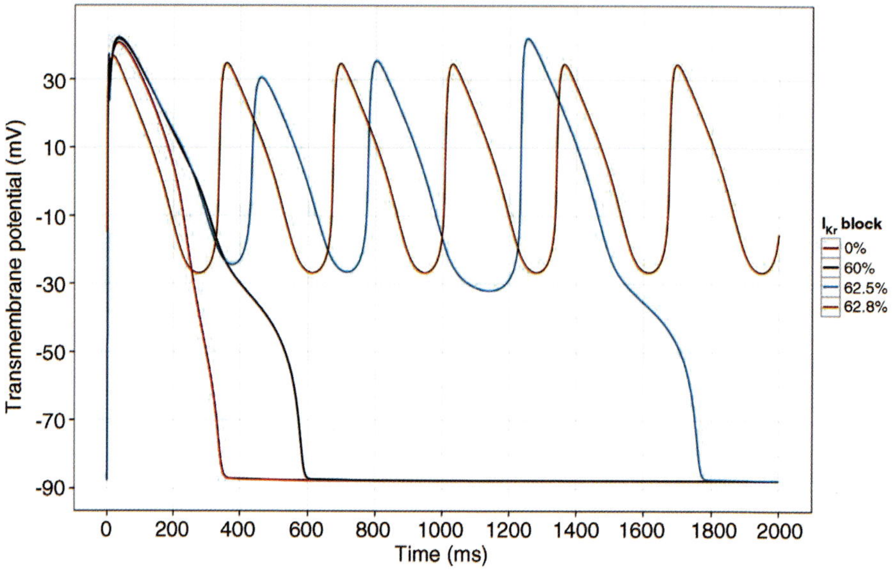

Figure 14.5 Simulated cardiac AP in M cells in the presence of critical hERG block results in aberrant $I_{Ca\text{-}L}$ currents and EADs (orange and cyan tracings). The normal AP tracing is shown in red and subcritical slowing of $-dV_m(t)/dt$ in black (noting that AP prolongation during phase 2 does not result in EADs in our simulations).

Abnormal EADs, the unique triggers for TdP arrhythmia, occur at a critical increase in $I_{Ca\text{-}L}$ (Figure 14.5) [31]. EADs occurred spontaneously during our simulations at a critical reduction of $I_{Kr(peak)}$, and were preceded by triangulation of the AP waveform (reflecting critical slowing of $-dV_m(t)/dt$ during phase 3). However, *EADs did not occur at milder I_{Kr} reductions in phase 2, despite the appearance of isomorphic prolongation.* Both forms of AP prolongation translate to indistinguishable forms of LQT (maximal prolongation being longer during phase 2 than phase 3), but reflect vastly different electrophysiological origins [11,12].

4) *Reduction in baseline I_K levels over supra-AP timescales caused by normal regulatory mechanisms exacerbate hERG dysfunction*

Mid to late repolarization is driven by the delicate balance between outward I_{Kr} and I_{Ks} currents and inward $I_{Ca\text{-}L}$ current, which vary throughout the AP as a function of $V_m(t)$ [3,25]. Additionally, *baseline* levels of I_{Kr} and I_{Ks} currents vary over supra-AP timescales in response to physiological modulation of channel gating properties [25]. In particular, hERG activation and inactivation slow and accelerate, respectively, with increasing catecholamine levels, whereas KCNQ1 activation accelerates with increasing heart rate and catecholamine levels [25,32]. β2-Adrenergic receptor agonists govern the degradation of phosphoinositol-4,5-bisphosphate (PIP_2), an endogenous pan-ion channel activator, and upregulate baseline I_{Ks} via protein kinase A-mediated KCNQ1 phosphorylation [33,34]. PIP_2 depletion results in transient knockdown of baseline I_{Kr} and I_{Ks} current levels and *enhanced vulnerability to ventricular arrhythmia* when superimposed on acquired or inherited hERG dysfunction [33,34].

Proarrhythmic sensitivity to I_{Kr} loss grows with increasing dysfunction of KCNQ1 or minK, reaching acute proportions in cases of extreme loss-of-function mutations (most notably, Jervell and Lange-Nielsen syndrome [35]).

5) *Effects of hERG dysfunction are nonuniformly manifest across the ventricular wall*

   Differences in hERG and KCNQ1 expression levels across the ventricular wall (endocardium, midmyocardium, and epicardium), mirrored by differences in I_{Kr}:I_{Ks} ratios, result in stratification of AP timings across these tissues (known as transmural dispersion of repolarization (TDR)) [36]. TDR underlies the torsional contraction of ventricular tissue (blood is wrung, rather than squeezed [37]), but when exaggerated by abnormal I_{Kr}:I_{Ks} ratios in the presence of hERG dysfunction, TDR facilitates the propagation of EADs from midmyocardium (M) into excitable epi- and endocardial layers ("substrates" for arrhythmogenesis) [25,36].

6) *Blocker-induced loss of baseline I_{Kr} can act alone to cause EADs, but may be exacerbated by genetic loss-of-function mutations in hERG or KCNQ1*

   Interindividual variation in baseline I_{Kr}, I_{Ks} or reserve levels thereof could conceivably arise from genetic diversity in pathways regulating hERG or KCNQ1 expression or trafficking, relatively mild loss-of-function mutations in the α- or β-channel subunits, or polymorphisms in channel modulation pathways (e.g., PIP_2 regulation). Inherited knockdown of baseline I_{Kr} or I_{Ks} levels could translate to increased sensitivity to hERG blockade and reduction in the EAD-causing occupancy level (which we refer to as γ_c). However, a recent study by Behr *et al.* [38] suggests that "common genomic variants do not contribute importantly to risk for drug-induced torsade de pointes across multiple [hERG blocking] drugs." As we will now demonstrate, hERG dysfunction/blockade is a sufficient condition for cellular EAD formation, which in combination with additional tissue/organ level contributions (not considered in the present work) significantly heightens TdP risk.

14.1.2
The Dynamics of hERG Blockade

Occupancy in static or quasi-static systems at equilibrium (which we refer to as γ) depends on the equilibrium constant (K_d) and free blocker concentration

($[\text{blocker}]_{\text{free}}$), as described by the Hill equation:

$$\gamma = [\text{blocker}]_{\text{free}}/([\text{blocker}]_{\text{free}} + K_{\text{d}}). \tag{14.1}$$

Starmer *et al.* observed long ago that blocker association and dissociation to/from voltage-gated ion channels is constrained to the open channel time period (which we denote as τ_{phys}) by fast channel gating under physiological conditions (which we denote as ν_{phys}) [19,20]. The effects of channel gating on binding diminish under *in vitro* conditions, as the gating frequency (denoted as ν_{exptl}) slows below ν_{phys}, and open channel times (which we denote as τ_{exptl}) increase beyond τ_{phys} in patch clamp, or to infinity in radioligand binding (RLB) assays. Bound lifetimes at the multisecond supraphysiological cycle lengths (CLs) used in standard patch clamp protocols are determined by blocker–channel interactions underlying k_{off}, and possibly extend to minutes or hours in *nongating* channels (which we refer to as "intrinsic lifetime"). However, at the fast ν_{phys}, intrinsic lifetimes are capped by τ_{phys} (which we refer to as the "extrinsic lifetime"). Intrinsic lifetimes longer than τ_{phys} are superseded, or "hijacked," by channel closure when the intrinsic $k_{\text{off}} \ll$ the true k_{off} at ν_{phys}. As we will demonstrate shortly, lifetimes ranging between τ_{phys} and τ_{exptl} converge to equivalent lifetime and potency under physiological conditions. However, not all blockers converge to the same lifetime, as observed by Starmer *et al.* for bound complexes in static versus gating channels (referred to by the authors as "tonic" and "phasic" blockade, respectively) [19–21]. Such differences were later referred to as "use-dependent" and "reverse use-dependent" blockade by Hondeghem and Snyders [10], and "frequency-dependent" and "frequency-independent" blockade by Stork *et al.* [22]. Frequency-dependent blockers dissociate prior to or during channel closing, whereas frequency-independent blockers are trapped behind the closed activation gate prior to subsequent channel reopening [19–22]. Blockers dissociate exclusively from the open state, which may vary throughout the channel closing period (the last ~150 ms of the AP) due to the dramatic changes in channel conformation (Figure 14.2).

Stork *et al.* compared the evolution of hERG blockade by eight drugs in patch clamp studies as a function of both CL (30, 100, 300, and 1000 ms) and number of cycles required to achieve maximal current reduction [22]. Steady-state blockade was achieved rapidly for haloperidol, cisapride, domperidone, amiodarone, bepridil, and droperidol (requiring ~1–3 pulses, depending on blocker and CL), suggesting fast on-rates for those blockers. Maximal reductions in steady-state current were achieved at the 1000 ms CL for haloperidol, cisapride, domperidone, amiodarone, and droperidol, consistent with slower intrinsic off-rates of those blockers at long open channel times. Currents caused by bepridil, E-4031, and terfenadine were insensitive to CL, suggesting that those blockers are trappable. Trappable blockers accumulate to equilibrium occupancy levels over time, whereas nontrappable blockers do not (occupancy by such blockers is refreshed during every AP cycle). The lifetimes of trappable and nontrappable blockers are capped to floors of CL and τ_{phys}, respectively, such that the trappable lifetime is ($\text{CL}/\tau_{\text{phys}}$)-fold longer than that of the nontrappable case (approximately threefold, given $\text{CL} = 1$ s and $\tau_{\text{true}} = 0.34$ s). Blocker off-rates may generally vary with

CL *in vivo* (determined by changes in heart rate) due to variation in the proportion of time spent in the open versus closed states. Hondeghem and Snyders observed for the trappable hERG blocker quinidine (which is nontrappable in $Na_v1.5$ channels): "quinidine causes both CL-dependent widening of the QRS-complex and lengthening of the action potential duration. However, whereas the sodium channel block is most marked at fast heart rates and nearly nonexistent at slow heart rates, prolongation of the action potential duration is most marked at slow heart rates" [10].

In this work, we revisit hERG blockade in a mechanistic context, treating channel occupancy as a dynamic phenomenon governed by both channel gating and binding contributions. We connect the work of Starmer *et al.* [19–21], Stork *et al.* [22], Hondeghem *et al.* [10,11,18], O'Hara *et al.* [23], and Redfern *et al.* [24] into a general hypothesis about the relationships between blocker binding kinetics, dynamic channel occupancy, and EAD formation at the cellular level (in both the *in vitro* and *in vivo* contexts).

14.1.3 Simulations of the Human Cardiac AP in the Presence of hERG Blockade

AP simulations were performed using the O'Hara–Rudy dynamic model of the non diseased human heart implemented in MatLab, which is available directly from the authors [23]. We replaced the hERG component of the model with a Markov representation previously reported by Silva and Rudy [39], and coupled the following dynamic equations for blocker association and dissociation to the Markov model for the purpose of calculating time- and state-dependent blocker occupancy (which we refer to as $\gamma(t)$):

$$d\gamma(t)/dt = \text{on-rate}-\text{off-rate} = k_{on}[\text{blocker}]_{free}(t)(1-\gamma(t)) - k_{off}\gamma(t), \tag{14.2}$$

Equation 14.2 was formulated for trappable blocker simulations as

$$d\gamma(t)/dt = k_{on}[\text{blocker}]_{free}(P_o + P_i)(1-\gamma(t)) - k_{off}(P_o + P_i)\gamma(t), \tag{14.3}$$

where P_o and P_i are the open and inactivated channel state probabilities, respectively.

Equation 14.2 was formulated for nontrappable blocker simulations as

$$d\gamma(t)/dt = k_{on}[\text{blocker}]_{free}(P_o + P_i)(1-\gamma(t)) - k_{off}(P_o + P_i)\gamma(t) - (\mu P_i + \beta_2 P_o)\gamma(t), \tag{14.4}$$

where μ and β_2 are the rate constants for channel deactivation from the inactive and open states, respectively.

I_{Kr} was then calculated from

$$I_{Kr} = g_{Kr}P_o(1-\gamma(t))(V(t) - E_K), \tag{14.5}$$

where g_{Kr} is the hERG channel conductance, $V(t)$ is the membrane potential, and E_K is the Nernst potential for potassium. We performed separate AP simulations for epi-, endo-, and midmyo (M)-cardial cells in the absence and presence of varying degrees of blockade and tested for EADs under different blocker binding kinetics regimes and intracellular exposures.

14.1.4
Estimation of Proarrhythmic hERG Occupancy Levels Based on AP Simulations

We simulated reduction in I_{Kr} as a function of escalating levels of trappable and non trappable hERG blocker occupancy (determined from blocker k_{on}, k_{off}, and intracellular exposure inputs) on AP duration and morphology using the *in silico* O'Hara–Rudy dynamic model [23] until reaching the EAD-causing level (γ_c). Trappable and nontrappable hERG blockers evoked EADs via decidedly different binding kinetics behavior and γ_c:

1) *Trappable blockers*
   AP duration in M, endo-, and epicardial cells was prolonged at occupancies >10% relative to the activated hERG channel population, becoming increasingly non uniform across the three cell types with escalating occupancy (the likely basis for abnormal enhancement of transmural dispersion in intact ventricles). AP phase 2 became increasingly prolonged with hERG occupancy (translating to increasingly shallow $-dV_m(t)/dt$), and by inference, extended the $Ca_v1.2$ reopening time window). Additionally, AP phase 3 became increasingly prolonged during the $Ca_v1.2$ opening $V_m(t)$ range, translating to increasing levels of $I_{Ca\text{-}L}$ conduction (as evidenced by a growing "shoulder" during phase 3 of the AP waveform) (Figure 14.4), ultimately reaching depolarizing levels of $I_{Ca\text{-}L}$ (i.e., EADs). Trappable blockers evoked EADs in M cells at ~62.8% of the open channel population at $I_{Kr(peak)}$ (~35% of the total hERG population) after hundreds of AP cycles, but at considerably higher occupancies in endo- and epicardial cells (~93 and >98%, respectively). EADs occurred abruptly at, but not prior to, reaching γ_c in both forms of the model, suggesting that γ_c constitutes a *tipping point* in the dynamic behavior of the system. We note that our predicted γ_c may or may not quantitatively capture the true EAD-causing occupancy in humans (and furthermore, γ_c may vary across individuals or over time.)
2) *Nontrappable blockers*
   We used the modified O'Hara–Rudy model to probe γ_c of nontrappable blockers as a function of on-rate at fixed $k_{off} = 2\,s^{-1}$, $k_{on} = 1 \times 10^6$, $k_{on(open)}$ $=1 \times 10_6$, 1×10^7, and $1 \times 10^8\,M^{-1}\,s^{-1}$, and intracellular concentrations ranging from 100 nM to 100 μM. EADs were evoked at concentrations in excess of 10 μM at $k_{on} = 1 \times 10^6$, 1 μM at $k_{on} = 1 \times 10^7$, and 100 nM at $k_{on} = 1 \times 10^8\,M^{-1}\,s^{-1}$, translating in all cases to an EAD-causing on-rate of ~$10\,s^{-1}$ (representing ~50% of the ~$20.3\,s^{-1}$ time-averaged hERG activation rate that we calculated using the O'Hara–Rudy model).

García-Ferreiro *et al.* observed that the on-rate of astemizole ($k_{on} = 4 \times 10^6$ $M^{-1} s^{-1}$), but not imipramine ($k_{on} = 2.5 \times 10^6 M^{-1} s^{-1}$), exceeds the rate of KCNH1 channel opening at a blocker concentration of 10 μM (corresponding to on-rates of 40 and 25 s^{-1} for the two blockers, respectively) [40]. Our results are in qualitative agreement with these experimental findings. Nontrappable blockers evoked EADs at ~83% of the maximal open channel population at $I_{Kr(peak)}$ (~45% of the total population at $I_{Kr(peak)}$) for nontrappable blockers, based on Equation 14.1 and K_d values derived from the EAD-causing k_{off} and k_{on} values and exposures.

14.1.5
Novel Insights about the Causes of Inadvertent hERG Binding Function

1) *Predicted solvation properties of the ion conduction pathway*
   Bulk-like and H-bond depleted water dominate the solvation network of the ion conduction pathway of the open hERG channel. The predicted solvation consists of the following:
   a) A single high occupancy, H-bond enriched solvation site ($\Delta G \approx -1.5$ kcal/mol) located near the base of the selectivity filter (Figure 14.6). This result is consistent with the following:
      i) The strong electrostatic potential within the channel needed for ion conduction, which would likely be attenuated by the screening effects of abundant high occupancy solvation.
      ii) A low barrier for blocker entry into the channel, translating to specific (i.e., saturable) but nonselective binding. The association barrier is likely predominated by blocker, rather than protein desolvation cost.
      iii) Accommodation of multiple blocker chemical configurations, conformations, and binding configurations (due to the lack of directional constraints imposed by water H-bond replacement). A distribution of docking poses was observed for all blockers docked to a hERG homology model by Farid *et al.* [41].
      iv) The above factors, coupled with the large, radially symmetric cavity, are consistent with high tolerance for structural and size diversity, and flat structure–activity relationships (i.e., the absence of activity "cliffs") observed for most hERG blocker series.
   b) A radially distributed band containing 22 H-bond depleted solvation sites around Tyr652 and Phe656 side chains lining the inner surface of the ion conduction pathway (Figure 14.7) (total $\Delta G \approx +72$ kcal/mol). This result is consistent with a high maximal intrinsic barrier for blocker dissociation. In previous work, we used WaterMap [42,43] to study the solvation networks of the ATP pocket in p38 kinase relative to a series of ATP-competitive inhibitors [44] and porin OmpC relative to a set of antibacterial substrates [45]. A large amount of H-bond

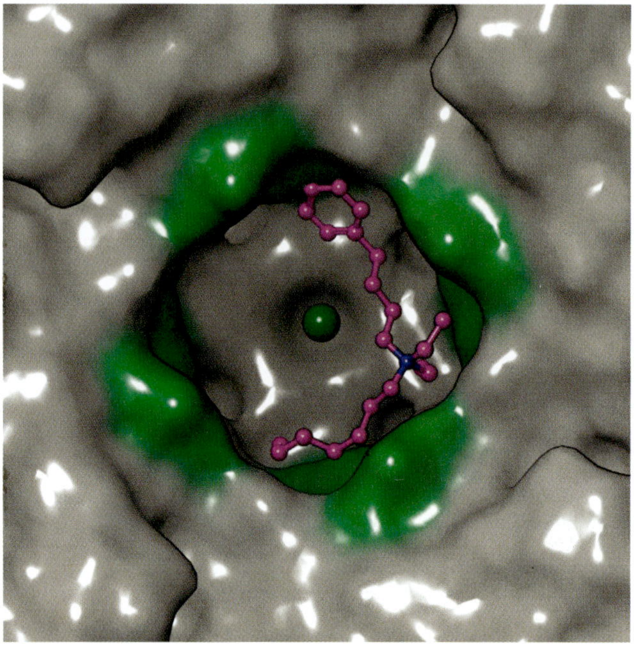

Figure 14.6 WaterMap of the ion conduction pathway of the Farid *et al.* hERG homology model, showing the single nonnegligible H-bond enriched hydration site predicted by WaterMap (predicted $\Delta G = -1.5$ kcal/mol) (green sphere). Induced fit docked clofilium (magenta) is overlaid on the structure for reference. The molecular surface of the ion conduction pathway is shown in gray, with Tyr652 and Phe656 residues in green. The view is from the intracellular direction looking toward the selectivity filter entrance.

depleted solvation is predicted within the ATP pocket of p38α. BIRB 796, the slowest off-rate inhibitor of the series (measured $t_{1/2} \approx 23$ h), transfers a large fraction of this water ($\Delta G \approx +67$ kcal/mol) from p38α to bulk solvent, whereas analogue 3, the fastest off-rate inhibitor of the series (measured $t_{1/2} \approx 800$ ms), transfers a comparatively smaller amount ($\Delta G \approx +21$ kcal/mol). Induced fit docked terfenadine [41] (a known trappable blocker) [22] is predicted to transfer 12 H-bond depleted water molecules solvating hERG (total $\Delta G \approx +26$ kcal/mol), from which we estimate $t_{1/2} \approx 8$ s (based on ~10,000-fold slower k_{off} suggested from the 5 kcal/mol difference with analogue 3 above). These results contrast measured antibacterial lifetimes on the order of 200 μs in porin OmpC, which is devoid of H-bond depleted solvation.

2) *Structure–kinetics-based blocker classification hypotheses*

The limited success of traditional structure–activity models in explaining the fundamental molecular causes of hERG blockade is largely attributable to two assumptions inherent to such models that break down for voltage-gated ion channels, namely, that binding is at equilibrium and

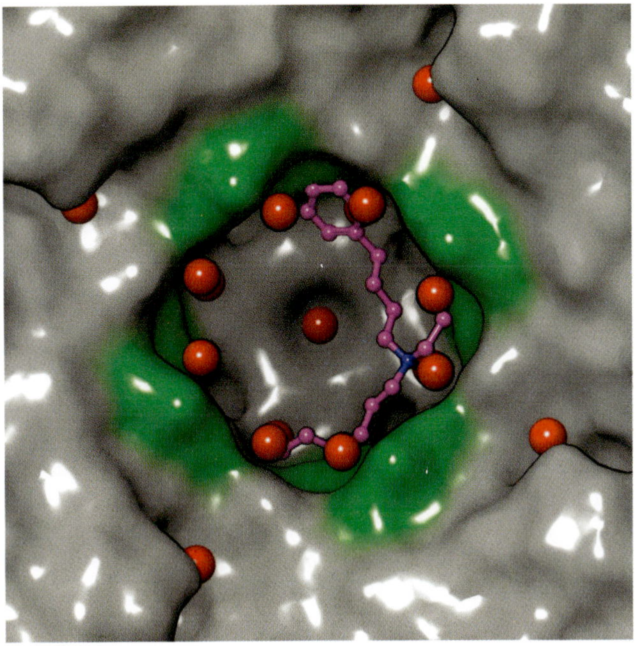

Figure 14.7 Same as Figure 14.6, but showing the locations of all H-bond depleted hydration sites predicted by WaterMap (red spheres).

governed by classical intermolecular interactions. IC_{50} values measured using RLB or conventional patch clamp assays performed at subphysiological gating frequencies are inherently biased toward the intrinsic binding contribution. The origin of this contribution is well explained by our WaterMap predictions.

a) A low maximal association barrier and fast maximal k_{on} stemming from the sparsity of H-bond enriched solvation. This is consistent with the following:
   i) Known lack of native binding function of the ion conduction pathway.
   ii) Specific (i.e., saturable), but nonselective (if not promiscuous) binding, stemming from limited molecular recognition capability.
   iii) A diminished role for blocker H-bond groups in achieving fast k_{on}.
b) A moderate to high maximal dissociation barrier and slow $k_{off(floor,intrinsic)}$ stemming from the presence of significant H-bond depleted solvation. Under physiological conditions, $k_{off(floor,intrinsic)}$ is hijacked, obviating the need for potent blockers to displace large amounts of such solvation.

Our findings underscore the decidedly nonequilibrium nature of hERG blockade under physiological conditions, in which high occupancy is achieved via fast on-rate and fast k_{off} (necessitating continuous refreshment of the bound state). The lower limit of k_{on} and upper limit of k_{off} among potent blockers are dictated by the following:

a) The plausible range of intracellular exposure (which we assume is <1 μM for the present purpose).
b) *Trappability*: $k_{on} > 1 \times 10^6\, M^{-1}\, s^{-1}$, $k_{off} \approx 0.69\, s^{-1}$ versus $k_{on} > 1 \times 10^7\, M^{-1}\, s^{-1}$, $k_{off} \approx 2\, s^{-1}$ for trappable and nontrappable blockers, respectively. Trappability is likely determined by shape complementarity with the closed channel state.

We now address the molecular and physicochemical properties governing high occupancy, as relates to the aforementioned kinetics behavior. The general susceptibility of potassium channels to blockade by small *quaternary* alkylamines (i.e., tetraethylammonium) was first demonstrated by Armstrong [46,47] and later for hERG by Ficker *et al.* [48]. However, whereas C_1 or C_2 is sufficient to block most other potassium channels, C_{10}-triethylammonium is the minimum configuration needed for blocking hERG (IC_{50} = 3.6 μM) [48]. To test the possible extension of these findings to the prevalent *basic* alkylamine hERG blocker class, we synthesized and tested four unsubstituted alkyl- and aryl-alkylamine analogues (denoted I1–I4) of the antiarrhythmic drug ibutilide (Table 14.1) in standard in-house Qpatch and RLB assays. We used these compounds to study the role of alkyl chain length, cyclization, aromaticity, and substitution on hERG activity (largely reflecting the intrinsic binding contribution), concluding that the activity of ibutilide is driven largely by the trialkylamine substructure, with only incremental contributions from the polar and aromatic substituents. Results for the quaternary amine blocker clofilium, induced fit docked in a homology model of the hERG pore domain by Farid *et al.*, suggest a multitude of binding modes that conform to the radial symmetry of the ion conduction pathway [41]. The authors proposed a "wheel-like" (hub–spokes–rim) binding paradigm for aryl-alkylamine-type blockers, in which the basic group serves as the "hub," *N*-alkyl groups as the "spokes," and aromatic groups as the "rim." This paradigm is consistent with the isopotentials of the binding site mapped by Farid *et al.*, which the authors described as a large "crown-shaped" hydrophobic region around the central axis of the pore (encompassing the H-bond depleted solvation around Tyr652 and Phe656), and "propeller-shaped" hydrophilic region sandwiched between the hydrophobic crown and intracellular face of the selectivity filter (encompassing the H-bond enriched solvating water molecule) [41] (Figure 14.6).

We manually visualized the two-dimensional chemical structures of 5895 nonacid compounds that were active (i.e., hERG inhibition ≥40% at 30 μM) in our in-house hERG Qpatch assay (filtered from a total of 6323 acidic + nonacidic compounds), looking specifically for non-alkylamine-type hERG blocking motifs that were not previously reported in other studies. We focused initially on the subset of smaller fragments, for which the hERG binding contribution could be isolated to a single substructure. In the course of this work,

Table 14.1 List of the model compounds synthesized in this work.

Compound	Structure	hERG RLB (IC_{50} μM)	hERG QPatch (IC_{50} μM)	Na_v1.5 QPatch (IC_{50} μM)	MW	C log *P*	pK_a (Moka)
Ibutilide	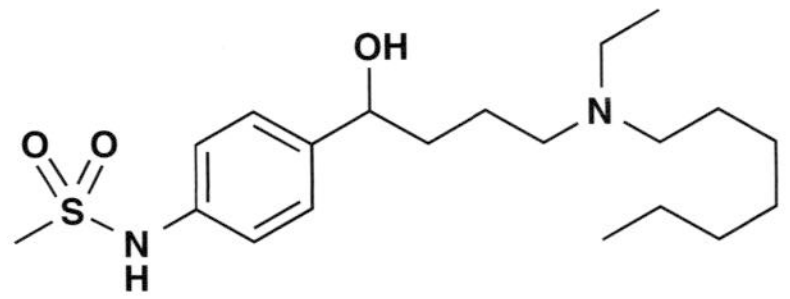	0.026 (1)	<0.4 (1)	>30	370.56	3.8	9.74
I1	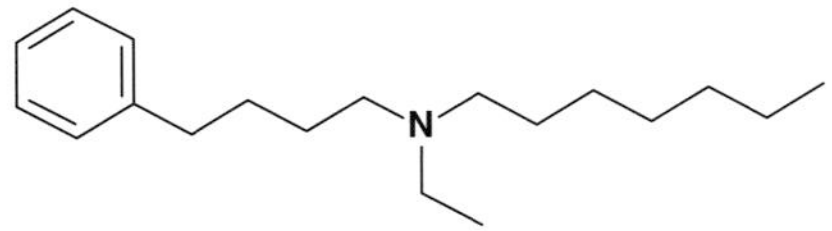	0.76 (30)	<0.4 (1)	5.3	275.47	6.7	9.99
I2[a)]	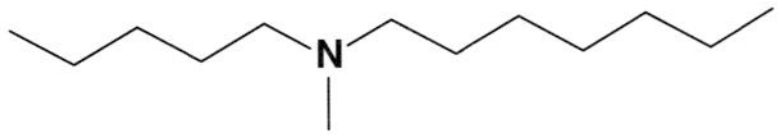	12.41 (477)	1.0 (2.5)	>30	199.38	5.3	10.05

(*continued*)

Table 14.1 (*Continued*)

Compound	Structure	hERG RLB (IC_{50} μM)	hERG QPatch (IC_{50} μM)	Na_v1.5 QPatch (IC_{50} μM)	MW	C log *P*	pK_a (Moka)
I3	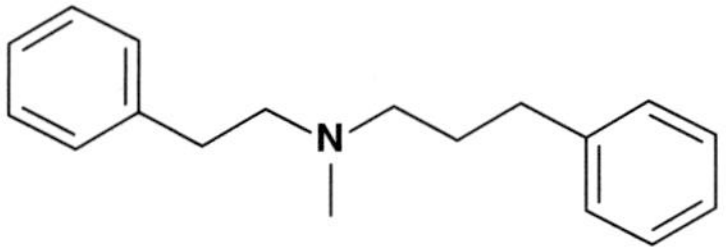	1.14 (44)	1.9 (5)	28.4	253.38	4.6	9.38
I4[b)]	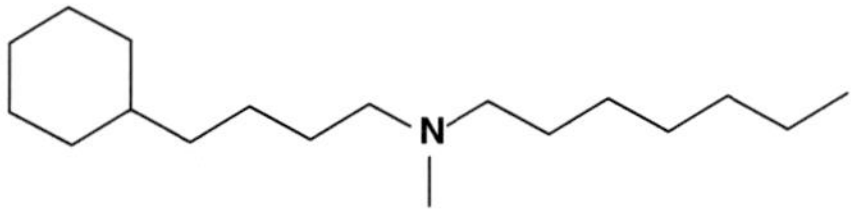	1.69 (65)	2.0 (5)	>30	267.49	7.4	10.19

Fold-differences in IC_{50} relative to ibutilide are shown in parentheses.

a) for ibutilide analogue I2 ($CDCl_3$, 400.3 MHz) δ 0.74–0.84 (m, 6H), 1.12–1.31 (m, 12H), 1.35–1.47 (m, 4H), 2.14 (s, 3H), 2.22–2.26 (m, 4H) ppm. ^{13}CNMR ($CDCl_3$, 100.7 MHz) δ 14.07, 14.08, 22.64, 22.67, 27.03, 27.36, 27.63, 29.31, 29.86, 31.86, 42.38, 57.95, 57.99 ppm.

b) for I4 ($CDCl_3$, 400.3 MHz) δ 0.75–0.82 (m, 5H), 1.02 (t, *J* = 8 Hz, 3H), 1.07–1.33 (m, 16H), 1.37–1.43 (m, 4H), 1.55–1.62 (m, 5H), 2.35 (t, *J* = 7.6 Hz, 4H), 2.47 (q, *J* = 6.8 Hz, 2H) ppm. ^{13}CNMR ($CDCl_3$, 100.7 MHz) δ 14.07, 22.61, 24.77, 26.42, 26.73, 27.48, 29.17, 31.81, 33.40, 37.32, 37.63, 47.27, 53.04 ppm.

we visually identified several active neutral bisaryl fragments (i.e., aryl–linker–aryl) containing variable length, chemically diverse linkers. We then performed two-dimensional substructure searching on our full Qpatch dataset using in-house proprietary software with queries containing different combinations of 5- and 6-rings and 6- and 6-rings connected by zero- to three-atom linkers. Atom-type matching criteria were set to [C, O, N, S] for all atoms in the search queries. We assigned formal charges to the hits generated from each query using the Epik [49] method in LigPrep (available in Schrödinger's Maestro software) with pH set to 7.0. The hits were comprised of compounds containing basic centers lacking bisaryl motifs (i.e., which we designate as type I blockers), neutral bisaryl motifs (i.e., which we designate as type II blockers), compounds lacking bisaryl motifs, compounds containing bisaryl motifs with basic centers (i.e., which we designate as type III blockers), and compounds containing neither bisaryl motifs nor basic centers. We made no attempt to expand the linker length in our queries beyond three atoms, although it appears that longer linkers are tolerated.

Neutral blockers have received considerably less notoriety than their basic counterparts, but have nonetheless been reported [50]. Examples include vesnarinone (see above) and a neutral analogue of sertindole (patch clamp hERG $IC_{50} = 1.5\,\mu M$) previously reported by Pearlstein *et al.* [51]. We analyzed the distribution of neutral versus charged hERG blockers in our in-house Qpatch dataset. To our surprise, bisaryl-containing (i.e., aryl–linker–aryl) compounds were present in a large proportion of the dataset and, more importantly, in an overwhelming proportion of both basic and neutral active and very active blockers (defined as >40 and >80% inhibition at 30 μM, respectively) (Table 14.2).

Overall, our findings suggest that hERG binding falls far outside the classical lock and key model, but rather is governed by structural and physicochemical properties that promote the following:

1) Fast k_{on}: Nontrappable blocker occupancy builds and decays within every AP cycle (exhibiting almost total dependence on fast k_{on} and high intracellular exposure to achieve EAD-causing occupancy), whereas trappable blocker occupancy builds and decays over multiple cycles (k_{on} determines the minimum exposure and number of cycles required to achieve EAD-causing occupancy). Blockers need not replace the H-bonds of favorable solvation to enter the ion conduction pathway, obviating the need for strategically positioned blocker H-bond groups. We postulate that basic blocker groups behave like "electrostatic mimetics" of potassium. In the absence of H-bond enriched solvation, electrostatic attraction between the unscreened negative field of the channel and positively charged blocker groups further accelerates k_{on} (possibly in some cases to the diffusion limit). The measured k_{on} of vesnarinone ($4.1 \times 10^5\,M^{-1}\,s^{-1}$) [52], a *neutral*, nontrappable hERG blocker, is far below the $1 \times 10^7\,M^{-1}\,s^{-1}$ needed to achieve the putative EAD-causing occupancy level.

Table 14.2 Distribution of compounds tested in Qpatch falling into type II (bisaryl), III (basic bisaryl), I (basic non-bisaryl), non-type II/III (other, including type I), and non-type I/II/III (other).

Type	Total number of nonacid compounds tested	Number of compounds in type	% of all compounds tested	Number of active compounds	% of active compounds	Number of very active compounds	% of very active compounds
II/III	5895	4463/5895	76	3250/4463	73	1211/4463	37
II	1712			1001/1712	58		
III	2682			2221/2682	83		
Non-type II/III	5895	1432/5895	24	942/1432	66	391/1432	27
I	1432	943/1432	66	675/943	72		
Non-type I/II/III	5895	462/5895	8	265/462	574		
				265/5895			

2) $k_{off} \approx k_{off(floor,true)}$: Achieved through displacement of a relatively small subset of H-bond depleted solvation. k_{off} is further slowed by trapping. Further work is needed to determine the specific structural requirements for trappability.

Such properties are present in three broad chemical classes of drug-like molecules:

a) *Type I*: Positively charged aromatic/aliphatic non-bisaryl blockers exhibiting high $\log P$ and high pK_a [53] (the familiar, canonical blocker class). We assume that proarrhythmic blockers of this nature bind via fast pK_a-dependent on-rates, with lifetimes approaching τ_{phys} (no examples of trappable type I blockers are currently known to us).
b) *Type II*: *Neutral* bisaryl blockers capable of displacing a subset of the H-bond depleted water solvating Tyr652 and/or Phe656. We assume that trappability is a prerequisite for proarrhythmic behavior of type II blockers (consistent with possibly slower k_{on} of neutral molecules).
c) *Type III*: Combination of types I and II. We assume that trappable type III blockers carry the greatest proarrhythmic risk due to fast k_{on}, together with slow $k_{off(open,true)}$ and/or trappability.

That comparatively few active compounds in our dataset fall outside of type I, II, and III classes (only 265/462 compounds tested) is noteworthy.

14.1.6 Implications of Our Findings for hERG Safety Assessment

1) *hERG blocker potency revisited*

   The results of our AP simulations suggest that hERG binding is governed by both intrinsic and extrinsic contributions. Our results suggest that the intrinsic off-rate is hijacked by the extrinsic contribution under physiological conditions. However, the hijacking effect is underestimated in conventional patch clamp protocols (and altogether neglected in RLB assays). This can be understood as follows. The bound lifetimes of trappable and nontrappable blockers are capped at τ_{phys} and CL (i.e., 0.34 and 1 s), respectively, compared with therapeutic drug–target lifetimes typically ranging from minutes to hours. Trappable and nontrappable blockers approach equilibrium occupancy as the channel gating frequency approaches zero (i.e., $\tau_{exptl} \rightarrow \infty$), irrespective of the relative weighting of k_{on} and k_{off} in K_d (i.e., equilibrium occupancy is kinetics agnostic). On the other hand, high occupancy is favored by k_{on}-weighted binding as channel gating approaches the physiological ~1 Hz physiological limit (i.e., $k_{off} < k_{off(floor,true)}$ has no impact on occupancy under such conditions). Physiologically relevant blocker potency is overestimated in conventional patch clamp experiments when K_d is weighted toward slow $k_{off(intrinsic)}$

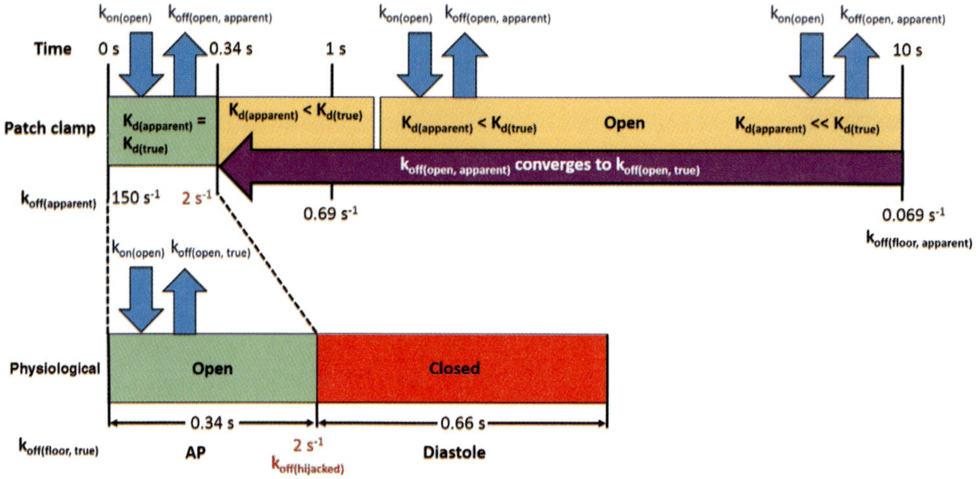

Figure 14.8 Transformations between measured $K_{d(apparent)}$ (top timeline) and physiological $K_{d(true)}$ (bottom timeline) for *nontrappable* blockers. Voltage-gated ion channels alternate in time between open and closed states at a frequency referred to in the text as ν_{phys} (the physiological frequency *in vivo*) and ν_{exptl} (subphysiological gating frequencies typically used in patch clamp assays). Channels spend far greater time in the open state under standard patch clamp protocols relative to the physiological timescale (referred to in the text as τ_{exptl} and τ_{phys}, respectively). Nontrappable blockers are incompatible with the closed state of hERG, and are expelled during the closing process (and therefore do not accumulate over time). The dissociation rate constant k_{off} is "hijacked" by channel closing at the fast ν_{phys} compared with the slower ν_{exptl}, such that blockers exhibiting k_{off} < the rate of channel closing converge to the rate of closing (i.e., $k_{off(open,\ intrinsic)} \rightarrow k_{off(open,\ true)} = k_{off(floor,\ true)}$ = rate of channel closing). Furthermore, occupancy depends on fast on-rates at ν_{phys} (i.e., higher exposure and/or faster k_{on}) compared with ν_{exptl}. As a result, blockers exhibiting slower k_{on}, accompanied by $k_{off(open,\ intrinsic)} << k_{off(open,\ true)}$, may appear far more potent in patch clamp experiments relative to their true potency *in vivo*. However, nontrappable blockers exhibiting fast on-rates gain potency at faster gating frequencies, where the channels spend more time on aggregate in the open state.

(irrespective of trappability), but may translate to the physiological case when weighted toward fast k_{on}. Since either scenario is plausible for a given blocker, true potency may or may not be reflected in *in vitro* IC_{50} measurements. This problem is compounded for nontrappable blockers, whose occupancy under physiological conditions is heavily on-rate dependent (whereas trappable blockers simply require longer times to reach equilibrium occupancy at slower on-rates). Unsurprisingly, many combinations of slow $k_{off(intrinsic)}$, slow k_{on} and fast $k_{off(intrinsic)}$, fast k_{on} equate to similar $k_{off(intrinsic)}/k_{on}$ ratios. As τ_{exptl} approaches τ_{phys}, k_{off} converges to a constant $k_{off(floor,true)}$ of $2\,s^{-1}$ (i.e., ln(2)/0.34 s) and $0.69\,s^{-1}$ (i.e., ln(2)/1 s) for nontrappable (Figure 14.8) and trappable (Figure 14.9) blockers, respectively. Under physiological conditions, occupancy is driven solely by fast on-rate in combination with fast k_{off} (capped on the bottom by $k_{off(floor,true)}$). However, unambiguous mapping from IC_{50} determined at

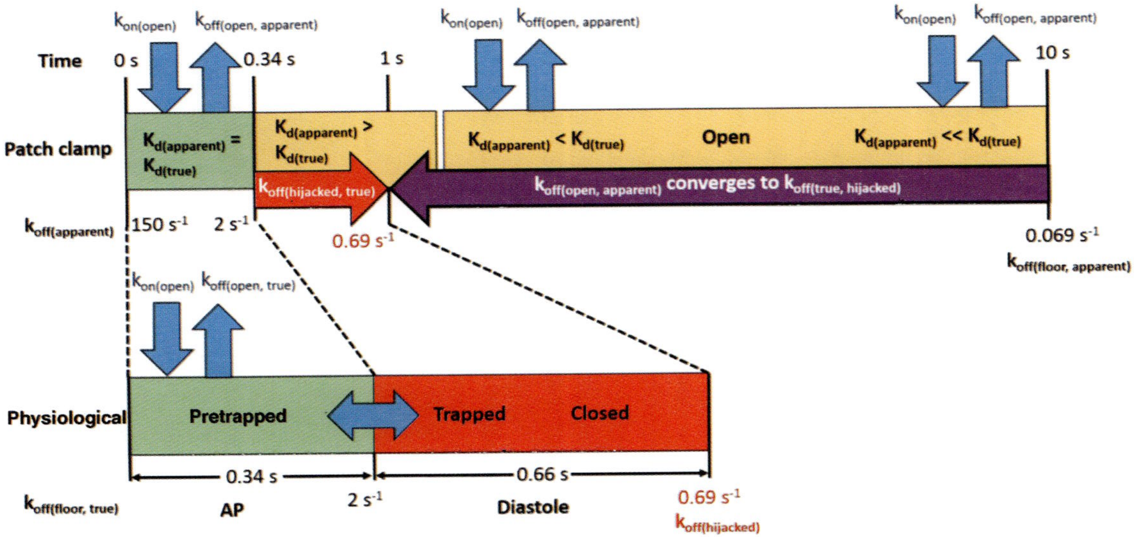

Figure 14.9 Transformations between measured $K_{d(\text{intrinsic})}$ (top timeline) and physiological $K_{d(\text{true})}$ (bottom timeline) for *trappable* blockers (see Figure 14.8 for variable definitions). Trappable and nontrappable blockers differ in their maximal bound lifetimes. As for nontrappable blockers, occupancy depends on fast on-rates at ν_{phys} (i.e., higher exposure and/or faster k_{on}) compared with ν_{exptl}. Blockers exhibiting slower k_{on}, accompanied by $k_{\text{off(open, intrinsic)}} << k_{\text{off (floor, true)}}$, may appear far more potent in patch clamp experiments relative to their true potency *in vivo*. Trappable blockers are compatible with the deactivated state of hERG, surviving expulsion during the closing process, and therefore accumulate over time. The dissociation rate constant $k_{\text{off(true)}}$ is hijacked by channel closing at the fast ν_{phys} compared with the slower ν_{exptl}, such that blockers exhibiting $k_{\text{off(open, intrinsic)}}$ slower than the rate of channel closing converge to the rate of closing (i.e., $k_{\text{off(open, intrinsic)}} \rightarrow k_{\text{off(floor, true)}}$.

$\tau_{\text{exptl}} > \tau_{\text{phys}}$ to $K_{\text{d(true)}}$ is precluded by the degeneracy of slow k_{off}/slow k_{on} and fast k_{off}/fast k_{on} scenarios. Furthermore, the minimum k_{on} needed to achieve EAD-causing occupancy levels differs between trappable and nontrappable cases ($k_{\text{on}} = 1 \times 10^5\,\text{M}^{-1}\,\text{s}^{-1}$ versus $1 \times 10^7\,\text{M}^{-1}\,\text{s}^{-1}$). At $k_{\text{on}} = 1 \times 10^5\,\text{M}^{-1}\,\text{s}^{-1}$, $K_{\text{d(intrinsic)}}$ maps to $K_{\text{d(true)}} = 6.9$ and $20\,\mu\text{M}$ for the two blocker subtypes, respectively, whereas at $k_{\text{on}} = 1 \times 10^7\,\text{M}^{-1}\,\text{s}^{-1}$, $K_{\text{d(intrinsic)}}$ maps to $K_{\text{d(true)}} = 69$ and 200 nM. From Equation 14.1, the EAD-causing level for nontrappable blockers (i.e., predicted $\gamma_c = 83\%$) is achieved at intracellular concentrations $\geq 5k_{\text{off(open,true)}}/k_{\text{on}}$ (e.g., a nontrappable blocker exhibiting $k_{\text{off(open,true)}}/k_{\text{on}} = 200\,\text{nM}$ requires $1\,\mu\text{M}$ intracellular concentration to achieve γ_c). On the other hand, trappable blockers reach the equilibrium level defined by $k_{\text{off(open,true)}}/k_{\text{on}}$ at intracellular concentrations ~1.6-fold above this ratio.

The limited success of conventional modeling and analysis methods in characterizing the true nature of hERG structure–activity and *in vitro–in vivo* relationships likely stems from the atypical nature of binding within the ion conduction pathway of voltage-gated channels:

a) Certain blockers are trapped within closed channels, while others are expelled (both subtypes may be present in the same dataset, and even within a single chemical series). Trappability is likely driven by steric compatibility with closing/closed channels, although the specific structural properties that promote trappability are currently unknown.
b) k_{on} is favored in K_{d} due to the existence of a frequency-dependent floor on k_{off} (a likely source of interlaboratory variability in measured IC_{50} values). Molecules bind to hERG via fast on-rates, dissociate slowly relative to the open channel time (the intrinsic contribution), and either exit from or remain bound during channel closure (the extrinsic contribution).
c) The lack of a defined cause–effect relationship between blocker potency and the proarrhythmic effects thereof.

Weak or inactive blockers exhibit either:

a) On-rate $\ll$ the rate of channel closing, or
b) $k_{\text{off}} \gg k_{\text{off(floor,true)}}$ and $k_{\text{on}} < 1 \times 10^7\,\text{M}^{-1}\,\text{s}^{-1}$, where similar behavior is expected irrespective of gating frequency. A special case consists of the second scenario combined with $k_{\text{on}} \geq 1 \times 10^7\,\text{M}^{-1}\,\text{s}^{-1}$, where significant potency is possible. The closed state does little to enhance the occupancy of trappable versus nontrappable blockers under this scenario (i.e., in both cases, γ_c is achieved transiently during each gating cycle at exposures $\geq 5k_{\text{off}}/k_{\text{on}}$). For example, $k_{\text{off(open,true)}} = 3 \times 10^1\,\text{s}^{-1}$ equates to $t_{1/2}$ of 23 ms (a mere 7% of the physiological open channel time). At $k_{\text{on}} = 1 \times 10^8\,\text{M}^{-1}\,\text{s}^{-1}$ (where $k_{\text{off}}/k_{\text{on}} = 300\,\text{nM}$), EAD-causing occupancy levels are expected at intracellular exposures $\geq 1.5\,\mu\text{M}$.

We argued previously that solvation energy contributions far outweigh classical intermolecular interactions (i.e., van der Waals, electrostatic, H-bond, etc.) to kinetic barriers and ΔG [44,45,54]. In particular, we proposed that ligand association and dissociation barrier heights predominantly consist of the cost of water transfer to/from a binding site and bulk solvent. Blocker binding under both physiological and nonphysiological conditions is well explained by this theory. As τ_{exptl} approaches ∞, $k_{\text{off(floor)}}$ approaches the intrinsic value (i.e., $k_{\text{off(floor,intrinsic)}}$) defined by the energetic cost of unfavorable water displacement. As τ_{exptl} approaches τ_{phys}, $k_{\text{off(floor)}}$ approaches $k_{\text{off(floor,true)}}$, which is defined by $\ln(2)/\tau_{\text{phys}}$ (nontrappable) or ln(2)/CL (trappable). It follows that the off-rate from conformationally dynamic channels is a function of two k_{off} terms:

a) $k_{\text{off(intrinsic)}}$, which depends on the total free energy of displaced unfavorable solvation (sufficient to promote bound lifetimes of τ_{phys}).
b) k_{off} from closed channels, which is assumed to be infinitely slow for trappable blockers, and approximately the rate of channel closing for nontrappable blockers (i.e., $k_{\text{off(hijacked)}}$).

Kinetic studies of hERG blockade are hampered by two major challenges in measuring k_{on} and $k_{\text{off(open,true)}}$:

a) Measured k_{off} is biased toward $k_{\text{off(intrinsic)}}$ under nonphysiological conditions (i.e., $\tau_{\text{exptl}} > \tau_{\text{phys}}$).
b) The rates of association and dissociation are not necessarily reflected in the time to maximal current reduction following extracellular blocker application and time to current recovery after washout, respectively (the typical approach used for measuring k_{on} and k_{off}) when the buildup and decay of intracellular blocker concentration serve as the rate-determining steps for binding.

2) *hERG safety index revisited*

Drug safety is traditionally gauged via the separation between toxic and therapeutic plasma exposure levels (which we refer to as the therapeutic index), or alternatively, plasma exposure relative to IC_{50} at the toxicity-inducing off-target(s) (which we refer to as the safety index):

$$IC_{50(\text{min})} = E_{\text{T}}N, \tag{14.6}$$

where $IC_{50(\text{min})}$ is the safe limit of off-target IC_{50}, E_{T} is the safe upper limit of therapeutic exposure, and N is the safety index (determined from known incursions of plasma exposure between the therapeutic and toxic levels in the patient population). Such incursions may arise from (a) intentional or inadvertent overdose; (b) drug–drug interactions; (c) genetic variability in drug metabolism; and (d) accumulation in cardiomyocytes. A widely used safety index (SI) for hERG was devised by Redfern *et al.* based on an analysis of the therapeutic exposure–

hERG IC_{50}–TdP relationships for 52 marketed drugs exhibiting a wide range of *in vitro* hERG activity and torsadogenic behavior [24]:

$$IC_{50(\text{min})} = (\text{free } C_{\text{max}}) \times 30, \tag{14.7}$$

where $IC_{50(\text{min})}$ is as defined above, and free C_{max} is the peak therapeutic plasma concentration of unbound drug (coinciding with maximal on-rate across the dosing interval). Based on the following reasoning, we hypothesize that the Redfern *et al.* dataset overwhelmingly consists of trappable blockers, and furthermore, that the k_{off} of such blockers is neither significantly faster nor slower than $k_{\text{off(open,true)}}$:

a) The proarrhythmic occupancy level differs between trappable and nontrappable blockers, as does the occupancy–exposure relationship and the nonequilibrium nature of nontrappable blocker binding. As such, both blocker subtypes cannot be represented using a single model.
b) Torsadogenic blockers are self-selecting for $k_{\text{off(open,true)}}$ in their measured IC_{50} values.

We studied the relationship between nonequilibrium occupancy and EAD formation versus the relationship between equilibrium occupancy (i.e., exposure relative to IC_{50}) and torsadogenicity studied by Redfern *et al.* Occupancy varies nonlinearly at exposures above and below the IC_{50} (i.e., the 50% occupancy level, by definition) in accordance with Equation 14.1 (plotted in Figure 4.10). Therefore, to facilitate comparison of our results, we expressed the Redfern SI in terms of occupancy. First, we devised an occupancy-based SI expression:

$$\text{SI} = \gamma_c - \gamma_{\text{ther}}, \tag{14.8}$$

where SI consists of the separation between the critical toxic occupancy (γ_c) and that at the therapeutic concentration (γ_{ther}). Next, we calculated γ_{ther} via substitution of $[\text{blocker}]_{\text{free}}$ in Equation 14.1 with free C_{max} in Equation 14.8 (assuming approximate equivalence between IC_{50} and K_d):

$$\gamma_{\text{ther}} = (IC_{50}/30)/((IC_{50}/30) + IC_{50}) \approx 3\%. \tag{14.9}$$

Assuming $\gamma_c = 50\%$ in the Redfern SI, we arrive at

$$\text{SI} = 50\% - 3\% = 47\%. \tag{14.10}$$

It is apparent from Equation 14.11 that the Redfern SI is not as much an SI as a complete intolerance for hERG occupancy at the therapeutic exposure (i.e., a ~47% cushion is needed to accommodate exposure-driven occupancy escalation to the putative TdP-causing level). Our results are well aligned with those of Redfern *et al.* for trappable blockers ($\gamma_c = 63\%$ versus 50%, equating to a 1.6-fold exposure difference relative to $K_{d(\text{true})}$), consistent with the causal relationship between EADs and TdP. The Redfern *et al.* dataset contains a small number of *known* trappable blockers distributed throughout the four blocker categories annotated by the authors [24] (see Figure 14.11), and likely harbors additional

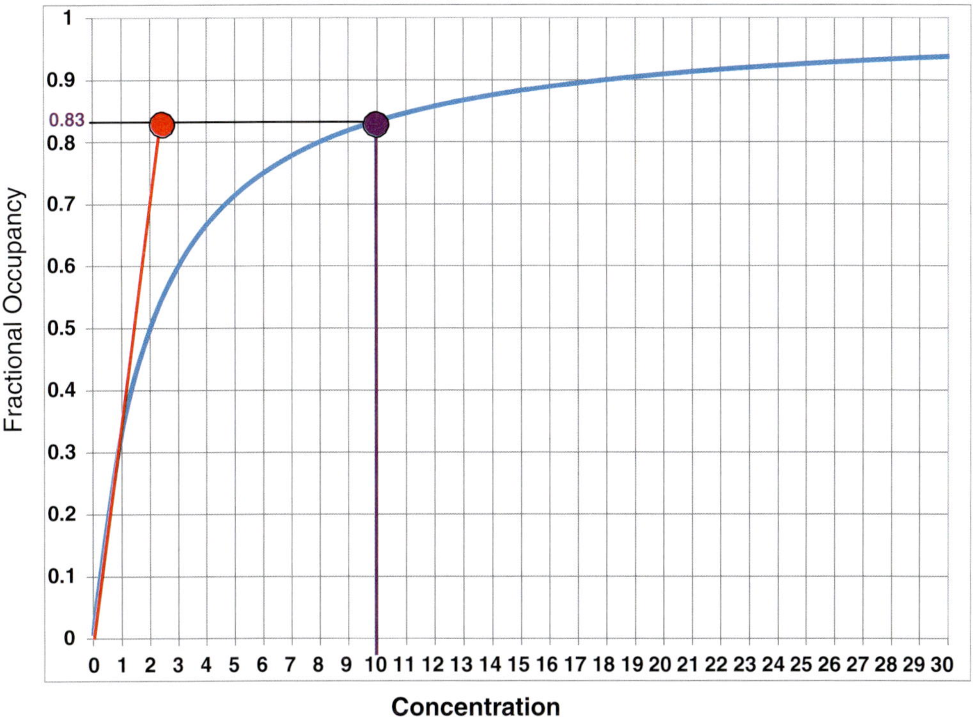

Figure 14.10 Occupancy is a hyperbolic function of concentration (Equation 14.1). Occupancy equates approximately to the concentration/K_d ratio only at concentrations $<< K_d$ (the linear region of the curve), diverging rapidly above, as illustrated for the nontrappable blocker cisapride. Cisapride achieves the putative 83% EAD-causing occupancy at an intracellular concentration of 10 nM, whereas this occupancy level is reached at ~2.5 nM based on a linear occupancy-concentration relationship. Nevertheless, 4.9 nM (the highest reported exposure for cisapride) extending to 10 nM represents a plausible gain in exposure due to higher dosing, or drug-drug interactions.

cases. Conversely, the Redfern SI makes little sense for nontrappable blockers whose EAD-causing occupancy is ~33% above $K_{d(true)}$ (exposure 5-fold above $K_{d(true)}$) versus ~13% for trappable blockers (exposure 1.6-fold above $K_{d(true)}$).

We calculated the occupancies of the 52 drugs in the Redfern *et al.* dataset at the highest reported free plasma exposure and lowest reported hERG IC_{50} using Equation 14.1 (data obtained from the supplementary information in Ref. [24]). The distribution of occupancies is shown in Figure 14.12, together with exposure gains required to reach γ_c for selected drugs. The estimated occupancies are well aligned with our putative γ_c values for trappable and nontrappable blockers. The reported IC_{50} values (Figure 19) fall within the expected ceiling and floor $K_{d(true)}$ values (Figures 14.8 and 14.9) among the known trappable and nontrappable cases (except cisapride). Although hERG dysfunction alone is sufficient to cause TdP, the SI may vary with the following:

a) Baseline I_{Kr} levels, including normal time-dependent fluctuations governed by adrenergic state, and permanent knockdown caused by genetic loss-of-function mutations in hERG or KCNQ1 [32,34].
b) I_{Kr} demand, as governed by heart rate [10] and changes in overall ion current balance (e.g., due to multi-ion channel blockade [55,56]).

The use of AP/QT prolongation as a torsadogenicity biomarker has been called into question by Hondeghem, who has long advocated the proarrhythmic nature of nonisomorphic AP changes (i.e., triangulation, reverse use dependence, and instability), together with organ level effects, collectively referred to as λ TRIaD [18]. The limitations of LQT as a proarrhythmia biomarker are exemplified by the trappable blocker terfenadine (hERG $IC_{50} = 20$ nM), which exhibits a significant disconnect in exposure levels required to cause triangulation in AP recordings (low nanomolar exposure) versus LQT [28]. This behavior is consistent with the results of our AP simulations, in which prolongation and EADs were induced by trappable blockers at far lower occupancy levels in M versus epi- and endocardial cells (~63% versus >90% in our simulations, respectively) due to significantly higher hERG populations in the latter cells.

Current hERG mitigation workflows center on modulation of pK_a and $\log P$ (applicable to type I blockers), and in many cases, "shots on goal" optimization toward greater hERG IC_{50}. Overall, our results suggest that new safety and mitigation criteria are needed to properly account for the kinetic nature of hERG binding and blockade:

a) Medium-throughput patch clamp assays are needed to identify trappable blockers based on frequency-dependent versus independent behavior. Based on our arguments, trappability rather than hERG IC_{50} is of critical importance for both safety assessment and mitigation.

Figure 14.11 Distribution of occupancies calculated from Equation 14.1 using the highest reported therapeutic plasma exposure and lowest reported hERG IC_{50} for 52 marketed drugs in the Redfern *et al.* data set. The bars are color-coded by the categories assigned by Redfern *et al.* (category 1: orange, category 2: red, category 3: magenta, category 4: blue, category 5: green). The Redfern (3%), trappable EAD-causing ($\gamma_c = 62.8\%$), and nontrappable EAD-causing ($\gamma_c = 83\%$) occupancy levels are shown as vertical lines (black, purple, and teal, respectively). Exposure gains above the highest reported therapeutic plasma levels needed to reach the respective EAD-causing level are annotated for the known trappable and nontrappable cases. These exposures equate to $1.6K_{d(true)}$ and $5K_{d(true)}$ for trappable and nontrappable blockers, respectively. A true safety margin would fall significantly below these occupancies, suggesting that the risk/benefit ratio is extremely large for trappable blockers.

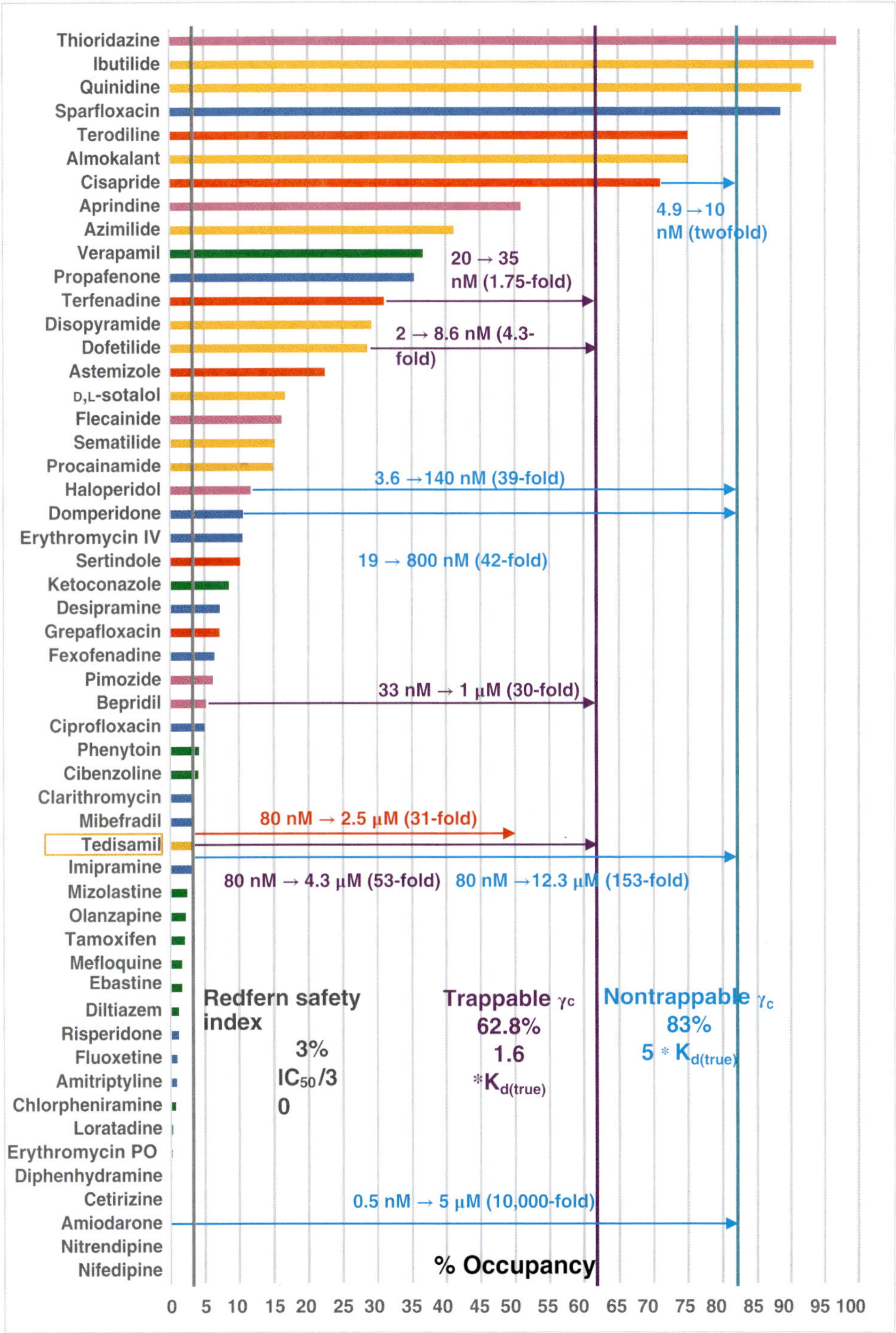
Thioridazine
Ibutilide
Quinidine
Sparfloxacin
Terodiline
Almokalant
Cisapride
Aprindine
Azimilide
Verapamil
Propafenone
Terfenadine
Disopyramide
Dofetilide
Astemizole
D,L-sotalol
Flecainide
Sematilide
Procainamide
Haloperidol
Domperidone
Erythromycin IV
Sertindole
Ketoconazole
Desipramine
Grepafloxacin
Fexofenadine
Pimozide
Bepridil
Ciprofloxacin
Phenytoin
Cibenzoline
Clarithromycin
Mibefradil
Tedisamil
Imipramine
Mizolastine
Olanzapine
Tamoxifen
Mefloquine
Ebastine
Diltiazem
Risperidone
Fluoxetine
Amitriptyline
Chlorpheniramine
Loratadine
Erythromycin PO
Diphenhydramine
Cetirizine
Amiodarone
Nitrendipine
Nifedipine
4.9 → 10 nM (twofold)
20 → 35 nM (1.75-fold)
2 → 8.6 nM (4.3-fold)
3.6 → 140 nM (39-fold)
19 → 800 nM (42-fold)
33 nM → 1 μM (30-fold)
80 nM → 2.5 μM (31-fold)
80 nM → 4.3 μM (53-fold)
80 nM → 12.3 μM (153-fold)
Redfern safety index 3% IC50/30
Trappable γc 62.8% 1.6 *Kd(true)
Nontrappable γc 83% 5 * Kd(true)
0.5 nM → 5 μM (10,000-fold)
% Occupancy
0 5 10 15 20 25 30 35 40 45 50 55 60 65 70 75 80 85 90 95 100

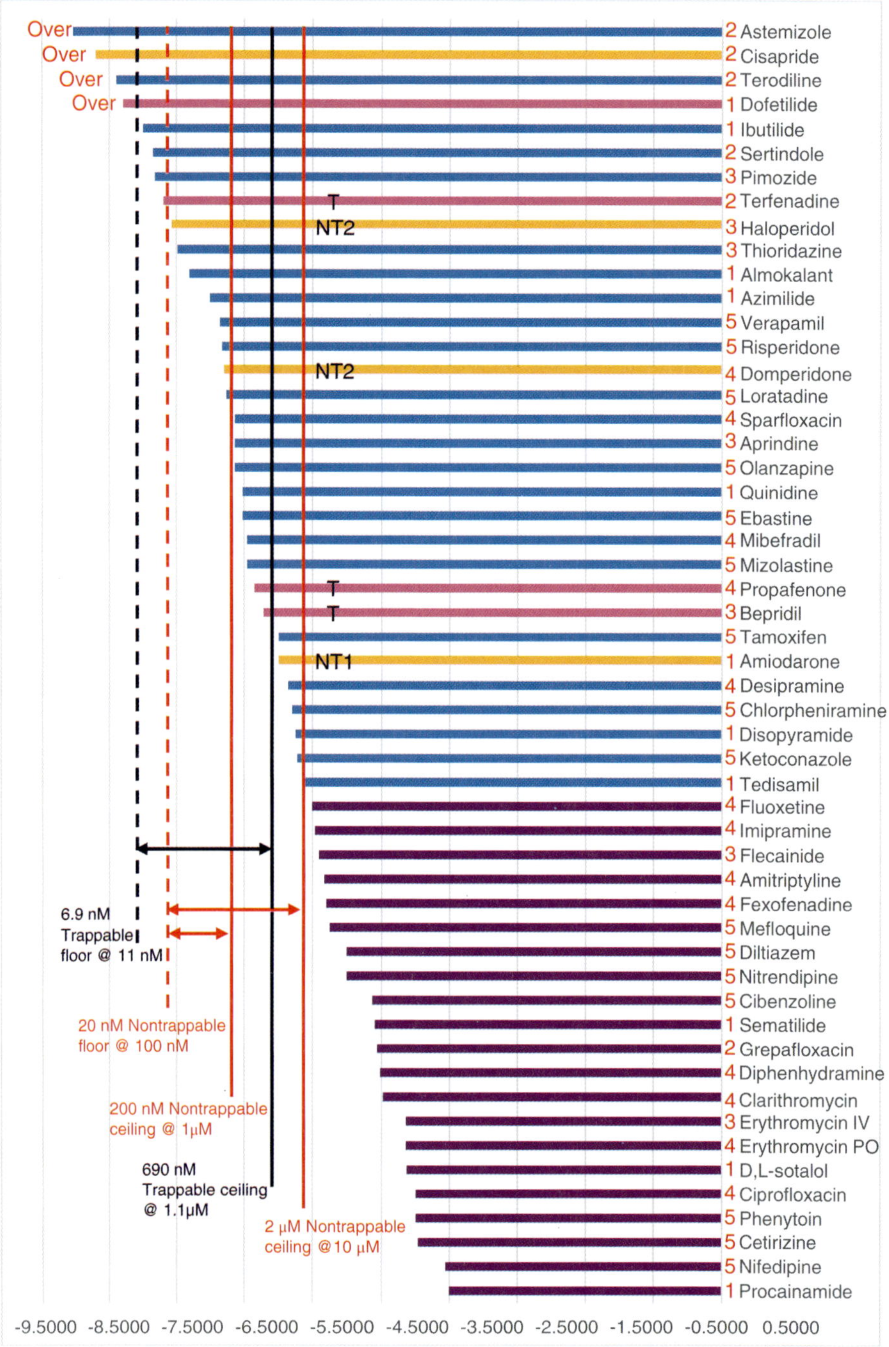

Figure 14.12 Distribution of the lowest reported log(hERG IC_{50}) of the 52 drugs in the Redfern *et al.* data set. The Redfern *et al.* categories are listed adjacent to the drug names. The bars for known trappable and nontrappable cases are color-coded magenta

b) Demonstration of a viable chemical route between trappability and nontrappability *prior to lead selection*: Trappable blockers should be assumed unsafe, with chemistry efforts focused on identifying nontrappable analogues. Windisch *et al.* synthesized five nontrappable analogues of the trappable blocker propafenone, which the authors attributed to differences in calculated pK_a [57]. However, experimental pK_a measurements of similarly substituted piperazines measured by Lacivita *et al.* [58] suggest that the calculated pK_a values were considerably overestimated (i.e., measured values of 7.59–8.39 for non-CF_3-containing substitutions compared with calculated values of 5.96–9.82). Both trappable and nontrappable propafenone blockers exhibited similarly fast on-rates (with times to steady-state block ranging between 440 and 2390 ms), likely due to the basic center present in these compounds. We hypothesize that susceptibility to trapping is conveyed by the bisaryl motif (type II/III blockers). However, it is likely that only a subset of bisaryl blockers is trappable, and the possibility that certain non-bisaryl motifs are trappable cannot be ruled out. The combination of positive charge and trappability may bring the best of both worlds to hERG blockers, promoting rapid buildup to the equilibrium γ_c level.
c) Optimization of nontrappable blockers toward slower k_{on} and lower therapeutic exposure: Our type I ibutilide analogues suggest that hERG activity lacks significant sensitivity to chemical modification, but is likely approachable via pK_a and $\log P$ modulation. Log P modulation may have little impact on k_{on} and IC_{50} when pK_a is >9 (Table 14.1), and furthermore, the overlapping contributions of pK_a and $\log P$ to solubility, permeability, pharmacokinetics, hERG binding, and on-target potency constrain these properties. For example, pK_a of 6–8 may reduce hERG binding, while maintaining solubility (provided $\log P$ is sufficiently low). Torsadogenic nontrappable blockers are known to exist (e.g., haloperidol, cisapride, domperidone, amiodarone, and droperidol) [22].

Figure 14.12 *(Continued)*

and orange, respectively. Vertical lines denoting $K_{d(true,\ ceiling)}$ (solid lines) and $K_{d(true,\ floor)}$ (dotted lines) are overlaid on the bar graph for reference (color-coded blue and red for trappable and nontrappable cases, respectively). Blockers exhibiting IC_{50} values above both the trappable and nontrappable ceilings are color-coded purple. Such blockers require high exposure to reach γ_c. Nontrappable drugs falling below the 2 μM ceiling (requiring at least 10 μM exposure to reach the EAD-causing occupancy), and those falling below the 200 nM ceiling (requiring at least 1 μM exposure to reach the EAD-causing occupancy) are annotated with "NT1" and "NT2," respectively. Drugs falling below the trappable and nontrappable floors such that $K_{d(true)}$ is underestimated (i.e., due to $k_{off(open,\ apparent)} < k_{off(floor,\ true)}$) are annotated with "Over." All of the known trappable and nontrappable drugs, except those with overestimated potency, fall within the ranges expected from the rationale described in Figures 14.8 and 14.9.

14.1.7 Conclusion and Future Directions

We studied the relationship between blocker binding and channel gating kinetics using the O'Hara–Rudy human AP model and showed that hERG blockade reaches a tipping point in both $I_{Kr(peak)}$ reduction and slowing of $-dV_m(t)/dt$ at AP phase 3 (abruptly at ~63% occupancy and ~83% for trappable and nontrappable blockers, respectively). We addressed putative structure–kinetic relationships of hERG blockers based on a previously published general theory of binding kinetics, in which the association and dissociation barriers are attributed to H-bond enriched and H-bond depleted solvation, respectively. We used WaterMap to calculate the solvation properties of a published homology model of the open form of hERG. The results suggest that the ion conduction pathway is solvated by a large amount of H-bond depleted water, which is sufficient to achieve intrinsic lifetimes far longer than the ~340 ms physiological open channel period. A different picture emerges under physiological conditions, wherein blocker off-rates are hijacked by channel closing, resulting in bound lifetimes equivalent to the open channel period or shorter (the extrinsic lifetime). Analysis of our in-house automated patch clamp data suggests that three molecular properties promote hERG binding: the combination of high $\log P$ and pK_a (present in many hydrophobic bases), neutral bisaryl motifs, and basic bisaryl motifs. We speculate that bisaryl groups slow $k_{off(open)}$, and may in some cases promote trapping due to packing with Tyr652 and/or Phe656 side chains deep within the ion conduction pathway. We conclude that the current approaches to evaluating structure–activity relationships of hERG blockers, trial-and-error mitigation, and safety assessment could benefit from a substantial overhaul. Efforts are needed to better understand blocker structure–kinetic relationships (particularly the structural requirements for trapping), to develop physiologically relevant hERG assays, and to determine reliable dynamic occupancy-based safety criteria.

References

1 Sanguinetti, M.C., Jiang, C., Curran, M.E., and Keating, M.T. (1995) A mechanistic link between an inherited and an acquired cardiac arrhythmia: hERG encodes the IKr potassium channel. *Cell*, **81**, 299–307.

2 Sanguinetti, M.C., Chen, J., Fernandez, D., Kamiya, K., Mitcheson, J., and Sanchez-Chapula, J.A. (2005) Physicochemical basis for binding and voltage-dependent block of hERG channels by structurally diverse drugs, in *The hERG Cardiac Potassium Channel: Structure, Function and Long QT Syndrome: Novartis Foundation Symposium, No. 266* (eds D.J. Chadwick and J. Goode), John Wiley & Sons, Inc., New York.

3 Sanguinetti, M.C. and Tristani-Firouzi, M. (2006) hERG potassium channels and cardiac arrhythmia. *Nature*, **440**, 463–469.

4 Mitcheson, J.S. (2008) hERG potassium channels and the structural basis of drug-induced arrhythmias. *Chemical Research in Toxicology*, **21**, 1005–1010.

5 Mitcheson, J.S., Chen, J., and Sanguinetti, M.C. (2000) Trapping of a

methanesulfonanilide by closure of the hERG potassium channel activation gate. *Journal of General Physiology*, **115**, 229–240.

6 Roy, M., Dumaine, R., and Brown, A.M. (1996) hERG, a primary human ventricular target of the nonsedating antihistamine terfenadine. *Circulation*, **94**, 817–823.

7 Brown, A.M. and Rampe, D. (2000) Drug-induced long QT syndrome: is HERG the root of all evil. *Pharma News*, 7, 15–20.

8 Rampe, D., Roy, M.L., Dennis, A., and Brown, A.M. (1997) A mechanism for the proarrhythmic effects of cisapride (Propulsid): high affinity blockade of the human cardiac potassium channel HERG. *FEBS Letters*, **417**, 28–32.

9 Rampe, D. and Brown, A.M. (2013) A history of the role of the hERG channel in cardiac risk assessment. *Journal of Pharmacological and Toxicological Methods*, **68**, 13–22.

10 Hondeghem, L.M. and Snyders, D.J. (1990) Class III antiarrhythmic agents have a lot of potential but a long way to go: reduced effectiveness and dangers of reverse use dependence. *Circulation*, **81**, 686–690.

11 Hondeghem, L.M., Carlsson, L., and Duker, G. (2001) Instability and triangulation of the action potential predict serious proarrhythmia, but action potential duration prolongation is antiarrhythmic. *Circulation*, **103**, 2004–2013.

12 Hondeghem, L.M. and Hoffmann, P. (2003) Blinded test in isolated female rabbit heart reliably identifies action potential duration prolongation and proarrhythmic drugs: importance of triangulation, reverse use dependence, and instability. *Journal of Cardiovascular Pharmacology*, **41**, 14–24.

13 Haverkamp, W., Breithardt, G., Camm, A.J., Janse, M.J., Rosen, M.R., Antzelevitch, C., Escande, D., Franz, M., Malik, M., Moss, A., and Shah, R. (2000) The potential for QT prolongation and proarrhythmia by non-antiarrhythmic drugs: clinical and regulatory implications. Report on a policy conference of the European Society of Cardiology. *European Heart Journal*, **21**, 1216–1231.

14 Pearlstein, R., Vaz, R., and Rampe, D. (2003) Understanding the structure–activity relationship of the human Ether-à-go-go-related gene cardiac K+ channel: a model for bad behavior. *Journal of Medicinal Chemistry*, **46**, 2017–2022.

15 Jamieson, C., Moir, E.M., Rankovic, Z., and Wishart, G. (2006) Medicinal chemistry of hERG optimizations: highlights and hang-ups. *Journal of Medicinal Chemistry*, **49**, 5029–5046.

16 Fermini, B. and Fossa, A.A. (2003) The impact of drug-induced QT interval prolongation on drug discovery and development. *Nature Reviews. Drug Discovery*, **2**, 439–447.

17 Farid, R., Day, T., Friesner, R.A., and Pearlstein, R.A. (2006) New insights about HERG blockade obtained from protein modeling, potential energy mapping, and docking studies. *Bioorganic and Medicinal Chemistry*, **14**, 3160–3173.

18 Hondeghem, LM. (2011) *QT Prolongation Is a Poor Predictor of Proarrhythmia Liability: Beyond QT Prolongation!*, Springer, Berlin, pp. 639–654.

19 Starmer, C.F. and Courtney, K.R. (1986) Modeling ion channel blockade at guarded binding sites: application to tertiary drugs. *American Journal of Physiology*, **251**, H848–H856.

20 Starmer, C.F. (1987) Theoretical characterization of ion channel blockade: competitive binding to periodically accessible receptors. *Biophysical Journal*, **52**, 405–412.

21 Starmer, C. and Grant, A.O. (1985) Phasic ion channel blockade: a kinetic model and parameter estimation procedure. *Molecular Pharmacology*, **28**, 348–356.

22 Stork, D., Timin, E.N., Berjukow, S., Huber, C., Hohaus, A., Auer, M., and Hering, S. (2007) State dependent dissociation of HERG channel inhibitors. *British Journal of Pharmacology*, **151**, 1368–1376.

23 O'Hara, T., Virág, L., Varró, A., and Rudy, Y. (2011) Simulation of the undiseased human cardiac ventricular action potential: model formulation and experimental validation. *PLoS Computational Biology*, **7**, 1–29.

24 Redfern, W.S., Carlsson, L., Davis, A.S., Lynch, W.G., MacKenzie, I., Palethorpe, S.,

Siegl, P.K., Strang, I., Sullivan, A.T., Wallis, R., Camm, A.J., and Hammond, T.G. (2003) Relationships between preclinical cardiac electrophysiology, clinical QT interval prolongation and torsade de pointes for a broad range of drugs: evidence for a provisional safety margin in drug development. *Cardiovascular Research*, **58**, 32–45.

25 Issa, Z.F., Miller, J.M., and Zipes, D.P. (2012) *Clinical Arrhythmology and Electrophysiology: A Companion to Braunwald's Heart Disease*, 2nd edn, Elsevier Saunders, Philadelphia, PA.

26 Hondeghem, L.M. (2006) Estimation of proarrhythmic hazards by QT prolongation/shortening: QT obsession? *Drug Information Journal*, **40**, 273–279.

27 Hondeghem, L.M. (2008) QT and TdP. QT: an unreliable predictor of proarrhythmia. *Acta Cardiologica*, **63**, 1–7.

28 Hondeghem, L.M. (2011) QTc prolongation as a surrogate for drug-induced arrhythmias: fact or fallacy? *Acta Cardiologica*, **66**, 685–689.

29 Zhou, Z., Gong, Q., Ye, B., Fan, Z., Makielski, J.C., Robertson, G.A., and January, C.T. (1998) Properties of HERG channels stably expressed in HEK 293 cells studied at physiological temperature. *Biophysical Journal*, **74**, 230–241.

30 Roden, D.M. (2008) Repolarization reserve: a moving target. *Circulation*, **118**, 981–982.

31 Weiss, J.N., Garfinkel, A., Karagueuzian, H.S., Chen, P.-S., and Qu, Z. (2010) Early after depolarizations and cardiac arrhythmias. *Heart Rhythm*, **7**, 1891–1899.

32 Viitasalo, M., Paavonen, K.J., Swan, H., Kontula, K., and Toivonen, L. (2005) Effects of epinephrine on right ventricular monophasic action potentials in the LQT1 versus LQT2 form of long QT syndrome: preferential enhancement of "Triangulation" in LQT1. *Pacing and Clinical Electrophysiology*, **28**, 219–227.

33 Thomas, D., Kiehn, J., Katus, H., and Karle, C. (2004) Adrenergic regulation of the rapid component of the cardiac delayed rectifier potassium current, IKr, and the underlying hERG ion channel. *Basic Research in Cardiology*, **99**, 279–287.

34 Woodcock, E.A., Kistler, P.M., and Ju, Y.-K. (2009) Phosphoinositide signalling and cardiac arrhythmias. *Cardiovascular Research*, **82**, 286–295.

35 Schwartz, P.J., Spazzolini, C., Crotti, L., Bathen, J., Amlie, J.P., Timothy, K., Shkolnikova, M., Berul, C.I., Bitner-Glindzicz, M., Toivonen, L., Horie, M., Schulze-Bahr, E., and Denjoy, I. (2006) The Jervell and Lange-Nielsen syndrome: natural history, molecular basis, and clinical outcome. *Circulation*, **113**, 783–790.

36 Wolk, R., Cobbe, S.M., Hicks, M.N., and Kane, K.A. (1999) Functional, structural, and dynamic basis of electrical heterogeneity in healthy and diseased cardiac muscle: implications for arrhythmogenesis and anti-arrhythmic drug therapy. *Pharmacology & Therapeutics*, **84**, 207–231.

37 Nakatani, S. (2011) Left ventricular rotation and twist: why should we learn? *Journal of Cardiovascular Ultrasound*, **19**, 1–6.

38 Behr, E.R., Ritchie, M.D., Tanaka, T., Kääb, S., Crawford, D.C., Nicoletti, P., Floratos, A., Sinner, M.F., Kannankeril, P.J., Wilde, A.A.M., Bezzina, C.R., Schulze-Bahr, E., Zumhagen, S., Guicheney, P., Bishopric, N.H., Marshall, V., Shakir, S., Dalageorgou, C., Bevan, S., Jamshidi, Y., Bastiaenen, R., Myerburg, R.J., Schott, J.-J., Camm, A.J., Steinbeck, G., Norris, Kris, Altman, R.B., Tatonetti, N.P., Jeffery, S., Kubo, M., Nakamura, Y., Shen, Y., George, A.L., Jr., and Roden, D.M. (2013) Genome wide analysis of drug-induced torsades de pointes: lack of common variants with large effect sizes. *PLoS One*, **8** (11), e78511.

39 Silva, J. and Rudy, Y. (2005) Subunit interaction determines I_{Ks} participation in cardiac repolarization and repolarization reserve. *Circulation*, **112**, 1384–1391.

40 García-Ferreiro, R.E., Kerschensteiner, D., Major, F., Monje, F., Stühmer, W., and Pardo, L.A. (2004) Mechanism of block of hEag1 K+ channels by imipramine and astemizole. *Journal of General Physiology*, **124**, 301–317.

41 Farid, R., Day, T., Friesner, R.A., and Pearlstein, R.A. (2006) New insights about HERG blockade obtained from protein modeling, potential energy mapping, and docking studies. *Bioorganic and Medicinal Chemistry*, **14**, 3160–3173.

42 Abel, R., Young, T., Farid, R., Berne, B.J., and Friesner, R.A. (2008) Role of the active-site solvent in the thermodynamics of factor Xa ligand binding. *Journal of the American Chemical Society*, **130**, 2817–2831.

43 Young, T., Abel, R., Kim, B., Berne, B.J., and Friesner, R.A. (2007) Motifs for molecular recognition exploiting hydrophobic enclosure in protein–ligand binding. *Proceedings of the National Academy of Sciences of the United States of America*, **104**, 808–813.

44 Pearlstein, R.A., Sherman, W., and Abel, R. (2013) Contributions of water transfer energy to protein–ligand association and dissociation barriers: Watermap analysis of a series of p38α MAP kinase inhibitors. *Proteins*, **81**, 1509–1526.

45 Tran, Q.-T., Williams, S., Farid, R., Erdemli, G., and Pearlstein, R. (2013) The translocation kinetics of antibiotics through porin OmpC: insights from structure-based solvation mapping using WaterMap. *Proteins*, **81**, 291–299.

46 Armstrong, C.M. (1969) Inactivation of the potassium conductance and related phenomena caused by quaternary ammonium ion injected in squid axon. *Journal of General Physiology*, **54**, 553–575.

47 Armstrong, C.M. (1971) Interaction of tetraethylammonium ion derivatives with the potassium channels of giant axons. *Journal of General Physiology*, **58**, 413–437.

48 Ficker, E., Jarolimek, W., and Brown, A.M. (2001) Molecular determinants of inactivation and dofetilide block in Ether-à-go-go (EAG) channels and EAG-related K(+) channels. *Molecular Pharmacology*, **60**, 1343–1348.

49 Shelley, J.C., Cholleti, A., Frye, L., Greenwood, J.R., Timlin, M.R., and Uchimaya, M. (2007) Epik: a software program for pK_a prediction and protonation state generation for drug-like molecules. *Journal of Computer-Aided Molecular Design*, **21**, 681–691.

50 Aronov, A.M. (2006) Common pharmacophores for uncharged human Ether-à-go-go-related gene (hERG) blockers. *Journal of Medicinal Chemistry*, **49**, 6917–6921.

51 Pearlstein, R.A., Vaz, R.J., Kang, J., Chen, X.L., Preobrazhenskaya, M., Shchekotikhin, A.E., Korolev, A.M., Lysenkova, L.N., Miroshnikova, O.V., Hendrix, J., and Rampe, D. (2003) Characterization of HERG potassium channel inhibition using CoMSiA 3D QSAR and homology modeling approaches. *Bioorganic and Medicinal Chemistry Letters*, **13**, 1829–1835.

52 Katayama, Y., Fujita, A., Ohe, T., Findlay, I., and Kurachi, Y. (2000) Inhibitory effect of vesnarinone on cloned cardiac delayed rectifier K^+ channels expressed in a mammalian cell line. *The Journal of Pharmacology and Experimental Therapeutics*, **294**, 339–346.

53 Shamovsky, I., Connolly, S., David, L., Ivanova, S., Nordén, B., Springthorpe, B., and Urbahns, K. (2008) Overcoming undesirable HERG potency of chemokine receptor antagonists using baseline lipophilicity relationships. *Journal of Medicinal Chemistry*, **51**, 1162–1178.

54 Pearlstein, R.A., Hu, Q.-Y., Zhou, J., Yowe, D., Levell, J., Dale, B., Kaushik, V.K., Daniels, D., Hanrahan, S., Sherman, W., and Abel, R. (2010) New hypotheses about the structure–function of proprotein convertase subtilisin/kexin type 9: analysis of the epidermal growth factor-like repeat A docking site using WaterMap. *Proteins*, **78**, 2571–2586.

55 Mirams, G.R., Cui, Y., Sher, A., Fink, M., Cooper, J., Heath, B.M., McMahon, N.C., Gavaghan, D.J., and Noble, D. (2011) Simulation of multiple ion channel block provides improved early prediction of compounds' clinical torsadogenic risk. *Cardiovascular Research*, **91**, 53–61.

56 Kramer, J., Obejero-Paz, C.A., Myatt, G., Kuryshev, Y.A., Bruening-Wright, A., Verducci, J.S., and Brown, A.M. (2013) MICE models: superior to the HERG

model in predicting Torsade de Pointes. *Science Reports*, **3**, 2100.

57 Windisch, A., Timin, E.N., Schwarz, T., Stork-Riedler, D., Erker, T., Ecker, G.F., and Hering, S. (2011) Trapping and dissociation of propafenone derivatives in HERG channels. *British Journal of Pharmacology*, **162**, 1542–1552.

58 Lacivita, E., Leopoldo, M., De Giorgio, P., Berardi, F., and Perrone, R. (2009) Determination of 1-aryl-4-propylpiperazine pK_a values: the substituent on aryl modulates basicity. *Bioorganic and Medicinal Chemistry*, **173**, 1339–1344.

Section 4
Kinase Antitargets

Antitargets and Drug Safety, First Edition. Edited by László Urbán, Vinod F. Patel, and Roy J. Vaz.

15
Introduction to Kinase Antitargets

Mark C. Munson

Kinases represent an important enzyme class in drug discovery. More than 400 human diseases have been connected either directly or indirectly to protein kinases [1]. At least 10 000 relevant patent applications have been filed in the last decade. Through the end of 2013, 26 small molecules (Table 15.1) and 7 large molecules (Table 15.2) have been approved by the US Food and Drug Administration (FDA), with the majority of these agents registered for use in oncology. Based on a recent global sales report of pharmaceutical and biotechnology companies focused on cancer [2], seven of these drugs achieved yearly sales of more than $1 billion and nearly $22 billion collectively in 2012: trastuzumab, $6.2 billion; bevacizumab, $6.2 billion; imatinib, $4.6 billion; erlotinib, $1.4 billion; sunitinib, $1.1 billion; cetuximab, $1.1 billion; sorafenib, and $1.0 billion. The kinase inhibitor sales market is expected to reach $40 billion by 2016 [3].

A survey of www.clinicaltrials.gov reveals further compelling statistics. Using the search term "kinase" returns >3500 hits (completed, ongoing, or recruiting). Refinement yields more than 50 unique small molecules targeting kinases in phase II or III clinical trials (Table 15.3; antibodies and proteins were not included in this analysis). Similar to the trend of approved agents, most of these drugs are under investigation in oncology, although fibrosis, rheumatoid arthritis (RA), pain, glaucoma, acute coronary syndrome (ACS), and transplant also appear in the list of indications. Analysis of the data using a dual search term "kinase" and "x," where x represents the acronym commonly reported for the kinase (e.g., EGFR (epidermal growth factor receptor)) generated Table 15.4. This search criterion was used to minimize false hits (unrelated acronyms) and likely underestimates results. Kinases returning five or more trials were reported along with a brief biological description of the class and number of isoforms. Thirty kinases were identified (Table 15.4, column 2). Not surprisingly, of those representing the highest frequency hits (top 13, more than 40 hits each), eight (EGFR, Abl, vascular endothelial growth factor receptor (VEGFR), mTOR, cKIT, Raf, ALK, and MEK) are targets that have been successfully drugged. Although there is no formal evidence that *selective* platelet-derived growth factor receptor (PDGFR) inhibition is clinically meaningful (no approved antibodies), based on

Antitargets and Drug Safety, First Edition. Edited by László Urbán, Vinod F. Patel, and Roy J. Vaz.

Table 15.1 Approved small-molecule inhibitors of kinases through December 2013: general information.

S. No.	Drug	Trade name	Company	Reported target kinases[a)] [4–7]	Approved indications	Approval date
1	Sirolimus	Rapamune	Wyeth	**mTOR**	Renal transplant	1999
2	Imatinib	Gleevec	Novartis	**BCR-Abl**, **cKit**, **PDGFR,** Abl1, Abl2, cFms, DDR2, Lck	CML, GIST, fibrosarcoma, HES, ALL, MPD, systemic mastocytosis	2001
3	Gefitinib	Iressa	AstraZeneca	**EGFR**, Gak, IRAK	NSCLC	2003
4	Erlotinib	Tarceva	OSI	**EGFR**, Gak, Lok, YSK4, Slk, Abl1	NSCLC, pancreatic cancer	2004
5	Everolimus	Afinitor	Novartis	**mTOR**	Transplant rejection: heart, kidney, and liver (registered); RCC, astrocytoma, neuroendocrine tumors of the pancreas (NT), angiomyolipoma, BC	2004
6	Sorafenib	Nexavar	Bayer	**PDGFR**, **VEGFR**, Raf, DDR1, HIPK4, Zak, DDR2, Flt3, cFms, cKit, Flt1	HCC, RCC, advanced thyroid cancer	2005
7	Dasatinib	Sprycel	Bristol Myers Squibb	**BCR-Abl**, Abl1, EphB6, EphA3, Abl2, Lck, Blk, Src, EphA5, EphA8	CML, lymphocytic leukemia	2006
8	Sunitinib	Sutent	Pfizer	**PDGFR**, **VEGFR2**, **Flt1**, cKit, Flt3, DRAK1, cFms, BIKE, PHKG1	RCC, GIST, NT	2006
9	Lapatinib	Tykerb	GlaxoSmithKline	**EGFR**, **ErbB2**, ErbB4	Metastatic BC	2007
10	Nilotinib	Tasigna	Novartis	**BCR-Abl**, Abl1, Zak, Abl2, cKit, DDR2, p38beta, EphA8, cFms	CML	2007
11	Temsirolimus	Torisel	Wyeth	**mTOR**	RCC	2007
12	Pazopanib	Votrient	GlaxoSmithKline	**Flt1**, **VEGFR2**, **PDGFR**, cKit, cFms, Flt4, TAOK3, DDR1, EphB6	RCC, soft tissue sarcomas	2009
13	Crizotinib	Xalkori	Pfizer	**Alk**, Met, MERTK, Ros1, EphB6, Axl, Ltk, Slk, MST1R, Lck	Alk+ NSCLC	2011
14	Vemurafenib	Zelboraf	Plexxikon	**CRaf, BRaf (V600E)**, Mek5, SRMS, Zak, Brk, Fgr	Metastatic melanoma with *BRAF*^{V600E} mutation	2011

15	Vandetanib	Caprelsa/ Zactima	AstraZeneca	**Ret**, RIPK2, EGFR, DDR1, Abl, Lck, Mek5, EphA6, STK35, VEGFR, Flt3	Medullary thyroid cancer	2011
16	Ruxolitinib	Jakafi	Incyte	**Jak1**, **Jak2**, **Jak3**, Tyk2, MAP3K2, CAM2A, ROCK2, ROCK1	Myelofibrosis	2011
17	Axitinib	Inlyta	Pfizer	**PDGFR**, **Flt1**, **VEGFR2**, AURC, cKit, Plk4, cFms, Abl1	RCC	2012
18	Bosutinib	Bosulif	Pfizer	**BCR-Abl**, Abl1, MAP4K5, Lck, ErbB3, Src, Gak, Frk, Abl2, STK35	CML	2012
19	Cabozantinib	Cometriq	Exelixis	**Met**, Ret, VEGFR, cKit, Trk, Flt3, Axl, DDR1, MERTK, HIPK4, Lok, Ret, Tie2, PDGFR, EphA3	Medullary thyroid cancer	2012
20	Tofacitinib	Xeljanz	Pfizer	**Jak**, Tyk2	Rheumatoid arthritis	2012
21	Regorafenib	Stivarga	Bayer	**VEGFR**, **PDGFR**, **FGFR**, BCR-Abl, BRaf, BRaf(V600E), cKit, Ret, Tie2, Eph2A, p38	Metastatic CRC and CRC, GIST	2012
22	Ibrutinib	Imbruvica	Pharmacyclics	**Btk**, Blk, Bmx, Csk, Fgr, Brk, Hck, EGFR, Yes, ErbB2, Itk, Jak3, Frk, Lck, Ret, Flt3	MCL	2013
23	Dabrafenib	Tafinlar	GlaxoSmithKline	**Braf, CRaf, BRaf (V600E)**	Metastatic melanoma	2013
24	Afatinib	Gilotrif	Boehringer Ingelheim	**EGFR, ErbB2**	Metastatic NSCLC	2013
25	Ponatinib	Iclusig	Ariad	**BCR-Abl**, **BCR-Abl (T315I)**, VEGFR, PDGFR, FGFR, Eph, Src, cKIT, Ret, Tie2, Flt3	CML, Philadelphia positive ALL	2013
26	Trametinib	Mekinist	GlaxoSmithKline	**MEK1**, **MEK2**	Metastatic melanoma	2013

ALL, acute lymphocytic leukemia; BC, breast cancer; CML, chronic myelogenous leukemia; CRC, colorectal cancer; GIST, gastrointestinal stromal tumors; HCC, hepatocellular carcinoma; HES, hypereosinophilic syndrome; MCL, mantle cell lymphoma; MPD, myeloproliferative disorders; NSCLC, non-small cell lung cancer; NT, neuroendocrine tumors.

a) Data based on reported enzyme activity <100 nM. Kinase(s) highlighted in bold are considered primary targets for respective disease indications. Relevance (efficacy and/or toxicology) in the clinic should be based on cellular potency (K_m for ATP of kinases vary significantly), plasma exposure *in vivo* (C_{max} versus AUC), and plasma protein binding, which is beyond the scope of this table.

Table 15.2 Approved large-molecule inhibitors of the kinase pathway [4].

S. No.	Drug	Trade name	Company	Target kinase pathway	Approved indication	Approval date
1	Trastuzumab	Herceptin	Genentech	ErbB2 monoclonal antibody	BC, metastatic BC, stomach and metastatic stomach cancer	1998
2	Cetuximab	Erbitux	ImClone Bristol Myers Squibb Merck	EGFR monoclonal antibody	CRC, squamous cell carcinoma of the head and the neck	2003
3	Bevacizumab	Avastin	Genentech	VEGFA monoclonal antibody	CRC, NSCLC, metastatic BC, RCC, GM, ovarian and fallopian tube cancer	2004
4	Pegaptanib	Macugen	Gilead	Pegylated anti-VEGF aptamer	Age-related macular degeneration	2004
5	Ranibizumab	Lucentis	Genentech	VEGFA monoclonal antibody	Age-related macular degeneration, diabetic macular edema, macular edema, chloroidal neovascularization	2006
6	Panitumumab	Vectibix	Amgen	EGFR monoclonal antibody	Metastatic CRC and CRC	2006
7	Pertuzumab	Perjeta	Genentech	ErbB2 monoclonal antibody	Metastatic BC and BC	2012

BC, breast cancer; CRC, colorectal cancer; GM, glioblastoma; NSCLC, non-small cell lung cancer; RCC, renal cell carcinoma.

its key role in pericyte function, its inhibition likely contributes to the efficacy of several drugs targeting VEGFR and angiogenesis [8].

Kinases control cellular communication via distinct signaling networks [10]. This is tightly regulated through transfer of phosphate from high-energy adenosine triphosphate (ATP) onto the hydroxyls of serine, threonine, or tyrosine residues in specific protein substrates. This leads to amplification of signals and control of downstream functions or activation of transcription factors, resulting in a cellular phenotypic response (proliferation, angiogenesis, migration, and differentiation). The kinome, a term coined by Manning *et al.* in 2002, encompasses this broad but related family of approximately 500 enzymes [11]. It phylogenetically organizes them based on evolutionary development, homology, and biological relationships and is described in detail in a number of review articles [12–15].

Table 15.3 Late-stage small-molecule inhibitors of kinases (phase II and III) [4].

S. No.	Names	Company	Primary target kinases	Clinical setting	Status
1	Nintedanib BIB1120 Vargatef	Boehringer Ingelheim	VEGFR, FGFR, PDGFR	NSCLC, ovarian, IPF	Preregistered
2	K115	D. Western Therapeutics Institute	Rho	Glaucoma	Preregistered
3	Masitinib AB1010	AB Science	FGFR3, Lyn, cKit, PDGFR	CRC	Phase III
4	Dinaciclib SCH727965	Merck	CDK1/2/5/9	Refractory CLL	Phase III
5	Idelalasib GS1101 CAL101	Gilead	PI3K delta	CLL	Phase III
6	Selumetinib AZD6244	AstraZeneca/ Array	MEK	NSCLC	Phase III
7	Dovitinib TKI258	Novartis	FGFR, PDGFR, VEGFR	RCC (did not meet endpoint) scirrhous gastric carcinoma	Phase III
8	Vatalanib PTK787/ZK 222584	Novartis	VEGFR	Metastatic colorectal cancer (did not meet primary endpoint) metastatic NT, sarcoma	Phase III
9	Linifanib ABT869	Abbott	VEGFR, PDGFR	HCC, NSCLC, CRC	Phase III
10	Apatinib YN968D1	Jiangsu Hengrui Medicine	VEGFR2, Ret	Gastric cancer, NSCLC	Phase III
11	Motesanib AMG706	Amgen/ Takeda	VEGFR, PDGFR, cKit	NSCLC	Phase III
12	Icotinib BPI2009H	Beta Pharma	EGFR	NSCLC, gastroesophageal	Phase III
13	Alisertib MLN8237	Millennium/ Takeda	AUR1	T-cell lymphoma	Phase III
14	Saracatinib AZD0530	AstraZeneca	Src, Abl, Yes	Ovarian, metastatic CRC	Phase III
15	Pacritinib ONX0803 SB1518	S*BIO	Jak2, CDK2, Flt3	Myelofibrosis	Phase III
16	Midostaurin	Novartis	cKit, Flt3, PKC	AML	Phase III
17	Neratinib HKI272 PB272 PF0528767	Pfizer Puma Biotechnology	EGFR, ErbB2, ErbB4	NSCLC, metastatic BC	Phase III
18	Dacomitinib	Pfizer	EGFR, ErbB2, ErbB4	GB, NSCLC	Phase III

(continued)

Table 15.3 (*Continued*)

S. No.	Names	Company	Primary target kinases	Clinical setting	Status
19	Brivanib Brivanib alaninate (prodrug) BMS58264	Bristol Myers Squibb	VEGFR, FGFR	Metastatic CRC, HCC	Phase III
20	Tivantinib ARQ197	ArQule	Met	HCC, metastatic BC	Phase III
21	Buparlisib BKM120 NVP-BKM120	Novartis	PI3K alpha	Metastatic BC, bladder cancer, esophageal	Phase III
22	ARRY162 MEK162	Array Novartis	MEK	Ovarian, melanoma	Phase III
23	XL647 EXEI7647	Exelixis Kadmon	VEGFR, Src family, EGFR, ErbB2, EphB4	NSCLC	Phase III
24	Lenvatinib E7080	Esai	VEGFR, PDGFR, cKit, FGFR	HCC, thyroid cancer	Phase III
25	Volasertib BI6727	Boehringer Ingelheim	PLK1	AML	Phase III
26	Baricitinib	Incyte Eli Lilly	JAK1/2	Rheumatoid arthritis	Phase III
27	Palbociclib PD-332991	Pfizer	CDK4/5	BC	Phase III
28	P-276-00	Piramal	CDK1/4/9	Mucositis, various cancers	Phase III
29	Seliciclib CYC-202	Cyclacel	CDK2/7/9	Nasopharyngeal, NSCLC	Phase III
30	Tandutinib MLN518	Millennium	Flt3	AML	Phase II
31	Alvocidib HL-275	Tolero	Pan CDK	CLL	Phase II
32	Semaxinib SU5416	Sugen	VEGFR	Melanoma, hematological cancers	Phase II
33	Milciclib PHA-848125	Nerviano	CDK1/2/4, TRKA	Thymoma	Phase II
34	LEE-011	Astex	CDK4/6	BC, melanoma	Phase II
35	LY-2835219	Lilly	CDK4/5	NHL	Phase II
36	BAY-1000394	Bayer	Pan-CDK	NSCLC	Phase II
37	MK2206	Merck	Akt	BC, melanoma	Phase II
38	Quizartinib AC220	Ambit	RET, cKit, cFms, Flt3	AML	Phase II
39	AT9283	Astex	AUR, Jak, Flt3, BCR-Abl	MM	Phase II

40	Tivozanib ASP4130 KRN951	AVEO/ Kyoma Hakko/ Kirin	VEGFR	BC, metastatic CRC	Phase II
41	Galunisertib LY2157299	Eli Lilly	Alk	HCC	Phase II
42	MGCD265	MethylGene	VEGFR, MST1R, Ron, Tie2, Met	NSCLC	Phase II
43	CT327	Creabilis	Trk	Dermatitis, pruritus (topical)	Phase II
44	Pelitinib	Pfizer	EGFR	NSCLC	Phase II
45	Canertinib PD183805	Pfizer	EGFR, ErbB2, ErbB4	Metastatic BC	Phase II
46	GLPG0634	Galapagos/ AbbVie	Jak	Rheumatoid arthritis, Crohn's	Phase II
48	Losmapimod GW856553	GlaxoSmithKline	P38	Acute coronary syndrome	Phase II
49	Fostamatinib R788	Rigel	Syk, Flt3	Thrombocytopenia	Phase II
50	Sonolisib PX866	Oncothyreon	Akt, PI3K	Castrate resistant PC, GB	Phase II
51	Danusertib PHA-739358	Pfizer/ Nerviano	Trk, AUR, Ret, Abl, FGFR	NSCLC	Phase II
52	ARRY797	Array	P38	Pain	Phase II
53	Pictilisib	Genentech	PI3K	Metastatic BC	Phase II
54	Momelotinib	Gilead	Jak1/2	Myelofibrosis	Phase II
55	Ceritinib LDK378	Novartis	Alk	NSCLC	Phase II
56	AR12286	Aerie	Rock	Glaucoma	Phase II
57	Poziotinib	Hanmi Pharmaceutical	EGFR/ErbB2/ ErbB4	Adenocarcinoma of lung	Phase II

AML, acute myeloid leukemia; BC, breast cancer; CLL, chronic lymphocytic leukemia; CRC, colorectal cancer; IPF, idiopathic pulmonary fibrosis; GB, glioblastoma multiforme; HCC, hepatocellular carcinoma; MM, multiple myeloma; NHL, non-Hodgkin's lymphoma NSCLC, non-small cell lung cancer; NT, neuroendocrine tumors; PC, prostate cancer; RCC, renal cell carcinoma.

Data taken from numerous preclinical studies of kinases (genetic mouse models, siRNA/shRNA-mediated inhibition, and protein or small-molecule inhibition) as well as years of clinical trials begin to build a picture around which signaling pathways are important for normal versus pathological functions. Inhibition of certain kinase pathways leads to signature preclinical and clinical toxicity that is now well documented [16]. More will be discussed in the following chapters.

Chapters 15–18 update the kinase state of the art, with a focus on selectivity and toxicity (preclinical and clinical). What ultimately matters to physicians and patients is clear: how well does the drug work (efficacy) in comparison with the side effect profile (safety). The authors of these chapters shed light on this balance based on significant experience in the field as well as extensive analysis of literature. We hope to leave the reader with a deeper appreciation for the

Table 15.4 Commonly targeted kinases in disease.

S. No.	Kinase	Isoforms [9]	Kinase name	ClinicalTrials.gov hits	Functions
1	EGFR	4	Epidermal growth factor receptor	616	Initiates several signal transduction cascades, principally the MAPK, Akt, and JNK pathways, leading to DNA synthesis and cell proliferation
2	Abl	2	Abelson murine leukemia viral oncogene homolog 1	280	Proto-oncogene encodes a cytoplasmic and nuclear protein tyrosine kinase implicated in cell differentiation, division, adhesion, and stress response
3	Aur	3	Aurora	194	Controls chromatid segregation
4	VEGFR	3	Vascular endothelial growth factor	155	Vasculogenesis (formation of the circulatory system) and angiogenesis (growth of blood vessels from preexisting vasculature)
5	PI3	4	Phosphatidylinositide 3-kinases	110	Involved in cellular functions such as cell growth, proliferation, differentiation, motility, survival, and intracellular trafficking
6	Akt	3	Protein kinase B	87	Glucose metabolism, apoptosis, cell proliferation, transcription, and cell migration
7	mTOR	1	Mammalian target of rapamycin	87	Cell growth, proliferation, motility, survival, protein synthesis, and transcription
8	PDGFR	2	Platelet-derived growth factor	81	Blood vessel formation (angiogenesis) and growth of blood vessels from already-existing blood vessel tissue
9	cKit	1	Mast/stem cell growth factor	78	Melanocyte physiology, influencing melanogenesis, proliferation, migration, and survival of the pigment-producing cells
10	Flt	4	FMS-like tyrosine kinase	57	Expressed by immature hematopoietic cells. Important for normal development of stem cells and the immune system
11	Raf	3	v-Raf murine sarcoma viral oncogene homolog B1	55	Participates in the RAS-RAF-MEK-ERK signal transduction cascade
12	MEK	2	Mitogen-activated protein kinase kinase	50	Involved in many cellular processes such as proliferation, differentiation, transcription regulation, and development
13	Alk	7	Anaplastic lymphoma kinase	46	Development of the brain. Exerts its effects on specific neurons in the nervous system

14	Src	2	Proto-oncogene tyrosine–protein kinase Src	44	Src family kinases (Src, Yes, Fyn, Fgr, Lck, Hck, Blk, Lyn) interact with many cellular cytosolic, nuclear and membrane proteins
15	CDK	20	Cyclin-dependent kinases	40	Cell cycle regulation. Involved in regulating transcription, mRNA processing, and the differentiation of nerve cells
16	p38	4	P38 mitogen-activated protein kinase	34	Mitogen-activated protein kinase responsive to stress stimuli, such as cytokines, ultraviolet irradiation, heat and osmotic shock. Involved in cell differentiation, apoptosis and autophagy
17	Met	1	MET tyrosine kinase	32	Essential for embryonic development and wound healing. A proto-oncogene that encodes hepatocyte growth factor receptor
18	PKC	9	Protein kinase C	32	A family of serine- and threonine-specific protein kinases that can be activated by calcium and the second messenger diacylglycerol
19	Jak	4	Janus kinase	32	Nonreceptor tyrosine kinases that transduce cytokine-mediated signals via the JAK-STAT pathway
20	Btk	1	Bruton's kinase	31	Role in B-cell maturation as well as mast cell activation through the high-affinity IgE receptor
21	Ret	1	Rearranged for transfection	23	Proto-oncogene encodes a receptor tyrosine kinase for members of the glial cell line-derived neurotrophic factor family of extracellular signaling molecules
22	FGFR	4	Fibroblast growth factor receptor	19	Family of receptors that bind to fibroblast growth factors
23	cFms	1	Colony-stimulating factor 1 receptor	19	Osteoclast and macrophage function
24	Fak	2	Focal adhesion kinase	14	Recruited at early stages to focal adhesions and mediates several downstream responses
25	IGFR	1	Insulin growth factor receptor	10	Role in growth and continues to have anabolic effects in adults. Activated by insulin-like growth factor
26	Tie	2	TEK tyrosine kinase endothelial	9	TEK signaling pathway important for endothelial cell-smooth muscle cell communication in venous morphogenesis

(*continued*)

Table 15.4 (*Continued*)

S. No.	Kinase	Isoforms [9]	Kinase name	ClinicalTrials.gov hits	Functions
27	Plk	4	Polo-like kinase	7	Formation of and changes in the mitotic spindle and in the activation of CDK/cyclin complexes during M-phase of the cell cycle
28	Chk	2	CSK-homologous kinase	5	A protein kinase that is activated in response to DNA damage and is involved in cell cycle arrest
29	Erk	6	Extracellular signal-related kinase	5	Regulation of meiosis, mitosis, and postmitotic functions is differentiated
30	Syk	1	Spleen tyrosine kinase	5	Primarily expressed in hematopoietic cells. Transmits signals from B cell receptors

complexity of the area and for those practicing drug discovery provide insights into identifying safer and more effective kinase drugs. While industry and academia have greatly advanced this field in the last decade, there is still much to learn about effectively drugging these targets. Since the majority of approved drugs and late-stage kinase agents are in oncology, there is an emphasis on this therapeutic setting. Although cost is also a key consideration, given the wide scope and rapidly changing economic landscape, this will not be discussed.

By definition, the term antitarget refers to a biological target (e.g., enzyme, receptor, and ion channel) that, when engaged by a drug, elicits an undesirable side effect. It is important to distinguish this from nonspecific effects. Toxicity due to membrane disruption or aggregation, redox or energy perturbation, and formation of reactive metabolites (e.g., glutathione depletion or nonspecific modification of proteins) are often a function of drug properties and not driven by mechanistically well-understood pharmacology [17]. These can be difficult to distinguish and identify structure–activity relationships (SAR).

Sometimes a disease target can also be the antitarget (on-mechanism-based toxicity). An example is the clinical observation of inhibition of the MEK/ERK pathway [18]. This highly selective class of kinase drugs (Table 15.1; epidermal growth factor receptor inhibitors, erlotinib and gefitinib; BRaf inhibitor, vemurafenib; and MEK inhibitor, trametinib) as well as EGFR antibodies (Table 15.2; cetuximab and panitumumab) can cause an acneiform rash displaying characteristic erythema (redness) and papules (Table 15.5). The mechanism is not fully understood, but inhibition of this pathway affects expression of genes that stimulate inflammation, apoptosis, and cell attachment [19]. The EGFR pathway plays an important role in rapidly dividing normal cells such as keratinocytes and the intestinal epithelium (primary sites of toxicity). Pharmacodynamics (PD) and efficacy (EGFR, Raf, and MEK inhibition) appear linked to dose-limiting toxicity (rash) [20]. The therapeutic index (TI) in cancer patients is managed by

Table 15.5 Approved small-molecule inhibitors of kinases: side effects.

S. No.	Drug	Trade name	Label warnings[a)]	Reference
1	Sirolimus	Rapamune	Increased risk of developing infections or certain cancers, especially lymphoma and skin cancers. Swelling in hands, feet, and various tissues. Impaired wound healing. Increased levels of cholesterol and triglycerides in blood. Increased protein in urine. Increased risk for viral infections. Potentially life-threatening lung or breathing problems. Common side effects: high blood pressure, pain (stomach and joint), diarrhea, headache, fever, urinary tract infection, anemia, nausea, and low platelet count	www.rapamune.com
2	Imatinib	Gleevec	Edema and serious fluid retention, cytopenias, severe congestive heart failure and left ventricular dysfunction. Hepatotoxicity, bleeding, severe gastrointestinal bleeding and perforation; in some cases fatal. Heart disease, skin reactions, such as fluid-filled blisters, hypothyroidism. Long-term use may result in potential liver, kidney, and/or heart toxicities, immune system suppression. Possible harm to an unborn child when administered to a pregnant woman. Growth retardation. Cases of tumor lysis syndrome (TLS), have been reported and can be life-threatening. Dizziness, blurred vision, or drowsiness	www.gleevec.com
3	Gefitinib	Iressa	Very common side effects: diarrhea, vomiting, nausea, skin reactions such as an acne-like rash, loss of appetite, weakness, dry, red, or sore mouth, increased liver enzymes. Common side effects: dry, red, or itchy eyes, red and sore eyelids, nail problems, hair loss, fever, bleeding, protein in urine, increase of bilirubin and aspartate aminotransferase, increase of creatinine levels, cystitis. Uncommon side effects: inflammation of the pancreas or liver. Rare side effects: inflammation of the blood vessels in the skin, hemorrhagic cystitis, gastrointestinal perforation	www.iressa.com
4	Erlotinib	Tarceva	Interstitial lung disease. Liver and kidney problems. Gastrointestinal (GI) perforation, which has led to death. Serious skin conditions. Blistering and skin peeling that may result in other serious skin disorders or death. Blood, bleeding, and clotting problems. These have led to heart attack, stroke, and death. Eye irritation and damage to the cornea. Unusual eyelash growth or swelling of the cornea. Tarceva can cause harm to an unborn baby	www.tarceva.com

(*continued*)

Table 15.5 (*Continued*)

S. No.	Drug	Trade name	Label warnings[a)]	Reference
5	Everolimus	Afinitor	Lung infections or breathing problems, kidney failure. Common side effects: feeling weak or tired, cough, shortness of breath, diarrhea and constipation, skin problems (e.g., rash, acne, dry skin, or itching), nausea and vomiting, fever, loss of appetite, weight loss, swelling of arms, hands, feet, ankles, face, or other parts of the body, abnormal taste or dry mouth, inflammation of the lining of the digestive system, headache, nose bleeding, absence of menstrual periods, pain in arms and legs, mouth and throat, back or joints, or abdomen, low red blood cells, white blood cells or platelets, increased blood cholesterol level, decreased blood phosphate level, increased blood sugar levels, high blood pressure, difficulty sleeping, hair loss, muscle spasms, dizziness, nail disorders, anxiety, aggression, and other abnormal behaviors	www.afinitor.com
6	Sorafenib	Nexavar	Hypertension, increased risk of bleeding, cardiac ischemia and/or myocardial infarction. Gastrointestinal perforation was an uncommon adverse reaction. Most common adverse reactions: diarrhea, fatigue, abdominal pain, weight loss, anorexia, nausea, hand–foot skin reaction, rash/desquamation, alopecia. Elevations in serum lipase and reductions in serum phosphate of unknown etiology	www.nexavar.com
7	Dasatinib	Sprycel	Anemia, neutropenia, thrombocytopenia, severe bleeding that can lead to death, fluid retention in the lining of the lungs, the sac around the heart or the stomach cavity. Abnormal heart rate, heart problems, or a heart attack that can lead to death and pulmonary arterial hypertension (PAH). Other common side effects: diarrhea, headache, cough, skin rash, fever, nausea, tiredness, vomiting, muscle pain, weakness, and infections	www.sprycel.com
8	Sunitinib	Sutent	Heart problems, abnormal heart rhythm changes, high blood pressure, bleeding sometimes leading to death, osteonecrosis, tumor lysis syndrome, hormone problems, including thyroid and adrenal gland problems. Common side effects: yellow skin, tiredness, weakness, fever, gastrointestinal symptoms, including diarrhea, nausea, vomiting, mouth sores, upset stomach, abdominal pain, and constipation, rash or other skin changes, including drier, thicker, or cracking skin, blisters or a rash on the palms of your hands and soles of your feet, taste changes, loss of appetite, pain or swelling in arms or legs, cough, shortness of breath, bleeding	www.sutent.com

9	Lapatinib	Tykerb	Decreased left ventricular ejection fraction, hepatotoxicity, diarrhea, interstitial lung disease and pneumonitis, QT prolongation, adverse reproductive effects, palmar-plantar erythrodysesthesia and rash, and fatigue. Common side effects when dosed with letrozole or capecitabine include: diarrhea, red, painful hands and feet, nausea, rash, vomiting, tiredness or weakness, mouth sores, loss of appetite, indigestion, unusual hair loss or thinning, nose bleeds, headache, dry skin, itching, nail disorders such as nail bed changes, nail pain, infection and swelling of the cuticles	www.tykerb.com
10	Nilotinib	Tasigna	Myelosuppression (grade 3/4 thrombocytopenia, neutropenia, and anemia), QT prolongation and sudden death. Elevated serum lipases, hepatotoxicity.	www.nilotinib.com
11	Temsirolimus	Torisel	Skin rash, weakness or fatigue, mouth sores, nausea, swelling and fluid retention. Serious (including a life-threatening or fatal) allergic reaction. Increased blood sugar levels, cholesterol and/or triglycerides, potential increased risk of infections, chronic inflammation of the lungs, which in rare cases may be fatal, and perforation of the bowels, improper wound healing, and increased risks of bleeding, and in the elderly, increased risks of edema and pneumonia	www.torisel.com
12	Pazopanib	Votrient	Irregular or fast heartbeat, fainting, heart failure, blood clots, thrombotic microangiopathy, including thrombotic thrombocytopenia purpura, bleeding problems, perforations of the bowel or stomach, reversible posterior leukoencephalopathy, high blood pressure, wound healing issues, protein in the urine, serious infections leading to sudden death, birth defects, collapsed lung (pneumothorax). Common side effects: diarrhea, high blood pressure, change in hair color, nausea or vomiting, loss of appetite, feeling tired, decreased weight, tumor, muscle, or bone pain, headache, taste changes, trouble breathing, and change in skin color	www.votrient.com
13	Crizotinib	Xalkori	Life threatening or fatal liver injury, yellowing of skin or whites of eyes, fatigue, nausea or vomiting, decreased appetite, right-side stomach pain, increased ease of bleeding or bruising, pneumonitis, QT prolongation. Common side effects: vision problems, nausea and diarrhea and vomiting, swelling of hands and feet, and constipation	www.xalkori.com

(*continued*)

Table 15.5 (*Continued*)

S. No.	Drug	Trade name	Label warnings[a)]	Reference
14	Vemurafenib	Zelboraf	Allergic reactions, rash or redness all over body, feeling faint, trouble breathing or swallowing, throat tightness or hoarseness, fast heartbeat, swelling of face, lips, or tongue, severe skin reactions, QT prolongation, abnormal liver function tests and eye problems. Most common side effects: joint pain, rash, hair loss, tiredness, sunburn or sun sensitivity, nausea, itching, and warts	www.zelboraf.com
15	Vandetanib	Caprelsa	Serious skin reactions, breathing problems (interstitial lung disease), stroke, bleeding, heart failure, diarrhea, thyroid hormone changes, hypertension, reversible posterior leukoencephalopathy syndrome (RPLS). Most common side effects: diarrhea, acne, nausea, high blood pressure, headache, feeling tired, upper respiratory tract infections, loss of appetite and stomach pain	www.caprelsa.com
16	Ruxolitinib	Jakafi	Thrombocytopenia, anemia, neutropenia. Serious bacterial, myobacterial, fungal, and viral infections. Progressive multifocal leukoencephalopathy. Use during pregnancy is not recommended and should only be used if the potential benefit justifies the potential risk to the fetus	www.jakafi.com
17	Axitinib	Inlyta	High blood pressure (hypertension), thyroid gland issues, blood clots in veins or arteries, bleeding (sometimes leading to death), tear in the stomach or intestinal wall (perforation), reversible posterior leukoencephalopathy syndrome, increased protein in the urine, changes in liver function. Most common side effects: diarrhea, high blood pressure, fatigue, decreased appetite, nausea, hoarseness, decreased weight, vomiting, constipation, rash, redness, or itching	www.inlyta.com
18	Bosutinib	Bosulif	Stomach pain, diarrhea, vomiting, low blood cell counts, including thrombocytopenia, anemia, and neutropenia, liver problems, fluid retention. Most common side effects: diarrhea, nausea, low blood counts, vomiting, stomach pain, rash, fever, and fatigue	www.bosulif.com
19	Cabozantinib	Cometriq	Hemorrhage, intestinal/stomach tears or fistulas, issues to an unborn baby, blood clots, stroke, heart attacks, chest pain, wound healing problems, hypertension, osteonecrosis, hand and foot skin reactions, reversible posterior leukoencephalopathy syndrome, protein in the urine and kidney problems. Most common side effects: redness, swelling, or pain in mouth or throat, mouth sore, diarrhea,	www.cometriq.com

			weight loss, decreased appetite, nausea and vomiting, tiredness and weakness, change in taste, hair color turning lighter, constipation, voice changes or hoarseness, change in liver function blood tests, low levels of calcium in your blood	
20	Tofacitinib	Xeljanz	Activation of hepatitis B or C infections in people who carry the virus in their blood. May increase the risks of certain cancers, perforations in the stomach or intestine, changes in laboratory tests (lymphocyte, neutrophil, and red blood cell count). Common side effects: upper respiratory tract infections, headache, diarrhea, nasal congestion	www.xeljanz.com
21	Regorafenib	Stivarga	Hepatotoxicity (sometimes severe or fatal), hemorrhage (respiratory, gastrointestinal, or genitourinary tracts), dermatological toxicity, palmar-plantar erythrodysesthesia (PPE) and severe rash, hypertension, cardiac ischemia and infarction, reversible posterior leukoencephalopathy syndrome, gastrointestinal perforation or fistulas, wound healing complications, embryo-fetal toxicity. The most frequently observed adverse drug reactions: asthenia/fatigue, decreased appetite and food intake, hand–foot skin reaction, PPE, diarrhea, mucositis, weight loss, infection, hypertension, and dysphonia	www.stivarga.com
22	Ibrutinib	Imbruvica	Bleeding problems, infections, decreased blood cell counts, kidney failure and death, second cancers. Most common side effects: low blood platelet count, diarrhea, low white blood cell count, low red blood cell count, fatigue, muscle and bone pain, swelling of legs and feet, upper respiratory tract infection, nausea, bruising, shortness of breath, constipation, rash, abdomen pain, vomiting, and decreased appetite	www.imbruvica.com
23	Dabrafenib	Tafinlar	Risks of new cancers (cutaneous squamous cell carcinoma). May cause fetal harm during pregnancy. Fever, blood sugar problems, eye pain, swelling or redness. Most common side effects: thickening of the outer layer of skin, headache, joint aches, warts, hair loss, redness, swelling, peeling or tenderness of hands and feet	www.tafinlar.com
24	Afatinib	Gilotrif	Diarrhea, bullous and exfoliative skin disorders, interstitial lung disease, hepatic toxicity, keratitis, embryo-fetal toxicity, ventricular dysfunction. Common adverse reactions: diarrhea, rash/dermatitis acneiform, stomatitis, paronychia, dry skin, decreased appetite, pruritus	www.gilotrif.com
25	Ponatinib	Iclusig	Vascular occlusion, heart failure (including fatalities) and hepatotoxicity (including liver failure and death), hypertension, pancreatitis, neuropathy,	www.iclusig.com

(continued)

Table 15.5 (Continued)

S. No.	Drug	Trade name	Label warnings[a)]	Reference
			ocular toxicity, hemorrhage, fluid retention, cardiac arrhythmias, myelosuppression, tumor lysis syndrome, compromised wound healing and gastrointestinal perforation, embryo-fetal toxicity. Most common non-hematologic adverse reactions: (≥20%) were hypertension, rash, abdominal pain, fatigue, headache, dry skin, constipation, arthralgia, nausea, and pyrexia. Hematologic adverse reactions included thrombocytopenia, anemia, neutropenia, lymphopenia, and leukopenia.	
26	Trametinib	Mekinist	Cardiomyopathy (defined as cardiac failure, left ventricular dysfunction, or decreased left ventricular ejection fraction (LVEF)), retinal pigment epithelial detachment, retinal vein occlusion, interstitial disease, serious skin toxicity, embryo-fetal toxicity. Most common side effects: diarrhea, swelling of face, arms and legs	www.mekinist.com

a) Data extracted from labels provided by respective company website. Although representative of primary adverse effects and side reactions, this is not an exhaustive list of warnings.

adjustments in dosing schedule and palliative treatment of the side-effect rash with steroids. Tissue distribution of the drug is also believed to affect the degree and severity of rash. Physicochemical properties (PSA, clog$P$, pK_a, and protein binding) adjusted during the drug design phase have been used to modulate ADME characteristics and tissue distribution [21]. Advanced molecules against these targets are making their way through late-stage clinical trials (Table 15.3). Whether increased TI can be achieved through subtle structural changes remains to be determined. In this pathway, there may well be inherent limitations to what can be improved in medicinal chemistry to impact this tight balance. The target class will be discussed in depth in a subsequent chapter.

More commonly, kinase drugs and/or the leads they derive from inhibit multiple targets affecting many downstream signaling pathways, unlike monoclonal antibodies. Modulation of this profile provides an opportunity to impact the selectivity and increase the probability of success (safety) before a drug candidate moves into the clinic. Reviewing Table 15.1, column five, a majority of approved agents fall into this less selective category. In particular, those agents that target the BCR-Abl pathway (e.g., imatinib, dasatinib, nilotinib, bosutinib, and ponatinib for the treatment of chronic myelogenous leukemia (CML)) or agents (e.g., sorafenib, sunitinib, pazopanib, and axitinib) targeting angiogenesis for the treatment of highly vascularized tumors such as renal cell carcinoma (RCC) and hepatocellular carcinoma (HCC) are relatively promiscuous. Accordingly, a variety of toxicities associated with these classes of molecules are observed (Table 15.5), some likely on target, others not. In the case of BCR-Abl inhibitors, literature implicates direct Abl inhibition and on-mechanism cardiotoxicity [22,23] and this risk has been reported for the entire class, irrespective of kinase antitarget profile or chemotype.

Inhibition of kinases involved in angiogenesis can negatively impact normal functions of the heart, wound healing, and vascularization [24,25]. There is strong evidence that targeting this pathway with a small molecule or selective antibody (e.g., VEGFR and PDGFR) plays a role in some of the observed clinical toxicities associated with several kinase inhibitors [26,27]. Drugs that target these pathways have warning labels reflecting potential adverse events (Table 15.5; sorafenib, sunitinib, pazopanib, vandetanib, axitinib, and cabozantinib). However, direct correlation of toxicology to any single kinase based on promiscuous small-molecule inhibitors can be misleading. In addition, the antibodies (bevacizumab and ranibizumab) target the ligand (VEGFR-A), not the receptor (VEGFR), making direct comparisons challenging (VEGF-A binds multiple receptors). Antibodies can induce antibody-dependent cell-mediated cytotoxicity (ADCC) and complement-dependent cytotoxicity (CDC) that often lead to unique cellular and/or tissue-specific toxicity based on differing expression profiles [28]. The major vasculature side effects are similar for both modalities of drugs supporting this on-mechanism relationship [29,30].

The selectivity question is more complex when directly comparing enzymatic kinase inhibition profiles, although this represents a major source of reported comparative data (Ambit, ProQinase data). Understanding the relevance of biochemical activity requires additional knowledge that is sometimes unavailable or difficult to obtain. For example, the differing K_m values for ATP of each kinase means that cellular potency can shift dramatically for one kinase but not another (similar biochemical activity, but multiple log order change in cellular potency) [31]. This is further complicated by the fact that often mechanistic readouts are performed in engineered cell lines, and apples to apples comparison is not always technically feasible (different cell types, sensitivity, and growth media requirements). Functional assays, particularly in oncology, employ proliferation or apoptosis readouts, as this is the desirable endpoint of cancer treatment. Results of these assays can be highly misleading. Interference of numerous cellular processes can impact cell integrity and survival and lead to nonspecific cell death. Without proper control cell lines and diligent scrutiny, interpretations can be dubious.

Additional key factors also influence the relevance of off-target activities. These include protein binding (while absolute shifts are equal, relative contribution to activity can be impacted), plasma levels required for efficacy *in vivo* (C_{max} versus trough, AUC, and time above threshold), and binding kinetics (slow off-rate, allosteric inhibition or irreversible binding, and tissue distribution and retention). See Table 15.6 for details and examples across the drug class. Compounds that demonstrate slow off-rates or bind an enzyme in an inactive form yield different potencies or effects (distal scaffolding or docking proteins). In turn, this can lead to alternative conclusions merely based on the conditions of

Table 15.6 Approved small-molecule inhibitors of kinases: properties.

S. No.	Drug	Structure	MW	PSA	clog*P*	Binding mode[a)] [32,33]	Reversible binding	Aqueous solubility[b)]	Dose (mg/day) [34][c)]	Human plasma binding[d)]	Human[e)] plasma ~C_{max} (dose)
1	Sirolimus	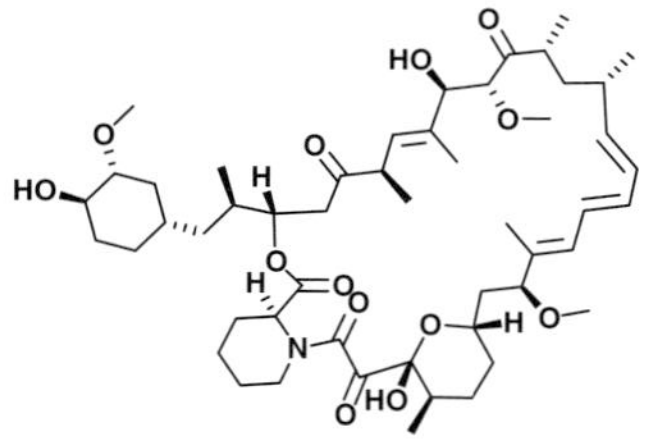	914	195	7.0	Allosteric	Yes	14	5–15 q.d.	92	10 ng/ml (4 mg) [35]
2	Imatinib	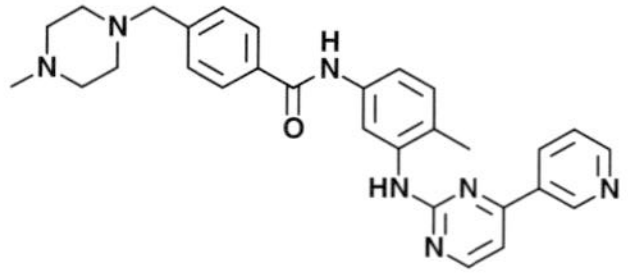	493	84	4.3	Type IIA	Yes	>500	400–800 q.d./b.i.d.	93	2600 ng/ml (400 mg) [36]
3	Gefitinib	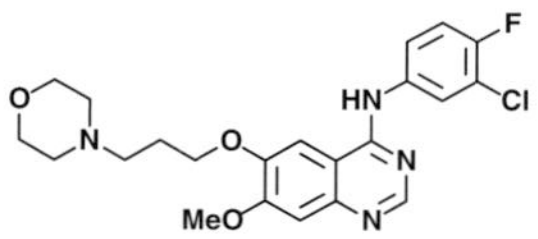	446	67	3.8	Type I	Yes	<0.3	250 q.d.	90	140 ng/ml (250 mg) [37]
4	Erlotinib	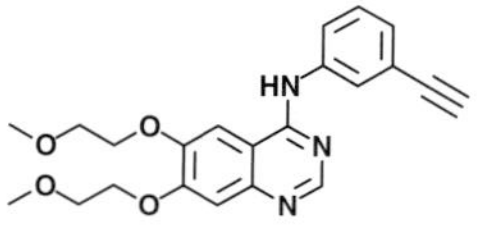	393	73	4.1	Type I	Yes	2	150 q.d.	94	1900 ng/ml (150 mg) [38]

5	Everolimus	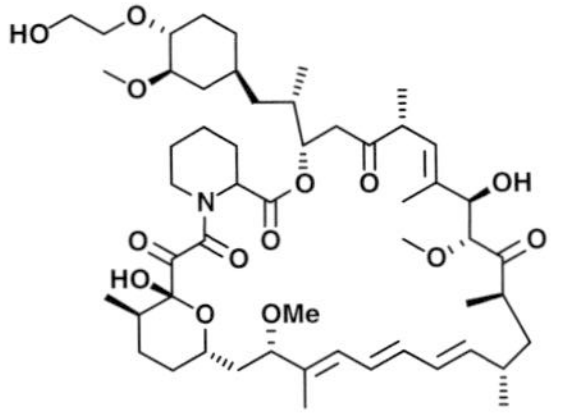	958	204	7.1	Allosteric	Yes	18	10 q.d.	74	90 ng/ml (10 mg) [39]
6	Sorafenib	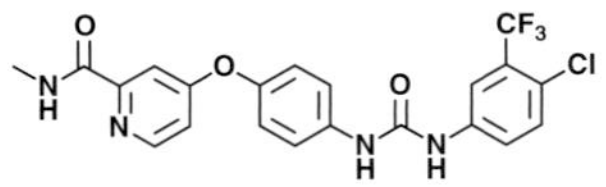	464	91	5.4	Type IIA	Yes	<0.3	200 b.i.d	>99	3600 ng/ml (200 mg) [40]
7	Dasatinib	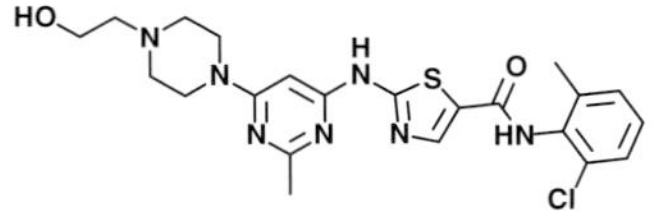	488	104	2.3	Type I	Yes	69	100 q.d.	94	100 ng/ml (100 mg) [41]
8	Sunitinib	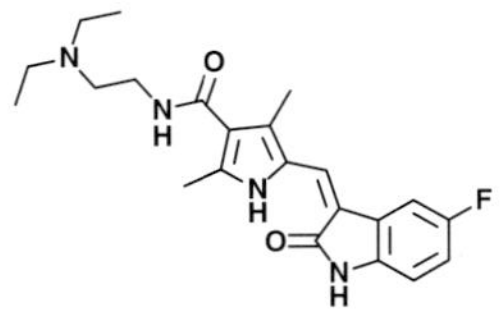	398	73	2.9	Type IIA	Yes	85	50 q.d.	95	26 ng/ml (50 mg) [42]
9	Lapatinib	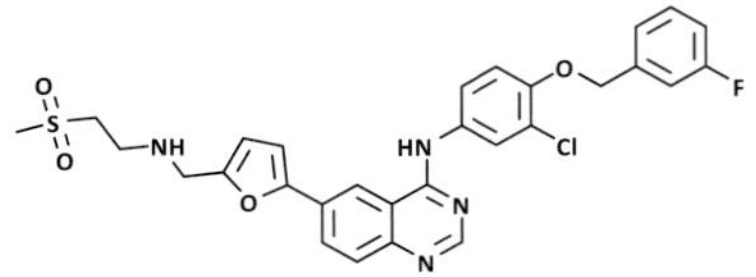	581	101	5.8	Type IIB	Yes	0.1	1250 q.d.	>99	2500 ng/ml (1250 mg) [43]

(*continued*)

Table 15.6 (Continued)

S. No.	Drug	Structure	MW	PSA	clog*P*	Binding mode[a] [32,33]	Reversible binding	Aqueous solubility[b]	Dose (mg/day) [34][c]	Human plasma binding[d]	Human[e] plasma ~C_{max} (dose)
10	Nilotinib	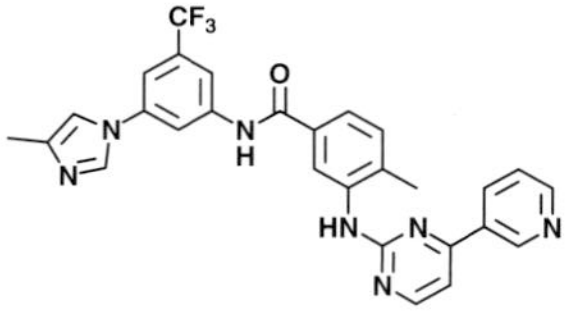	529	93	5.5	Type IIA	Yes	<0.1	400 b.i.d.	99	2000 ng/ml (400 mg) [44]
11	Temsirolimus	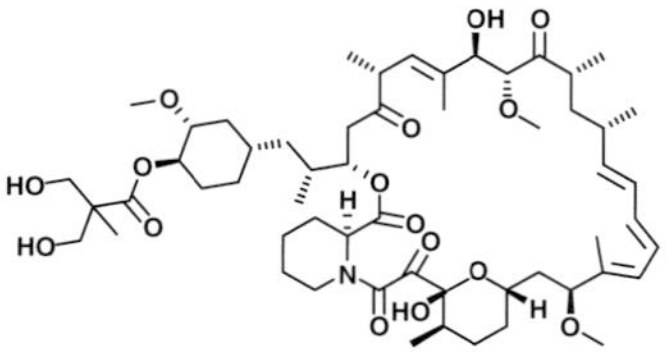	1030	241	7.4	Allosteric	Yes	12	25 1/week infused	85	600 ng/ml (25 mg) [45]
12	Pazopanib	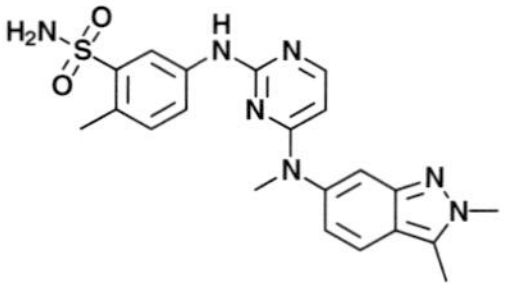	437	115	3.5	Type I	Yes	<0.3	800 q.d.	>99	45 000 ng/ml (800 mg) [46]
13	Crizotinib	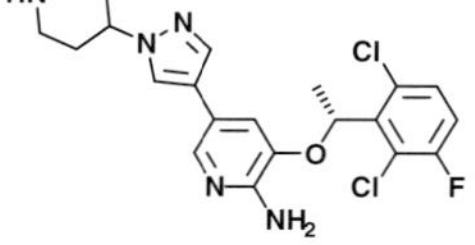	450	75	4.2	Type I	Yes	71	250 b.i.d.	91	61 ng/ml (100 mg) [47]

14	Vemurafenib	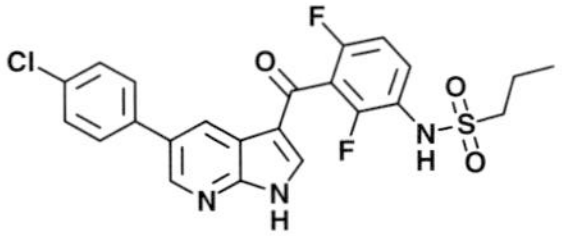	489	87	4.1	Type IIB	Yes	<0.3	960 b.i.d.	>99	62 000 ng/ml (960 mg) [48]
15	Vandetanib	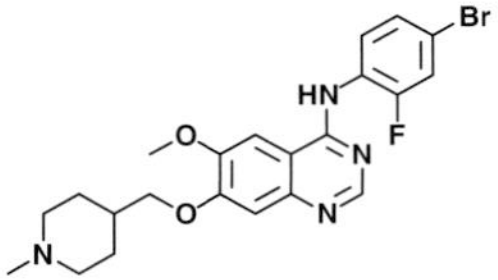	474	58	5.6	Type I	Yes	>500	300 q.d.	>99	1000 ng/ml (300 mg) [49]
16	Ruxolitinib	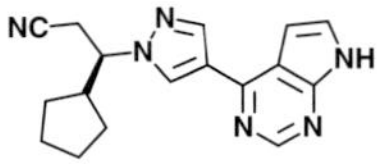	306	76	2.2	Type I	Yes	200	15–20 b.i.d.	97	640 ng/ml (10 mg) [50]
17	Axitinib	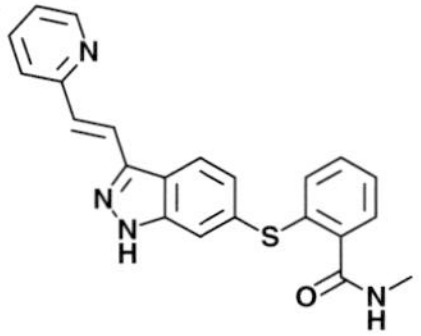	485	87	4.3	Type IIA	Yes	1	5 b.i.d.	>99	50 ng/ml (5 mg) [51]
18	Bosutinib	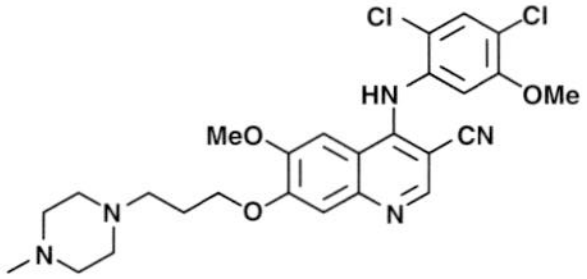	530	82	4.9	Type IIA	Yes	20	500 q.d.	94	125 ng/ml (500 mg) [52]

(continued)

Table 15.6 (*Continued*)

S. No.	Drug	Structure	MW	PSA	clog*P*	Binding mode[a)] [32,33]	Reversible binding	Aqueous solubility[b)]	Dose (mg/day) [34][c)]	Human plasma binding[d)]	Human[e)] plasma ~C_{max} (dose)
19	Cabozantinib	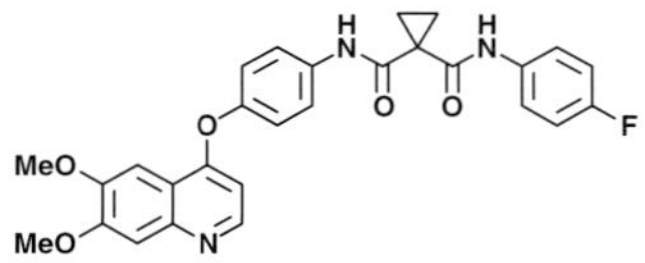	501	98	4.9	Type IIA	Yes	0.1	140 q.d.	>99	70 ng/ml (160 mg) [53]
20	Tofacitinib	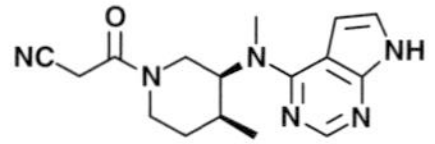	312	84	1.5	Type I	Yes	>500	5 b.i.d.	40	360 ng/ml (30 mg) [54]
21	Regorafenib	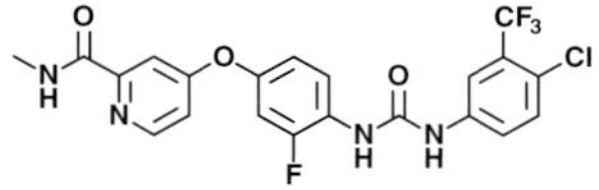	482	91	5.1	Type IIA	Yes		160 q.d.	99.5	3100 ng/ml (160 mg) [55]
22	Ibrutinib	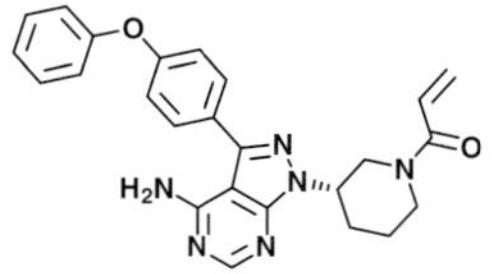	440	95	4.0	Type IIB	Covalent	19	560 q.d.	97.3	420 ng/ml (420 mg) [56]
23	Dabrafenib	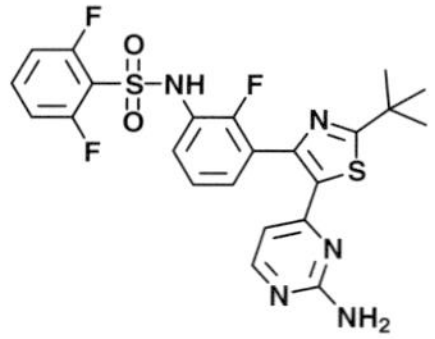	519	109	4.6	Type IIB	Yes	3	150 b.i.d.	99.7	2500 ng/ml (150 mg) [57]

24	Afatinib	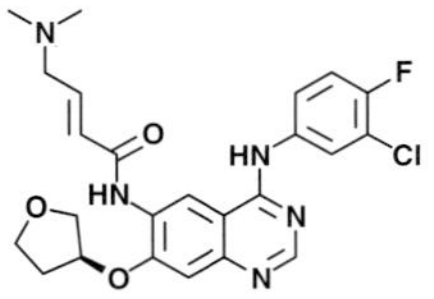	485	87	4.3	Type I	Covalent	75	40 q.d.	95	60 ng/ml (40 mg) [58]
25	Ponatinib	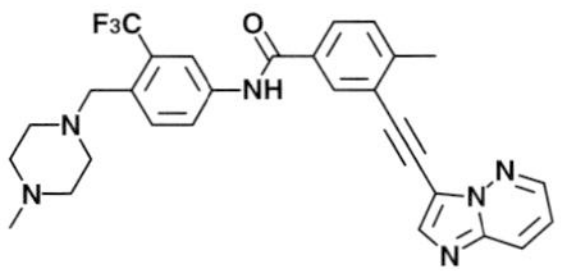	532	63	5.7	Type IIA	Yes	<0.3	45 q.d.	>99	15 ng/ml (15 mg) [59]
26	Trametinib	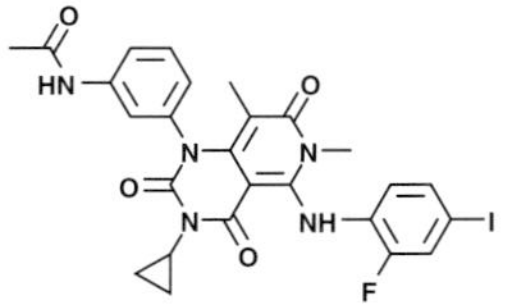	615	102	4.8	Allosteric	Yes	<0.3	2 q.d.	97.4	20 ng/ml (2) [60]

a) Binding modes: type I DFG-in α-C-helix-in, type IIA DFG-out α-C-helix-in, type IIB DFG-in α-C-helix-out, allosteric non-ATP competitive.
b) Solubility measured in-house at pH 7.4 using dried solid from a fresh DMSO stock and units in ug/mL.
c) www.rxlist.com (last accessed January 2014).
d) www.druginformation.com (last accessed January 2014).
e) Since C_{max}, AUC and plasma levels vary significantly dependent on numerous factors (fed versus fasted, age, healthy versus diseased, etc.), values presented provide a representative exposure at a clinically relevant dose.

the assay (ATP concentration, enzyme activation state, timing of assay readout, enzyme construct, etc.). It is not uncommon to observe changes of 10–100-fold in potency dependent on these subtle factors. The details of assays often vary between laboratories or even researchers and calibrating results to the literature is difficult.

Covalent inhibitors targeting an accessible cysteine (e.g., neratinib and recently approved ibrutinib) offer unique advantages, especially in oncology, but cloud the kinetics. Irreversible binding makes interpretation of potency and therapeutic index more challenging [61]. Potency is time dependent with irreversible inhibitors (affinity versus inactivation of protein versus resynthesis rate) and in a dynamic *in vivo* setting, reversible binding to antitargets may rapidly decrease between dosing (high C_{max}, high clearance compounds). In a static *in vitro* environment, this is not true unless the assay is carefully adapted (washout and timing studies). Here, potential off-target reversible effects can be overestimated from *in vitro* studies. Even fine-tuned reactive acrylamides (the common electrophilic motif used to weaponize the drug toward the cysteine thiol moiety) can lead to both nonspecific and antitarget effects if the cysteine is conserved across other kinases [62]. Highly activated weaponized molecules can nonspecifically react with proteins or glutathione and lead to direct or idiosyncratic toxicity unrelated to kinase inhibition.

These are cautionary notes that researchers must keep in mind when making decisions about advancing a compound or stopping its progression. Enzymatic as well as functional cell assays are notorious for leading to misinterpretations in the kinase field. Direct mechanistic readouts in matched pair cell lines provide the most relevant method of determining a true selectivity index, although this is not always practical. For classes of compounds that show significant promiscuity and where primary binding energy is derived from a kinome-conserved bi- or tridentate hinge interaction or general lipophilicity, this can require a major investment in resources, time, and money to improve the selectivity profile. A rule of thumb in medicinal chemistry is where your lead starts is close in structure to where your drug ends up. In this author's experience, templates that begin with a high rate of kinase promiscuity tend to be very difficult to engineer into selective drugs unless there is a unique structural component to the target that can be exploited. If selectivity is a primary goal, then numerous chemotypes should be evaluated early in the program. Absolute potency biases selection from an HTS at the expense of selectivity and can lead down a long and unproductive path.

Many of the targets inhibited by drugs are passengers and their inhibition has no relevance to the original target disease – what one might call "passenger kinases." Given the complexity of biological systems and disease, the probability that random passenger kinase(s) will fortuitously impact disease to a greater extent than elicit undesirable side effects is low. For example, there is little compelling evidence to suggest that inhibition of cKIT or PDGFR with imatinib in CML patients contributes to its clinical benefit [63]. This is supported by the fact that bosutinib, an effective second-line treatment in CML, is not active against either of these kinases. Passenger kinases can carry unknown risks and/or consequences for safety while adding questionable value or limiting the necessary dose to achieve maximal on-target activity. In some cases, there is a dearth of literature around these off-target kinases and secondary cellular assays are unavailable for further interrogation. For example, sunitinib is a very potent inhibitor of the DRAK1 kinase, although there is scant literature reported on the function and relevance of its blockade. There are dozens of kinases that fall into this well of limited knowledge.

On the other hand, passenger kinases have proven invaluable for treatment of cancer. For example, cKit activity by imatinib led to approval in GIST treatment and ALK activity in the cMet inhibitor, Crizotinib, gave rise to hope for non-small cell lung cancer patients. In these cases the drug's activities arrived prior to the biological relevance of targets driving disease.

Understanding subtle SAR that drives selectivity and its function on cells is highly valuable. Strong systems biology and an array of selective inhibitors can prove indispensable in shedding light on these questions. What targets are critical for efficacy? What antitargets limit effective plasma concentration due to safety? What targets impact neither parameter? In the absence of a complete *in vitro* picture, which is often the case in kinase discovery, gathering *in vivo* efficacy and a preliminary exploration of liabilities can be instructive. If ill-defined antitarget activity cannot be eliminated or reduced, making a risk to benefit assessment before entering the clinic is challenging. Sometimes surrogate markers can be used to monitor the relationship between pharmacodynamic engagement and adverse events. Rash and EGFR/BRaf/MEK or VEGFR and hypertension are good examples. In most cases these relationships are unknown and were not identified in preclinical species. When safety is paramount (non-life-threatening diseases), widening the index against antitargets should be prioritized and cellular context and selectivity should be placed early in the discovery flow scheme. With a deeper understanding of the kinome, research will be better positioned to make more informed decisions [64]. SciFinder returns nearly a million hits when the term kinase is entered, although we are only scratching the surface of the complex biology and interrelated signaling cascades they regulate. Clinically, there are only a handful of kinases we understand the liabilities of inhibition. The consequences of selective knockdown of hundreds of others (*in vitro* or *in vivo*) remain unknown and we will continue to face this dilemma for some time.

Inertia has pushed kinase research down to two divergent paths: polypharmacology [65] and high selectivity. The former lends itself to faster early lead advancement, since an often challenging hurdle has been reduced. It is also biased toward a more phenomenological approach (potential for serendipitous discovery of additivity or synergy). It also generates more safety risks. Polypharmacology, by definition, means more biological targets are impacted. Gathering early *in vivo* efficacy and toxicology, at exposures that cover each of the targets, is therefore even more important. In many ways, it takes a holistic view of the profile and harkens back to the way drugs were advanced decades earlier. This is often favored by smaller organizations where resources are limited, budgets are smaller, and where quickly demonstrating proof of concept (POC) in the clinic is a high priority. Some of these are driven by financial pressures from venture companies looking for return on investment. There have been a handful of examples of highly selective drugs discovered by small biotechs: vemurafenib for BRaf by Plexxikon, ruxolitinib for JAK by Incyte, and several advanced clinical compounds by Array BioPharma (selumetinib for MEK and ARRY382 for cFMS).

The more selective strategy tends toward longer commitment in discovery (optimization for selectivity takes time) and a rigorous credentialing of the target. It is favored by more conservative and larger pharmaceutical organizations, where confidence in mechanism, translation to the clinic, and safety remain a primary concern. A good example is tofacitinib from Pfizer, the only kinase inhibitor approved outside of oncology, aside from analogues of the natural product rapamycin. Its path to market in rheumatoid arthritis was expensive and challenging, but the opportunities are great for an oral therapy given the tens of billions of dollars in revenue generated from antibodies and proteins targeting cytokines and other pathways in this disease area.

There is a biological consequence and limitation to targeting a selective-mechanism in cancer. This has become evident the past decade with drugs like crizotinib and vemurafenib. Tumors evolve to survive and it is rare that a particular cancer, especially in a more advanced metastatic stage, can be eradicated or even effectively controlled by inhibition of any single pathway [66,67]. Polypharmacological or selective targeting strategy – there are pros and cons with each [68] and it is becoming clear that magic bullet (targeted) curative treatments in cancer are elusive and will require complementary strategies.

Sorafenib was originally identified as an inhibitor of BRaf and targeted for treatment of melanoma, where the pathway is implicated (Table 15.1; vemurafenib and trametinib are both approved for melanoma). Sorafenib's potency against this tumor type via inhibition of a key BRaf mutation (V600E) identified in a subset of patients was ultimately insufficient to demonstrate compelling efficacy in the clinic. It was observed that sorafenib blocks targets involved in angiogenesis: VEGFR and PDGFR [69]. Based on serendipity, persistence, and pursuing a novel angle, sorafenib was approved in renal cell carcinoma (RCC) in 2005, and then in hepatocellular carcinoma (HCC) [70]. For the latter indication, it still remains unclear what target(s) drive clinical efficacy since *in vitro* growth inhibition is insufficient to explain its *in vivo* effects. Sorafenib's antiangiogenic properties are likely driving activity, but this is yet to be proven. In HCC, where therapeutic options are limited, fortuitous kinase polypharmacology is likely a contributing factor in its modest benefit in the clinic. The drug has proceeded to generate over $1 billion per year in sales and remains the only targeted molecular therapeutic approved in HCC.

Imatinib, discovered by Novartis and approved in 2001 (Table 15.1), was rationally identified and successfully developed as a targeted agent toward a unique translocation, the Philadelphia chromosome BCR-Abl. This mutation drives a very specific and deadly form of blood cancer, chronic myelogenous leukemia. Its compelling story has been thoroughly reviewed and the reader is referred to two excellent accounts that place imatinib's development and importance as a cancer drug in historical context [71,72]. In CML and what has turned out to be the exception than the rule in cancer, direct and specific blockade of the single hyperactivated BCR-Abl mutation is sufficient to control disease long term. The 10-year survival rate is an impressive 68% for patients taking this drug in the early staging of disease [73] and who tolerate its long-term use. For a variety of reasons, including a relatively indolent mutation rate in the chronic phase of disease and impressive duration of response, even though the disease is rare, with an *incidence* rate of approximately 4800 in the United States (based on 2010 statistics), *prevalence* is far higher at nearly 70 000 [74]. This has led to one of the most successful oncology drug stories in recent history, not only in financial terms (nearly $5 billion in global sales in 2012) but also from a patient benefit perspective. Like the current AID's cocktail for HIV-positive patients, it has been transformative to the lives of patients with CML and their families.

Imatinib is active against a handful of other kinases, including cKIT and PDGFR. It happens that a subset of gastrointestinal stromal tumors (GISTs) is driven by mutations of cKIT and that imatinib is effective as frontline treatment in this disease. Similarly, patients with hypereosinophilic syndrome (HES) that have a translocation mutation (FIP1L1/PDGFRA) are responsive to imatinib, due to effective inhibition of PDGFR. Imatinib has therefore captured multiple indications (CML, GIST, and HES) from both a design perspective (BCR-Abl) and an opportunistic one (cKIT and PDGFR).

Efficacy like that seen with imatinib in CML continues to be the holy grail to which new oncology programs are compared in this era of targeted therapeutics. Its effectiveness remains unparalleled in the kinase field more than a decade after its approval and 30 years of research in the field. Recently, approved targeted agents, such as vemurafenib in melanoma (BRaf V600E mutation) and crizotinib in non-small cell lung carcinoma (EML4-ALK fusion), demonstrated impressive response rates. Unfortunately, these drugs show rapid resistance to therapy through various mechanisms [75]. This appears to be the rule for kinase inhibitors in oncology and has focused the industry on two major strategies: next-generation kinase inhibitors treating resistance mutations [BCR-Abl (T315I) in CML; EML4-ALK (C1156Y and L1196M) in NSCL; cKIT (D816V) in GIST] and combination therapy. Conceptually, the former offers the possibility of selectively targeting mutations driving disease while sparing normal homeostatic functions of wild-type enzyme (e.g., EGFR mutations and better safety profiles). Both offer promise from a patient stratification and efficacy perspective, but increased challenges in drug design

From a practical standpoint, treatment of resistance mutations is less complex if disease continues to be driven exclusively through the same pathway and structural biology can be exploited. CML (BCR-Abl; first-line imatinib, second-line dasatinib, nilotinib, or bosutinib, and third-line ponatinib) and GIST (mutant-cKIT; first-line imatinib, second-line sunitinib, and third-line regorafenib) are good examples, where second- and third-generation inhibitors have been successfully brought to market. After decades of patient biopsies, genomic/proteomic phenotyping, and advances in translational medicine, it is clear that single driving mutations in cancer may be a limited well from which to draw water. While the idea of personalized medicine in oncology is scientifically attractive, niche indications treating late-stage cancer patients to extend survival a few months has led the health industry to reassess the cost-to-benefit ratio. Approval agencies (NICE, FDA) and insurance companies are scrutinizing this complex math carefully. With costs of many cancer drugs rising precipitously, transformative treatment remains a key but lofty goal [76,77].

The evidence for combination therapy is compelling [78] and dates back to the early days of chemotherapy [72]. If you can attack multiple nodes in a tumor, including those of early resistance, more profound (sometimes cures) and longer duration of benefit can be achieved. But combining agents also compounds distinct and/or overlapping toxicities. Promiscuous inhibitors carrying unnecessary kinase baggage decrease the probability that they can be combined safely, especially in oncology where patients have comorbidities and are already on palliative medications. The many permutations of treatment in combination settings go up rapidly and make identifying optimal protocols lengthy and expensive and also require long-term commitment.

When multiple kinase nodes impact or drive tumor biology (e.g., MEK/ERK, PI3K, and EGFR), blockade of any single one is often not profoundly effective or long-lasting. The groundbreaking angiogenesis paper by Judah Folkman in 1971 was anticipated to be the next major breakthrough in oncology [79] in hopes of avoiding the recurring theme of resistance – strangle the support network of tumors where mutations are infrequent. While several drugs targeting this concept have partly realized this hope (Tables 15.1 and 15.2; inhibitors of VEGFR/VEGF-A and PDGFR), most of these agents have shown only modest single agent activity. The clinical development of multiple novel agents in parallel is relatively unprecedented, but the oncology field recognizes that targeted therapeutics in the right combination or setting may lead to more profound and early responses in the clinic. This is clear as an increasing number of trials are being conducted using classical cytotoxics combined with one or more targeted agents, antiangiogenics, and, more recently, the highly impressive immunotherapeutics – BMS antibody drugs ipilimumab against CTLA-4 and nivolumab against PD-1.

Safety remains a major challenge for either strategy. As disease progresses, tumors inherently become more aggressive, genomically unstable, and metastasize to other tissues and organs. Patients grow weaker as a result of both disease progression and compounded treatment side effects. Safety is a relative term in oncology, where, historically, many treatments were and still are chemical poisons combined and titrated carefully through trial and error to more selectively kill rapidly proliferating tumor cells over normal tissue. It is a therapeutic area in which patients accept a far greater amount of risk and side effects since cancer by its very nature is life-threatening. In this regard, imatinib is comparatively very well tolerated. As referenced in Table 15.5, treatment with this drug can lead to serious or even fatal adverse events and often it cannot be combined due to interactions with the metabolism of other drugs. The former may be inherent to the target class (Abl inhibition) required to achieve efficacy, whereas the latter is clearly molecule specific.

If we turn the clock back 20 years, it was not clear that this vast and untapped area of kinase biology could be exploited to identify drugs. The flat and ubiquitous hinge recognition pocket where ATP binds, the most obvious druggable site within kinases, suggested homology across the kinome that would predispose against identifying highly selective inhibitors. Staurosporine, a natural product originally isolated in 1977 from the bacterium *Streptomyces staurosporeus*, was the poster child for this argument. It demonstrated high affinity (<100 nM) for much of the kinome [80] and it was clearly indiscriminate in its effects on killing numerous cell types. Since kinases play such a dramatic role in many cellular processes and since achieving selectivity was a major challenge, many believed that identifying a drug with an acceptable therapeutic index would be highly unlikely. Genetic models where targets had been knocked out or down in animals demonstrated the potential for profound toxicology, at least from a drug developmental standpoint.

Fortunately, thanks to the power of structural biology and an underestimation of the persistence of biologists and medicinal chemists, a compelling retort to the skeptics was only a few years away. First examples of preclinical inhibitors with selectivity and potency were realized from the EGFR quinazoline era. Imatinib (Gleevec) was a breakthrough in the kinase field when it was approved in 2001. It demonstrated that molecules could be identified and modified, through a rationale design approach, to target-specific kinases with very good selectivity and an acceptable safety profile in the clinic. Interestingly, the drug binds its targets in a DFG-out protein confirmation, which is an inactive form of the protein, and leads to interesting time-dependent kinetics. Additional drugs have also been designed around this unique binding mode (Table 15.6, column 7). More recently, several true allosteric inhibitors have been reported for the kinases MEK, AKT, and TRK [5,81]. These chemotypes tend to be exquisitely selective for their target since they bind a part of the protein that is not conserved across other classes. Design elements of kinase inhibitors will be discussed in greater detail in chapter 18 of this book. Unlike the GPCR field, kinases have provided an area of deep understanding for subtle structure–activity relationships based on thousands of X-rays of structures against dozens of different kinase constructs.

The field has come a long way in a short time. Fifteen years ago, there were no drugs approved in the kinase area. The onus was on those arguing selectivity would not prohibit this class from being safely drugged. Now, through the end of 2013, we have seen 26 small molecules approved against more than a dozen targets. Six antibodies and one aptamer are on the market. Recently, tofacitinib was given the go ahead by the FDA for treatment of rheumatoid arthritis, the first approval outside of oncology (excluding analogues of rapamycin in transplant). In many ways, this is a major landmark for the field as the hurdle for safety in rheumatic disease is much higher than oncology. Does this indicate that drugs in this class will be mainly restricted to the oncology field? Treatment for oncology patients is much shorter than for other indications. Only time will tell. This raises the interesting question of the safety of these drugs in a truly chronic setting. Based on the current trajectory, one would anticipate approvals to continue in this area for years to come. We are still developing a greater appreciation for the vast biology of this class of enzymes, including functions in disease as well as the potential liabilities for inhibition and the expectations remain high. The author hopes that the subsequent chapters will help advance this field even further over the next decade.

References

1 Melnikova, I. and Golden, J. (2004) Targeting protein kinases. *Nature Reviews. Drug Discovery*, **3**, 993–994.

2 Decision Resources (2013) Pharmaview Commercial Landscape Report Series: Oncology, September.

3 Palaia, J. (2014) Global Information. www.prnewswire.com/news-releases/kinase-inhibitors-market-to-reach-116-billion-in-us-403-billion-globally-by-2016-161937715.html (last accessed January 2014).

4 Thomson Reuters (2014) http://integrity.thomson-pharma.com/integrity (last accessed January 2014).

5 Uitdehaag, J., Verkaar, F., Alwan, H., de Man, J., Buijsman, R., and Zaman, G. (2012) A guide to picking the most selective kinase inhibitor tool compounds for pharmacological validation of drug targets. *British Journal of Pharmacology*, **166** (3), 858–876.

6 Selleck (2104) http://www.selleckchem.com (last accessed January 2104).

7 Davis, M., Hunt, J., Herrgard, S., Ciceri, P., Wodicka, L., Pallares, G., Hocker, M., Treiber, D., and Zarrinkar, P. (2011) Comprehensive analysis of kinase inhibitor selectivity. *Nature Biotechnology*, **29** (11), 1046–1052.

8 Ribatti, D., Nico, B., and Crivellato, E. (2011) The role of pericytes in angiogenesis. *The International Journal of Developmental Biology*, **55** (3), 261–268.

9 ProQinase (2014) http://www.proqinase.com/content/view/82 (last accessed January 2014).

10 Hubbard, S. and Till, J. (2000) Protein tyrosine kinase structure and function. *Annual Review of Biochemistry*, **69**, 373–398.

11 Manning, G., Whyte, D., Martinez, R., Hunter, T., and Sudarsanam, S. (2002) The protein kinase complement of the human genome. *Science*, **298**, 1912–1934.

12 Hartmann, J., Haap, M., Kopp, H.G., and Lipp, H.P. (2009) Tyrosine kinase inhibitors: a review on pharmacology, metabolism and side effects. *Current Drug Metabolism*, **10**, 470–481.

13 Bradbury, R. (2010) Kinase inhibitors: approved drugs and clinical candidates, in *Burger's Medicinal Chemistry, Drug Discovery, and Development*, 7th edn (eds D. Abraham and R. Rotella), John Wiley & Sons, Inc., pp. 295–344.

14 Devron, R., Shah, D., Shah, R., and Morganroth, J. (2013) Tyrosine kinase inhibitors: their on-target toxicities as potential indicators of efficacy. *Drug Safety*, **36** (6), 413–426.

15 O'Brien, Z. and Moghaddam, M. (2013) Small molecule kinase inhibitors approved by the FDA from 2000 to 2011: a systematic review of preclinical ADME data. *Expert Opinion on Drug Metabolism and Toxicology*, **9** (12), 1597–1612.

16 Lussier, Y. (2011) Kinase inhibitor toxicities imputed from kinome and clinical trial data. ASCPT AAPS Symposium, Washington, DC.

17 Guengerich, F. (2011) Mechanisms of drug toxicity and relevance to pharmaceutical development. *Journal of Drug Metabolism and Pharmacokinetics*, **26** (1), 3–14.

18 Roberts, P. and Der, C. (2007) Targeting the Raf-MEK-ERK mitogen-activated protein kinase cascade for the treatment of cancer. *Oncogene*, **26**, 3291–3310.

19 Dy, G. and Adjei, A. (2013) Understanding, recognizing, and managing toxicities of targeted anticancer therapies. *CA: A Cancer Journal for Clinicians*, **63**, 249–279.

20 Segaert, S. and Cutsem, E. (2005) Clinical signs, pathophysiology and management of skin toxicity during therapy with epidermal growth factor receptor inhibitors. *Annals of Oncology*, **16**, 1425–1433.

21 Akinleye, A., Furqan, M., Mukhi, N., Ravella, P., and Delong Liu, D. (2013) MEK and the inhibitors: from bench to bedside. *Hematological Oncology*, **6** (27), 1–11.

22 Orphanos, G., Ioannidis, G., and Ardavanis, A. (2009) Cardiotoxicity induced by tyrosine kinase inhibitors. *Acta Oncologica*, **48**, 964–970.

23 Cheng, H. and Force, T. (2010) Molecular mechanisms of cardiovascular toxicity of targeted cancer therapeutics. *Circulation Research*, **106**, 21–34.

24 Curigliano, G., Mayer, E., Burstein, H., Winer, E., and Goldhirsch, A. (2010) Cardiac toxicity from systemic cancer therapy: a comprehensive review. *Progress in Cardiovascular Diseases*, **53**, 94–104.

25 Verheul, H. and Pinedo, H. (2007) Possible molecular mechanisms involved in the toxicity of angiogenesis inhibition. *Nature Reviews. Cancer*, **7**, 475–485.

26 Gupta, R. and Maitland, M. (2011) Sunitinib, hypertension, and heart failure: a model for kinase inhibitor-mediated cardiotoxicity. *Current Hypertension Reports*, **13**, 430–435.

27 Mellor, H., Bell, A., Valentin, J.P., and Roberts, R. (2011) Cardiotoxicity associated with targeting kinase pathways in cancer. *Toxicological Sciences*, **120** (1), 14–32.

28 Natsume, A., Niwa, R., and Satoh, M. (2009) Improving effector functions of antibodies for cancer treatment: enhancing ADCC and CDC. *Drug Design Development and Therapy*, **3**, 7–16.

29 Imai, K. and Takaoka, A. (2006) Comparing antibody and small-molecule therapies for cancer. *Nature Reviews. Cancer*, **6**, 714–727.

30 Gerber, D. (2008) Targeted therapies: a new generation of cancer treatments. *American Family Physician*, **77** (3), 311–319.

31 Hafenbradl, D., Baumann, M., and Neumann, L. (2011) Part One: hit finding and profiling for protein kinases – assay development and screening, libraries, in *Protein Kinases as Drug targets* (eds B. Klebl and M. Hamacher) Wiley-VCH Verlag GmbH, Weinheim, pp. 1–44.

32 Blanc, J., Geney, R., and Menet, C. (2013) Type II kinase inhibitors: an opportunity in cancer for rational design. *Anticancer Agents in Medicinal Chemistry*, **13** (5), 731–747.

33 Wang, X. and Schleicher, K. (2013) Conformation-specific inhibitors of Raf kinases, in *The Enzymes: Inhibitors of the Ras Superfamily G-Proteins Part B*, vol. **34** (eds F. Tamanoi and C.J. Der), Academic Press, Waltham, MA, pp. 41–61.

34 Micromedex®, Cerner Multum™, and Wolters Kluwer™ (2014) www.drugs.com (last accessed January 2014).

35 Cohen, E., Sharma, M., Janisch, L., Llobrera, M., House, L., Wu, K., Ramirez, J., Fleming, G., Stadler, W., and Ratain, M. (2011) A phase I study of sirolimus and bevacizumab in patients with advanced malignancies. *European Journal of Cancer*, **47**, 1484–1489.

36 Peng, B., Hayes, M., Resta, D., Racine-Poon, A., Druker, B., Talpaz, M., Sawyers, C., Rosamilia, M., Ford, J., Lloyd, P., and Capdeville, R. (2004) Pharmacokinetics and pharmacodynamics of imatinib in a phase I trial with chronic myeloid leukemia patients. *Journal of Clinical Oncology*, **22** (5), 935–942.

37 Swaisland, H., Smith, R., Laight, A., Kerr, D., Ranson, M., Wilder-Smith, C., and Duvauchelle, T. (2005) Single-dose clinical pharmacokinetic studies of gefitinib. *Clinical Pharmacokinetics*, **44** (11), 1165–1177.

38 Mita, A., Papadopoulos, K., de Jonge, M., Schwartz, G., Verweij, J., Mita, M., Ricart,

A., Chu, Q., Tolcher, A., Wood, L., McCarthy, S., Hamilton, M., Iwata, K., Wacker, B., Witt, K., and Rowinsky, E. (2011) Erlotinib 'dosing-to-rash': a phase II intrapatient dose escalation and pharmacologic study of erlotinib in previously treated advanced non-small cell lung cancer. *British Journal of Cancer*, **105**, 938–944.

39 Fury, M., Sherman, E., Haque, S., Korte, S., Lisa, D., Shen, R., Wu, N., and Pfister, D. (2012) A phase I study of daily everolimus plus low-dose weekly cisplatin for patients with advanced solid tumors. *Cancer Chemotherapy and Pharmacology*, **69** (3), 591–598.

40 Siu, L., Awada, A., Takimoto, C., Piccart, M., Schwartz, B., Giannaris, T., Lathia, C., Petrenciuc, O., and Moore, M. (2006) Phase I trial of sorafenib and gemcitabine in advanced solid tumors with an expanded cohort in advanced pancreatic cancer. *Clinical Cancer Research*, **12** (1), 144–151.

41 Takahashi, N., Miura, M., Scott, S., Niioka, T., and Sawada, K. (2012) Pharmacokinetics of dasatinib for Philadelphia-positive acute lymphocytic leukemia with acquired T315I mutation. *Hematological Oncology*, **15**, 5–23.

42 Khosravan, R., Toh, M., Garrett, M., La Fargue, J., Ni, G., Marbury, T., Swan, S., Lunde, N., and Bello, C. (2010) Pharmacokinetics and safety of sunitinib maleate in subjects with impaired renal function. *Journal of Clinical Pharmacology*, **50** (4), 472–481.

43 Chu, Q., Cianfrocca, M., Goldstein, L., Gale, M., Murray, N., Loftiss, J., Arya, N., Koch, K., Pandite, L., Fleming, R., Paul, E., and Rowinsky, E. (2008) A phase I and pharmacokinetic study of lapatinib in combination with letrozole in patients with advanced cancer. *Clinical Cancer Research*, **14**, 4484–4490.

44 Tanaka, C., Yin, O., Sethuraman, V., Smith, T., Wang, X., Grouss, K., Kantarjian, H., Giles, F., Ottmann, O., Galitz, L., and Schran, H. (2010) Clinical pharmacokinetics of the BCR-Abl tyrosine kinase inhibitor nilotinib. *Clinical Pharmacology and Therapeutics*, **87** (2), 197–203.

45 Hidalgo, M., Buckner, J., Erlichman, C., Pollack, M., Boni, J., Dukart, G., Marshall, B., Speicher, L., Moore, L., and Rowinsky, E. (2006) A phase I and pharmacokinetic study of temsirolimus (CCI-779) administered intravenously daily for 5 days every 2 weeks to patients with advanced cancer. *Clinical Cancer Research*, **12**, 5755–5763.

46 Hurwitz, H., Dowlati, A., Saini, S., Savage, S., Suttle, A., Gibson, D., Hodge, J., Merkle, E., and Pandite, L. (2009) Phase I trial of pazopanib in patients with advanced cancer. *Clinical Cancer Research*, **15**, 4220–4227.

47 Yamazaki, S., Skaptason, J., Romero, D., Vekich, S., Jones, H., Tan, W., Wilner, K., and Koudriakova, T. (2011) Prediction of oral pharmacokinetics of cMet kinase inhibitors in humans: physiologically based pharmacokinetic model versus traditional one-compartment model. *Drug Metabolism and Disposition: The Biological Fate of Chemicals*, **39**, 383–393.

48 Roche (2014) www.roche-australia.com/content/dam/internet/corporate/roche/en_AU/files/oncology/zelboraf-pi.pdf (January 2014).

49 de Boer, R., Humblet, Y., Wolf, J., Nogová, L., Ruffert, K., Milenkova, T., Smith, R., Godwood, A., and Vansteenkiste, J. (2009) An open-label study of vandetanib with pemetrexed in patients with previously treated non-small-cell lung cancer. *Annals of Oncology*, **20** (3), 486–491.

50 Shi, J., Chen, X., Emm, T., Scherle, P., McGee, R., Lo, Y., Landman, R., McKeever, E., Jr., Punwani, N., Williams, W., and Yeleswaram, S. (2012) The effect of CYP3A4 inhibition or induction on the pharmacokinetics and pharmacodynamics of orally administered ruxolitinib (INCB018424 phosphate) in healthy volunteers. *Journal of Clinical Pharmacology*, **52**, 809–818.

51 Pithavala, Y., Tortorici, M., Toh, M., Garrett, M., Hee, B., Kuruganti, U., Ni, G., and Klamerus, K. (2010) Effect of rifampin on the pharmacokinetics of axitinib (AG-013736) in Japanese and Caucasian healthy volunteers. *Cancer Chemotherapy and Pharmacology*, **65**, 563–570.

52 Daud, A., Krishnamurthi, S., Saleh, M., Gitlitz, B., Borad, M., Gold, P., Chiorean, E., Springett, G., Abbas, R., Agarwal, S., Bardy-Bouxin, N., Hsyu, P., Leip, E., Turnbull, K., Zacharchuk, C., and Messersmith, W. (2012) Phase I study of bosutinib, a Src/Abl tyrosine kinase inhibitor, administered to patients with advanced solid tumors. *Clinical Cancer Research*, **18**, 1092–1100.

53 Kurzrock, R., Sherman, S., Ball, D., Forastiere, A., Cohen, R., Mehra, R., Pfister, D., Cohen, E., Janisch, L., Nauling, F., Hong, D., Ng, C., Ye, L., Gagel, R., Frye, J., Müller, T., Ratain, M., and Salgia, R. (2006) A phase I dose-escalation study of the safety and pharmacokinetics of a XL184, a VEGFR and Met kinase inhibitor, administered orally to subjects with advanced malignancies. *European Journal of Cancer Supp*, **4** (12), Abstract 405.

54 Cohen, S., Zwillich, S., Chow, V., Labadie, R., and Wilkinson, B. (2009) Co-administration of the JAK inhibitor CP-690,550 and methotrexate is well tolerated in patients with rheumatoid arthritis without need for dose adjustment. *British Journal of Clinical Pharmacology*, **69** (2), 143–151.

55 Strumberg, D., Scheulen, M., Schultheis, B., Richly, H., Frost, A., Büchert, M., Christensen, O., Jeffers, M., Heinig, R., Boix, O., and Mross, K. (2012) Regorafenib (BAY 73–4506) in advanced colorectal cancer: a phase I study. *British Journal of Cancer*, **106**, 1722–1727.

56 Byrd, J., Furman, R., Coutre, S., Flinn, I., Burger, J., Blum, K., Grant, B., Sharman, J., Coleman, M., Wierda, W., Jones, J., Zhao, W., Heerema, N., Johnson, A., Sukbuntherng, J., Chang, B., Clow, F., Hedrick, E., Buggy, J., James, D., and O'Brien, S. (2013) Targeting BTK with ibrutinib in relapsed chronic lymphocytic leukemia. *The New England Journal of Medicine*, **369**, 32–34.

57 Denton, C., Minthorn, E., Carson, S., Young, G., Richards-Peterson, L., Botbyl, J., Han, C., Morrison, R., Blackman, S., and Ouellet, D. (2013) Concomitant oral and intravenous pharmacokinetics of dabrafenib, a BRAF inhibitor, in patients with BRAF V600 mutation-positive solid tumors. *Journal of Clinical Pharmacology*, **53** (9), 955–961.

58 Yap, T., Vidal, L., Adam, J., Stephens, P., Spicer, J., Shaw, H., Ang, J., Temple, G., Bell, S., Shahidi, M., Uttenreuther-Fischer, M., Stopfer, P., Futreal, A., Calvert, H., de Bono, J., and Plummer, R. (2010) Phase I trial of the irreversible EGFR and HER2 kinase inhibitor BIBW 2992 in patients with advanced solid tumors. *Journal of Clinical Oncology*, **28** (25), 3965–3972.

59 Narasimhan, N., Dorer, D., Niland, K., Haluska, F., and Sonnichsen, D. (2013) Effects of ketoconazole on the pharmacokinetics of ponatinib in healthy subjects. *Journal of Clinical Pharmacology*, **53** (9), 974–981.

60 Infante, J., Fecher, L., Falchook, G., Nallapareddy, S., Gordon, M., Becerra, C., DeMarini, D., Cox, D., Xu, Y., Morris, S., Peddareddigari, V., Le, N., Hart, L., Bendell, J., Eckhardt, G., Kurzrock, R., Flaherty, K., Burris, H., 3rd, and Messersmith, W. (2012) Safety, pharmacokinetic, pharmacodynamic, and efficacy data for the oral MEK inhibitor trametinib: a phase 1 dose-escalation trial. *The Lancet Oncology*, **13**, 773–781.

61 Kalgutkar, A. and Dalvie, D. (2012) Drug discovery for a new generation of covalent drugs. *Expert Opinion on Drug Discovery*, **7** (7), 561–581.

62 Liu, Q., Sabnis, Y., Zhao, Z., Zhang, T., Buhrlage, S., Jones, L., and Gray, N. (2013) Developing irreversible inhibitors of the protein kinase cysteinome. *Chemistry & Biology*, **20**, 146–159.

63 Remsing, R., Rix, U., Colinge, J., Hantschel, O., Bennett, K., Stranzl, T., Müller, A., Baumgartner, C., Valent, P., Augustin, M., Till, J., and Superti-Furga, G. (2009) Global target profile of the kinase inhibitor bosutinib in primary chronic myeloid leukemia cells. *Leukemia*, **23** (3), 477–485.

64 Graves, L., Duncan, J., Whittle, M., and Johnson, G. (2013) The dynamic nature of the kinome. *Biochemistry*, **450**, 1–8.

65 Knight, Z., Lin, H., and Shokat, K. (2010) Targeting the cancer kinome through polypharmacology. *Nature Reviews. Cancer*, **10**, 130–137.

66 Zhang, J., Yang, P., and Gray, N. (2009) Targeting cancer with small molecule kinase inhibitors. *Nature Reviews. Cancer*, **9**, 28–39.
67 Holohan, C., Van Schaeybroeck, S., Longley, D., and Johnston, P. (2013) Cancer drug resistance: an evolving paradigm. *Nature Reviews. Cancer*, **13**, 714–726.
68 Kamb, A., Wee, S., and Lengauer, C. (2007) Why is cancer drug discovery so difficult? *Nature Reviews. Drug Discovery*, **6**, 115–120.
69 Wilhelm, S., Adname, L., Newell, P., Villanueva, A., Llovet, J.M., and Lynch, M. (2008) Preclinical overview of sorafenib, a multikinase inhibitor that targets both Raf and VEGF and PDGF receptor tyrosine kinase signaling. *Molecular Cancer Therapeutics*, **7**, 3129–3140.
70 Iver, R., Fetterly, G., Lugade, A., and Thanaval, Y. (2010) Sorafenib: a clinical and pharmacologic review. *Expert Opinion on Pharmacotherapy*, **11** (11), 1943–1955.
71 Leaf, C. (2013) *The Truth in Small Doses: Why We're Losing the War on Cancer and How to Win It*, Simon and Schuster, New York, NY.
72 Mukherjee, S. (2010) *The Emperor of All Maladies: A Biography of Cancer*, Scribner, a Division of Simon and Schuster, New York, NY.
73 Kantarjian, H., O'Brien, S., Garcia-Manero, G., Faderl, S., Ravandi, F., Jabbour, E., Shan, J., and Cortes, J. (2012) Very long-term follow-up results of imatinib mesylate therapy in chronic phase chronic myeloid leukemia after failure of interferon alpha therapy. *Cancer*, **118** (12), 3116–3122.
74 Huang, X., Cortez, J., and Kantarjian, H. (2012) Estimations of the increasing prevalence and plateau prevalence of chronic myeloid leukemia in the era of tyrosine kinase inhibitor therapy. *Cancer*, **118** (12), 3123–3127.
75 Doebele, R., Pilling, A., Aisner, D., Kutateladze, T., Le, A., Weickhardt, A., Kondo, K., Linderman, D., Heasley, L., Franklin, W., Varella-Garcia, M., and Camidge, D.R. (2012) Mechanisms of resistance to crizotinib in patients with *ALK* gene rearranged non-small cell lung cancer. *Clinical Cancer Research*, **18** (5), 1472–1482.
76 Lewis, J., Lipworth, W., Kerridge, I., and Dav, R. (2013) The economic evaluation of personalised oncology medicines: ethical challenges. *The Medical Journal of Australia*, **199** (7), 471–473.
77 Ebara, T., Ohno, T., and Nakano, T. (2013) Quantitative medical cost-effectiveness analysis of molecular-targeting cancer drugs in Japan. *Daru*, **21** (1), 21–40.
78 Li, F., Zhao, C., and Wang, L. (2013) Molecular-targeted agents combination therapy for cancer: developments and potentials. *International Journal of Cancer*, **7**, 1–13.
79 Folkman, J. (1971) Tumor angiogenesis: therapeutic implications. *The New England Journal of Medicine*, **285** (21), 1182–1186.
80 Gani, O. and Engh, R. (2010) Protein kinase inhibition of clinically important staurosporine analogues. *Natural Product Reports*, **27** (4), 489–498.
81 Lamba, V. and Ghosh, I. (2012) New directions in targeting protein kinases: focusing upon true allosteric and bivalent inhibitors. *Current Pharmaceutical Design*, **18** (20), 2936–2945.

16
Clinical and Nonclinical Adverse Effects of Kinase Inhibitors

Douglas A. Keller, Richard J. Brennan, and Karen L. Leach

16.1
Introduction

Protein kinases are enzymes that catalyze the transfer of the phosphate from adenosine triphosphate (ATP) to target proteins at serine, threonine, tyrosine, or histidine residues. Phosphorylation may alter the function of the target protein by increasing or decreasing its activity, stabilizing it or marking it for degradation, changing its subcellular localization, or altering its interaction with other proteins. Over 500 distinct protein kinases are encoded by the human genome [1], and are involved in the regulation of a wide variety of cellular regulatory processes, including apoptosis, survival, proliferation, and differentiation.

Mutations and dysregulation of protein kinases are recognized to play causal roles in a wide variety of human diseases, and kinases have emerged over the last 20 years as a major drug target class. Kinase signaling is involved in all stages of tumorigenesis through modulation of transformation and differentiation, cell cycle progression, and motility [2], and kinase inhibition has shown particular success in treating both hematological and solid tumors, with 24 of 26 USFDA-approved small-molecule kinase inhibitors (KIs) (Table 15.1) addressing oncologic indications.

All drugs cause adverse effects and, although they are largely considered targeted therapies, KIs are no exception. As KIs have primarily been developed to inhibit specific kinases in known pathways of cellular function, it was an implicit assumption that there would be less toxicity than seen with drugs with a less well-defined biological foundation [3], in particular a radically improved safety profile compared with cytotoxic chemotherapeutic agents. In general, while a broad range of adverse effects is seen with kinase inhibitors (Table 16.1), the most common adverse effects are generally tolerable [4–6].

Adverse effects of drugs can be typically ascribed to off-target pharmacology or specific chemical interactions between the drug (or drug metabolite) and a cellular macromolecule. Often the nature of these interactions is unknown and some adverse effects are referred to as "idiosyncratic," meaning that the

Antitargets and Drug Safety, First Edition. Edited by László Urbán, Vinod F. Patel, and Roy J. Vaz.

Table 16.1 Summary of adverse effects observed with small-molecule kinase inhibitor drugs.

Compound (targets)	Gastro-intestinal	Hemat-opoietic and lymphoid	Hepatic	Cardio-vascular	Skin, bone, teeth	Thyroid	Ocular	Neuro-logical	Lung	Renal	Repro-ductive system	Other toxicity
Afatinib (EGFR)	H[a], R, M		H		H, R		H, M		H, R, M	R	R, M	R: embryo-fetal
Axitinib (VEGFR1/2/3, AURB/C, Kit, Flt1, cFms, PLK4)	H		H	H, R	R	H	H	H		H	R, D	R: embryo-fetal
Bosutinib (BCR-Abl, Src, Lyn, Hck)	H, R, D	H, R	H	H, D								H: fluid retention R: embryo-fetal
Cabozantinib (RET, Met, VEGFR1/2/3, Kit, Trk, Flt3, Axl, DDR1, MERTK, HIPK4, LOK, RET, Tie1/2, Flt3, PDGFR, EphA3)	H, R, D	R, D	H, R, D	H	H, R, D			H		H, R, D	R, D	R: embryo-fetal
Crizotinib (ALK, c-Met, Ros)	R, D		H, R, D	H, R, D	R		H, R		H			R: embryo-fetal
Dabrafenib (B-Raf)				H, D	H, R, D		H	H			R, D	H: new malignancies R: embryo-fetal

Dasatinib (BCR-Abl, Src, Lck, Yes, Fyn, Kit, EphA2, PDGFR, Lyn, EphA2, DDR2, BTK)	H, R, P	H, R, P	R, P	H, R, P	H			H	H		R, P	H: fluid retention R: embryo-fetal
Erlotinib (EGFR)	H, D		H, R	H	H, R, D		H, D		H	H, R, D	R	R: adrenal
Everolimus (mTOR)	R, P	H, R, P		P	H, P		R		H, R	H, R	R, P	R: embryo-fetal P: pancreatic, adrenal
Gefitinib (EGFR)	H		H, R	D	H, R, D		H, R, D		H	R		R: embryo-fetal
Ibrutinib (BTK, Lyn, Lck)	H, R, D	H, R, D		H	H, R		D	H		H		H: secondary malignancies R: pancreatic, embryo-fetal
Imatinib (BCR-Abl, Kit, PDGFR, cFms, DDR2)	H, D, P	H, R, D, P	H, D	H		H	H		H	R, D, P	R, D, P	H: fluid retention R: embryo-fetal
Lapatinib (EGFR, ErbB2)	H, R, D		H	H	H, R, D				H			R: neonatal
Nilotinib (BCR-Abl, PDGFR, DDR1/2)	H	H	H, D, P	H	H	D, P	R	H				H, D, P: pancreatic R: embryo-fetal
Pazopanib (VEGFR1/2/3, PDGFR, FGFR1/3, Kit, Lck, cFms, DDR1, EphB6)	H, P	H, R	H	H	H, R	H		H		H	R	R: embryo-fetal

(continued)

Table 16.1 (Continued)

Compound (targets)	Gastro-intestinal	Hemat-opoietic and lymphoid	Hepatic	Cardio-vascular	Skin, bone, teeth	Thyroid	Ocular	Neuro-logical	Lung	Renal	Repro-ductive system	Other toxicity
Ponatinib (BCR-Abl, BCR-Abl T315I, VEGFR, PDGFR, FGFR, Eph, Src family kinases, Kit, RET, Tie2, Flt3)		H, R, P	H, P	H, P	H, R	P	H	H		R		H, P: pancreas H: fluid retention R: embryo-fetal
Regorafenib (VEGFR1/2/3, BCR-Abl, B-Raf, B-Raf(V600E), Kit, PDGFR, RET, FGFR1/2, Tie2, Eph2A, p38)	H, D	H, R, D	H	H, R	H, R, D	R, D		H		R, D	R, D	R: embryo-fetal
Ruxolitinib (Jak1/2/3, TYK2)		H, R, D		D								
Sirolimus (mTOR)	H, P	H, P		H, R	H, R		R	H	H	H	R	H: secondary malignancies; fluid retention R: embryo-fetal
Sorafenib (C-Raf, B-Raf, B-Raf (V600E), Kit, Flt3, RET, VEGFR2/3, PDGFR)	H, R, D	H, R, D	H, R, D	H	H, R, D	H			H	H, R, D	R, D	R: pancreatic, adrenal, embryo-fetal

Sunitinib (PDGFR, VEGFR1/2/3, Kit, Flt3, cFms, RET, cFms)	H, R, P	H, R, P	H, R, P	H, R, P	H, R, P	H				H	P	R, P: pancreatic, adrenal R: embryo-fetal
Temsirolimus (mTOR)	H, P	H, R, P	R	R	H				H	H, R	R, P	H: hyperglycemia R: embryo-fetal
Tofacitinib (Jak1/2/3, TYK2)	H, R	H, R, P										R: embryo-fetal
Trametinib (MEK1/2)	R, D	R	R	H, R	H, R, D		H	H	H, D		R	H: secondary malignancies Rabbits: embryo-fetal
Vandetanib (RIPK2, EGFR, DDR1 Abl, Lck, RET, MEK5, EphA6, STK35, VEGFR2/3, Flt3)	R, D			H, R, D	H, R	H	H		H, R	R		R: pancreatic; embryo-fetal; masses in long-term study
Vemurafenib (A/B/C-Raf, B-Raf[V600E])		H	H, D	H, D	H		H					H: phototoxicity

Adverse effects listed were described in the public literature, drug labels, or FDA reviews. (*Source:* http://www.accessdata.fda.gov/scripts/cder/drugsatfda/index.cfm, last accessed August 5, 2014).

a) H, human; R, rodent; D, dog; P, nonhuman primate; M, mini-pig.

biological makeup of the patient is the determining factor in the initiation of toxicity [7].

The first small-molecule KI drug was approved by FDA in 1999, but over half of the available drugs in this class were approved in the past 4 years (Table 15.1). A review from 2009 [8] contained 9 small-molecule KIs, while the number is now 26. The limited amount of time since approval for most KIs means that there is little postapproval experience with these drugs and a relatively small amount of published literature on their adverse effects. Since a significant proportion of known adverse effects is not recognized until a drug has been on the market for several years [9], it is highly likely that the spectrum of adverse effects attributed to KI will become broader in coming years. The use of approved drugs for new indications may also give rise to new adverse effects, as different patient populations are exposed for different time periods.

Kinases as drug targets and antitargets are introduced in Chapter 15. Characterization of drug binding to a target as "selective" is relative, as the activity of the drug is due to the nature of the binding as well as the concentration of the drug at the binding site. Initial KI drugs were considered selective, but as additional kinases and intracellular pathways were discovered, in many cases the extent of selectivity was found to be reduced. A good example of this is imatinib, which when discovered was profiled against the panel of 27 kinases known and available at the time and considered to be highly selective for Abl kinases [3]. The only other significant activity was against PDGFR. As the kinase literature increased and new screens became available, imatinib was profiled against additional targets and found to also interact with Kit, cFms, and DDR2.

Due to the use of ATP as the phosphate donor substrate, all protein kinases share a conserved kinase active site core. Almost all small-molecule inhibitors of protein kinases target the ATP binding domain of the enzyme and, while high inhibitory potency is often readily achievable, target specificity is effectively impossible due to the highly conserved nature of the ATP binding domain. In a screen of 20 KIs, including 16 that were approved drugs or in clinical development, against a panel of 119 protein kinases (less than 24% of the human kinome), Fabian *et al.* demonstrated that target specificity was highly variable and did not correlate with chemical structure or the identity of the targeted kinase [10]. It should be noted that the active site of kinase proteins can be highly flexible upon binding, whereby the inhibitor induces a fit by causing the protein amino acids to be displaced and reposition. In these cases, for example, the DFG out motif, the protein active site becomes highly dissimilar to other kinases and a high degree of specificity can be attained (e.g., Imatinib/Abl). More recent, broader ranging studies have shown the same lack of specificity and unpredictability of activity spectra for small-molecule inhibitors [11,12]. To muddy the waters further, kinases themselves can be promiscuous, phosphorylating many different proteins [13] and a single protein may be phosphorylated by multiple kinases [14]. As a result, it is challenging to design a molecule to modulate a single biological function via inhibition of a particular kinase, and polypharmacology may be the rule rather than the exception for KI.

16.2 Perspectives on the Clinical Safety of Kinase Inhibitor Therapy

The first approved small-molecule drugs specifically designed to target kinases were inhibitors of the BCR-ABL fusion protein (imatinib) and epidermal growth factor receptor (EGFR) (erlotinib and gefitinib). These drugs have been on the market for over 10 years now and there is a reasonable amount of clinical experience in their use. Myelosuppression is the most common side effect of agents targeting the BCR-ABL fusion protein in chronic myelocytic leukemia (CML) and can be managed clinically by dose reduction or pausing therapy, or by treatment with platelet and red blood cell transfusions, growth factors, and antibiotic prophylaxis [5]. Similarly, one of the most common adverse effects following treatment of advanced lung, pancreatic, colorectal, and head and neck cancers with inhibitors of EGFR is acneiform rash [6,15], which, although it can impact quality of life and lead to treatment cessation, is non-life-threatening [16].

Some adverse effects of KI can be attributed to the biological functions of the targeted enzymes. For example, EGFR-related skin toxicities are dose dependent, and thought to result from blockade of the receptor's activity in follicular and interfollicular epidermal growth signaling. Indeed, skin rash has been suggested as a surrogate biomarker of clinical response, and a "dose to rash" protocol adopted in dose escalation clinical trials with some EGFR inhibitors, and aggressive treatment of the symptoms is recommended to prevent treatment cessation [15,17]. Similarly, secondary hypertension and vascular thrombosis are commonly associated with the antiangiogenic KIs such as sunitinib, sorafenib, and axitinib [18].

Both the pattern and severity of observed adverse effects are dependent on the particular spectrum of target activities of KI. Imatinib, nilotinib, and dasatinib, used in the treatment of CML, are all inhibitors of ABL and PDGFR kinases. They each demonstrate a distinct inhibitory spectrum across multiple kinases, which impacts the toxicities observed with each in clinical use. For example, although myelosuppression is a common side effect of treatment with each of these agents, the severity of the effect may be related to the relative potency for inhibition of c-KIT. Peripheral edema is a common side effect in imatinib-treated patients (55.5%) and to a lesser extent dasatinib (18%), but is relatively rare in nilotinib (<4%). This is thought to reflect, at least in part, their relative potencies for PDGFR [5]. The severe adverse effect of pleural effusion, on the other hand, is rare in imatinib or nilotinib treatment, but is a relatively common occurrence (14–30%) in clinical trials with dasatinib [5,19]. Dasatinib is a multikinase inhibitor with potent activity against a wide range of kinases in addition to BCR-ABL, including several kinases implicated in angiogenesis and vascular integrity such as PDGFR-β and Src family kinases. The particular mechanism of dasatinib-induced pleural effusions is as yet unclear, but may be multifactorial [19–21].

Another promiscuous KI, sunitinib, approved for the treatment of renal cell carcinoma (RCC) and imatinib-resistant gastrointestinal stromal tumor (GIST), has been associated with severe cardiovascular adverse effects. In a phase I/II clinical trial with 75 patients, 8 experienced a cardiovascular event and 6 suffered congestive heart failure [22]. Sunitinib cardiotoxicity involves mitochondrial dysfunction and cardiomyocyte cytotoxicity, and is likely related to off-target inhibition of AMPK [23].

While a degree of severe toxicity may be acceptable in treatments for life-threatening diseases such as cancer, kinases are increasingly being targeted for chronic diseases such as rheumatoid arthritis and ulcerative colitis [24–26]. Tolerance of severe adverse effects in such indications is lower, and a more thorough understanding of the causal links between kinase inhibition profiles and adverse outcomes will be increasingly important in successful drug discovery and development for these indications. Compounds with cleaner safety profiles will be both more likely to gain regulatory approval and be competitive in the marketplace.

16.3 Adverse Effects of Kinase Inhibitor Drugs

Specific adverse effects of small-molecule KI drugs are described in this section. Biologics that are inhibitors of kinase function are not addressed in this chapter, but many of these molecules have similar adverse effects, if they affect the same molecular target as the small molecule. Some biologics are more specific in their kinase interactions than small molecules, and have fewer side effects. There is more published literature on clinical adverse effects of KI than there is on nonclinical adverse effects. Due to the relatively recent development of most approved KIs and the lack of published literature, the information in this section is taken from the following sources: published literature, when available, as well as drug labels and clinical medical and nonclinical pharmacology reviews published on the FDA website (http://www.accessdata.fda.gov/scripts/cder/drugsatfda/index.cfm) and accessed between May 1 and 9, 2014. Tissues with toxicities that are not clearly kinase mediated are mentioned first, followed by tissue where at least some of the toxicities are target related.

16.3.1 Hepatic Toxicity

Drug-induced liver injury (DILI) is a major cause of hepatic failure, and is also the most common cause of failure of drugs during both preclinical and clinical development. The manifestation of DILI is covered extensively in Chapters 5–9. A wide variety of drugs can result in liver injury, including KI, antibiotics, CNS drugs, and nonsteroidal anti-inflammatory drugs (NSAIDS) [27]. In general, the overall risk of serious hepatotoxicity across all drug treatments is quite low, and has been estimated at 10–15 cases per 100 000 patient-years. Because of the low incidence, idiosyncratic DILI is not expected to be observed in clinical trials [28].

Hepatotoxicity of tyrosine kinase inhibitors has been observed in both preclinical and clinical settings. In a meta-analysis, PubMed was reviewed for phase III randomized trials with axitinib, pazopanib, sorafenib, sunitinib, regorafenib, or vandetanib. Results from 3689 patients in phase III trials during 2006–2012 showed that hepatotoxicity is fairly common and occurs in 23–40% of treated patients [29]. Only 5% of treated patients, however, had grade 3–4 hepatotoxicity. Hepatotoxicity was characterized by increases in ALT (34% treated versus 24.3% control), AST (39.2% treated versus 24% control), and bilirubin (21.8% treated versus 11.2% control). One complicating aspect of these levels, however, is that increased serum transaminases are often present in patients with liver metastases and thus biopsy is required to confirm drug-related hepatotoxicity. In another meta-analysis, phase II and III trial results from over 3000 patients treated with gefitinib, lapatinib, pazopanib, erlotinib, imatinib, sorafenib, and vandetanib were scored. Patients treated with a KI were four times more likely to experience a high grade (≥3) hepatic event [30]. In this analysis, the increase in odds of hepatotoxicity was due to increased odds of elevation of AST and ALT, but not bilirubin levels. These statistics of hepatotoxicity frequency may be an underestimate of the true prevalence, since a meta-analysis approach is dependent on the reporting of the hepatic adverse events in the literature, as opposed to a direct review of patient records.

Sixteen of the 26 of the marketed KI have prescribing information requiring monitoring of liver function during clinical use, including all of the relatively selective EGFR inhibitors, the VEGFR inhibitors, and the BCR-ABL inhibitors with the exception of dasatinib. Dasatinib did, however, cause hepatotoxicity in animals. Time to onset of hepatic injury varies from several days to months following treatment, and for the most part, the hepatotoxicity is described as hepatocellular necrosis [31,32]. The toxicity is usually reversible upon discontinuation of the drug, but for seven of the marketed KIs, fatal cases of hepatic failure have been reported. The majority of the marketed KIs are used to treat cancer, and thus due to the severity of the disease, some degree of hepatotoxicity is considered acceptable because of the overall drug benefit. As newer KIs come to market especially for nononcology indications, the requirements for safety will likely be more stringent. Since it may take some time for broader patient use to reveal adverse effects of very low incidence, hepatotoxicity of recently marketed KI may not be recognized for several years.

16.3.1.1 **Role of Metabolism and Clearance Pathways in Hepatotoxicity**

CYP-mediated metabolism is a predominant mechanism contributing to DILI, including KI-induced hepatotoxicity. Erlotinib-induced hepatotoxicity is thought to be the result of CYP-mediated bioactivation via CYP3A4/5 and CYP1A2. Li demonstrated the formation of erlotinib–GSH adducts and proposed that both epoxide and quinone-imine intermediates are generated that can react with cellular nucleophiles [33]. Erlotinib treatment has also been associated with

Stevens–Johnson syndrome and epidermal necrolysis, which is consistent with metabolic activation and reactive intermediates [34]. Lapatinib was approved for use by the FDA in 2007, but in 2008 a black-boxed warning was issued due to reports of hepatotoxicity, including rare cases of liver toxicity-related deaths. Lapatinib undergoes CYP-mediated metabolism and causes mechanism-based inactivation of CYP3A4 and CYP3A5 via covalent modification of the apoprotein and/or the heme moiety, likely contributing to liver toxicity [35].

Pazopanib also inhibits multiple CYP enzymes, and the contribution of this inhibition to metabolism of CYP-specific probe drugs was investigated in a clinical trial in patients with advanced renal cell carcinoma [36]. Pazopanib inhibited the metabolism of dextromethorphan by CYP2D6 as evidenced by an increase in urine dextromethorphan levels. There was no effect on metabolism of drugs specific for CYP1A2, CYP2C9, or CYP2C19. Coadministration of midazolam (CYP3A specific) and pazopanib 800 mg once daily resulted in a ~30–35% increase in midazolam AUC and C_{max}, consistent with pazopanib acting as a weak inhibitor of CYP3A enzymes. In another study, administration of once-daily pazopanib 800 mg and weekly paclitaxel (a CYP3A4 and CYP2C8 substrate) increased the mean paclitaxel AUC (40%) and C_{max} (30%), relative to treatment with weekly paclitaxel alone [37].

These results demonstrate a contribution of CYP metabolism to KI-induced liver injury and suggest that coadministration of KI with strong CYP3A4 inhibitors may increase serum KI concentrations, increasing the risk for toxicity. Conversely, strong CYP3A4 inducers may decrease serum concentrations, potentially leading to reduced efficacy.

UGT1A1 is a UDP-glucuronosyltransferase, an enzyme important in clearing bilirubin from the systemic circulation. It is the major isoform responsible for glucuronidation of bilirubin, and thus deficiencies of this enzyme result in increased levels of bilirubin, one of the hallmarks of hepatotoxicity. Gilbert's syndrome patients carry a common genetic variant, *UGT1A1*28*, and have increased levels of bilirubin and mild jaundice without overt liver disease [38]. A number of KIs, including regorafenib, erlotinib, nilotinib, sorafenib, and pazopanib, are UGT1A1 inhibitors. Drug-induced increases in bilirubin resulting from enzyme inhibition can be exacerbated in patients with Gilbert's syndrome, resulting in even higher levels of unconjugated bilirubin, an effect that has been noted for lapatinib and pazopanib [28].

UDP-glucuronosyltransferase 1A9 is another glucuronosyltransferase isozyme, and is the predominant enzyme responsible for acetaminophen glucuronidation. Clinically, coadministration of drugs with acetaminophen can result in lower acetaminophen clearance, thus increasing the risk of acetaminophen toxicity. In fact, coadministration of acetaminophen with imatinib and sunitinib has resulted in liver failure [39,40]. This inhibition can be detected preclinically, as nine different KIs were shown to inhibit UGT1A9 activity in human liver microsomes [41] suggesting that *in vitro* assays are a useful part of a screening strategy to assess potential toxicity resulting from inhibition of glucuronidation.

Many KIs are substrates for ATP-binding cassette subfamily B member 1 (MDR1, P-gp) and ATP-binding cassette subfamily G member 2 (ABCG2, BCRP), and several others also inhibit the hepatic organic anion-transporting polypeptide 1B t(OATP1B1) [42]. Pazopanib inhibits OATP1B1, and is a substrate for MDR1 and ABCG2, activities also shared by the statins, which are widely used to treat hypercholesterolemia [43]. A summary analysis of pazopanib trials involving 976 patients showed that incidence of elevated ALT (three or more times ULN) was 21% in patients who received both pazopanib and any statin and 14% in patients who received only pazopanib [44]. An accompanying pharmacogenetic analysis demonstrated that the ABCG2 421C>A polymorphism may be associated with ALT elevation in patients taking pazopanib and simvastatin. Those with the variant allele had a higher incidence of ALT $\geq 3\times$ ULN (5/7, 71%) compared with patients with wild-type genotype (2/21, 10%; odds ratio = 19.6). This polymorphism was not associated with ALT elevations in pazopanib-treated patients without concurrent use of statins. This study showed that concomitant use of pazopanib and simvastatin increased the risk of transaminase elevations in patients with cancer, and suggests that discontinuation of simvastatin may be required to manage the risk of liver injury. Many KIs are metabolized via the same mechanisms as pazopanib, and thus coadministration with the statins is considered a risk for hepatotoxicity, which is shared across the class.

16.3.1.2 Genetic Risk Factors for Hepatotoxicity

Besides the increased hepatic risks resulting from genetic polymorphisms in transport proteins already described, additional genetic risk factors have been linked to increased ALT levels during KI therapy. Human leukocyte antigen (HLA) variants have been associated with a variety of drug hypersensitivity responses [45], and the HLA variants DQA1/DRB1 have been linked to ximelagatran-induced hepatotoxicity [46]. Genetic analysis from two separate studies of patients treated with lapatinib showed the association of these two HLA variants (*DQA1**02:01 and *DRB1**07:01) with lapatinib-induced increases in serum ALT [28,47,48]. Indeed, all 11 patients that had ALT increases more than fivefold ULN were carriers of these alleles. These results suggest the involvement of immune system-mediated mechanisms in lapatinib-induced hepatotoxicity, and it has been suggested that the inactivation of CYP3A isoforms by lapatinib may result in hapten formation leading to the hypersensitivity response in patients carrying these HLA variants. Not all lapatinib-treated patients carrying these variants have liver injury however, suggesting that additional factors contribute to the hepatotoxicity phenotype, consistent with other findings on the role of HLA in drug hypersensitivity [49]. A nonimmune system gene polymorphism associated with pazopanib ALT elevations is in the HFE gene, indicating a potential relationship to iron homeostasis. Further associations of hepatotoxicity with genetic loci and immune system genes are likely to be identified in the future.

16.3.1.3 Preclinical Evaluation of Hepatotoxicity

In preclinical animal models, the major liver finding observed is usually an increase in ALT and/or AST levels, with histopathology confirming the effect. Animal *in vivo* studies, however, are not completely predictive of human hepatotoxicity. A joint study involving 12 pharmaceutical companies with data compiled from 150 compounds showed that translation from rodent and nonrodent species to humans was 71%. When considering hepatotoxic drugs only, the translation fell to 55% [50,51]. This is thought to be due, at least in part, to the insensitivity of aminotransferase enzyme levels as biomarkers in animal models [52]. In addition to these species-specific differences, patient-related risk factors such as underlying disease, age, comedications, activation of the innate immune system, and genetic predispositions are not captured in animal studies.

For KI specifically, animal studies have not been highly predictive of human hepatotoxicity. Of the 26 KIs approved in the United States, 16 have hepatotoxicity as a warning or precaution in the label, and there is some evidence that dasatinib can cause clinical hepatotoxicity (Table 16.1). Of these 17 clinically important hepatotoxicants, only 10 were also hepatotoxic in animal studies. Seven of the 17 compounds were hepatotoxic in rats. Not all 17 compounds were tested in dogs and nonhuman primates (NHP); however, of the 11 tested in dogs, only 6 showed hepatotoxicity, and of the 6 tested in NHP, 3 showed hepatotoxicity in that species. There were only a few false-positive signals from animal studies where two of the nine KIs negative for clinical hepatotoxicity showed hepatotoxicity in the rat, and no false-positive signals in dog or primates. Before making conclusions about the predictive power of these animal models, however, it is important to recognize that in many cases the animal exposures were lower than the human exposures achieved in the clinic, due to the higher sensitivity of animals to some KIs.

Multiple mechanisms are thought to contribute to DILI. Formation of reactive oxygen species (ROS) and mitochondrial dysfunction play key roles [45,53]. Acetominophen-induced hepatotoxicity has been well studied, revealing several key steps leading to liver injury. Reactive metabolite formation, following saturation of the major sulfation and glucoronidation detoxification pathways, results in mitochondrial glutathione depletion, covalent binding to cellular proteins, and disruption of mitochondrial function. ROS are subsequently generated leading to mitochondrial DNA damage and opening of the mitochondrial transition pore, leading to cell injury and death. A number of kinases are implicated in the development of acetaminophen-induced DILI, including JNK, GSK3β, and ASK. JNK inhibition, either through siRNA or via small-molecule inhibitors, protects against acetaminophen hepatotoxicity *in vivo* [54,55]. It is possible that off-target inhibition of other kinases involved in defense, repair, or inflammatory pathways could have positive or negative effects on hepatotoxic liabilities. For example, inhibition of GSK-3β protects against ischemia reperfusion injury in the liver through an immune modulatory mechanism [56], although gene knockouts of GSK-3β in mice are embryo-lethal due to hepatocyte apoptosis during development [57].

A number of cell-based systems, including primary hepatocyte cultures, have been used to model hepatotoxicity *in vitro*. In comparison with immortalized and hepatocellular cancer cell lines, such as HepG2, primary hepatocyte cultures have a higher capacity for metabolic activation, which is a key component of liver injury. Dasatinib, a KI targeting BCR-ABL and Src family kinases for the treatment of chronic myeloid leukemia (CML) and Philadelphia chromosome-positive acute lymphoblastic leukemia (ALL), causes hepatotoxicity in some patients. Hepatocyte degeneration is also observed in Sprague-Dawley rats treated with dasatinib. Treatment of primary hepatocytes results in increased reactive oxygen species generation, decreased mitochondrial membrane potential, and activation of apoptotic proteins leading to LDH release and reduced cell viability, suggesting that a reactive metabolite mechanism of action is responsible for dasatinib hepatotoxicity [58].

Newer models using two or three-dimensional cocultures, flow-based cocultures, or induced stem cell cultures may provide a more "liver-like" model with better predictivity of *in vivo* hepatotoxic liability. These more complex systems may also offer opportunities to investigate in more detail the mechanisms by which the KIs induce liver injury [51,59,60].

16.3.2
Thyroid Toxicity

Thyroid hormones are important for the normal development and function of a variety of organs. There are two forms of thyroid hormone: 3,3′,5,5′-tetraiodothyronine (T4) and 3,3′,5-triiodothyronine (T3), which are produced and secreted from the thyroid gland. T4 undergoes deiodination to T3, which binds to nuclear thyroid receptors. These receptors act as a transcription factor to induce a variety of genes, which regulate protein, fat, and carbohydrate metabolism. In the general population, the incidence of hypothyroidism is ~3–4% [61,62].

Treatment with KI can lead to thyroid dysfunction with a reported prevalence of 14% to as high as 85%, although the severity is usually low, with 2% at Grade 3 or 4 [63,64]. The KIs that have been associated most with hypothyroidism are sunitinib, sorafenib, axitinib, pazopanib, vandetanib, and imatinib. Symptoms of hypothyroidism include anorexia, fatigue, and cold intolerance. Clemons *et al.* [64] carried out a retrospective chart analysis of patients treated with sunitinib or sorafenib from 2005 to 2011. Among patients with normal baseline thyroid function, 15 (44%) of 34 patients treated with sunitinib and 6 (27%) of 22 patients treated with sorafenib developed hypothyroidism. These results agree with other summarized data demonstrating that patients treated with sunitinib have a twofold increased risk of requiring thyroid hormone replacement therapy compared with sorafenib [65,66]. The development of hypothyroidism was associated with a longer progression-free survival of 18.2 months (treated) versus 10.1 months (untreated).

16.3.2.1 Mechanistic Basis of Thyroid Toxicity

The exact molecular mechanisms leading to hypothyroidism are not known, but KI-mediated inhibition of VEGFR, PDGFR, RET, and BRAF are thought to be major contributors. VEGF plays an essential role in embryonic development and, in the adult VEGF is a survival factor for some tumor blood vessels, thus explaining the efficacy of VEGFR KI in inhibiting angiogenesis and halting tumor growth. The majority of adult normal vasculature does not depend on VEGF for survival; however, certain organs, including thyroid, pancreas, pituitary, and adrenal cortex are VEGF dependent. Thyroid gland is well vascularized and shows the highest blood flow rates per unit weight of any tissue in the body [67]. Treatment of normal mice with the VEGFR inhibitor AG-013736 for 21 days resulted in a 68% regression of thyroid capillaries, as measured by CD31 immunoreactivity, and serum TSH levels were increased 19-fold compared with the control group [68]. Vascular regression in mouse thyroids after treatment with AG-013736 was completely reversed within 2 weeks after treatment by the regrowth of capillaries. Similarly, hypothyroidism in patients resulting from VEGFR KI treatment is usually reversible following drug withdrawal.

Besides the effects on capillaries, additional mechanisms may contribute to KI-induced hypothyroidism. Increased hepatic deiodinase (D3) activity was demonstrated in rats administered sunitinib for 8 days [69]. A corresponding decrease in serum levels of both T3 and T4 was observed, reflecting this increase in T4/T3 metabolism. In the same report, clinical translation of this mechanism was noted in a retrospective analysis of patients treated with sunitinib for 10 weeks. Forty-two percent of the patients developed elevated TSH levels with a decreased T3/rT3 ratio, consistent with increased metabolism. Similarly, decreased T3/T4 and T3/rT3 ratios were noted in patients treated with sorafenib, also suggesting increased type 3 deiodination [70].

Decreased iodine uptake may be another contributory mechanism. In a study of 24 sunitinib-treated patients, no antithyroid autoantibodies or changes in thyroglobulin levels were detected, and thyroid gland echography was normal, all of which suggests a lack of direct effect on thyroid cells [71]. In five out of six patients tested however, ^{123}Iodine uptake was below the lower normal limit of radioiodine uptake (15–45%).

16.3.2.2 Clinical Management of Thyroid Toxicity

Several studies have demonstrated a correlation between KI-induced hypothyroidism and improved progression-free survival [66,72]. Although not validated, this may suggest that TSH can be a biomarker of treatment efficacy. Thyroid hormones however may themselves promote tumor growth by stimulating growth factors, and thus the observed hypothyroidism may contribute to KI efficacy. One of the symptoms of hypothyroidism is fatigue, and it is not known whether this is the primary mechanism for KI-induced fatigue. Although a clear consensus appears to be lacking, patients with overt hypothyroidism and suffering from associated symptoms are treated with levothyroxine [65]. Further clinical trials are needed to address the importance of hypothyroidism and the role of thyroid replacement in KI therapy.

16.3.3 Bone and Tooth Toxicity

Clinical evidence of the effects of KI on bone is scarce, but several marketed compounds are reported to cause changes in bone metabolism [8]. Dasatinib increases trabecular bone volume in rats [73], and decreases markers of bone resorption in humans [74]. Mechanisms responsible for this effect are inhibition of SRC kinases and cFms, resulting in osteoclast activity inhibition. Hypophosphatemia in imatinib patients led to the speculation that bone formation and resorption were being inhibited [75], but more recently it was shown that imatinib can increase bone formation in patients [76]. In healthy, normal rats, however, imatinib treatment did not result in an increase in bone volume [77]. The kinases c-KIT and PDGFR-A are expressed on osteoclasts and osteoblasts, which may contribute to the potential for KI bone effects, and bone changes may result in a secondary hyperparathyroidism in patients [78]. In addition, the antiangiogenic properties of some KI may lead to an exacerbation of osteonecrosis of the jaw from bisphosphonate treatments [78]. Preclinically, the inhibitors of VEGFR, PDGFR, and FGFR appear to cause bone effects in rats and dogs, particularly at the growth plates.

Tooth development is divided into three stages: initiation, bud stage, and morphogenesis. This process occurs as a result of interactions between epithelium and mesenchymal cells. The tooth has been considered one of the simplest organs in the body, but its developmental regulation is quite complex and is controlled by four major groups of signaling molecules: FGF, bone morphogenetic proteins (BMPs), Wnt signaling, and Sonic hedgehog [79–82]. The corresponding signaling pathways contain a number of kinases, accounting for the deleterious effects of KI on teeth.

Growth factors induce epithelial cell proliferation during the initiation stage of tooth formation. This is followed by further proliferation and epithelial migration into areas of mesenchymal cells during the budding stage. Mesenchymal cells, in turn, play a role in the later stages of tooth formation and tooth buds differentiate in response to further molecular signals to form the final tooth organ [81].

FGF, VEGF, and PDGF are involved in several aspects of tooth development and are expressed in both epithelial and mesenchymal cells. At least 12 of the 22 members of the FGF family have been shown to play a role in the process, from initiation of tooth development to maintaining the final mineralized tissue [83]. In rodents, the incisors continuously grow throughout the life of the animal, and FGF is required to maintain the stem cells that support this process. FGF family members regulate the function of both epithelial and mesenchymal cells. In FGF-$3^{-/-}$, FGF-$10^{+/-}$ mutant mice, for example, the enamel layer of teeth is either thin or absent [83,84]. The brown color of rodent teeth is a result of iron-containing pigments in ameloblastic epithelial cells, and treatment of rats with VEGFR/FGFR inhibitors results in white teeth due to the inhibition of these epithelial cells [85].

Given the importance of FGF and VEGFR as critical players in tooth development, it is not surprising that KIs inhibiting these kinases have been associated with tooth toxicity in preclinical studies, especially in rodent (Table 16.1). These inhibitors include sunitinib, sorafenib, vandetanib, pazopanib, and regorafenib. In clinical studies, however, dental effects have not been a major adverse effect associated with compound treatment and generally are not reported in the list of significant adverse reactions [86–89]. Although effects on teeth appear to be an on-target mechanism, it is normally not manifested to any appreciable level in the patient population, perhaps due to a lower proliferative index in humans compared with rodents.

16.3.4 Cardiovascular Toxicity

Cardiovascular effects have been serious and dose limiting for many approved KIs and undoubtedly have prevented other compounds from reaching the market. The types of cardiovascular effects observed with these compounds range from blood pressure alterations to myocardial necrosis and valvular effects. For a thorough discussion of the cardiovascular effects of KI, refer to Chapter 17.

16.3.5 Cutaneous Toxicity

Treatment with any of the EGFR inhibitors (gefitinib, erlotinib, and lapatinib) as well as multikinase inhibitors of VEGFR, B-raf, and PDGFR (sorafenib, sunitinib, pazopanib, and vandetanib) results in cutaneous toxicities of any grade in 50–100% of patients, with grade 3 or above in 5–30% of patients [90]. These skin effects are often the second most common adverse effect following GI effects, and the toxicities manifest as rash, abnormalities in hair growth, dry and itchy skin (xerosis), and nail inflammation.

Rash is the most common cutaneous toxicity and presents as an acne-like rash with papulopustules of the face, scalp, and trunk. It differs from acne in that it is sometimes itchy and is not accompanied by comedones (blackheads or whiteheads). The rash is early in onset following KI treatment, usually occurring after 1 week, and for patients with grade 3 or higher, the rash can be quite painful, requiring dose reduction or drug holiday [91]. The occurrence of the rash is often considered as a positive correlation with antitumor activity; however, the severity is not consistently linked to efficacy, so it is not considered a biomarker [92]. Hand–foot skin reaction is a more severe toxicity that is characterized by painful blisters on pressure or friction areas such as palms, fingertips, and sides of the feet. These lesions can progress to thickened, hyperkeratotic skin, and VEGFR and PDGFR inhibition is the proposed underlying mechanism [93].

Xerosis (dry skin) and changes in head and body hair are additional cutaneous toxicities associated with EGFR inhibitors. These side effects gradually develop over several weeks or months of treatment. Alopecia and changes in hair texture are the most frequent observation, and in women, facial hypertrichosis has been noted. In some patients treated with sunitinib, hair depigmentation can occur, which has been hypothesized to be the result of c-kit inhibition leading to decreased melanogenesis [91,94].

16.3.5.1 Mechanistic Basis of Cutaneous Toxicity

KI-related cutaneous toxicities are thought to be a direct reflection of the on-target activity of EGFR inhibitors, because of the critical roles that EGFR plays in the epidermis [90]. The skin is composed of three layers: the epidermis, which is the most superficial layer, and underneath the dermis and hypodermis. Keratinocytes, which make up ~90% of the epidermis, normally undergo differentiation and migration toward the skin surface, followed by a final stage of apoptosis and formation of the stratum corneum, the skin layer that forms a protective barrier. EGFR is a master regulator of all these processes, and inhibition of EGFR signaling induces growth arrest, apoptosis, and premature differentiation (Figure 16.1). EGFR inhibitors decrease expression of cytoskeletal proteins such as vinculin and inhibit cell migration, all of which contribute to the rash phenotype. Impairment of the epidermal barrier results in a secondary inflammatory response that results in an increase in cytokine production and chemokines such as CCL18, CXCL9, and CXCL1, all of which contribute to the skin inflammation that accompanies treatment with EGFR inhibitors. Mutant mice with decreased/nonfunctional EGFR have a number of epidermal defects such as thin skin and abnormal hair follicles, including an inflammatory component, providing genetic evidence for the central role of EGFR in skin physiology [95,96].

The hair growth cycle consists of three phases: growth (anagen), involution (catagen), and resting (telogen). Epidermal growth factor receptor is localized into the outer root sheath of the hair follicle, and activation of EGFR controls the progression from anagen to catagen. Inhibition of this mechanism results in the reversible, late-onset alopecia commonly seen in patients treated with EGFR inhibitors [91].

16.3.5.2 Preclinical Evaluation of Cutaneous Toxicity

Rats and dogs both demonstrate skin lesions when treated with multiple doses of EGFR inhibitors. As already stated, mouse genetic models have demonstrated the role of EGFR in skin physiology. EGFR-deficient mice die prematurely, but show abnormalities in epidermis and hair follicles [97]. Mice expressing a dominant negative EGFR have altered hair characteristics leading to alopecia. They show epidermal hyperplasia and infiltration of the skin with inflammatory elements. Furthermore, in isolated skin keratinocytes from mutant mice, EGFR autophosphorylation was markedly decreased following EGF stimulation [97].

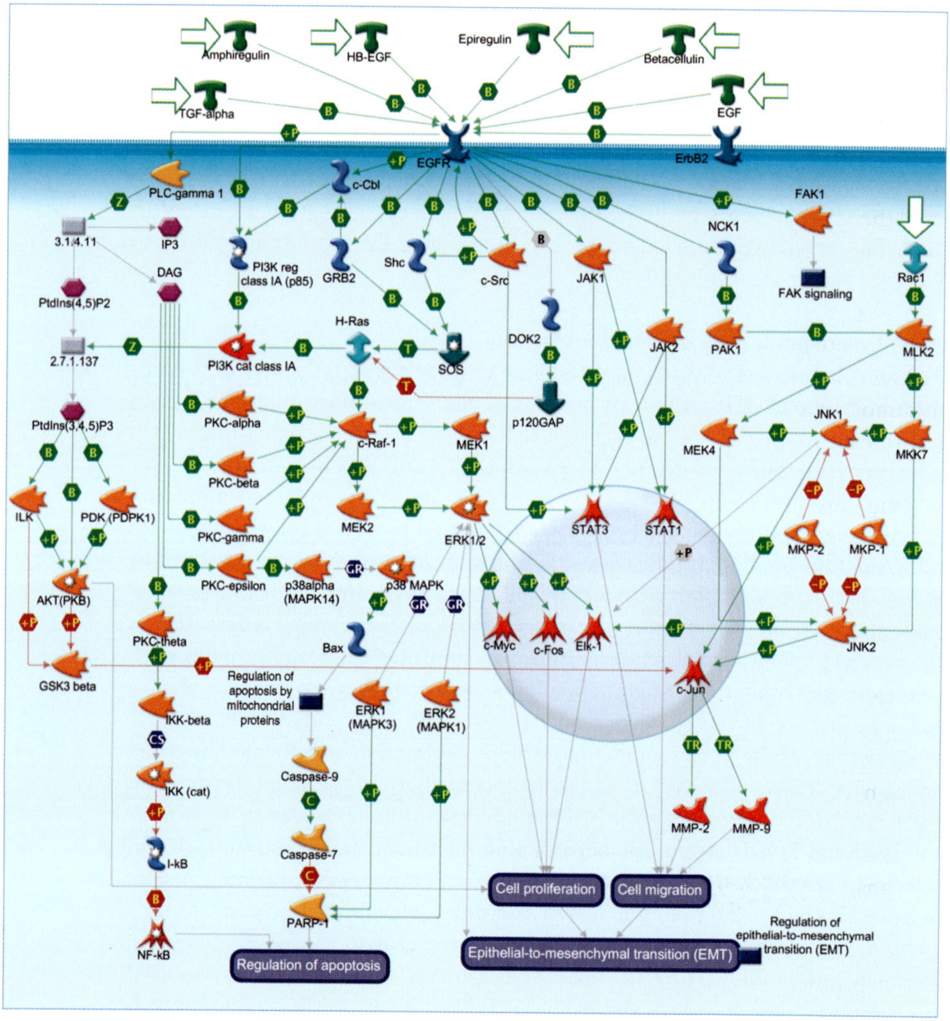

Figure 16.1 EGFR signaling impacts cell proliferation and migration and apoptosis through interactions with other kinases, including JAK1/2, Src, MEK, and ERK1/2. Compounds are represented by hexagons, proteins by solid shapes representing different classes of compound, and enzymatic reactions by gray rectangles. Protein–protein, compound–protein, and compound–reaction interactions are shown as unidirectional arrows, and a mechanism of interaction represented by letters in hexagonal boxes over the arrows. Red color of interactions and mechanisms represents a negative effect (inhibition and downregulation) and green a positive effect (activation and upregulation). (Reprinted with permission from Thomson Reuters (MetaCore™). Full legend available at https://ftp.genego.com/files/MC_legend.pdf.)

Nude mice treated with erlotinib develop skin lesions, including the recruitment of inflammatory cells [98]. The role of EGFR signaling has also been shown in cultured normal human kertatinocytes, and treatment with EGFR inhibitors induces apoptosis, and expression of the differentiation markers keratin 1 (KRT1) and KRT10 can be followed in these cultures. The contribution of EGFR signaling to the inflammatory component of skin reactions has also been studied in epithelial cells, where treatment with an EGFR inhibitor increased CCL2, CCL5, and CXCL10 levels [99].

16.3.5.3 Clinical Management of Cutaneous Toxicity

Systemic treatment with tetracycline derivatives, usually doxycycline, is the most effective treatment for the cutaneous toxicity and does not interfere with the antitumor activity of the KI [100]. In a clinical trial with 60 patients, treatment with tetracycline reduced the intensity but not the incidence of rash, but also improved the quality of life of the patients [101]. If skin lesions are severe, reducing drug dose may be necessary. For less severe cases of rash, topical antibiotics and corticosteroid creams have shown efficacy in relieving symptoms [94].

16.3.6 Developmental and Reproductive Toxicity

Because of the critical role of kinases in cell cycle, apoptosis, proliferation, and developmental processes, the potential for affecting fetal development is particularly high. Indeed, of the 33 FDA-approved KIs (Tables 15.1 and 15.2), all but one are given an FDA pregnancy classification of C (animal reproduction studies have shown an adverse effect on the fetus and there are no adequate and well-controlled studies in humans, but potential benefits may warrant use of the drug in pregnant women despite potential risks) or D (there is positive evidence of human fetal risk based on adverse reaction data from investigational or marketing experience or studies in humans, but potential benefits may warrant use of the drug in pregnant women despite potential risks). The exception is the VEGF inhibitory RNA aptamer pegaptanib, which is indicated for wet macular degeneration. Pegaptinib has a pregnancy category of B (animal reproduction studies have failed to demonstrate a risk to the fetus and there are no adequate and well-controlled studies in pregnant women). The use of pegaptinib in a generally older patient population and its particular method of delivery by intraocular injection mean that the risk of systemic exposure during pregnancy is very low for this KI.

The extraordinary success of imatinib and other BCR-ABL-directed KIs in treating CML means that patients diagnosed in the chronic phase can now reasonably anticipate a normal life expectancy. In the 11 years since the marketing approval of this drug, a reasonable body of data has been generated regarding its effects on fertility and fetal development. Over 150 conceptions have been reported by men during treatment with imatinib, of which all but two resulted in normal deliveries [102]. In women treated with imatinib, the picture is less rosy. In a recent publication, of the 167 women exposed to imatinib during the organogenesis period of pregnancy, 128 pregnancies and deliveries were uneventful (77%), while 24 ended in spontaneous abortion (14%), a slightly higher percentage than the normal population, and 15 (9%) presented with abnormalities [102]. Abnormalities consist mainly of skeletal malformations, soft tissue abnormalities involving abnormal vessel and organ formation, and low birth weights. Similar toxicities are described in animal studies [103]. Fewer data are available for the newer BCR-ABL targeting KIs nilotinib and dasatinib. In the investigators brochure for nilotinib, 45 cases of exposure during pregnancy are reported with one case of fetal abnormalities and a second case of twins with congenital heart defects, one of which was fatal.

While cases of pregnancy in other cancers treated with KI are yet too sporadic to draw firm conclusions, a recent study of transplant organ recipients treated with the mTOR inhibitor sirolimus reported results from 30 pregnancies with exposure during pregnancy. Nineteen live births and 11 spontaneous abortions resulted. Among the 19 live births, 47% were premature and two infants had birth defects. One infant suffered multiple malformations, including cleft lip and palate and microtia (in this case the mother was concomitantly exposed to mycophenolic acid, also a known teratogen). The second suffered Tetralogy of Fallot. The remaining 17 children were reported normal and based on the very limited data set, sirolimus was not considered to be associated with an increased risk or a pattern of birth defects [104].

16.3.6.1 Preclinical Evaluation of Reproductive Toxicity

Many of the approved KI drugs exhibit reproductive or embryo-fetal toxicity in preclinical studies (Table 16.1). Angiogenesis plays a key role in embryo-fetal development and KIs targeting angiogenic pathways such as VEGF signaling cause embryo-fetal developmental toxicity in rats and rabbits at clinically relevant dose levels [105]. Inhibition of VEGFR itself leads to impaired vascularization of both maternal placenta and fetal organs [106]. EGF signaling is critically involved in the development of several organs, and EGFR knockout mice suffer impaired epithelial development in several organs, including the kidney, and die at midgestation or shortly after birth [107]. The EGFR inhibitor erlotinib, when given during organogenesis, caused embryo-fetal lethality and abortion in rabbits at doses approximately three times the recommended human daily dose. Another EGFR-target KI, gefitinib, caused a reduced number of offspring and reduced fetal weight in rats and rabbits. Generally, developmental toxicity of KI is well predicted in preclinical species.

16.3.6.2 Clinical Management of Reproductive Toxicity

Because of the high potential for developmental toxicity, the use of KI therapy during pregnancy is not recommended. Due to the high potential for exposure to KI during reproductive age in patients with CML, specific recommendations have been made for these patients, whereby KI therapy should be considered only when treatment with interferon-alpha, leukophoresis, or hydroxyurea has been unsuccessful, and then only after the first trimester if at all possible [108,109]. As KI therapy develops for more diseases beyond cancer, careful management of the risks of exposure during pregnancy will be necessary.

16.3.7
Gastrointestinal Toxicity

Gastrointestinal toxicity is commonly seen with KIs as a consequence of their activity on rapidly proliferating cells. Since many cell types in the GI tract replicate at a high rate, through activation of the same pathways used by cancer cells to replicate, they are susceptible to inhibition of the same targets as cancer cells. GI toxicity can result from inhibiting a number of these proliferative mechanisms. A therapeutic index is achieved when targeted cells overexpress these pathways and become dependent on them for continued proliferation, thereby also making them particularly sensitive to pathway inhibition. As shown in Table 16.1, most of the approved KI drugs show GI toxicity in animals as well as in humans.

16.3.8
Hematopoietic Toxicity

Many KI drugs target cancers of the hematopoietic system, others are immunosuppressive, and clinical hematopoietic toxicity is observed with a large number of these drugs (Table 16.1). Some of these compounds are inhibitors of kinases involved in cell cycle regulation through ABL, MEK, JAK/Stat, and related pathways [110]. Other pathways associated with hematopoietic toxicity involve VEGFR, c-kit, and Flt-3 [111]. Effects seen in the bone marrow are often target related and therefore are expected and closely monitored. With promiscuous KIs such as ponatinib, sorafenib, and dasatinib, the multiplicity of targets makes an effect on the rapidly proliferating bone marrow a likely event.

Clinical manifestations of hematopoietic toxicity can be seen at frequencies as high as 72% for neutropenia [111] and 44% for thrombocytopenia [112] with sunitinib. Neutropenia, thrombocytopenia, and anemia are commonly observed adverse events with inhibitors of ABL, BTK, and JAK, and sometimes with VEGFR inhibitors. VEGFR and mTOR inhibitors often exert an immunosuppressive effect on bone marrow, leading to impaired wound healing or susceptibility to infection.

16.3.8.1 Mechanistic Basis of Hematopoietic Toxicity

An examination of the pathways targeted by drugs that affect the hematopoietic system reveals clear indications of the mechanisms behind the effects, in most cases. As the bone marrow tissue is constantly and rapidly proliferating, inhibition of pathways that limit the ability of the tissue to proliferate would be expected to decrease the number of cells produced, leading to the various penias. Inhibition of JAK, ABL, MEK, c-kit, and related targets will have direct effects on cell growth in rapidly proliferating tissues (Figure 16.2). VEGF receptors are

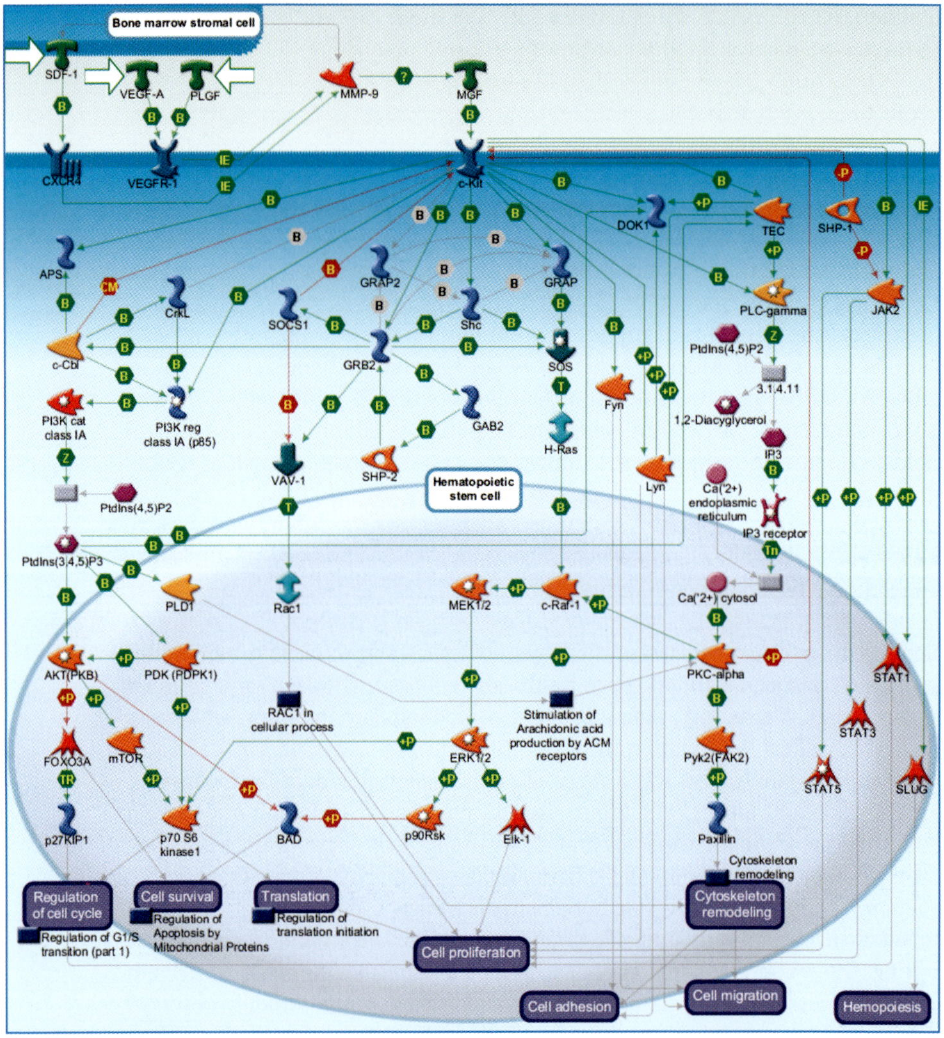

Figure 16.2 Pathways and networks associated with cell survival, proliferation, and cycle regulation in hematopoietic stem cells. Multiple interactions between pathways are shown being mediated through c-Kit and other kinases. Compounds are represented by hexagons, proteins by solid shapes representing different classes of compound, and enzymatic reactions by gray rectangles. Protein–protein, compound–protein, and compound–reaction interactions are shown as unidirectional arrows, and a mechanism of interaction represented by letters in hexagonal boxes over the arrows. Red color of interactions and mechanisms represents a negative effect (inhibition and downregulation) and green a positive effect (activation and upregulation). (Reprinted with permission from Thomson Reuters (MetaCore^{TM}). Full legend available at https://ftp.genego.com/files/MC_legend.pdf.)

known to be expressed on cells in the bone marrow, as well as on circulating monocytes and platelets [113]. Hematopoietic stem cells secrete VEGF, stimulating the growth of myeloid and erythroid lines [114]. Inhibition of vascular function in the bone marrow would also decrease cell maturation and release into the circulation. As shown in Figure 16.1, there is a high level of overlap between the JAK, ABL, MEK, c-kit, and VEGF pathways, so it is not surprising that hematopoiesis can be affected by so many targets.

There is also evidence that inhibition of VEGFR can affect T cell function [115]. Rapamycin was shown to possess anti-lymphangiogenic properties, through mTOR-mediated impairment of VEGF-A and VEGF-C signaling [116]. While not proven, this mechanism can be extrapolated to other mTOR inhibitors such as sirolimus and temsirolimus that cause hematopoietic and lymphatic effects.

16.3.8.2 Preclinical Evaluation of Hematopoietic Toxicity

Rapidly proliferating tissues such as bone marrow are affected by many KIs and hematopoietic toxicity is commonly observed in preclinical safety studies. In general, inhibitors of ABL, BTK, c-met, MEK, JAK, VEGFR, and mTor that cause hematopoietic effects in humans also cause the same effects in preclinical model species. Rats, dogs, and nonhuman primates all seem to be sensitive to these effects. There are a few examples where animals appear to be more sensitive to effects of these compounds than humans, although this may be a function of dose. Cabozantinib, tofacitinib, and trametinib all cause hematopoietic effects in the dog, NHP, and/or rat, while not showing these effects in humans.

16.3.9 Ocular Toxicity

KI may cause disturbances of the visual system, ranging from periorbital edema to central serous retinopathy, and many different mechanisms are involved [88]. Outside of the MEK inhibitors, the ocular effects seen are rarely severe or dose limiting. Conjunctivitis is often observed in patients treated with erlotinib, gefitinib, imatinib, afatinib, and vandetanib, and many of these compounds also cause keratitis. Serious effects of the posterior ocular segment such as hemorrhage, retinopathy, and retinal vessel occlusion are unusual, but have been observed with axitinib, trametinib, imatinib, and vemurafenib. Visual disturbances have been reported in up to 60% of patients treated with crizotinib in a phase 3 clinical trial. Ocular adnexa abnormalities are observed with almost all of the marketed KIs. In general, however, ocular toxicity with KI is less severe than that seen with cytotoxic cancer chemotherapy drugs.

16.3.9.1 Mechanistic Basis of Ocular Toxicity

Inhibitors of EGFR are particularly prone to causing ocular effects due to the relatively high expression of EGFR in the basal epithelia of the eye [117,118], resulting in susceptibility of the conjunctiva and cornea to damage. Posterior segment effects may result from inhibition of pathways related to MEK, MAPK,

PI3K, and intersections of these. Retinal vein occlusion (RVO) is seen clinically with the MEK inhibitor trametinib, and also with the investigational agent PD0325901, a MAPK kinase inhibitor [119], and can be replicated in a rabbit model [120]. The proposed mechanisms involve increased oxidative stress and inflammatory response, endothelium and blood–retinal barrier damage, and prothrombotic effects. It is also now understood that FGFR and MAPK are critical in maintaining the function of the retinal pigment epithelium [121], such that interfering with these pathways could lead to visual effects. Overall, perturbation of any of the pathways mentioned above has the potential to cause ocular effects, but evidence to date indicates that potency is a factor in the development of toxicity, with less potent agents being less toxic.

16.3.9.2 Preclinical Evaluation of Ocular Toxicity

As discussed above, RVO can be replicated in a rabbit model, but was not seen in rats or dogs treated with PD0325901. This could be due to the higher level of similarity between the rabbit and human eyes, compared with the rat and dog eyes. EGFR inhibitors have produced corneal thinning in rats and dogs, and opacification in dogs [118], indicating that preclinical models can be effective for screening of some types of ocular effects. The mTor inhibitors everolimus and sirolimus also cause lens opacities, in rats, while ibrutinib, a BTK, Lck, Lyn inhibitor, causes this effect in dogs. It is always good practice to check that this effect is not due to plasma glucose changes. Nilotinib causes anterior chamber exudates, keratitis, and retrobulber hemorrhage in rats only. In general, the effect of "visual disturbance" recorded in clinical trials cannot be detected in animals, since they cannot convey the nature of the effect to observers, and the changes cannot be detected by histopathology. An electroretinogram study was conducted in rats treated with crizotinib, with the results indicating changes in light/dark adaptation. There was also a high concentration of crizotinib-derived material deposited in eye structures in rats, with a long residence time.

16.3.10 Pulmonary Toxicity

Interstitial lung disease (ILD) was first reported with gefitinib therapy in Japan [122]. ILD has now also been reported following erlotinib, afatinib, crizotinib, imatinib, lapatinib, sirolimus, temsirolimus, trametinib, and vandetanib therapy. Sorafenib has also been associated with ILD-like effects, and everolimus is considered to cause noninfectious pneumonitis. Risk factors for ILD are preexisting pulmonary fibrosis, male gender, and smoking [123]. The prevalence of ILD is also higher in Japanese patients than in Caucasians, for at least some of the EGFR inhibitors [124] and imatinib [125].

Originally thought to be a rare event caused by EGFR inhibitors, ILD has since been observed with mTOR inhibitors and some MEK, ALK, and broad-spectrum KIs. Not surprisingly, the pathways involved all overlap to some extent and are integral to cell replication. One hypothesis for the mechanism of EGFR inhibition-related ILD is that, since EGFR is important in the stimulation of epithelial repopulation and restoration of barrier integrity in the lung after damage, interference with this pathway could inhibit the response to lung injury [123]. ILD diagnosis in humans is complex, with CT imaging being an important component of the conclusion. Thus, an identical syndrome has not been observed in preclinical safety studies. The rat does seem to be susceptible to lung injury with treatment by some of the compounds causing ILD in humans, but mechanistic comparisons between species are not available.

16.3.11 Renal Toxicity

Several KIs affect the kidney, typically through VEGFR or EGFR inhibition. Axitinib, cabozantinib, erlotinib, ibrutinib, pazopanib, sorafenib, and sunitinib have renal effects in humans [126,127, FDA reviews]. mTor inhibitors also exhibit renal toxicity in the clinic, although the adverse effects of sirolimus may be due to potentiation of coadministered cyclosporine, via TGF-β1-mediated mechanisms [128]. A preeclampsia-like syndrome of hypertension and proteinuria is seen with some VEGFR inhibitors, likely due to expression of VEGF in podocytes and tubular epithelial cells, as well as VEGFR in glomerular and peritubular endothelial cells [113].

The relationship between VEGFR inhibition and renal toxicity is supported by studies in genetically altered mice, and in normal rodents treated with anti-VEGF antibodies [129–131]. EGFR signaling is important in maintaining electrolyte balance, and EGFR expression has been found in glomeruli and tubules of human kidney [132]. There is however little correlation between animals and humans for renal toxicity, other than for mTor inhibitors that show kidney toxicity in humans and rats. There are several examples of compounds that cause renal effects in animals but not in humans, as shown in Table 16.1.

16.4 Derisking Strategies for Kinase Inhibitor Toxicity

One of the challenges in derisking KI is that it can be difficult to determine whether adverse events are mediated by kinase or nonkinase targets. Furthermore, for kinase-mediated effects, these may be due to on-target or off-target kinase inhibition. Since it is challenging to prevent adverse events resulting from primary pharmacology, most drug discovery efforts have been aimed at developing compounds with high kinase selectivity in the assumption that the risk of toxicity will decrease as selectivity increases.

A number of commercial companies provide wide-scale, high-throughput screening assays against most of the kinases in the kinome. These assays are biochemical in nature and utilize peptide substrates and purified, catalytically active kinases. The assays are usually conducted at concentrations of ATP close to the

K_m of each enzyme. A screening strategy incorporating these assays provides a maximal view of kinase promiscuity. Physiological levels of ATP are, however, much higher than typically used in biochemical assays, ~1–3 mM, and the Cheng–Prusoff equation predicts that the IC_{50} values for ATP-competitive KI will be right-shifted, resulting in lower potency at higher cellular ATP concentrations. Biochemical assays may therefore overestimate the promiscuity of KI. Several commercial assay formats are now offered using 1 mM ATP, which may better replicate the kinase selectivity of a compound under physiological conditions. A typical first pass assessment, although a binding assay with nonphysiological substrates, is an abbreviated protein construct possessing the kinase domain and low ATP concentrations, applied using the Ambit screen. Hits can be followed up in detail with a more physiological system (cells).

In the context of a more native biological system, chemical proteomic approaches have been useful in identifying kinase targets. Activity-based protein profiling (ABPP) is a useful strategy for determining the promiscuity of a KI. ABPP uses small-molecule probes that covalently label the active site of an enzyme and the technology has been applied to a wide variety of gene families, including serine hydrolases, cysteine proteases, and glycosidases [133]. In the case of kinases, the technology has taken advantage of the reactivity of a conserved lysine present in all but a few protein kinases. This lysine is located in the ATP binding loop, close to the β- and γ-phosphates of ATP, where it reacts electrostatically with the phosphate backbone. ABPP probes have been designed with a biotinylated acyl group at the terminal phosphate of ATP, which reacts with the conserved lysine to form a stable amide bond. The biotin-labeled kinases can be isolated using streptavidin, followed by protease digestion, and the biotinylated peptides are analyzed by liquid chromatography–mass spectrometry (LC-MS). These nucleotide-based probes have been shown to label at least 75% of human kinases in crude cell lysates. Control versus KI-treated cell lysates or tissues can be compared in these experiments, and thus reactivity in a biologically relevant system can be assessed [134].

Other probes take advantage of different reactive amino acids. Approximately 46 kinases (9% of the kinome) have a reactive cysteine in their active site. Hypothemycin is a resorcylic acid lactone that is susceptible to Michael addition by a cysteine thiolate, resulting in time-dependent inactivation of the kinase that is competitive with ATP. Kinobeads are a bead matrix to which several mixed KIs are attached and are shown to capture a substantial portion of the kinome expressed in cell lysates. Addition of a KI to the cell lysates results in the inhibitor binding to its targets, preventing those kinases from binding to the beads, while nontarget kinases still bind. Subsequent digestion and mass spectrometry is used to identify those kinases to which the inhibitor bound.

The "gold standard" for assessing kinase selectivity is the measurement of functional kinase activity directly in cells or tissues. Activity is measured in a background that contains physiological levels of ATP, full-length protein substrates, and any scaffolding proteins. Commercial assay formats include ELISA where the phosphorylation of the direct substrate can be followed, reporter assays that measure downstream readouts of kinase activation, and enzyme fragment complementation assays that utilize fragments of β-galactosidase fused to a portion of the kinase, or SH2 peptides, that are reconstituted upon activation of kinase activity.

16.5 Concluding Remarks

Kinase enzymes are attractive targets for drug discovery programs, as they control many critical cellular processes, and alteration in their activities is associated with the development and progression of many diseases. Although it was initially assumed that targeted therapy against specific disease-causing kinase activities would lead to high treatment efficacy with minimal adverse effects, this has not been fully realized. Marketed KIs for oncology indications do have both efficacy and safety advantages over traditional cytotoxic chemotherapeutic agents, however the treatment of non-life-threatening chronic diseases with KI therapy will require the development of drugs with more benign side effect profiles.

Target selectivity plays a role in the spectrum of adverse effects seen with KI, but it is not the sole determinant. Also important are the pathways and networks in which the affected kinases participate, and the range of biological functions controlled via these networks. Some highly selective (as far as we know) KIs have few adverse effects (e.g., ruxolitinib), while others (e.g., dabrafenib and erlotinib) have many. As more kinases are characterized, and the roles and interplay of the signaling networks in which they participate more completely understood, it should become possible to design KI drugs with improved efficacy and adverse effect profiles.

References

1 Manning, G., Whyte, D.B., Martinez, R., Hunter, T., and Sudarsanam, S. (2002) The protein kinase complement of the human genome. *Science*, **298**, 1912–1934.

2 Zhang, J. and Hochwald, S.N. (2013) Targeting receptor tyrosine kinases in solid tumors. *Surgical Oncology Clinics of North America*, **22**, 685–703.

3 Druker, B.J., Tamura, S., Buchdunger, E., Ohno, S., Segal, G.M., Fanning, S., Zimmerman, J., and Lydon, N.B. (1996) Effects of a selective inhibitor of the Abl tyrosine kinase on the growth of Bcr–Abl positive cells. *Nature Medicine*, **2**, 561–566.

4 Vokes, E.E. and Chu, E. (2006) Anti-EGFR therapies: clinical experience in colorectal, lung, and head and neck cancers. *Oncology*, **20**, 15–25.

5 Quintás-Cardama, A., Cortés, J.E., and Kantarjian, H. (2008) Practical management of toxicities associated with tyrosine kinase inhibitors in chronic myeloid leukemia. *Clinical Lymphoma Myeloma and Leukemia*, **8**, S82–S88.

6 Hu, J.C., Sadeghi, P., Pinter-Brown, L.C., Yashar, S., and Chiu, M.W. (2007) Cutaneous side effects of epidermal growth factor receptor inhibitors: clinical presentation, pathogenesis, and

management. *Journal of the American Academy of Dermatology*, **56**, 317–326.
7 Guengerich, F.P. and MacDonald, J.S. (2007) Applying mechanisms of chemical toxicity to predict drug safety. *Chemical Research in Toxicology*, **20**, 344–369.
8 Hartmann, J.T., Haap, M., Kopp, H.-G., and Lipp, H.-P. (2009) Tyrosine kinase inhibitors: a review on pharmacology, metabolism and side effects. *Current Drug Metabolism*, **10**, 470–481.
9 Lasser, K.E., Allen, P.D., Woodhandler, S.J., Himmelstein, D.U., Wolfe, S.M., and Bor, D.H. (2002) Timing of new black box warnings and withdrawals for prescription medications. *The Journal of the American Medical Association*, **287**, 2215–2220.
10 Fabian, M.A., Biggs, W.H., III, Treiber, D.K., Atteridge, C.E., Azimioara, M.D., Bendetti, M.G., Carter, T.A., Ciceri, P., Edeen, P.T., Floyd, M., Ford, J.M., Galvin, M., Gerlach, J.L., Grotzfeld, R.M., Herrgard, S., Insko, D.E., Insko, M.A., Lai, A.G., Leilias, J.-M., Mehta, S.A., Milanov, Z.V., Velasco, A.M., Wodicka, L.M., Patel, H.K., Zarrinkar, P.P., and Lockhart, D.J. (2005) A small molecule–kinase interaction map for clinical kinase inhibitors. *Nature Medicine*, **23** 329–336.
11 Anastassiadis, T., Deacon, S.W., Devarajan, K., Ma, H., and Peterson, J.R. (2011) Comprehensive assay of kinase catalytic activity reveals features of kinase inhibitor selectivity. *Nature Biotechnology*, **29**, 1039–1045.
12 Gao, Y., Davies, S.P., Augustin, M., Woodward, A., Patel, U.A., Kovelman, R., and Harvey, K.J. (2013) A broad activity screen in support of a chemogenomic map for kinase signalling research and drug discovery. *The Biochemical Journal*, **451**, 313–328.
13 Ptacek, J., Devgan, G., Michaud, G., Zhu, H., Zhu, X., Fasolo, J., Guo, H., Jona, G., Breitkreutz, A., Sopko, R., McCartney, R.R., Schmidt, M.C., Rachidi, N., Lee, S.J., Mah, A.S., Meng, L., Stark, M.J., Stern, D.F., De Virgilio, C., Tyers, M., Andrews, B., Gerstein, M., Schweitzer, B., Predki, P.F., and Snyder, M. (2005) Global analysis of protein phosphorylation in yeast. *Nature*, **438**, 679–684.
14 Bardswell, S.C., Cuello, F., Kentish, J.C., and Avkiran, M. (2012) cMyBP-C as a promiscuous substrate: phosphorylation by non-PKA kinases and its potential significance. *Journal of Muscle Research and Cell Motility*, **33**, 53–60.
15 Saif, M.W., Merikas, I., Tsimboukis, S., and Syrigos, K. (2008) Erlotinib-induced skin rash: pathogenesis, clinical significance and management in pancreatic cancer patients. *Journal of the Pancreas*, **9**, 267–274.
16 Jatoi, A. and Nguyen, P.L. (2008) Do patients die from rashes from epidermal growth factor receptor inhibitors? A systematic review to help counsel patients about holding therapy. *Oncologist*, **13**, 1201–1204.
17 Melosky, B., Burkes, R., Rayson, D., Alcindor, T., Shear, N., and Lacouture, M. (2009) Management of skin rash during EGFR-targeted monoclonal antibody treatment for gastrointestinal malignancies: Canadian recommendations. *Current Oncology*, **16**, 16–26.
18 Mouhayar, E., Durand, J.B., and Cortes, J. (2013) Cardiovascular toxicity of tyrosine kinase inhibitors. *Expert Opinion on Drug Safety*, **12**, 687–696.
19 Quintás-Cardama, A., Kantarjian, H., O'Brien, S., Borthakur, G., Bruzzi, J., Munden, R., and Cortes, J. (2007) Pleural effusion in patients with chronic myelogenous leukemia treated with dasatinib after imatinib failure. *Journal of Clinical Oncology*, **25**, 3908–3914.
20 Masiello, D., Gorospe, G., 3rd, and Yang, A.S. (2009) The occurrence and management of fluid retention associated with TKI therapy in CML, with a focus on dasatinib. *Journal of Hematology & Oncology*, **2**, 46.
21 Valent, P. (2011) Severe adverse events associated with the use of second-line BCR/ABL tyrosine kinase inhibitors: preferential occurrence in patients with comorbidities. *Haematologica*, **96**, 1395–1397.
22 Chu, T.F., Rupnick, M.A., Kerkela, R., Dallabrida, S.M., Zurakowski, D., Nguyen, L., Woulfe, K., Pravda, E., Cassiola, F., Desai, J., George, S., Morgan,

J.A., Harris, D.M., Ismail, N.S., Chen, J.H., Schoen, F.J., Van den Abbeele, A.D., Demetri, G.D., Force, T., and Chen, M.H. (2007) Cardiotoxicity associated with tyrosine kinase inhibitor sunitinib. *Lancet*, **370** 2011–2019.

23 Kerkela, R., Woulfe, K.C., Durand, J.B., Vagnozzi, R., Kramer, D., Chu, T.F., Beahm, C., Chen, M.H., and Force, T. (2009) Sunitinib-induced cardiotoxicity is mediated by off-target inhibition of AMP-activated protein kinase. *Clinical and Translational Science*, **2**, 15–25.

24 Cohen, S. and Fleischmann, R. (2010) Kinase inhibitors: a new approach to rheumatoid arthritis treatment. *Current Opinion in Rheumatology*, **22**, 330–335.

25 Sandborn, W.J., Ghosh, S., Panes, J., Vranic, I., Su, C., Rousell, S., and Niezychowski, W. (2012) Tofacitinib, an oral Janus kinase inhibitor, in active ulcerative colitis. *The New England Journal of Medicine*, **367**, 616–624.

26 Norman, P. (2014) Selective JAK inhibitors in development for rheumatoid arthritis. *Expert Opinion on Investigational Drugs*, **12**, 1–11.

27 Chitturi, S. and George, J. (2002) Hepatotoxicity of commonly used drugs: nonsteroidal anti-inflammatory drugs, antihypertensives, antidiabetic agents, anticonvulsants, lipid-lowering agents, psychotropic drugs. *Seminars in Liver Disease*, **22**, 169–183.

28 Spraggs, C.F., Xu, C.F., and Hunt, C.M. (2013) Genetic characterization to improve interpretation and clinical management of hepatotoxicity caused by tyrosine kinase inhibitors. *Pharmacogenomics*, **14**, 541–554.

29 Spraggs, C.F., Budde, L.R., Briley, L., Bing, P.N., Cox, C.J., King, K.S., Whittaker, J.C., Mooser, V.E., Preston, A.J., Stein, S.H., and Cardon, L.R. (2011) HLA-DQA1∗02:01 is a major risk factor for lapatinib-induced hepatotoxicity in women with advanced breast cancer. *Journal of Clinical Oncology*, **29**, 667–673.

30 Iacovelli, R., Palazzo, A., Procopio, G., Santoni, M., Trenta, P., de Benedetto, A., Mezi, S., and Cortesi, E. (2014) Incidence and relative risk of hepatic toxicity in patients treated with antiangiogenic tyrosine kinase inhibitors for malignancy. *British Journal of Clinical Pharmacology*, **77**, 929–938.

31 Teo, Y.L., Ho, H.K., and Chan, A. (2013) Risk of tyrosine kinase inhibitors-induced hepatotoxicity in cancer patients: a meta-analysis. *Cancer Treatment Reviews*, **39**, 199–206.

32 Shah, D.R., Shah, R.R., and Morganroth, J. (2013) Tyrosine kinase inhibitors: their on-target toxicities as potential indicators of efficacy. *Drug Safety*, **36**, 413–426.

33 Li, X., Kamenecka, T.M., and Cameron, M.D. (2010) Cytochrome P450-mediated bioactivation of the epidermal growth factor receptor inhibitor erlotinib to a reactive electrophile. *Drug Metabolism and Disposition*, **38**, 1238–1245.

34 Wnorowski, A.M., de Souza, A., Chachoua, A., and Cohen, D.E. (2012) The management of EGFR inhibitor adverse events: a case series and treatment paradigm. *International Journal of Dermatology*, **51**, 223–232.

35 Teng, W.C., Oh, J.W., New, L.S., Wahlin, M.D., Nelson, S.D., Ho, H.K., and Chan, E.C. (2010) Mechanism-based inactivation of cytochrome P450 3A4 by lapatinib. *Molecular Pharmacology*, **78**, 693–703.

36 Goh, B.C., Reddy, N.J., Dandamudi, U.B., Laubscher, K.H., Peckham, T., Hodge, J.P., Suttle, A.B., Arumugham, T., Xu, Y., Xu, C.F., Lager, J., Dar, M.M., and Lewis, L.D. (2010) An evaluation of the drug interaction potential of pazopanib, an oral vascular endothelial growth factor receptor tyrosine kinase inhibitor, using a modified Cooperstown 5+1 cocktail in patients with advanced solid tumors. *Clinical Pharmacology and Therapeutics*, **88**, 652–659.

37 Tan, A.R., Jones, S.F., Dowlati, A., Levinson, K., Beatty, K., Suttle, B., Gibson, D., Arumugham, T., Lager, J., and Burris, H.A., III (2008) Phase I study of the safety, tolerability, and pharmacokinetics (PK) of weekly paclitaxel administered in combination with pazopanib (GW786034). *Journal of Clinical Oncology*, **26**, 3552.

38 Bosma, P.J., Chowdhury, J.R., Bakker, C., Gantla, S., de Boer, A., Oostra, B.A., Lindhout, D., Tytgat, G.N., Jansen, P.L., Oude Elferink, R.P.J., and Chowdhury, N.R. (1995) The genetic basis of the reduced expression of bilirubin UDP-glucuronosyltransferase 1 in Gilbert's syndrome. *The New England Journal of Medicine*, **333**, 1171–1175.
39 Ridruejo, E., Cacchione, R., Villamil, A.G., Marciano, S., Gadano, A.C., and Mando, O.G. (2007) Imatinib-induced fatal acute liver failure. *World Journal of Gastroenterology*, **13**, 6608–6111.
40 Weise, A.M., Liu, C.Y., and Shields, A.F. (2009) Fatal liver failure in a patient on acetaminophen treated with sunitinib malate and levothyroxine. *Annals of Pharmacotherapy*, **43**, 761–766.
41 Liu, Y., Ramirez, J., and Ratain, M.J. (2011) Inhibition of paracetamol glucuronidation by tyrosine kinase inhibitors. *British Journal of Clinical Pharmacology*, **71**, 917–920.
42 Polli, J.W., Humphreys, J.E., Harmon, K.A., Castellino, S., O'Mara, M.J., Olson, K.L., John-Williams, L.S., Koch, K.M., and Serabjit-Singh, C.J. (2008) The role of efflux and uptake transporters in [*N*-{3-chloro-4-[(3-fluorobenzyl)oxy] phenyl}-6-[5-({[2-(methylsulfonyl)ethyl] amino }methyl)-2-furyl]-4-quinazolinamine (GW572016, lapatinib) disposition and drug interactions. *Drug Metabolism and Disposition*, **36**, 695–701.
43 Neuvonen, P.J., Niemi, M., and Backman, J.T. (2006) Drug interactions with lipid-lowering drugs: mechanisms and clinical relevance. *Clinical Pharmacology and Therapeutics*, **80**, 565–581.
44 Xu, C.F., Xue, Z., Bing, N., King, K.S., McCann, L.A., de Souza, P.L., Goodman, V.L., Spraggs, C.F., Mooser, V.E., and Pandite, L.N. (2012) Concomitant use of pazopanib and simvastatin increases the risk of transaminase elevations in patients with cancer. *Annals of Oncology*, **23**, 2470–2471.
45 Yuan, L. and Kaplowitz, N. (2013) Mechanisms of drug-induced liver injury. *Clinics in Liver Disease*, **17**, 507–518, vii.
46 Daly, A.K. (2010) Drug-induced liver injury: past, present and future. *Pharmacogenomics*, **11**, 607–611.
47 Spraggs, C.F., Budde, L.R., Briley, L.P., Bing, N., Cox, C.J., King, K.S., Whittaker, J.C., Mooser, V.E., Preston, A.J., Stein, S.H., and Cardon, L.R. (2011) HLA-DQA1*02:01 is a major risk factor for lapatinib-induced hepatotoxicity in women with advanced breast cancer. *Journal of Clinical Oncology*, **29**, 667–673.
48 Spraggs, C.F., Parham, L.R., Hunt, C.M., and Dollery, C.T. (2012) Lapatinib-induced liver injury characterized by class II HLA and Gilbert's syndrome genotypes. *Clinical Pharmacology and Therapeutics*, **91**, 647–652.
49 Bharadwaj, M., Illing, P., Theodossis, A., Purcell, A.W., Rossjohn, J., and McCluskey, J. (2012) Drug hypersensitivity and human leukocyte antigens of the major histocompatibility complex. *Annual Review of Pharmacology and Toxicology*, **52**, 401–431.
50 Olson, H., Betton, G., Robinson, D., Thomas, K., Monro, A., Kolaja, G., Lilly, P., Sanders, J., Sipes, G., Bracken, W., Dorato, M., Van Deun, K., Smith, P., Berger, B., and Heller, A. (2000) Concordance of the toxicity of pharmaceuticals in humans and in animals. *Regulatory Toxicology and Pharmacology*, **32**, 56–67.
51 Atienzar, F.A., Novik, E.I., Gerets, H.H., Parekh, A., Delatour, C., Cardenas, A., Macdonald, J., Yarmush, M.L., and Dhalluin, S. (2013) Predictivity of dog co-culture model, primary human hepatocytes and HepG2 cells for the detection of hepatotoxic drugs in humans. *Toxicology and Applied Pharmacology*, **275**, 44–61.
52 Igarashi, T., Nakane, S., and Kitagawa, T. (1995) Predictability of clinical adverse reactions of drugs by general pharmacology studies. *The Journal of Toxicological Sciences*, **20**, 77–92.
53 Jaeschke, H., McGill, M.R., and Ramachandran, A. (2012) Oxidant stress, mitochondria, and cell death mechanisms in drug-induced liver injury: lessons learned from acetaminophen

hepatotoxicity. *Drug Metabolism Reviews*, **44**, 88–106.
54 Gunawan, B.K., Liu, Z.X., Han, D., Hanawa, N., Gaarde, W.A., and Kaplowitz, N. (2006) c-Jun *N*-terminal kinase plays a major role in murine acetaminophen hepatotoxicity. *Gastroenterology*, **131**, 165–178.
55 Shinohara, M., Ybanez, M.D., Win, S., Than, T.A., Jain, S., Gaarde, W.A., Han, D., and Kaplowitz, N. (2010) Silencing glycogen synthase kinase-3beta inhibits acetaminophen hepatotoxicity and attenuates JNK activation and loss of glutamate cysteine ligase and myeloid cell leukemia sequence 1. *The Journal of Biological Chemistry*, **285**, 8244–8255.
56 Ren, F., Duan, Z., Cheng, Q., Shen, X., Gao, F., Bai, L., Liu, J., Busuttil, R.W., Kupiec-Weglinski, J.W., and Zhai, Y. (2011) Inhibition of glycogen synthase kinase 3 beta ameliorates liver ischemia reperfusion injury by way of an interleukin-10-mediated immune regulatory mechanism. *Hepatology*, **54**, 687–696.
57 Hoeflich, K.P., Luo, J., Rubie, E.A., Tsao, M.-S., Jin, O., and Woodgett, J.R. (2000) Requirement for glycogen synthase kinase-3β in cell survival and NF-κ-B activation. *Nature*, **406**, 86–90.
58 Xue, T., Luo, P., Zhu, H., Zhao, Y., Wu, H., Gai, R., Wu, Y., Yang, B., Yang, X., and He, Q. (2012) Oxidative stress is involved in Dasatinib-induced apoptosis in rat primary hepatocytes. *Toxicology and Applied Pharmacology*, **261**, 280–291.
59 Novik, E., Maguire, T.J., Chao, P., Cheng, K.C., and Yarmush, M.L. (2010) A microfluidic hepatic coculture platform for cell-based drug metabolism studies. *Biochemical Pharmacology*, **79**, 1036–1044.
60 Sirenko, O., Hesley, J., Rusyn, I., and Cromwell, E.F. (2014) High-content assays for hepatotoxicity using induced pluripotent stem cell-derived cells. *Assay and Drug Development Technologies*, **12**, 43–54.
61 Leese, G.P., Flynn, R.V., Jung, R.T., Macdonald, T.M., Murphy, M.J., and Morris, A.D. (2008) Increasing prevalence and incidence of thyroid disease in Tayside, Scotland: the Thyroid Epidemiology Audit and Research Study (TEARS). *Clinical Endocrinology*, **68**, 311–316.
62 Vanderpump, M.P. (2011) The epidemiology of thyroid disease. *British Medical Bulletin*, **99**, 39–51.
63 Torino, F., Corsello, S.M., Longo, R., Barnabei, A., and Gasparini, G. (2009) Hypothyroidism related to tyrosine kinase inhibitors: an emerging toxic effect of targeted therapy. *Nature Reviews. Clinical Oncology*, **6**, 219–228.
64 Clemons, J., Gao, D., Naam, M., Breaker, K., Garfield, D., and Flaig, T.W. (2012) Thyroid dysfunction in patients treated with sunitinib or sorafenib. *Clinical Genitourinary Cancer*, **10**, 225–231.
65 Bianchi, L., Rossi, L., Tomao, F., Papa, A., Zoratto, F., and Tomao, S. (2013) Thyroid dysfunction and tyrosine kinase inhibitors in renal cell carcinoma. *Endocrine-Related Cancer*, **20**, R233–R245.
66 Schmidinger, M., Vogl, U.M., Bojic, M., Lamm, W., Heinzl, H., Haitel, A., Clodi, M., Kramer, G., and Zielinski, C.C. (2011) Hypothyroidism in patients with renal cell carcinoma: blessing or curse? *Cancer*, **117**, 534–544.
67 Wang, J.F., Milosveski, V., Schramek, C., Fong, G.H., Becks, G.P., and Hill, D.J. (1998) Presence and possible role of vascular endothelial growth factor in thyroid cell growth and function. *The Journal of Endocrinology*, **157**, 5–12.
68 Kamba, T., Tam, B.Y.Y., Hashizume, H., Haskell, A., Sennino, B., Mancuso, M.R., Norberg, S.M., O'Brien, S.M., Davis, R.B., Gowen, L.C., Anderson, K.D., Thurston, G., Joho, S., Springer, M.L., Kuo, C.J., and McDonald, D.M. (2006) VGEF-dependent plasticity of fenestrated capillaries in the normal adult microvasculature. *The American Journal of Physiology*, **290**, H560–H576.
69 Kappers, M.H., van Esch, J.H., Smedts, F.M., de Krijger, R.R., Eechoute, K., Mathijssen, R.H., Sleijfer, S., Leijten, F., Danser, A.H., van den Meiracker, A.H., and Visser, T.J. (2011) Sunitinib-induced hypothyroidism is due to induction of

type 3 deiodinase activity and thyroidal capillary regression. *The Journal of Clinical Endocrinology and Metabolism*, **96**, 3087–3094.

70 Abdulrahman, R.M., Verloop, H., Hoftijzer, H., Verburg, E., Hovens, G.C., Corssmit, E.P., Reiners, C., Gelderblom, H., Pereira, A.M., Kapiteijn, E., Romijn, J.A., Visser, T.J., and Smit, J.W. (2010) Sorafenib-induced hypothyroidism is associated with increased type 3 deiodination. *The Journal of Clinical Endocrinology and Metabolism*, **95**, 3758–3762.

71 Mannavola, D., Coco, P., Vannucchi, G., Bertuelli, R., Carletto, M., Casali, P.G., Beck-Peccoz, P., and Fugazzola, L. (2007) A novel tyrosine-kinase selective inhibitor, sunitinib, induces transient hypothyroidism by blocking iodine uptake. *The Journal of Clinical Endocrinology and Metabolism*, **92**, 3531–3534.

72 Riesenbeck, L.M., Bierer, S., Hoffmeister, I., Kopke, T., Papavassilis, P., Hertle, L., Thielen, B., and Herrmann, E. (2011) Hypothyroidism correlates with a better prognosis in metastatic renal cancer patients treated with sorafenib or sunitinib. *World Journal of Urology*, **29**, 807–813.

73 Vandyke, K., Dwar, A.L., Diamond, P., Fitter, S., Schultz, C.G., Sims, N.A., and Zannettino, A.C.W. (2010) The tyrosine kinase inhibitor dasatinib dysregulates bone remodeling through inhibition of osteoclasts *in vivo*. *Journal of Bone and Mineral Research*, **25**, 1759–1770.

74 Yu, E.Y., Wilding, G., Posadas, E., Gross, M., Culine, S., Massard, C., Morris, M.J., Hudes, G., Calabro, F., Cheng, S., Trudel, G.C., Paliwal, P., and Sternberg, C.N. (2009) Phase II study of dasatinib in patients with metastatic castration-resistant prostate cancer. *Clinical Cancer Research*, **15**, 7241–7248.

75 Berman, E., Nicolaides, M., Maki, R.G., Fleischer, M., Chanel, S., Scheu, K., Wilson, B., Heller, G., and Sauter, N.P. (2006) Altered bone and mineral metabolism in patients receiving imatinib mesylate. *The New England Journal of Medicine*, **354**, 2006–2013.

76 Fitter, S., Dewar, A.L., Kostakis, P., To, L.B., Hughes, T.P., Roberts, M.M., Lynch, K., Vernon-Roberts, B., and Zanettino, A.C.W. (2008) Long-term imatinib therapy promotes bone formation in CML patients. *Blood*, **111**, 2538–2547.

77 O'Sullivan, S., Naot, D., Callon, K.E., Watson, M., Gamble, G.D., Ladefoged, M., Karsdal, M.A., Browett, P., Cornish, J., and Grey, A. (2011) Imatinib mesylate does not increase bone volume *in vivo*. *Calcified Tissue International*, **88**, 16–22.

78 Lodish, M.B. (2013) Kinase inhibitors: adverse effects related to the endocrine system. *The Journal of Clinical Endocrinology and Metabolism*, **98**, 1333–1342.

79 Jheon, A.H., Seidel, K., Biehs, B., and Klein, O.D. (2013) From molecules to mastication: the development and evolution of teeth. *Wiley Interdisciplinary Reviews: Developmental Biology*, **2**, 165–183.

80 Li, Z., Yu, M., and Tian, W. (2013) An inductive signaling network regulates mammalian tooth morphogenesis with implications for tooth regeneration. *Cell Proliferation*, **46**, 501–508.

81 Zhang, Y.D., Chen, Z., Song, Y.Q., Liu, C., and Chen, Y.P. (2005) Making a tooth: growth factors, transcription factors, and stem cells. *Cell Research*, **15**, 301–316.

82 Miletich, I. and Sharpe, P.T. (2003) Normal and abnormal dental development. *Human Molecular Genetics*, **12**, R69–R73.

83 Itoh, N. and Ornitz, D.M. (2011) Fibroblast growth factors: from molecular evolution to roles in development, metabolism and disease. *Journal of Biochemistry*, **149**, 121–130.

84 Li, C.Y., Prochazka, J., Goodwin, A.F., and Klein, O.D. (2014) Fibroblast growth factor signaling in mammalian tooth development. *Odontology*, **102**, 1–13.

85 Fletcher, A.M., Bregman, C.L., Woicke, J., Salcedo, T.W., Zidell, R.H., Janke, H.E., Fang, H., Janusz, W.J., Schulze, G.E., and Mense, M.G. (2010) Incisor degeneration in rats induced by VEGF/FGF receptor tyrosine kinase inhibition. *Toxicologic Pathology*, **38**, 267.

86 Thornton, K., Kim, G., Maher, V.E., Chattopadhyay, S., Tang, S., Moon, Y.J., Song, P., Marathe, A., Balakrishnan, S., Zhu, H., Garnett, C., Liu, Q., Booth, B., Gehrke, B., Dorsam, R., Verbois, L., Ghosh, D., Wilson, W., Duan, J., Sarker, H., Miksinski, S.P., Skarupa, L., Ibrahim, A., Justice, R., Murgo, A., and Pazdur, R. (2012) Vandetanib for the treatment of symptomatic or progressive medullary thyroid cancer in patients with unresectable locally advanced or metastatic disease: U.S. Food and Drug Administration Drug approval summary. *Clinical Cancer Research*, **18** 3722–3730.

87 Pick, A.M. and Nystrom, K.K. (2012) Pazopanib for the treatment of metastatic renal cell carcinoma. *Clinical Therapeutics*, **34**, 511–520.

88 Huillard, O., Boissier, E., Blanchet, B., Thomas-Schoemann, A., Cessot, A., Boudou-Rouquette, P., Durand, J.P., Coriat, R., Giroux, J., Alexandre, J., Vidal, M., and Goldwasser, F. (2014) Drug safety evaluation of sorafenib for treatment of solid tumors: consequences for the risk assessment and management of cancer patients. *Expert Opinion on Drug Safety*, **13**, 663–673.

89 Iyer, R., Fetterly, G., Lugade, A., and Thanavala, Y. (2010) Sorafenib: a clinical and pharmacologic review. *Expert Opinion on Pharmacotherapy*, **11**, 1943–1955.

90 Lacouture, M.E. (2006) Mechanisms of cutaneous toxicities to EGFR inhibitors. *Nature Reviews. Cancer*, **6**, 803–812.

91 Bianchini, D., Jayanth, A., Chua, Y.J., and Cunningham, D. (2008) Epidermal growth factor receptor inhibitor-related skin toxicity: mechanisms, treatment, and its potential role as a predictive marker. *Clinical Colorectal Cancer*, **7**, 33–43.

92 Baas, J.M., Krens, L.L., Guchelaar, H.J., Ouwerkerk, J., de Jong, F.A., Lavrijsen, A.P., and Gelderblom, H. (2012) Recommendations on management of EGFR inhibitor-induced skin toxicity: a systematic review. *Cancer Treatment Reviews*, **38**, 505–514.

93 Lacouture, M.E., Wu, S., Robert, C., Atkins, M.B., Kong, H.H., Guitart, J., Garbe, C., Hauschild, A., Puzanov, I., Alexandrescu, D.T., Anderson, R.T., Wood, L., and Dutcher, J.P. (2008) Evolving strategies for the management of hand-foot skin reaction associated with the multitargeted kinase inhibitors sorafenib and sunitinib. *Oncologist*, **13**, 1001–1011.

94 Robert, C., Sibaud, V., Mateus, C., and Cherpelis, B.S. (2012) Advances in the management of cutaneous toxicities of targeted therapies. *Seminars in Oncology*, **39**, 227–240.

95 Miettinen, P.J., Berger, J.E., Meneses, J., Phung, Y., Pedersen, R.A., Werb, Z., and Derynck, R. (1995) Epithelial immaturity and multiorgan failure in mice lacking epidermal growth factor receptor. *Nature*, **376**, 337–341.

96 Murillas, R., Larcher, F., Conti, C.J., Santos, M., Ullrich, A., and Jorcano, J.L. (1995) Expression of a dominant negative mutant of epidermal growth factor receptor in the epidermis of transgenic mice elicits striking alterations in hair follicle development and skin structure. *The EMBO Journal*, **14**, 5216–5223.

97 Threadgill, D.W., Dlugosz, A.A., Hansen, L.A., Tennenbaum, T., Lichti, U., Yee, D., LaMantia, C., Mourton, T., Herrup, K., Harris, R.C., Barnard, J.A., Yuspa, S.H., Coffey, R.J., and Magnuson, T. (1995) Targeted disruption of mouse EGF receptor: effect of genetic background on mutant phenotype. *Science*, **269**, 230–234.

98 Higgins, B., Kolinsky, K., Smith, M., Beck, G., Rashed, M., Adames, V., Linn, M., Wheeldon, E., Gand, L., Birnboeck, H., and Hoffmann, G. (2004) Antitumor activity of erlotinib (OSI-774, Tarceva) alone or in combination in human non-small cell lung cancer tumor xenograft models. *Anticancer Drugs*, **15**, 503–512.

99 Mascia, F., Mariani, V., Girolomoni, G., and Pastore, S. (2003) Blockade of the EGF receptor induces a deranged chemokine expression in keratinocytes leading to enhanced skin inflammation. *The American Journal of Pathology*, **163**, 303–312.

100 Hirsh, V. (2011) Managing treatment-related adverse events associated with EGFR tyrosine kinase inhibitors in

advanced non-small-cell lung cancer. *Current Oncology*, **18**, 126–138.

101 Jatoi, A., Rowland, K., Sloan, J.A., Gross, H.M., Fishkin, P.A., Kahanic, S.P., Novotny, P.J., Schaefer, P.L., Johnson, D.B., Tschetter, L.K., and Loprinzi, C.L. (2008) Tetracycline to prevent epidermal growth factor receptor inhibitor-induced skin rashes: results of a placebo-controlled trial from the North Central Cancer Treatment Group (N03CB). *Cancer*, **113**, 847–853.

102 Abruzzese, E., Trawinska, M.M., Perrotti, A.P., and De Fabritiis, P. (2014) Tyrosine kinase inhibitors and pregnancy. *Mediterranean Journal of Hematology and Infectious Diseases*, **6**, e2014028.

103 Choudhary, D.R., Mishra, P., Kumar, R., Mahapatra, M., and Choudry, V.P. (2006) Pregnancy on imatinib: fatal outcome with meningocele. *Annals of Oncology*, **17**, 178–179.

104 Constantinescu, S., Coscia, L., Moritz, M., McGrory, C., Ramirez, C., and Armenti, V. (2013). Pregnancy outcomes in solid organ transplant recipients with exposure to sirolimus. American Transplant Congress Meeting Abstracts, Abstract Number 417.

105 Patyna, S., Haznedar, J., Morris, D., Freshwater, K., Peng, G., Sukbuntherng, J., Chmielewski, G., and Matsumoto, D. (2009) Evaluation of the safety and pharmacokinetics of the multi-targeted receptor tyrosine kinase inhibitor sunitinib during embryo-fetal development in rats and rabbits. *Birth Defects Research Part B: Developmental and Reproductive Toxicology*, **86**, 204–213.

106 Wada, Y., Ozaki, H., Abe, N., Nagamitsu, T., Ohta, H., Nakahara, T., and Ishii, K. (2010) Effects of KRN633, an inhibitor of vascular endothelial growth factor receptor-2 tyrosine kinase, on vascular development of placenta and fetus of mid-pregnancy mice. *Journal of Pharmaceutical Sciences*, **112**, 290–298.

107 Threadgill, D.W., Dlugosz, A.A., Hansen, L.A., Tennenbaum, T., Lichti, U., Yee, D., LaMantia, C., Mourton, T., Herrup, K., Harris, R.C., Barnard, J.A., Yuspa, S.H., Coffey, R.J., and Magnuson, T. (1995) Targeted disruption of mouse EGF receptor: effect of genetic background on mutant phenotype. *Science*, **269**, 230–234.

108 Shapira, T., Pereg, D., and Lishner, M. (2008) How I treat acute and chronic leukemia in pregnancy. *Blood Reviews*, **22**, 247–259.

109 Kumar, S., Apostolova, M., and Woolley, P.V. (2011) A case of chronic myelogenous leukemia in pregnancy characterized by a complex translocation t(9;22;11)(q34;q11.2;q13). *Hematology Reports*, **3**, e27.

110 Steelman, L.S., Pohnert, S.C., Shelton, J.G., Franklin, R.A., Bertrand, F.E., and McCubrey, J.A. (2004) JAK/STAT, Raf/MEK/ERK, PI3K/Akt and BCR-ABL in cell cycle progression and leukemogenesis. *Leukemia*, **18**, 189–218.

111 Kumar, R., Crouthamel, M.-C., Rtominger, D.H., Gontarek, R.R., Tummino, P.J., Levin, R.A., and King, A.G. (2009) Myelosuppression and kinase selectivity of multikinase angiogenesis inhibitors. *British Journal of Cancer*, **101**, 1717–1723.

112 Funakoshi, T., Latif, A., and Galsky, M.D. (2013) Risk of hematologic toxicities in cancer patients treated with sunitinib: a systematic review and meta-analysis. *Cancer Treatment Reviews*, **39**, 818–830.

113 Verheul, H.M.W. and Pinedo, H.M. (2007) Possible molecular mechanisms involved in the toxicity of angiogenesis inhibition. *Nature Reviews. Cancer*, **7**, 475–485.

114 Larrivee, B., Lane, D.R., Pollet, I., Olive, P.L., Humphries, R.K., and Karsan, A. (2003) Vascular endothelial growth factor receptor-2 induces survival of hematopoietic progenitor cells. *The Journal of Biological Chemistry*, **278**, 22006–22013.

115 Terme, M., Pernot, S., Marcheteau, E., Sandoval, F., Benhamouda, N., Colussi, O., Dubreuil, O., Carpentier, A.F., Tartour, E., and Taieb, J. (2013) VEGFA-VEGFR pathway blockade inhibits tumor-induced regulatory T-cell proliferation in colorectal cancer. *Cancer Research*, **73**, 539–549.

116 Huber, S., Bruns, C.J., Schmid, G., Hermann, P.C., Conrad, C., Niess, H., Huss, R., Graeb, C., Jauch, K.-W., Heeschen, C., and Guba, M. (2007) Inhibition of the mammalian target of rapamycin impedes lymphangiogenesis. *Kidney International*, **71**, 771–777.

117 Liu, Z., Carvajal, M., Carraway, C.A., Carraway, K., and Pflugfelder, S.C. (2001) Expression of the receptor tyrosine kinases, epidermal growth factor receptor, ErbB2, and ErbB3, in human ocular surface epithelia. *Cornea*, **20**, 81–85.

118 Tullo, A.B., Esmaeli, B., Murray, P.I., Bristow, E., Forsythe, B.J., and Faulkner, K. (2005) Ocular findings in patients with solid tumours treated with the epidermal growth factor receptor tyrosine kinase inhibitor gefitinib ('Iressa', ZD1839) in phase I and II clinical trials. *Eye*, **19**, 729–738.

119 LoRusso, P.M., Krishnamurthi, S.S., Rinehart, J.J., Nabell, L.M., Malburg, L., Chapman, P.B., DePrimo, S.E., Bentivegna, S., Wilner, K.D., Tan, W., and Ricart, A.D. (2010) Phase I pharmacokinetic and pharmacodynamic study of the oral MAPK/ERK kinase inhibitor PD-0325901 in patients with advanced cancers. *Clinical Cancer Research*, **16**, 1924–1937.

120 Huang, W., Yang, A.H., Matsumoto, D., Collette, W., Marroquin, L., Ko, M., Aguirre, S., and Younis, H.S. (2009) PD0325901, a mitogen-activated protein kinase kinase inhibitor, produces ocular toxicity in a rabbit animal model of retinal vein occlusion. *Journal of Ocular Pharmacology and Therapeutics*, **25**, 519–530.

121 Van der Noll, R., Leijen, S., Neuteboom, G.H.G., Beijnen, J.H., and Schellens, J.H.M. (2013) Effect of inhibition of the FGFR-MAPK signaling pathway on the development of ocular toxicities. *Cancer Treatment Reviews*, **39**, 664–672.

122 Inoue, A., Saijo, Y., Maemondo, M., Gomi, K., Tokue, Y., Kimura, Y., Ebina, M., Kikuchi, T., Moriya, T., and Nukiwa, T. (2003) Severe acute interstitial pneumonia and gefitinib. *Lancet*, **361**, 137–139.

123 Min, J.H., Lee, H.Y., Lim, H., Ahn, M.-J., Park, K., Chung, M.P., and Lee, K.S. (2011) Drug-induced interstitial lung disease in tyrosine kinase inhibitor therapy for non-small cell lung cancer: a review on current insight. *Cancer Chemotherapy and Pharmacology*, **68**, 1099–1109.

124 Cohen, M.H., Williams, G.A., Sridhara, R., Chen, G., and Pazdur, R. (2003) FDA drug approval summary: Gefitinib (ZD1839) (Iressa®) tablets. *The Oncologist*, **8**, 303–306.

125 Ohnishi, K., Sakai, F., Kudoh, S., and Ohno, R. (2006) Twenty-seven cases of drug-induced interstitial lung disease associated with imatinib mesylate. *Leukemia*, **20**, 1162–1164.

126 Hayman, S.R., Leung, N., Grande, J.P., and Garovic, V.D. (2012) VEGF inhibition, hypertension and renal toxicity. *Current Oncology Reports*, **14**, 285–294.

127 Patel, T.V., Morgan, J.A., Demitri, G.D., George, S., Maki, R.G., Quigley, M., and Humphreys, B.D. (2008) A preeclampsia-like syndrome characterized by reversible hypertension and proteinuria induced by multitargeted kinase inhibitors sunitinib and sorafenib. *Journal of the National Cancer Institute*, **100**, 282–284.

128 Shihab, F.S., Bennett, W.M., Yi, H., Choi, S.-O., and Andoh, T.F. (2004) Sirolimus increases transforming growth factor-β expression and potentiates chronic cyclosporine nephrotoxicity. *Kidney International*, **65**, 1262–1271.

129 Eremina, V., Jefferson, J.A., Kowalewska, J., Hochster, H., Haas, M., Weisstuch, J., Richardson, C., Kopp, J.B., Golan-Kabir, M., Backx, P.H., Gerber, H.-P., Ferrara, N., Barisoni, L., Alpers, C.E., and Quaggin, S.E. (2008) VEGF inhibition and renal thrombotic microangiopathy. *The New England Journal of Medicine*, **358**, 1129–1136.

130 Hara, A., Wada, T., Furuichi, K., Sakai, N., Kawachi, H., Shimizu, F., Shibuya, M., Matsushima, K., Yokoyama, H., Egashira, K., and Kaneko, S. (2006) Blockade of VEGF accelerates proteinuria, via decrease in nephrin expression in rat

crescentic glomerulonephritis. *Kidney International*, **69**, 1986–1995.

131 Sugimoto, H., Hamano, Y., Charytan, D., Cosgrove, D., Kieran, M., Sudhakar, A., and Kalluri, R. (2003) Neutralization of circulating vascular endothelial growth factor (VEGF) by anti-VEGF antibodies and soluble VEGF receptor 1 (sFlt-1) induces proteinuria. *The Journal of Biological Chemistry*, **278**, 12605–12608.

132 Melenhorst, W.B.W.H., Mulder, G.M., Xi, Q., Hoenderop, J.G.J., Kimura, K., Eguchi, S., and van Goor, H. (2008) Epidermal growth factor receptor signaling in the kidney: key roles in physiology and disease. *Hypertension*, **52**, 987–993.

133 Cravatt, B.F., Wright, A.T., and Kozarich, J.W. (2008) Activity-based protein profiling: from enzyme chemistry to proteomic chemistry. *Annual Review of Biochemistry*, **77**, 383–414.

134 Patricelli, M.P., Szardenings, A.K., Liyanage, M., Nomanbhoy, T.K., Wu, M., Weissig, H., Aban, A., Chun, D., Tanner, S., and Kozarich, J.W. (2007) Functional interrogation of the kinome using nucleotide acyl phosphates. *Biochemistry*, **46**, 350–358.

17
Cardiac Side Effects Associated with Kinase Proteins and Their Signaling Pathways

Roy J. Vaz and Vinod F. Patel

17.1
A Case Study

Cardiotoxicity of kinase inhibitors is described in the case report [1] of a 27-year-old athletic female who was diagnosed with Philadelphia-positive acute lymphoblastic leukemia (ALL) in June 2004. She was treated, according to the Cancer and Leukemia Group B (CALGB) protocol, with daunorubicin and cyclophosphamide. She was then enrolled in a phase II trial of sequential chemotherapy and imatinib, and subsequently underwent an autologous stem cell transplant. Her left ventricular (LV) ejection fraction (LVEF) prior to the transplant was recorded to be 60%. The hospitalization for the myeloablative conditioning regimen, administered in December 2004, was complicated by infections that required vasopressor support. The patient was restarted on imatinib maintenance therapy at 400 mg twice daily after count recovery. In November 2005, the patient developed a persistent headache and was diagnosed with central nervous system relapse. No marrow involvement was detected. Imatinib was discontinued after 17 months of therapy and the patient was treated by cranial irradiation followed by reinduction with high-dose cytarabine and mitoxantrone. The treatment was again complicated by septic shock and infection that required vasopressor support for a day. Three days later, a diastolic murmur prompted examination by an echocardiogram that revealed an LVEF of 20–25%. Cardiac enzymes were within normal limits but brain natriuretic peptide (BNP) was elevated at 470 pg/ml (normal range is 0–100 pg/ml). The patient was placed under observation and recovered dramatically with an LVEF of 50% and discharged 2 weeks later in stable condition. Maintenance nilotinib (400 mg twice daily) therapy was started in January 2006 for 3 months after which the patient underwent a human leukocyte antigen-matched unrelated donor transplant and the conditioning regimen included fludarabine and melphalan. Severe mucositis required intubation and ventilator support for 1 week. Upon extubation, the patient required bilevel positive airway pressure for another week when she was reintubated for increasing shortness of breath related to congestive heart failure. An echocardiogram showed an LVEF of 30% with a highly elevated BNP of

Antitargets and Drug Safety, First Edition. Edited by László Urbán, Vinod F. Patel, and Roy J. Vaz.

3725 pg/ml. Cardiac enzymes revealed minor increases in the creatinine kinase muscle–brain fraction and in troponin I. The patient was treated with invasive hemodynamic monitoring-guided use of vasopressors and nicardipine. She was fully extubated 8 days later with normalization of the LVEF to 55% and BNP at 84 pg/ml. She was discharged 3 weeks after extubation. In August 2006, the patient was initiated on maintenance dasatinib oral dose of 70 mg twice daily. Skin and gastrointestinal graft versus host disease required immunosuppressive therapy including steroids. Ten months after initiation of dasatinib therapy, the patient was admitted with worsening bilateral pleural effusions and progressive shortness of breath. Dasatinib was discontinued on admission. However, on the fourth day of hospitalization, the patient became unresponsive with pulseless electrical activity. Aggressive cardiopulmonary resuscitation included emergent intubation. On arrival at the intensive care unit, an echocardiogram revealed an LVEF of 10–15%. A dobutamine infusion was initiated and then a nicardipine drip was added while monitoring other hemodynamic parameters. Her cardiac output tripled over 3 days and filling pressures returned toward normal. The patient was also treated with high doses of corticosteroids and extubated 11 days later. A repeat echocardiogram 4 days later showed an LVEF of 55%. The patient was discharged after 4 weeks. Shortly thereafter, she developed recurrent central nervous system relapse and expired suddenly.

This case study highlights the severe reversible cardiomyopathy a patient endures when treated with approved tyrosine kinase inhibitors (TKIs) imatinib (17 months), nilotinib (3 months), and dasatinib (10 months). The episodes occurred 2 weeks, 3 weeks, and 4 days, respectively, after discontinuation of these therapies with rapid reversibility after treatment. All of the medications, including the anthracyclines and mitoxantrone that result in cell death, added further complications. The tracking of LVEF for this patient over the relevant time period (Figure 17.1) shows the potential for this parameter to be a predictive biomarker for congestive heart failure (CHF) when using TKIs.

17.2 Introduction

The heart is considered a terminally differentiated organ with no potential for regeneration or repair, unlike tumor cells. However, the adult heart retains a limited population of cardiac stem cells that migrate to damaged regions of the heart and generate new cardiomyocytes. A recent study [2] using the integration of carbon-14 into the DNA of test subjects showed that cardiomyocytes renew with a gradual decrease from 1% annual turnover at the age of 25 to 0.45% at the age of 75. This led to a hypothesis [3] that cancer chemotherapy induces cardiotoxicity by targeting cardiac stem cells, interrupting the homeostasis of these cells, and depleting the pool, thereby losing the capability of regeneration and repair and hence displaying the symptoms of cardiotoxicity. This would suggest that a younger population, who possess more cardiac stem cells, would be

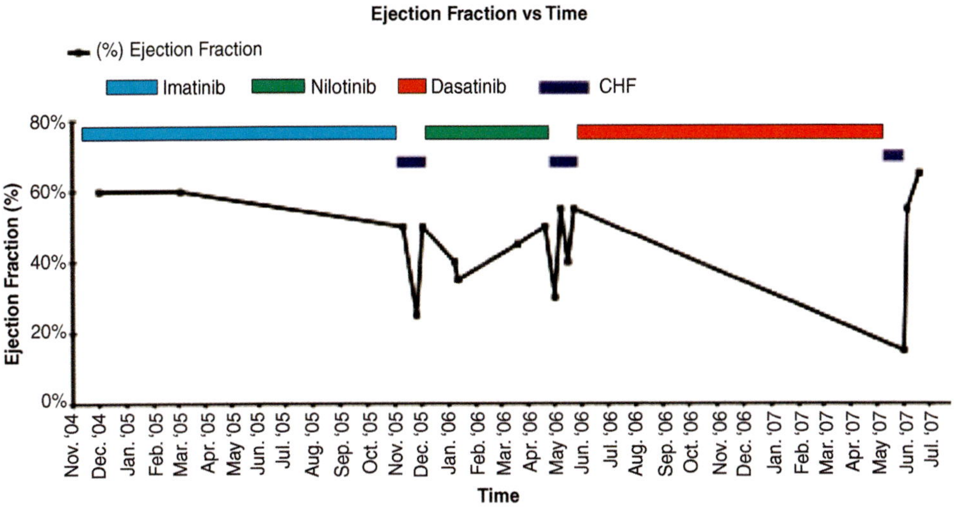

Figure 17.1 The patient's LVEF in relation to therapy with KIs described in the case [1].

more susceptible to chemotherapy-induced cardiotoxicity, which seems to be supported by the high incidence in pediatric cancer patients. Direct injection of cardiac stem cells into heart rescued anthracycline-induced cardiomyopathy [4].

In the treatment of cancers, some traditional cytotoxics, such as doxorubicin and cyclophosphamide, are known to be cardiotoxic. These drugs disrupt the replicative and signaling processes necessary for cell proliferation and survival. Unfortunately, due their lack of discrimination between tumor cells and normal proliferating cells, their therapeutic index is narrow. Treatment options for cancer patients have radically changed over the past decade with the advent of "targeted therapeutics." This approach was hypothesized to target tumor cells while sparing normal cells, thereby creating a wider therapeutic window. Since the success of imatinib (Gleevec) in treating chronic myeloid leukemia (CML) and fewer toxic side effects, a number of approved targeted drugs have followed to greatly improve management of cancers, including breast cancer, gastrointestinal stromal tumor (GIST), renal cell carcinoma (RC), colon carcinoma, non-small cell lung cancer (NSCLC), and metastatic melanoma (see Table 15.1). However, recent findings have revealed unanticipated cardiac side effects of the new therapeutics, including QT prolongation, reduction in LVEF, symptomatic CHF and acute coronary syndromes, and myocardial infarction (MI). In general, these have been managed medically and have not prevented their use. Administration of TKIs on a longer term basis (non-oncology indications) will require avenues for mitigating these risks and therefore an understanding of the mechanism of toxicity. It is known that not all TKIs exert the same toxicity on the heart, so it is not a class effect.

A subset of these adverse events is pharmacologically related to inhibition of cardiac ion channels (e.g., nilotinib induces QTc prolongation and sudden death due to blockade of the hERG current (see Table 15.5)), which affect the action potential of cardiomyocytes. Herein, we will focus on the observed and potential risk of cardiotoxicity induced by targeted therapy involving kinase signaling pathways for oncogenesis and survival of normal cardiomyocytes.

There are two primary modalities of kinase inhibitors – monoclonal antibodies (mAbs) and small molecules (SMs). Monoclonal antibodies are an effective modality for extracellular targets (growth factor receptors and ligands), while SMs are utilized to engage intracellular targets (catalytic activity of receptor and nonreceptor kinases). Due to the challenges associated with designing highly selective SM kinase inhibitors, safety profiles will be governed by on-mechanism (intended kinase target) and off-mechanism (unintended kinase target) effects. Conversely, a mAb therapeutic is highly selective and generally only displays on-mechanism side effects, thereby providing insight into mechanisms underlying cardiac safety signals, while SM safety pharmacology can be complex and difficult to interpret. Cardiac side effect profiles observed with mAbs and SMs will be described and molecular mechanisms that underlie those risks will be discussed in this chapter.

17.3 Cardiac-Specific Kinase Antitargets

17.3.1 Preclinical Findings in Genetically Modified or KI-Treated Mice

Force and Kolaja [5] have published a comprehensive overview of the role of kinases in the heart and vasculature in mouse models (Figure 17.2). From a genetics perspective, despite some differences in phenotype of the KO mouse being inconsistent with the equivalent human phenotype, the ability to generate cardiac-specific conditional KO mice and inducible knockdown models in addition to KO animals has allowed deciphering the role of kinases in the heart.

17.3.2 Clinical Findings of Kinase Inhibitors on the Heart and Their Mechanistic Understandings

17.3.2.1 ErbB2 Inhibition

The classic example of on-mechanism cardiotoxicity may be the cardiac effects of ErbB2-positive breast anti-ErbB2 mAb, trastuzumab. It has proven to be an effective treatment for ErbB2-positive metastatic breast cancer in combination with anthracycline leading to heart failure in 27% of the patients [6]. Recently, it was reported [7] that there is a 20% risk of left ventricular dysfunction in patients treated with trastuzumab after anthracycline therapy.

Kinase	Mouse model(s)	Role of kinase in heart/vasculature	Other notes
RAF1/BRAF	KO:DNTG	Anti-apoptotic:preserves LV function under stress. KO: LV dysfunction and HF in the absence of additional stress: DNTG: reduced hypertrophy but LV dysfunction due to cell death	KO:effects mediated by ASK1;RAF inhibits ASK1 via a non-kinase-dependent mechanism. RAF mutations account for some cases of Noonan syndrome (HCM phenocopy)
PI3K (p110α)	CATG:DNTG	Physiological heart growth; cardiomyocyte survival	Greater LV dysfunction after TAC in DNTG and improved LV function in CATG mouse
PI3K (p110γ)	KO	Regulates contractility and pathological hypertrophy	Mice protected from isoproterenol-induced injury
PDK1	KO	Cardiomyocyte survival and β-adrenergic responsiveness	Cardiac-specific KO displayed HF and DCM
AKT1, 2, or 3	CATG; DNTG; KO	Regulators of cardiomyocyte survival, growth, and metabolism	AKT1 promotes physiological hypertrophy and suppresses pathological hypertrophy: AKT2 promotes survival and insulin sensitivity
mTOR	Kinase inhibitor (KI) administered	mTORC1 regulates protein synthesis. inhibition leads to energy preservation under stress: mTORC2 regulates AKT activation	Rapamycin is well-tolerated and blocks cardiac hypertrophy. It will be used in combination regimens in cancer (long-term administration inhibits mTORC2 and AKT)
AMPK	Transgenic: KO	Sensor of energy stress: inhibits mTORC1. preserving energy stores. KO of AMPKa2 increased hypertrophy and LV dysfunction after TAC	Activated by tumor suppressor LKB1 or CAMKKβ. Activated mutant leads to glycogen storage hypertrophic cardiomyopathy
GSK3α/β	Transgenic: knock-in: KO	Together with AMPK. inhibits mTORC1: deletion of GSKβ protective in post-MI remodelling: deletion of GSK3α leads to HF in setting of stress	GSKα important in β-adrenergic responsiveness. Deletion leads to HF with stress
GDKs	Conditional KO:KO	CDK2 inhibiton reduces ischacmia–reperfusion injury. mediated via effects on retinoblastoma protein	Deletion of CDK2 and CDK4 during development leads to HF. but conditional deletion of CDK2 in adult mice lacking CDK4 does not lead to abnormalities
Aurora kinases	Kinase inhibitor administered	M phase regulators	KIs expected to disrupt CPC proliferation. karyokinesis, and any cytokinesis of cardiomyocytes resulting in cell death: associated with cardiotoxicity
PLKs	Kinase inhibitor administered	PLK1 involved in activation of CDC2. chromosome segregation. centrosome maturation. bipolar spinadle formation, and cytokinesis	As above
PDGFRs	KO	β isoform is crucial in angiogenesis and heart's response to PO	Conditional KO: HF with pressure overload
VEGFRs	VEGF trap: (monoclonal antibody): KO: kinase inhibitor administered	Crucial in angiogenesis and the heart's response to PO: antihypertensive effects	Heart-specific KO of VEGFR1 or VEGFR2 showed impaired respnse to ischaemia
EGFR (ERBB1)	Kinase inhibitor administered	Helps to maintain LV function in setting of chronic catecholamine stimulation: mediates pro-survival signaling	HF uncommon in clinical use
ERBB2 ERBB4	KO: conditional KO: transgenic	Cardiomyocyte survival and homeostasis: maintenance of LV function	KOs of HBEGF (ERBB ligand). neuregulin. ERBB2, and ERBB4 each develop DCM and HF. Neuregulin 1 KOs are more sensitive to doxorubicin-induced cardiotoxicity
KIT	*W/W′* mouse. kinase inhibitor administered	Promotes CSC and immature cardiomyocyte differentiation: promotes homing to sites of MI. promoting repair.	Imatinib reduced restenosis after arterial injury: *W/W′* mouse protected versus HF induced by PO
ABL/ARG	Kinase inhibitor administered	Maintains ER homeostasis. LV dysfunction is seen in rodents treated with imatinib	Minimal HF with ABL inhibitors noted in clinical use
JAK2	Transgenic: KO	JAK2 and STAT3 protective in many pathological settings	KO: displayed decreased ischemia–reperfusion injury. PO hypertrophy and peripartum cardiomyopathy
FAK	KO	Antihypertrophic and antifibrotic in heart	Eccentric hypertrophy and dilated cardiomyopathy with PO or angiotensin II

Figure 17.2 Kinases of importance in the heart and vasculature [5].

Kinase	Mouse model(s)	Role of kinase in heart/vasculature	Other notes
DMPK	Transgenic	Myotonic dystrophy type 1 is caused by excess repeats of the 3′ UTR region of DMPK	Overexpression in mouse heart leads to hypertrophic cardiomyopaty with dysrthymia
LTK	Transgenic	Activation of LTK results in cardiac hypertrophy and cardiomyocyte degeneration	Overexpression led to severe cardiac concentric hypertrophy
ROCK	Transgenic:KO	Pro-fibrotic and pro-apoptotic in the setting of PO	KO is protected from fibrosis. whereas transgenic shows accelerated hypertrophic cardiac decompensation
LKB1	KO	Activates AMPK, which is pro-angiogenic in heart	Cardiac-specific deletion leads to LV dysfunction. atrial fibrillation, and death
LDB3. ZASP, and/or Cypher	Conditional KO	Mutations in ZASP are associated with skeletal muscle myopathies	Deletion in cardiomyocytes leads to a DCM
ERK1/2	KO:transgenic	Generally promotes survival and may modulate physiological (but not pathological) hypertrophy	Activation of this pathway protects aginst cardiac ischemic injury: inactivation promotes LV dysfunction after PO
PKCα	KO:kinase inhibitor administered	Adverse effects on heart in setting of PO	PKCα KO (as opposed to PKCβ or PKCγ) protects against TAC-induced CHF. Ruboxistaurin protects against TAC-induced CHF
cGMP-dependent PK	KO	One of the four nodal kinases in HF: activated by PDE5 inhibitors: inhibits apoptosis. hypertrophy, and β-adrenergic responses	Clinical trial with sildenafil in HF showed improved LV function
PIM kinase	KO	Pro-survival: activated by AKT: regulated at level of gene expression	Promotes cardiac resident stem cell proliferation and survival
CAMKII	KO	Nodal kinase in HF: pro-hypertrophic: promotes decompensation in setting of PO	Mechanism of cardiotoxicity involves regulation of CAMKII gene expression and Ca^{2+} handling
GRK2 and/or GRK5	KO	Downregulates β-adrenergic signaling through recruitment of β-arrestin	Peptide inhibitor protects against HF
ASK1	KO	Promotes pathological hypertrophy and remodelling: pro-apoptotic	KO protected from PO and MI-induced remodeling
PTEN phosphatese	KO	Antihypertrophic impairs cardiomyocyte survival with stress, and antagonizes PI3K signaling	PO in PTEN KO mice reduced pathological hypertrophy. interstitial fibrosis, and apoptosis with preservation of LV function

Figure 17.2 *(Continued)*

Mechanistically, ErbB2-activating ligand neuregulin (Nrg1) induces ErbB2-promoted proliferation and survival of cardiomyocytes. Deletion of ErbB2 [8] or Nrg1 [9] in mice is lethal and leads to failure of ventricles to form properly. As in cancer cells, activation of receptor in cardiomyocytes activates the Erk and PI3/Akt pathways that promote survival [10].

17.3.2.2 EGFR Inhibition

To date, there is no direct evidence of implicating EGFR (ErbB1) in inducing heart failure or left ventricular dysfunction based on the use of mAbs (cetuximab and panitumumab) and small-molecule inhibitors (gefitinib and erlotinib) targeting this receptor signaling.

17.3.2.3 Dual EGFR/ErbB2 Inhibition

Interestingly, small-molecule dual ErbB2/EGFR inhibitor, lapatinib, showed limited depression of cardiac function. Clinical studies [11] revealed a low incidence of symptomatic heart failure (0.2%) or asymptomatic cardiac events (1.4%). The lower rate compared with trastuzumab is attributed to differences in the pharmacokinetics as well as the kinetics of interactions toward ErbB2 for the two drugs [12]. AMP-activated protein kinase (AMPK) is an important regulator of cellular energy metabolism and is required to maintain normal cardiac contractility [12]. Lapatinib has been shown to activate AMPK in an ErbB2- and calcium-dependent manner, protecting human cardiomyocytes, which could also account for the different toxicological profiles [13]. The pathway activated by trastuzumab and lapatinib leading to apoptosis or caspase activation in breast cancer cells and cardiomyocytes is discussed in Ref. [14] and in Figure 1 of Ref. [14]. ErbB2 is an upstream trigger for the induction of mitochondrial apoptosis, Bax/BAK activation, mitochondrial permeability transition pore opening, and cytochrome *c* release into the cytosol.

17.3.2.4 **Raf Inhibition**

Rapidly accelerated fibrosarcoma (Raf) kinase is a family of cytoplasmic serine/threonine kinases consisting of Raf-1, A-Raf, and B-Raf. Raf-1 plays a protective role in the heart in settings of pressure overload stress [15]. Deletion of Raf-1 in mouse heart led to dilated, hypocontractile heart with enhanced cardiomyocyte apoptosis and fibrosis [16]. The roles of A-Raf and B-Raf are not known. Sorafenib, a nonselective Raf inhibitor, approved for the treatment of RCC/HCC/advanced thyroid cancer, caused cardiac ischemia and myocardial infarction (Sorafenib prescribing information, http://www.unigraph.com/bayer/inserts/nexavar.pdf.). Vemurafenib (Zelboraf) was developed to address tumors driven by B-Raf mutation V900E and is approved to treat metastatic melanomas. This agent is more selective than sorafenib, but remains a pan-Raf inhibitor. Patients treated with vemurafenib presented with serious adverse effects including fast heartbeat (see Table 15.5). Dabrafenib, which was approved in 2013 as a highly selective kinase inhibitor of Raf, has been devoid of any cardiac issues (see Table 15.5), possibly due to its limited use to date. Conversely, gain-of-function mutations in Raf have been linked to hypertrophic cardiomyopathy (Noonan and LEOPARD syndromes) [17]. Heart-specific knockdown of Raf-1 [18] resulted in significant heart enlargement and reduced contractility, further supporting the on-target mechanism of cardiotoxicity.

17.3.2.5 **MEK Inhibition**

MEK inhibitor trametinib (Mekinist) achieves a high level of selectivity through its allosteric binding. On approval, precaution was provided on several side effects including cardiomyopathy defined as cardiac failure, left ventricular dysfunction, or decreased LVEF with onset in 63 days in 7% (14/211) of the patients in one of the trials (see Table 15.5). Subsequently, additional agents have advanced to late-stage development: selumetinib and ARRY162; however, there have been no reports of adverse cardiac events.

17.3.2.6 **JAK/STAT Inhibition**

The Janus kinase (JAK) family of NRTKs regulates cellular responses to numerous growth factors and cytokines. JAK signaling serves as a protective mechanism in the heart supported by evidence that mice lacking cardiac STAT3 have enhanced susceptibility to myocardial ischemia and age-related heart failure [19]. To date, however, ruxolitinib (Jakafi), the only JAK inhibitor approved, has not raised any concerns over cardiotoxicity.

17.3.2.7 **Bcr–Abl Inhibition**

The revolution in the treatment of Philadelphia-positive CML with Bcr–Abl inhibitor, imatinib (Gleevec), has gained widespread use. Its cross-reactivity with c-Kit and PDGFR has proven useful for the treatment of GIST. Severe congestive heart failure and left ventricular dysfunction, although not common, have been observed in patients receiving imatinib [20]. In mice, imatinib causes modest but consistent decline in left ventricular dysfunction and a more severe loss of myocardial mass. At the cellular level, cardiomyocytes treated with drug led to apoptotic and necrotic cell death [1]. Cell death was mediated by induction of a stress response-activated c-Jun N-terminal kinase (JNK) pathway in the endoplasmic reticulum (ER). Evidence points to inhibition of Abl kinase as the target responsible for cardiotoxicity. Dasatinib has also been implicated in the development of heart failure (4% CHF) (see Table 15.5) and, although an Abl inhibitor, is nonselective and other kinases such Src may play a role as well.

17.3.2.8 **PDGFR and c-Kit Inhibition**

Cardiomyocytes also express PDGFRs; however, their role in cardiac effects remains unclear. PDGF ligand is reported to be protective in the ischemic heart of mice [19]. c-Kit, although not expressed on cardiomyocytes, serves for proper housing of bone marrow-derived proangiogenic stem/progenitor cells to regions of infarction. This housing, in turn, is required to prevent adverse modeling after myocardial infarction. These data suggest caution in the use of c-Kit inhibitors in patients with a history of coronary heart disease.

17.3.2.9 **VEGFR Inhibition**

VEGF ligand, expressed by many tumors, and its receptor VEGFR2, which resides on endothelial cells, regulate tumor-associated angiogenesis. Blockade of the pathway with mAbs and small-molecule inhibitors of the catalytic kinase activity has led to approved drugs, bevacizumab (colorectal cancer) and sunitinib (renal cell carcinoma), respectively. Bevacizumab (Avastin), which blocks the VEGF receptor, is reported to induce hypertension in up to 23% of the patients in some of the clinical trials [21]. Hypertension has emerged as an on-mechanism side effect due to impaired nitric oxide production leading to EC dysfunction [19]. In addition, large vessel thrombosis has been observed with the use of bevacizumab. Studies with a "VEGF trap" demonstrated that pressure overload resulted in reduction of myocardial density, contractile dysfunction, cardiac fibrosis, and eventually heart failure [19]. VEGF induces a dose-dependent decrease in blood pressure by stimulating the secretion of vasodilators including NO and prostacyclin from vascular endothelial cells. Consistent with this, bevacizumab and small-molecule VEGFR KIs, such as sunitinib and sorafenib, are associated with the development of PAH. A direct link between PAH and subsequent LVEF has not been clearly established in the clinic [12].

17.4 Current and Future Directions

17.4.1 Preclinical Safety and Clinical Outcome Predictions

Incorporating both cultured cardiomyocyte-based assays and perfused heart methodology into chronic/subchronic rodent studies or including echocardiography in chronic large animal toxicity studies is suggested to possibly improve the gap between preclinical testing and clinical outcomes [22].

In addition, newer instrumentation such as speckle tracking imaging and cardiac magnetic resonance in addition to older echocardiography and nuclear medicine techniques should help evaluate the onset and progression of cardiotoxic effects, improving the therapeutic management and final outcome for the patient [23].

TKIs have been found to evoke cardiac dysfunction in cancer patients, which was not predicted based on preclinical safety evaluations of these agents. Due to the lack of predictability, early clinical trials omitted predefined cardiac endpoints such as measurement of LVEF at baseline and during treatment. Identification of congestive heart failure was mainly based on medical history and physical examination that are unreliable and insensitive. The available cardiotoxicity data on TKIs, therefore, are likely underestimated. The need for more regular use of preclinical tools to assess cardiotoxicity is clearly warranted. Myocyte damage, measured through detection of LDH release from neonatal rat cardiac myocytes, has proven a valuable method to predict cardiotoxicity [24]. It has been shown that lapatinib, imatinib, sorafenib, and sunitinib all increased LDH levels in this assay. Furthermore, plasma concentrations at which drugs induced cardiotoxicity in animals were within the ranges *in vitro*. The sensitive cardiac-specific troponin I is easily detected in cultured myocytes; therefore, cardiac troponin assays are suitable for detecting TKI-induced cardiotoxicity [25]. Application of induced pluripotent stem cells and stem cells derived from human cardiomyocytes for safety profile screening has increased over recent years [26]. Also, *in vitro* cell-based and *in vivo* assays are being developed for cardiotoxicity itself. The use of human stem cell-derived cardiomyocytes together with other cell systems [5] is being widely explored for their use and appears quite promising. Again there are services available for these assays (www.vistagen.com/.). A particular readout on these cells that seem to be promising is cell impedance. The assay seems to be validated and extended to 125 compounds whose kinome selectivity profile was included [26,27]. *In silico* models based on machine learning and recursive partitioning are yet another tool that has the potential for screening agents for their cardiotoxic potential (http://www.cellulardynamics.com/sot/posters/CDI140325SOT02pdf.pdf.).

The use of zebrafish in cardiotoxicity studies also seems applicable [28], whereby embryos with a green fluorescent protein stain have been utilized. Again, there seem to be services offered to assess KI cardiotoxicity using imaging together with zebrafish embryos (http://www.biobide.com/biobide-general-services/biobide-general-services/cardiotox-assay.html.).

Acute *in vivo* studies may be insufficient time for development of TKI-induced cardiac toxicity. Right and left ventricular functions were impaired by 10–30% in sunitinib-treated monkeys; however, such changes were not detected in rats [22]. For pharmacological effects of TKI, duration of target modulation is an important parameter; therefore, an *ex vivo* Langendorff heart or working heart models may be more appropriate [22]. Although not a common practice, echocardiography assessment in chronic rodent and nonrodent animal safety studies has been used by some companies. Toxicity studies in animal models of disease are economical on time and cost. In addition to assessment of gross endpoints (body weight gain), assessment of cardiovascular safety endpoints should be considered.

17.5 Conclusions

Kinases play a crucial role in normal cardiovascular development and during cardiovascular stress responses. From the growing wealth of information that is now emerging from the use of approved targeted kinase inhibitors, the cardiotoxicity observed can be mechanistically rationalized based on the inhibition of specific kinases.

Although cardiac side effects of present drugs are manageable, longer term safety and use in non-oncology settings remain unclear.

It is, therefore, imperative that future drug discovery efforts diligently profile compounds across the kinome (www.discoverx.com/.) and strive for a high level of kinase selectivity, especially against the cardiac antitargets identified, in order to minimize cardiovascular toxicities.

In addition to biochemical characterization, follow-up with cellular endpoints using cardiomyocyte cultures to determine drug-induced cardiotoxicity is important. Any alerts can be followed up in a rodent isolated perfuse heart model. Although safety studies are generally conducted in nondiseased animals, the therapeutic index can be estimated from chronic animal efficacy studies by including safety endpoints. Implementation of echocardiography in a large animal should also be considered on a case-by-case basis [22].

Scrutiny at the preclinical level for cardiac effects coupled with measurement of defined endpoints in the clinic should serve to improve the safety/quality of future kinase inhibitor drugs.

References

1 Francis, J., Ahluwalia, M.S., Wetzerl, M., Wang, E., Paplham, P., Smiley, S., McCarthy, P.L., Cohen, I.L., Spangenthal, E., and Battiwalla, M. (2010) Reversible cardiotoxicity with tyrosine kinase inhibitors. *Clinical Advances in Hematology & Oncology*, **8**, 128–132.

2 Bergmann, O., Bhardwaj, R.D., Bernard, S., Zdunek, S., Barnabe-Heider, F., Walsh, S., Zupicich, J., Alkass, K., Buchholz, B.A., Druid, H., Jovinge, S., and Frisen, J. (2009) Evidence for cardiomyocyte renewal in humans. *Science*, **324**, 98–102.

3 Li, Y.-M., Guo, Y.-P., and Liu, Y. (2010) Cancer chemotherapy induces cardiotoxicity by targeting cardiac stem cells. *Journal of Cellular and Molecular Medicine*, **14** (11), 2630–2632.

4 De Angelis, A., Piegari, E., Cappetta, D., Marino, L., Filippelli, A., Berrino, L., Ferreira-Martins, J., Zheng, H., Hosoda, T., Rota, M., Urbanek, K., Kajstura, J., Leri, A., Rossi, F., and Anversa, P. (2010) Anthracycline cardiomyopathy is mediated by depletion of the cardiac stem cell pool and is rescued by restoration of progenitor cell function. *Circulation*, **121**, 276–292.

5 Force, T. and Kolaja, K.L. (2011) Cardiotoxicity of kinase inhibitors: the prediction and translation of preclinical models to clinical outcomes. *Nature Reviews. Drug Discovery*, **10**, 111–126.

6 Slamon, D.J., Leylans-Jons, B., Shak, S., Fuchs, H., Bajamonde, A., Fleming, T., Eiermann, W., Wolter, J., Pegram, M., Baselga, J., and Norton, I. (2001) Use of chemotherapy plus a monoclonal antibody against HER2 for metastatic breast cancer that overexpresses HER2. *The New England Journal of Medicine*, **344**, 783–792.

7 Seidman, A., Hudis, C., Pierri, M.K., Shak, S., Paton, V., Ashby, M., Murphy, M., Stewart, S.J., and Keefe, D. (2002) Cardiac dysfunction in the trastuzumab clinical trials experience. *Journal of Clinical Oncology*, **20** (5), 1215–1221.

8 Lee, K.F., Simon, H., Chen, H., Bates, B., Hung, M.C., and Hauser, C. (1995) Requirement for neuregulin receptor ErbB2 in neural and cardiac development. *Nature*, **378**, 394–398.

9 Meyer, D. and Birchmeier, C. (1995) Multiple essential functions of neuregulin in development. *Nature*, **378**, 386–390.

10 Zhao, Z.Z., Sawyer, D.R., Baiga, R.R., Opel, D.J., Han, X., Marchionni, M.A., and Kelly, R.A. (1998) Neuregulins promote survival and growth of cardiac myocytes. *The Journal of Biological Chemistry*, **273**, 10261–10269.

11 Perez, E.A., Koehler, M., Byrne, J., Preston, A.J., Rappold, E., and Ewer, M.S. (2008) Cardiac safety of lapatinib: pooled analysis of 3689 patients enrolled in clinical trials. *Mayo Clinic Proceedings*, **83**, 679–686.

12 Mellor, H.R., Bell, A.R., Valentin, J.P., and Roberts, R.R.A. (2011) Cardiotoxicity associates with targeting kinase pathways in cancer. *Toxicological Sciences*, **120** (1), 14–32.

13 Spector, N.L., Yarden, Y., Smith, B., Lyass, L., Trusk, P., Pry, K., Jill, J.E., Xia, W., Seger, R., and Bacus, S.S. (2007) Activation of AMP-activated protein kinase by human EGF receptor 2/EGF receptor tyrosine kinase inhibitor protects cardiac cells. *Proceedings of the National Academy of Sciences of the United States of America*, **104**, 10607–10612.

14 Force, T., Krause, D.S., and R.A., VanEtten. (2007) Molecular mechanisms of cardiotoxicity of tyrosine kinase inhibition. *Nature Reviews Cancer*, **7**, 332–344.

15 Harris, I.S., Zhang, S., Treskov, I., Kovacs, A., Weinheimer, C., and Muslin, A. (2004) Raf-1 kinase is required for cardiac hypertrophy and cardiomyocytes survival in response to pressure overload. *Circulation*, **110**, 718–723.

16 Yamaguchi, O., Watanabe, T., Nishida, K., Kashiwase, K., Higuchi, Y., Takeda, T., Hikoso, S., Hirotani, S., Asahi, M., Taniike, M., Nakai, A., Tsujimoto, I., Matsumura, Y., Miyazaki, J., Chien, K.R., Matsuzawa, A., Sadamitsu, C., Ichijo, H., Baccarini, M., Hori, M., and Otsu, K. (2004) Cardiac specific disruption of the c-raf 1 gene induces cardiac dysfunction and apoptosis.

The Journal of Clinical Investigation, **114**, 937–943.

17 Pandit, B., Sarkozy, A., Pennacchio, L.A., Carta, C., Oishi, K., Martinelli, S., Pogna, E.A., Schackwitz, W., Ustaszewska, A., Landstrom, A., Bos, J.M., Ommen, S.R., Esposito, G., Lepri, F., Faul, C., Mundel, P., López Siguero, J.P., Tenconi, R., Selicorni, A., Rossi, C., Mazzanti, L., Torrente, I., Marino, B., Digilio, M.C., Zampino, G., Ackerman, M.J., Dallapiccola, B., Tartaglia, M., and Gelb, B.D. (2007) Gain-of-function RAF-1 mutations cause Noonan and LEOPARD syndromes with hypertrophic cardiomyopathy. *Nature Genetics*, **39**, 1007–1012.

18 Yamaguchi, O., Watanabe, T., Nishida, K., Kashiwase, K., Higuchi, Y., Takeda, T., Hikoso, S., Hirotani, S., Asahi, M., Taniike, M., Nakai, A., Tsujimoto, I., Matsumura, Y., Miyazaki, J., Chien, K.R., Matsuzawa, A., Sadamitsu, C., Ichijo, H., Baccarini, M., Hori, M., and Otsu, K. (2004) Cardiac-specific disruption of the c-raf-1 gene induces cardiac dysfunction and apoptosis. *The Journal of Clinical Investigation*, **114**, 937–943.

19 Chen, M.H., Kerkela, R., and Force, T. (2008) Mechanisms of cardiac dysfunction associated with tyrosine kinase inhibitor cancer therapeutics. *Circulation*, **118**, 84–95.

20 Kerkela, R., Grazette, L., Yacobi, R., Iliescu, C., Patten, R., and Beahm, C. (2006) Cardiotoxicity of cancer therapeutic agent imatinib mesylate. *Nature Medicine*, **12**, 908–916.

21 Ranpura, V., Pulipati, B., Chu, D., Zhu, X., and S., Wu. (2010) Increased risk of high-grade hypertension with bevacizumab in cancer patients: a meta-analysis. *American Journal of Hypertension*, **23**, 460–468.

22 Yang, B. and Papoian, T. (2012) Tyrosine kinase inhibitor induced cardiotoxicity: approaches to narrow the gaps between preclinical safety evaluation and clinical outcome. *Journal of Applied Toxicology*, **32**, 945–951.

23 Pizzuno, F., Vizzari, G., Bomzer, C.A., Qamar, R., Carerj, S., Zito, C., and Khandheria, B.K. (2014) Diagnosis of chemotherapy-induced cardiotoxicity. *Journal of Patient-Centered Research and Reviews*, **1**, 121–127.

24 Hasinoff, B.B. (2010) The cardiotoxicity and myocyte damage caused by small molecule anticancer tyrosine kinase inhibitors is correlated with lack of target specificity. *Toxicology and Applied Pharmacology*, **244**, 190–195.

25 Lindahl, B., Venge, B., and James, S. (2010) The new high-sensitivity cardiac troponin T assay improves risk assessment in acute coronary syndromes. *Journal of the American Heart*, **160**, 224–229.

26 Scott, C.W., Zhang, X., Abi-Gerges, N., Lamore, S.D., Abassi, Y.A., and Peters, M.F. (2014) An impedance-based cellular assay using human iPSC-derived cardiomyocytes to quantify modulators of cardiac contractility. *Toxicological Sciences*. doi: 10.1093/toxsci/kfu186.

27 Davis, M.I., Hunt, J.P., Herrgard, S., Ciceri, P., Wodicka, L.M., Pallares, G., Hocker, M., Treiber, D.K., and Zarrinkar, P.P. (2011) Comprehensive analysis of kinase inhibitor selectivity. *Nature Biotechnology*, **29** (11), 1046–1051.

28 Cheng, H., Kari, G., Dicker, A.P., Rodeck, U., Koch, W., and Force, T. (2011) A novel pre-clinical strategy for identifying cardiotoxic kinase inhibitors and mechanisms of cardiotoxicity. *Circulation Research*, **109** (12), 1401–1409.

18
Case Studies: Selective Inhibitors of Protein Kinases – Exploiting Demure Features

Ellen R. Laird

18.1
Introduction

The approval of 26 protein kinase inhibitors since 1999 has fully validated this target class for the treatment of human diseases, particularly in oncology (Chapter 15). Indeed, several of these agents are among the top 100 drugs [1]. The success of these compounds has ensured continued interest in kinase inhibitors as therapeutic agents; however, the lack of selectivity among kinases for several of the best-known compounds (e.g., imatinib, sunitinib, sorafenib, and dasatinib) [2] leads to adverse events that prevent dosing to their fullest potential for efficacy [3,4]. Additionally, kinase involvement in pathways that drive chronic diseases ensures that the desire for enhanced selectivity will continue and likely escalate [5–7]. Fortunately, exceptional selectivity within a tightly defined family of kinases has been demonstrated to be possible with the successful launch of the Janus kinase inhibitors tofacitinib for the treatment of rheumatoid arthritis (RA) [8,9], and the more recent approval of ruxolitinib for myelofibrosis [10]. Tofacitinib is described as demonstrating "significant selectivity versus a panel of >300 kinases"; [11] ruxolitinib has been reported to enjoy similar selectivity [12].

Selective inhibition of kinases has been the subject of numerous publications; discussions typically focus on dramatic differences in kinase sequence or conformation [13,14]. Examples include exploitation of a hydrophobic pocket that exists in kinases that harbor a relatively small residue at the beginning of the hinge sequence (the aptly named "gatekeeper" residue) [15], or the ability to capture an inactive fold of some kinases where a channel is opened between the C-helix and the activation loop (generally referred to as a "DFG-out" conformation, where DFG denotes the highly conserved residues at the beginning of the activation loop) [16]. Unfortunately, these features and folds are available to enough kinases that inhibitors designed to access them remain stubbornly promiscuous [17].

Antitargets and Drug Safety, First Edition. Edited by László Urbán, Vinod F. Patel, and Roy J. Vaz.

It has become evident that achieving a superior selectivity profile often requires identification and utilization of much subtler features. Fortunately, patterns are beginning to emerge that provide a framework for investigators seeking to enhance selectivity for a given kinase versus one or more antitarget kinases. It must be emphasized that access to multiple X-ray crystal structures of kinases in complex with relevant ligands is essential for formulating and testing hypotheses, especially when seeking differences in, for example, the position of observed solvent or side chain rotamers.

Recent reports where selectivity has been achieved reveal a remarkable variation in features that are hypothesized to provide the key. Notable examples include differences in the P-loop sequence [18] or conformation [19], dimensions of the ATP cleft [20], influence of residues beyond those that contact ATP or line the "DFG-out" channel [21], solvation effects [22,23], residues surrounding the exit from the ATP cleft [24], or intrinsic flexibility of the hinge residues [25].

In the sections that follow, three case studies from our experiences at Array BioPharma describing the achievement of selectivity versus challenging kinase antitargets are discussed, with particular emphasis on the identification and exploitation of demure structural features. In each instance, the inhibitors are contained within the ATP cleft, and involve selectivity tuning of very familiar molecular templates, that is, quinazolines and pyridinylpyrazoles. It is notable that although each case involves optimization of inhibitors targeting cancer pathways, the antitargets are known or expected to have effected dose limitations, with accompanying diminished opportunity for achieving efficacy. These cases will also rely on presenting *in vitro* enzyme inhibition data, as this provides clarity in interpretation of the influence of structural features on binding. For full discussions of the overall lead optimization process and structure–activity relationship (SAR), including cellular potency, *in vitro* and *in vivo* ADME, and pharmacological efficacy data, the reader is referred to the primary literature cited for each section.

18.2
Case I: Indane Oximes as Selective B-Raf Inhibitors [26]

The Ras/Raf/MEK/ERK (MAPK) signal transduction pathway is crucial for cell survival, growth, differentiation, and proliferation. Evaluation of various cancer cell lines and primary tumor samples has shown constitutive activation of the MAPK pathway in cancers of the lung, colon, pancreas, kidney, and ovary [27]. The Raf kinases function downstream of Ras and are responsible for activation of MEK and ERK. Mutations of the BRAF gene lead to amplification of the MAPK pathway via constitutive activation of B-Raf. Mutant B-Raf is present in ~7% of all cancers [28], with particular dominance in melanoma [29]. The mutation in which Valine 600 is substituted by glutamate (V600E) constitutes over 90% of B-Raf mutants [28], results in a 500-fold increase in catalytic activity over wild type [30], and is correlated with increases in malignancy and diminished response to chemotherapy [31]. Explicit targeting of B-Raf^{V600E} has been clinically validated recently by the effectiveness of the selective inhibitors vemurafenib [32] and dabrafenib [33].

One of the earliest series evaluated comprised a pyridinylimidazole scaffold, represented by **1** (Table 18.1). X-ray crystal structures of Raf isoforms were not yet available, and this template proved attractive owing to the limited conformational possibilities, and a well-established general binding mode reported for close analogues such as SB-203580 [34]. It was expected that **1** and close analogues would exhibit substantial p38 inhibition, and it emerged as the primary antitarget. Although inhibition of p38 MAP kinases has been broadly studied for the treatment of immunological and inflammatory disorders [35], the role of p38 in diverse cellular processes raises the possibility of substantial adverse events from significant inhibition [36]. Indeed, several diverse chemotypes have entered clinical trials and have been discontinued owing to elevation of liver transaminases and adverse neurological effects [35].

As expected, **1** exhibited significant p38α inhibition (Table 18.1); despite a 10-fold preference for both wild-type B-Raf and the activating mutant (B-Raf^{V600E}), the modest affinity for ATP known for p38 ($K_m = 25\,\mu M$) [37] ensured cellular activity sufficient for concern [38]. Analogues of **1** remained obstinately potent inhibitors of p38α. During the optimization process, we explored the possibility of incorporating an indanone oxime moiety as a surrogate for the chlorophenol of **1** [39], with the hypothesis that the fused ring might provide a starting point for exploration of a type II inhibitor. The resulting compounds exhibited a substantial improvement in potency on all Raf isoforms, with simultaneous loss of inhibition on p38α. Table 18.1 illustrates the consistent activity and selectivity for representative analogues: The simply adorned prototype **2**, the advanced analog **3** for which an X-ray structure was determined,[1] and the eventual early development candidate **4** [26] show comparable inhibition profiles.

The X-ray crystal structures for compound **1** in p38α and compound **3** in B-Raf are illustrated in Figure 18.1. The binding modes appear comparable (Figure 18.1a), and show the features that are typically observed for this class of inhibitors: A propeller-like conformation exists about the central heterocycle, and a single hydrogen bond is formed between the pyridyl nitrogen and a backbone NH from the hinge sequence. The hydrophobic aryl ring occupies a pocket proximal to the hinge that is made accessible by virtue of a small gatekeeper residue (Thr106 in p38α; Thr529 in B-Raf). Both compounds bind in a type I fashion, with the enzyme folded conventionally, that is, with a DFG-"in" conformation of the activation loop.

Given the SAR trends, the oxime functionality was the obvious choice for driving the potency and selectivity enhancements in favor of the Raf isoforms. This selectivity extended far beyond a preference over p38α: Compound **4** was assayed at a concentration of 1 μM against a panel of 212 kinases, and failed to

1) PDB accession code # 3D4Q

Table 18.1 Enzyme inhibition data for representative B-Raf inhibitors.

Enzyme	IC_{50} (nM) 1	IC_{50} (nM) 2	IC_{50} (nM) 3	(GDC-0879) IC_{50} (nM) 4
	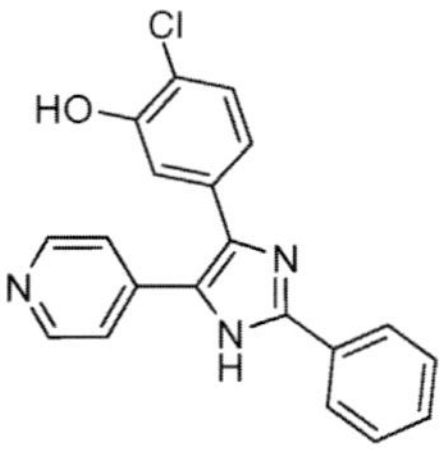	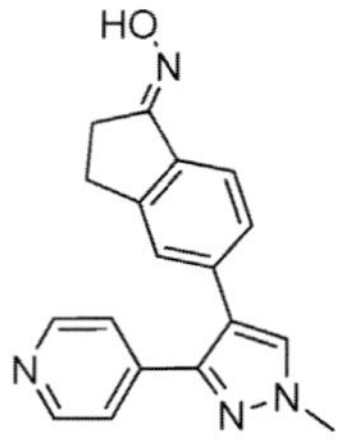	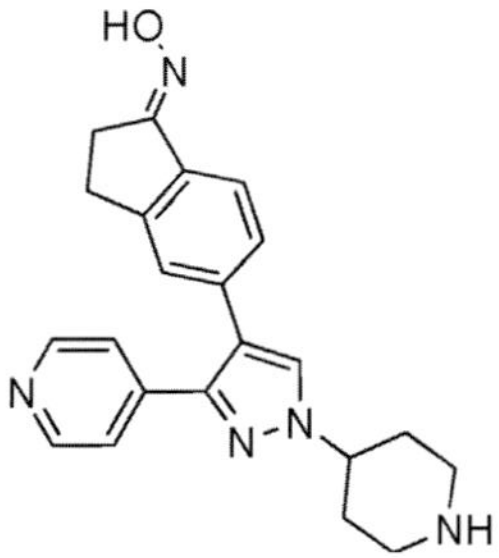	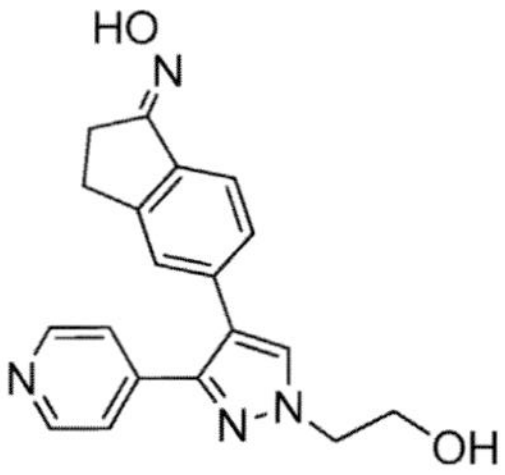
C-Raf	9	0.55	0.10	0.58
B-Raf	3	0.03	0.03	0.23
B-Raf (V600E)	3	0.02	0.03	0.13
p38α	30	>1000	>1000	>1000

The oxime-bearing analogues show consistent potency and selectivity for B-Raf over p38α.

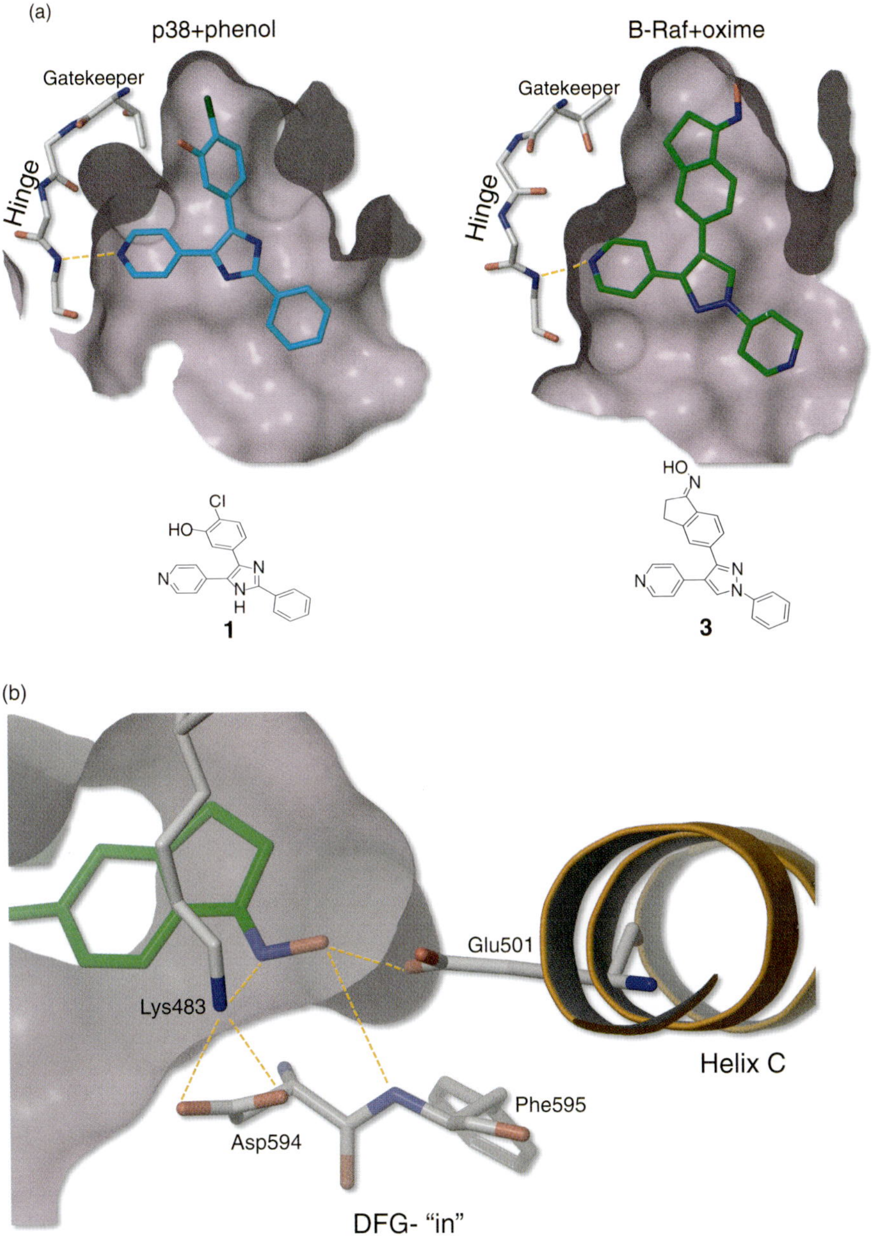

Figure 18.1 (a) X-ray crystal structures of p38::**1** and B-Raf::**3** suggest comparable binding modes. The hydrogen bonds to the hinge are shown as dashed orange lines, and the surfaces of the respective kinases are illustrated in plum. The side chains of the hinge sequence are not displayed for clarity. (b) The X-ray crystal structure of B-Raf in complex with compound **3** shows several explicit interactions for the oxime moiety. The indane ring makes substantial hydrophobic interactions with the gatekeeper pocket, while the oxime makes several hydrogen bonding interactions, which are illustrated with orange dotted lines.

inhibit any by at least 50%. A detailed view of the interactions involving the indanone oxime illustrates an efficiency of polar and hydrophobic contacts (Figure 18.1b). The indane ring fully occupies the hydrophobic regions of the gatekeeper pocket, the sp2 nitrogen of the oxime participates in a hydrogen bond with the catalytic lysine, and the oxime hydroxyl donates a second hydrogen bond to the glutamate residue from the C-helix. The hydroxyl oxygen is also poised to accept a hydrogen bond from the backbone NH of Phe595 of the activation loop.

Those familiar with kinase structure and function, however, will note that the glutamate and lysine residues are invariant among kinases, and that the main chain of the D**X**G sequence[2)] is also held in proximity. The oxime interactions cannot be directly responsible for the exquisite selectivity. A closer comparison of the complexes reveals a significant difference in the compound position. Figure 18.2a provides two views for the relative orientation of the inhibitors when the p38α::**1** and B-Raf::**3** X-ray structures are superimposed on the protein coordinates. The hinge-interacting pyridine nitrogen provides an anchor point, while a substantial shift exists in both plane and centroid between the two inhibitors. Consideration of the residues that line the floor of the ATP cleft provides a rationale: Ala157 and Leu167 of p38 correspond to Phe583 and Gly593 in B-Raf (Figure 18.2b). In each case, the larger hydrophobic residue provides the contact surface upon which the central heterocycle of the inhibitor rests. In the case of B-Raf::**3**, the combination of contacting the hinge and providing a hydrophobic surface for the pyrazole serves to thrust the oxime directly into the path of the lysine–glutamate pair (Figure 18.2c). Conversely, in p38α and other kinases, the indane oxime will be driven into sterically and electronically incompatible locations.

Sequence comparisons for members of the human kinome [40] indicate that only KSR1/2, MYT1, and SCYL1/3 share both the phenylalanine/glycine floor residues and a threonine at the gatekeeper position, which is consistent with observed screening panel data (see below). Further lead optimization of this series led to the early development of candidate GDC-0879 (**4**) [26], and further work enabled replacement of the oxime moiety with heterocyclic mimics [41].

This case study highlights the importance of identifying residues that are frequently neglected in the evaluation of kinase binding sites – qualitatively the floor of the ATP cleft in all kinases is comprised of nondescript bumps formed by hydrophobic side chains. Variation in the landscape can enable shifting of templates such that the bond vectors bearing substituents may be directed into unusual spaces.

A second observation warrants attention: B-Raf and p38α share only 27% sequence identity in the kinase domain. In the ATP cleft, of the approximately

2) While a Phe is the most common residue to comprise the central residue of the triad at the beginning of the activation loop, there are exceptions, for example, CDK8 contains a methionine in the corresponding position.

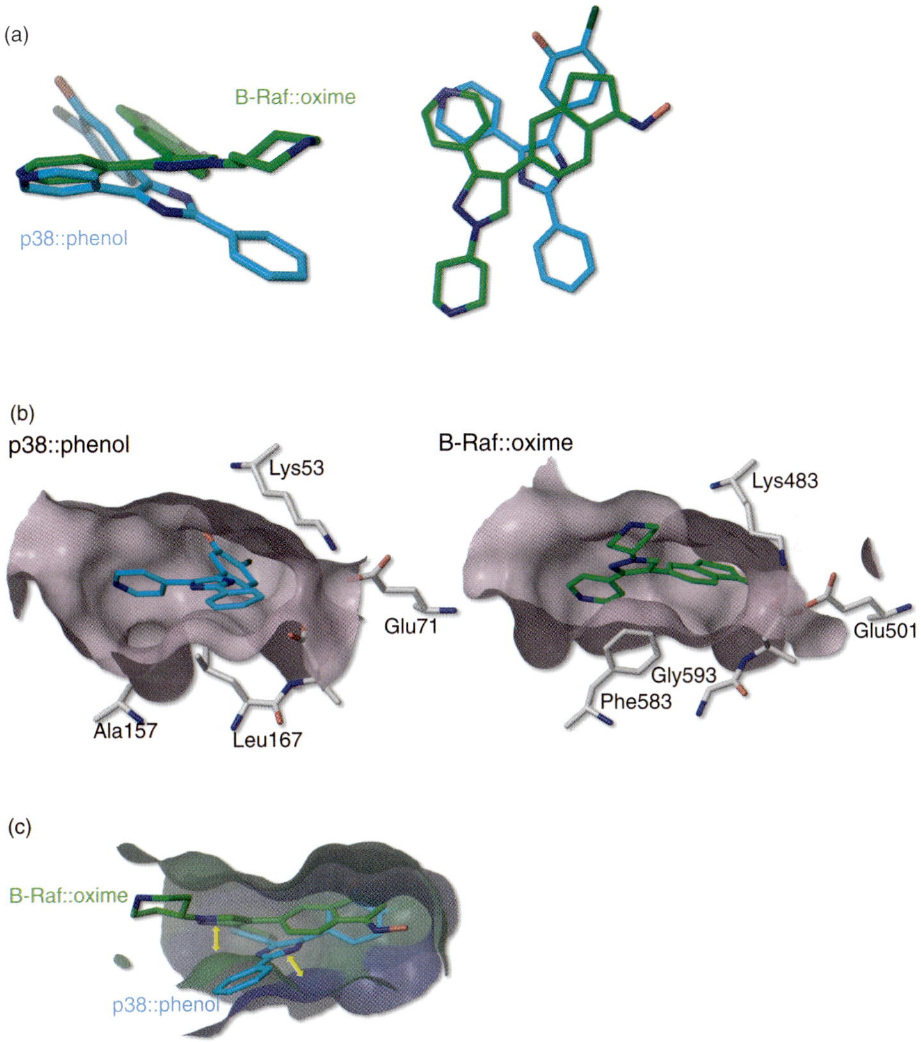

Figure 18.2 (a) Direct comparison of the relative positions for compounds **1** (blue carbon atoms) and **3** (green carbon atoms) in X-ray complexes with p38α and B-Raf, respectively. The structures are superimposed on the backbone atoms of the protein structures, which are not displayed for clarity. Although the hinge-binding pyridine nitrogens are nearly superimposable, the remaining features of the compounds are shifted dramatically. (b) The shift in compound positions illustrated in Figure 18.2a can be attributed to different residues that comprise the floor of the ATP cleft: Ala157/Leu167 in p38α are replaced with Phe583/Gly593 in B-Raf, with a concomitant shift in the hydrophobic surface. (c) Surfaces for the two proteins are shown matched to the inhibitors (p38α and **1** in blue, B-Raf and **3** in green), which are again superimposed on the protein backbone atoms. Yellow arrows indicate the dominant hydrophobic surfaces of Leu167 (p38α) and Phe583 (B-Raf) upon which the central heterocycle of the inhibitors rest.

20 residues whose side chains contact type I inhibitors, only half are identical. However, significant cross-binding occurs even with type II inhibitors [42]. Indeed, although sorafenib was originally approved as an inhibitor of B-Raf, it exhibits substantially higher binding affinity to p38α as well as to other targets. Such observations should give pause to the notion that relatives on the kinome dendrogram [43] or clustering of kinases based on their ATP site similarity [44] is the most practical means of identifying troublesome activities, and the importance of large-scale profiling is beginning to emerge [12].

18.3
Case II: ARRY-380 (ONT-380) – an ErbB2 Agent that Spares EGFR [45]

The ErbB (HER) family of receptor tyrosine kinases consists of four closely related members, of which EGFR (ErbB1/HER1) and ErbB2 (HER2) are the most studied isoforms [46]. Binding of growth factor ligands induces dimerization and kinase activation. Cellular signaling that is controlled by ErbB members includes the phosphatidylinositol 3-kinase/Akt protein kinase B (PKB) pathway, the Ras/Raf/MEK/ERK1/2 pathway, and the phospholipase C (PLCγ) pathway. Several malignancies are associated with increased expression or mutation of members of the ErbB family and include lung, breast, stomach, colorectal, head and neck, pancreatic carcinomas, and glioblastoma. The monoclonal antibody trastuzumab was the first agent to validate receptors of growth factors as molecular targets for cancer therapy [47], and several agents targeting the ErbB family have been approved as pan or dual agents. With the exception of lapatinib, which is a true dual inhibitor, most ErbB agents show a significant preference for inhibition of EGFR versus ErbB2 [48], with resulting side effects such as GI issues and severe rash [49].

The heterodimer formed by ErbB2 and ErbB3 is a remarkably sturdy signaling complex. Owing to the impaired kinase function of ErbB3, ErbB2 has become widely recognized as a clinically validated, high-value target for various cancers, especially breast cancer [50,51]. An additional appeal of selective inhibition of ErbB2 arises from the observed trastuzumab resistance [52], in particular the p95 truncated HER2 receptor [53], which leads to hyperactive ErbB2 activity.

Wishing to leverage our pan ErbB program toward an ErbB2 selective agent, we were intrigued by the observed selectivity for a potential metabolite of the lead quinazoline series (Figure 18.3). Compounds represented by generic structure **5** typically exhibited a modest sevenfold preference for ErbB2 versus EGFR, but were plagued by several PK issues. During the evaluation of potential metabolites such as the *N*-oxide **6**, a significant enhancement in selectivity for ErbB2 was notable. Indeed, fused heterocycles that maintained both the hydrogen bond acceptor and the expected van der Waals contact of the methyl group retained potency and selectivity; ARRY-380 (ONT-380) emerged as the eventual candidate.

Little structural data for the ErbB family existed during the course of these efforts: The sole X-ray available for EGFR in complex with erlotinib [54]

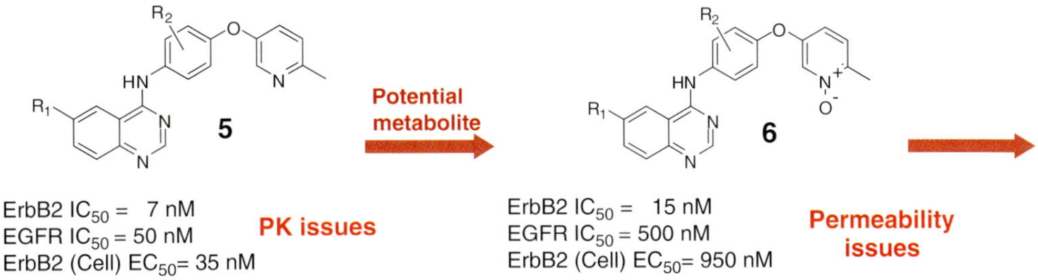

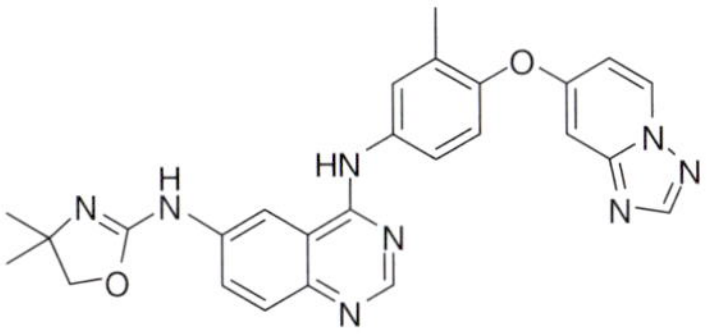

ARRY-380 (ONT-380)

	ErbB2	EGFR	ErbB4
K_i(nM)	1.8	72	276

Figure 18.3 The optimization path to ARRY-380 (ONT-380). Quinazolines related to **5** show encouraging potency, but insufficient selectivity versus EGFR as well as poor PK. The *N*-oxide metabolite **6** shows remarkable selectivity, which is largely driven by decreased activity in EGFR inhibition.

provided a satisfactory template for generation of a homology model for ErbB2, as the two isoforms share an overall sequence identity in the catalytic domain of 80%. Naturally, the high sequence similarity would result in scant differences between EGFR and ErbB2 in the ATP binding cleft (Figure 18.4). Of the residues

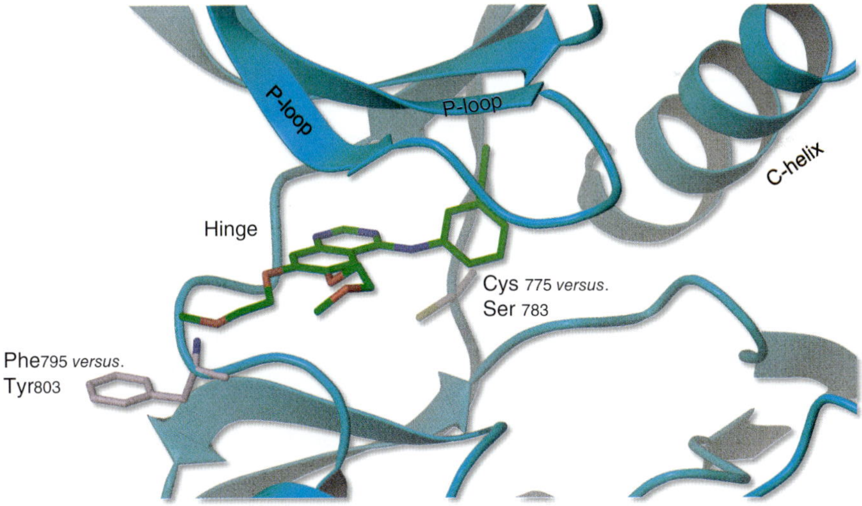

Figure 18.4 The X-ray crystal structure of EGFR in complex with Tarceva (PDB: 1M17). The backbone is illustrated as a blue ribbon, and the inhibitor is shown in green. Only two residues differ in the ATP site between EGFR and ErbB2, and are shown explicitly: Phe795 in EGFR corresponds to Tyr803 in ErbB2, and faces away from the binding cleft. Cys775 (EGFR) corresponds to Ser783 (ErbB2).

in van der Waals contact of typical type I inhibitors, only two differences exist: Phe795$^{(EGFR)}$/Tyr803$^{(ErbB2)}$ reside at the beginning of the C-lobe and face away from the ATP cleft, whereas Cys775$^{(EGFR)}$/Ser783$^{(ErbB2)}$ exist deep in the cleft at the beginning of strand β-4, and form part of the cleft floor while making contact to the C-helix. It was anticipated that the large phenoxypyridine moiety in analogues of **5** might occupy space near the C-helix; hence, the Cys/Ser difference warranted evaluation.

Consideration of side chain rotamer statistics [55] suggested that the seemingly modest residue difference might exhibit a significant conformational preference. A serine residue with the same backbone dihedral angles as Cys775 is expected to favor placement of the side chain ~180° from that observed for the cysteine. We hypothesized that Ser783 in ErbB2 would be poised for interaction with the triazolopyridine of ONT-380 and similar analogues. The standard rotamer population for Cys775 of EGFR favors the observed conformation in the X-ray crystal structure. The rotamer available to Ser783$^{(ErbB2)}$ is likely less sampled by Cys775$^{(EGFR)}$ owing to a required gauche dihedral angle that is sterically disfavored by the larger sulfur atom. The resulting loss in activity for ONT-380 as an inhibitor of EGFR is hypothesized to arise from an unsatisfied hydrogen bond and desolvation penalty for the triazolopyridine. The proposed binding modes and interactions are illustrated in Figure 18.5.

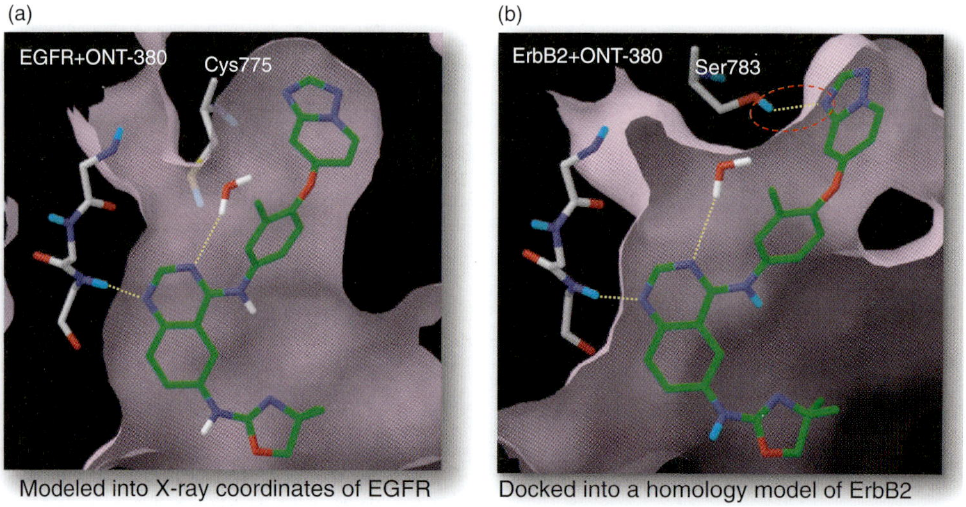

Figure 18.5 Proposed binding mode for ARRY-380 modeled into the X-ray coordinates of EGFR (PDB: 1M17) (a) and docked into a homology model of ErbB2 (b). Hydrogen bonding interactions are shown as dotted yellow lines. The quinazoline N1 forms a hydrogen bond to the hinge, while N3 is expected to coordinate to a bound water molecule. The position of Cys775 in EGFR is observed crystallographically; the orientation of Ser783 is predicted from known rotamer preferences and is able to interact with the triazolopyridine of ARRY-380.

Table 18.2 Kinases with minimal inhibition by ARRY-380 (ONT-380) at a concentration of 10 μM.

Kinase	% Inhibition (10 μM ARRY-380)
PKCmu	55
CK1_y	59
EphA1	66
EphA2	58
Flt4	62
KIT	52
Lck	69
Mer	61

It is notable that this rationale is further supported by an even larger loss in activity against ErbB4 (Figure 18.3), which bears a valine residue in the position corresponding to Ser783$^{(ErbB2)}$. Furthermore, in most kinases this position is occupied by a branched hydrophobic residue. Consistent with this observation, a larger panel screen of 100 kinases showed no activity for ONT-380 at 1 μM, and minimal activity for a few kinases at 10 μM (Table 18.2).

Several X-ray crystal structures of the ErbB family have become available since the conclusion of this work; in particular, our hypothesis regarding the preferred side chain position of Ser783 has been confirmed [56]. An additional structural feature cannot be ruled out as a contributor to potency and selectivity: The original X-ray crystal structure of EGFR in complex with erlotinib [54] includes nearly 40 residues beyond the defined kinase domain, which occupy the substrate binding site of a crystallographic neighbor. More recent structures confirm that this sequence can reside along the face of the kinase, with a small helix resting adjacent to the ATP cleft [57]. Kinases that contain additional C-proximal sequences present a variety of positions and secondary structural features; hence, the explicit influence of such residues in ErbB2 versus EGFR and in other kinases is yet to be clarified.

The clinical effect of achieving selectivity for ErbB2 versus EGFR is clear: ONT-380 is well tolerated in multiple preclinical tumor models and demonstrates significant dose-related tumor growth inhibition superior to trastuzumab and lapatinib [45]. The maximum tolerated dose of ONT-380 established in a phase 1 clinical trial is 600 mg b.i.d. Because ONT-380 spares EGFR, there is low incidence and severity of GI effects, rash, and fatigue. A phase 1b dose escalation trial of ONT-380 in combination with Kadcyla® in patients with metastatic HER2+ breast cancer is currently ongoing,[3] and a second phase 1b study is underway to evaluate the combination of ONT-380 with Xeloda and Herceptin.[4]

3) ClinicalTrialsgov. Identifier: NCT01983501.
4) ClincalTrialsgov. Identifier: NCT02025192.

Table 18.3 Enzyme inhibition data for representative AKT inhibitors.

	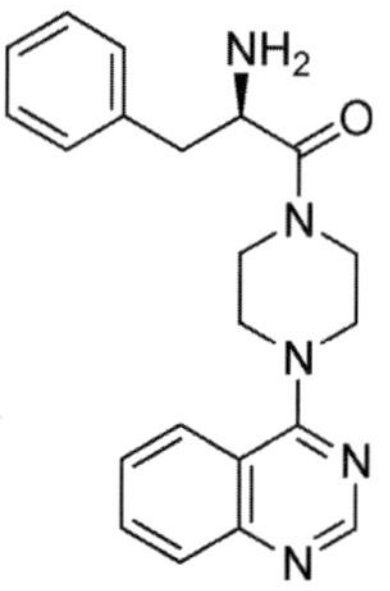 IC_{50} (nM) 7	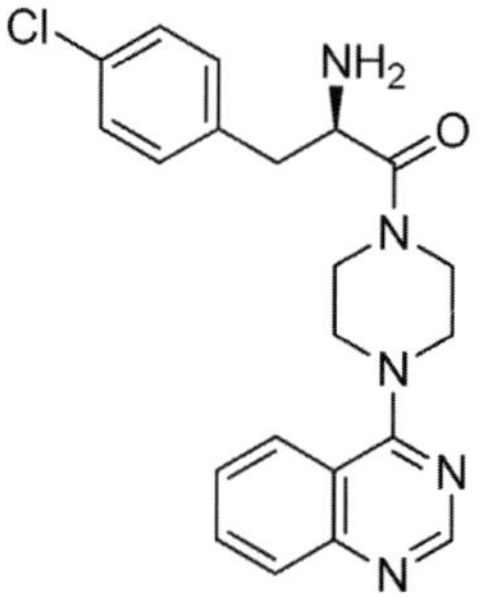 IC_{50} (nM) 8	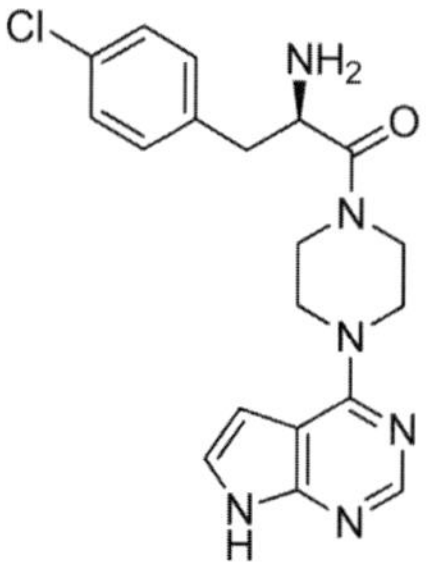 IC_{50} (nM) 9
Akt1	884	20	5

18.4
Case III: Discovery of GDC-0068 (Ipatasertib), a Potent and Selective ATP-Competitive Inhibitor of AKT [58]

Akt/PKB is a serine–threonine kinase that exists in three closely related isoforms (Akt1, Akt2, and Akt3) and that is activated by the PI3K pathway. Akt is a central node in the PI3K–Akt–mTOR pathway, and upon activation controls key processes in apoptosis, translation, transcription, and cell cycle progression [59]. Its activity is elevated in a wide variety of cancers, including prostate, colon, ovarian, breast, and melanoma. Activation can occur via loss of regulatory PTEN activity [60], amplification or mutation of PI3K, or Akt overexpression or mutation. shRNA knockdown of Akt in PTEN-null xenograft models has demonstrated significant antitumor effects when all three isoforms are inhibited [61]. These factors contribute to the appeal of a small-molecule inhibitor of Akt as a cancer therapy.

Evaluation of a high-throughput screening hit led to quinazoline **7** (Table 18.3) as a submicromolar inhibitor of Akt1 [62]; the proposed binding mode is shown in Figure 18.6. The quinazoline was expected to provide the sole hydrogen bond to the hinge, and the primary amine was poised for interaction with two glutamate residues near the exterior of the ATP cleft, which would allow the benzyl group to reach a small pocket under the P-loop. Substitutions on the benzylic group, particularly in the 4-position, led to significant potency improvements, represented by **8**. Because the key binding features emerge from the pyrimidine moiety, replacement of the quinazoline by a pyrrolopyrimidine template (**9**) was readily accommodated and the predicted binding mode was confirmed by an X-ray crystal structure of an advanced compound.[5] Close analogues, however, were plagued with poor

5) PDB accession # 3OCB.

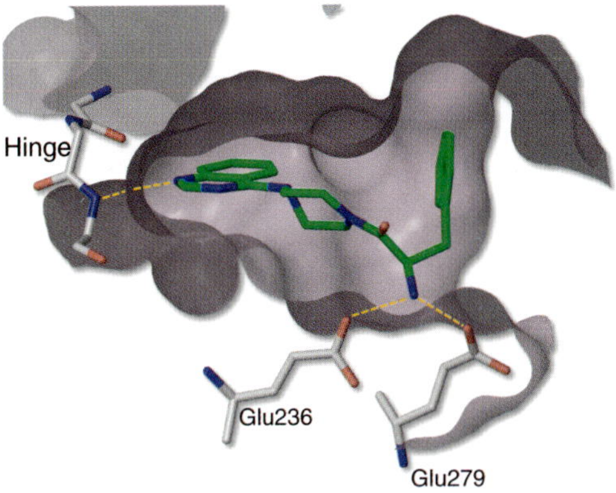

Figure 18.6 Proposed binding mode of quinazoline **7** in Akt1. The compound is illustrated in green carbons; the protein in contact with **6** is portrayed as a plum surface, with atoms involved in hydrogen bonds (dashed orange lines) explicitly shown. Side chains of the hinge are not displayed for clarity. The quinazoline functions as the hinge-binding template, while the amine serves to anchor the compound to the side chains of Glu236 and Glu279. The benzyl group is thus poised to fit into a shallow pocket under the P-loop.

selectivity in a large panel of kinases that correlated with poor tolerability, for example, PKA and ROCK1/2 [63,64], and which precluded advancement into proof-of-concept efficacy studies [62]. Selectivity versus the closely related PKA proved particularly difficult to achieve, and this kinase was identified as the primary antitarget.

During the course of evaluation of substitutions on the pyrrolopyrimidine core, it was noted that analogues with increased steric bulk near the gatekeeper residue (Met227 in Akt; Met120 in PKA) showed modest selectivity (Table 18.4). Analysis of a series of X-ray crystal structures of inhibitors bound to Akt1 and PKA revealed several residue differences near the hinge that result in a narrower and less polar cavity in PKA (Figure 18.7). Additionally, a frequently observed bound water in Akt1 near Ala230 (valine in PKA) was coordinated by the backbone and side chain of Glu228, as well as the side chain of Thr211. PKA, owing to the valine residue in corresponding space, presents no room for bound water. Consideration of the kinome sequences [40] indicates that only Akt1 possesses both Ala230 and Thr211. It was hypothesized that hydrophilic substituents positioned near Thr211 and directed toward the bound water could improve selectivity over PKA as well as over most other kinases.

A partially saturated core was designed in order to access this space. A relatively small number of substitutions around the cyclopentane were evaluated (Table 18.5), with distinct SAR, particularly with respect to selectivity versus PKA. While a number of analogues exhibited significant potency as Akt inhibitors, **10** (R^1 = methyl, R^2 = hydroxyl) also demonstrated excellent selectivity, and eventually emerged as the clinical candidate GDC-0068

Table 18.4 Enzyme inhibition and selectivity ratio for pyrrolopyridine analogues with added bulk near the gatekeeper residue show an encouraging preference for Akt.

	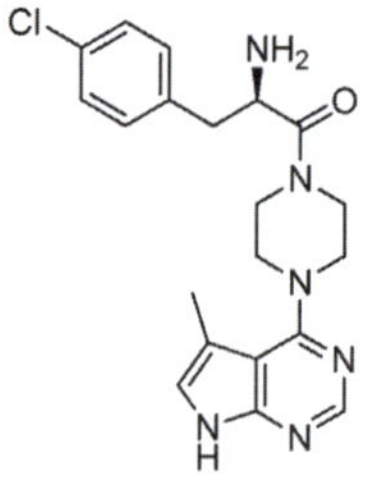	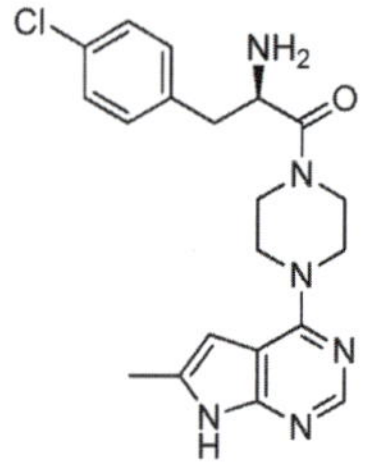	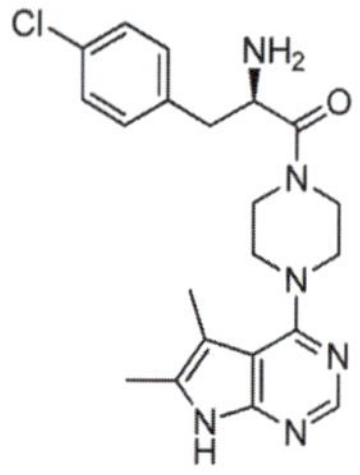
Akt1 IC_{50} (nM)	1.2	52	21
PKA IC_{50} (nM)	1.5	223	278
PKA/Akt1	1.2	4.3	13

Residue	Akt1	PKA
211	Thr	Val
230	Ala	Val
281	Met	Leu

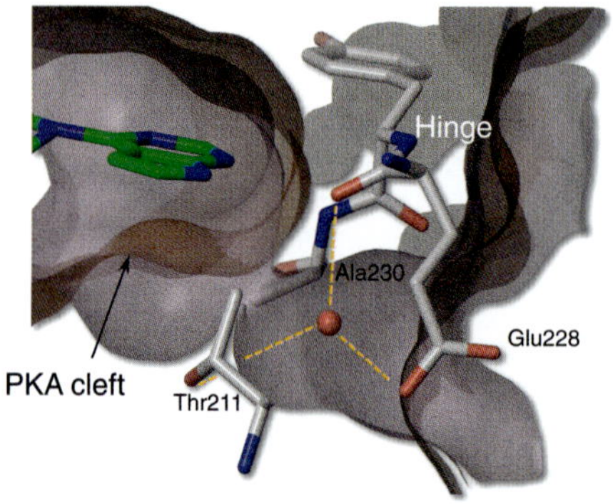

Figure 18.7 The residue differences and structural consequences for Akt1 selectivity are portrayed. The X-ray crystal structure of GDC-0068 illustrates the stereoelectronic selectivity elements in comparison with the X-ray structure of the antitarget PKA. The surface of Akt1 near the hinge-binding pyrrolopyrimidine (green) is illustrated in plum, while the truncated cleft in PKA is colored tan; the closure of the PKA cleft is indicated by a black arrow. The bound water is illustrated as a red sphere, and its hydrogen-bonding contacts to Thr211 and Glu228 are shown as orange dashed lines.

(ipatasertib).[6] In a panel of 230 kinases, ipatasertib inhibited only 3 kinases by greater than 70% at 1 μM concentration (PRKG1a, $IC_{50} = 98$ nM; PRKG1b, $IC_{50} = 69$ nM; and p70S6K, $IC_{50} = 860$ nM). An X-ray crystal structure of ipatasertib in complex with Akt1 is illustrated in Figure 18.8.[7] The role of the

6) ClinicalTrialsgov. identifier: NCT02063581.
7) PDB accession # 4EKL.

Table 18.5 Enzyme inhibition and selectivity data for a small set of dihydroindene analogues.

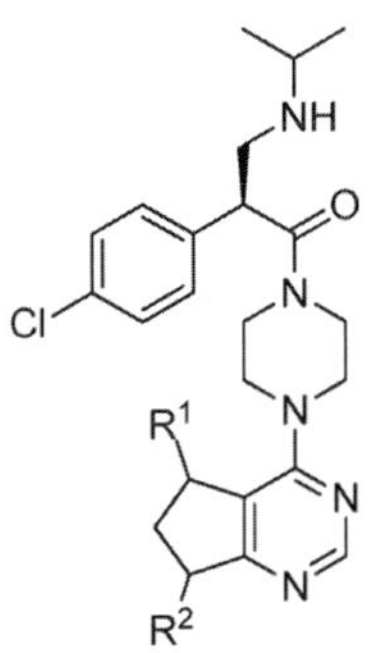

R^1	R^2	IC_{50} (nM) Akt1	IC_{50} (nM) Akt2	IC_{50} (nM) Akt3	IC_{50} (nM) Akt *p*-PRAS40 LNCaP	IC_{50} (nM) PKA
(*R*)-CH_3	H	6	12	5	287	33
Dimethyl	H	>2000	>2000	>2000	ND	>10 000
(*S*)-Vinyl	H	2	6	1	176	10
(*R*)-CH_2OH	H	81	356	83	846	957
(R)-CH_3	*(R)-OH*	*5*	*18*	*8*	*157*	*3100*
(*R*)-CH_3	(*S*)-OH	68	249	73	740	1552
(*R*)-CH_3	(*R*)-F	4	14	10	152	17
(*R*)-CH_3	(*S*)-F	12	35	23	901	541
(*R*)-CH_3	diF	1169	4177	4160	8548	>10 000
(*R*)-CH_2F	H	3	6	5	123	35

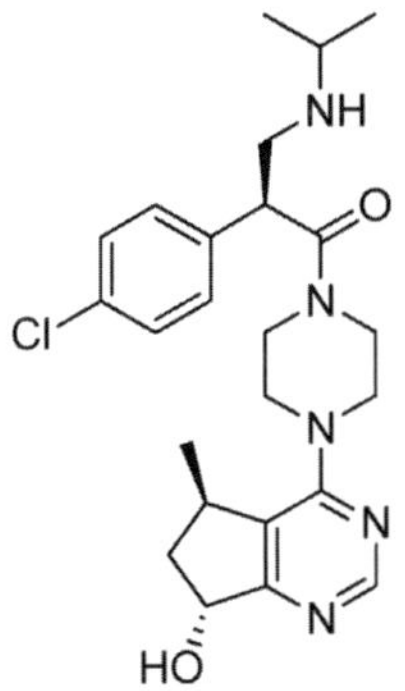

10 (GDC-0068; ipatasertib)

The data for compound **10** (GDC-0068) are given in italics.

hydroxyl group is evident, as it forms hydrogen bonds to the backbone carbonyl of Glu228 as well as to the bound water, which in turn bridges to the side chain of Glu228.

The influence of this superb selectivity is evidenced by its clinical status: ipatasertib is well tolerated in healthy volunteers, with a single agent MTD of 600 mg, and robust PD effects at and below the MTD. Ipatasertib is currently being studied in phase 1 as a single agent in patients with refractory solid tumors,[8] as well as recruiting for several combination trials.[9]

8) ClinicalTrialsgov. identifier: NCT01090960.
9) ClinicalTrialsgov. identifiers: NCT01562275, NCT01485861, NCT01896531, and NCT01362374.

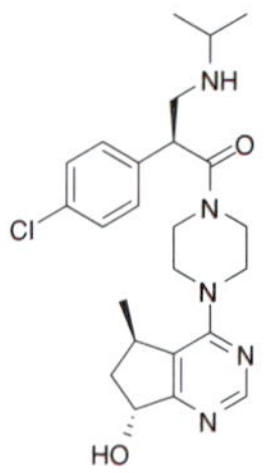

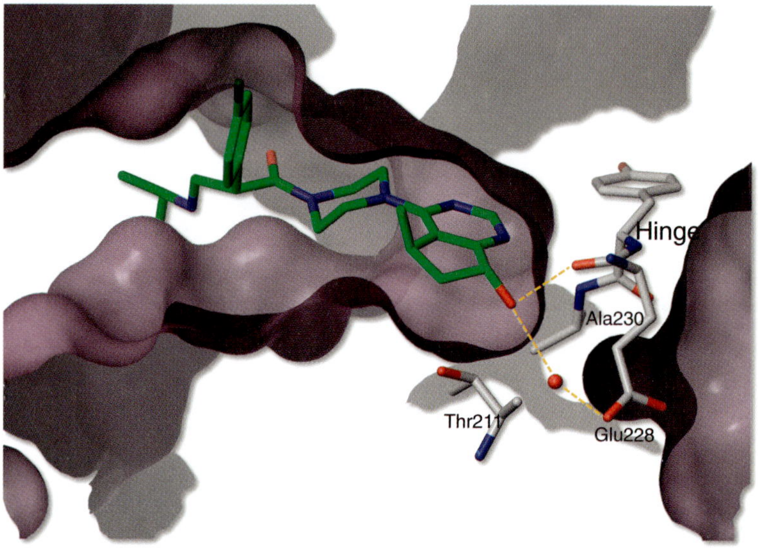

Figure 18.8 The X-ray crystal structure of Akt1::GDC-0068 confirms the design features. The compound is illustrated with green carbons, the protein surface is rendered in plum, and select side chains are shown in white. The hydroxyl group interacts with a bound water and Glu228 in a space made accessible by the small side chain of Ala230.

18.5 Concluding Remarks

The examples described here all achieved clinically relevant selectivity derived from very subtle, and easily overlooked, structural features, that is, a change in the shape of the ATP cleft, a side chain conformational preference, and a small pocket near the hinge. In each case, the selectivity arises from differences in sequence that are ultimately expressed as a change in shape or electronics. Selectivity can also arise from a variety of even less visible sources, such as differences in the K_m for ATP or other thermodynamic and kinetic parameters [38], the availability of truly allosteric sites [65,66], the ability to utilize covalent modifiers [67], and differences in protein scaffolding and cellular localization [68], none of which are necessarily "visible" at the outset of new target exploration.

The optimization of selectivity in these cases was driven in part by (i) the recognition of the appropriate antitarget from the outset of the program, and by (ii) the observation of nascent selectivity during the early screening or lead optimization stages. Clearly, devising a rationale for even modest selectivity is a valuable exercise that leads to a more sophisticated design strategy, and provides valuable insights into formulating hypotheses for each new target. These case studies also illustrate that imaginative possibilities exist even for time-worn templates such as quinazolines.

Although our emphasis in this chapter is on development of selective kinase inhibitors, the ongoing vigorous debate regarding multikinase inhibitors versus exquisite selectivity is appropriate. Emerging drug resistance mechanisms suggest that multitargeted therapies may provide prolonged efficacy in some cases [69,70]. It is likely that each disease indication and choice of pathway intervention will need to be suitably tailored, making the understanding of structural subtleties a vital part of developing new therapeutic agents.

References

1 Brooks, M. (2014) Top 100 Selling Drugs of 2013. http://wwwmedscapecom/viewarticle/820011.

2 Karaman, M.W., Herrgard, S., Treiber, D.K., Gallant, P., Atteridge, C.E., Campbell, B.T., Chan, K.W., Ciceri, P., Davis, M.I., Edeen, P.T., Faraoni, R., Floyd, M., Hunt, J.P., Lockhart, D.J., Milanov, Z.V., Morrison, M.J., Pallares, G., Patel, H.K., Pritchard, S., Wodicka, L.M., and Zarrinkar, P.P. (2008) A quantitative analysis of kinase inhibitor selectivity. *Nature Biotechnology*, **26** (1), 127–132.

3 Brazzelli, V., Grasso, V., and Borroni, G. (2013) Imatinib, dasatinib, and nilotinib: a review of adverse cutaneous reactions with emphasis on our clinical experience. *Journal of the European Academy of Dermatology and Venereology*, **27** (12), 1471–1480.

4 Mouhayar, E., Durand, J.-B., and Cortes, J. (2013) Cardiovascular toxicity of tyrosine kinase inhibitors. *Expert Opinion Drug Safety*, **12** (5), 687–696.

5 Rokosz, L.L., Beasley, J.R., Carroll, C.D., Lin, T., Zhao, J., Appell, K.C., and Webb, M.L. (2008) Kinase inhibitors as drugs for chronic inflammatory and immunological diseases; progress and challenges. *Expert Opinion on Therapeutic Targets*, **12** (7), 883–903.

6 Cohen, P. and Alessi, D.R. (2013) Kinase drug discovery: what's next in the field? *ACS Chemical Biology*, **8**, 96–104.

7 Tell, V. and Hilgeroth, A. (2013) Recent developments of protein kinase inhibitors as potential AD therapeutics. *Frontiers in Cellular Neuroscience*, **7**, 189.

8 Changelian, P.S., Flanagan, M.E., Ball, D.J., Kent, C.R., Magnuson, K.S., Martin, W.H., Rizzuti, B.J., Sawyer, P.S., Perry, B.D., Brissette, W.H., McCurdy, S.P., Kudlacz, E.M., Conklyn, M.J., Elliott, E.A., Koslov, E.R., Fisher, M.R., Strelevitz, T.J., Yoon, K., Whipple, D.A., Sun, J., Munchhof, M.J., Doty, J.L., Casavant, J.M., Blumenkopf, T.A., Hines, M., Brown, M.F., Lillie, B.M., Subramanyam, C., Chang, S.-P., Milici, A.J., Beckius, G.E., Moyer, J.D., Su, C., Woodworth, T.G., Gaweco, A.S., Beals, C.R., Littman, B.H., Fisher, D.A., Smith, J.F., Zagouras, P., Magna, H.A., Saltarelli, M.J., Johnson, K.S., Nelms, L.F., Des Etages, S.G., Hayes, L.S., Kawabata, T.T., Finco-Kent, D., Baker, D.L., Larson, M., Si, M.-S., Paniagua, R., Higgins, J., Holm, B., Reitz, B., Zhou, Y.-J., Morris, R.E., O'Shea, J.J., and Borie, D.C. (2003) Prevention of organ allograft rejection by a specific Janus kinase 3 inhibitor. *Science*, **302**, 879–878.

9 Flanagan, M.E., Blumenkopf, T.A., Brissette, W.H., Brown, M.F., Casavant, J.M., Chang, S.-P., Doty, J.L., Elliott, E.A., Fisher, M.B., Hines, M., Kent, C., Kudlacz, E.M., Lillie, B.M., Magnuson, K.S., McCurdy, S.P., Munchhof, M.J., Perry, B.D., Sawyer, P.S., Strelevitz, T.J., Subramanyam, C., Sun, J., Whipple, D.A., and Changelian, P.S. (2010) Discovery of CP-690,550: a potent and selective Janus kinase (JAK) inhibitor for the treatment of autoimmune diseases and organ transplant rejection. *Journal of Medicinal Chemistry*, **53**, 8468–8484.

10 Verstovsek, S., Kantarjian, H., Mesa, R.A., Pardanani, A.D., Cortes-Franco, J., Thomas, D.A., Estrov, Z., Fridman, J.S., Bradley, E.C., Erickson-Viitanen, S., Vaddi,

K., Levy, R., and Tefferi, A. (2010) Safety and efficacy of INCB018424, a JAK1 and JAK2 inhibitor, in myelofibrosis. *NEW England Journal of Medicine*, **363**, 1117–1127.

11 Chrencik, J.E., Patny, A., Leung, I.K., Korniski, B., Emmons, T.L., Hall, T., Weinberg, R.A., Gormley, J.A., Williams, J.M., Day, J.E., Hirsch, J.L., Kiefer, J.R., Leone, J.W., Fischer, H.D., Sommers, C.D., Huang, H.-C., Jacobsen, E.J., Tenbrink, R.E., Tomasselli, A.G., and Benson, T.E. (2010) Structural and thermodynamic characterization of the TYK2 and JAK3 kinase domains in complex with CP-690550 and CMP-6 *Journal of Molecular Biology*, **400**, 413–433.

12 Anastassiadis, T., Deacon, S.W., Devarajan, K., Ma, H., and Peterson, J.R. (2011) Comprehensive assay of kinase catalytic activity reveals features of kinase inhibitor selectivity. *Nature Biotechnology*, **29**, 1039–1045.

13 Liao, J.J.-L. (2007) Molecular recognition of protein kinase binding pockets for design of potent and selective kinase inhibitors. *Journal of Medicinal Chemistry*, **50** (3), 409–424.

14 Thaimattan, R., Banerjee, R., Miglani, R., and Iqbal, J. (2007) Protein kinase inhibitors: structural insights into selectivity. *Current Pharmaceutical Design*, **13** (27), 2751–2765.

15 Tong, L., Pav, S., White, D.M., Rogers, S., Crane, K.M., Cywin, C.L., Brown, M.L., and Pargellis, C.A. (1997) A highly specific inhibitor of human p38 MAP kinase binds in the ATP pocket. *Nature Structural Biology*, **4**, 311–316.

16 Liu, Y. and Gray, N.S. (2006) Rational design of inhibitors that bind to inactive kinase conformations. *Nature Chemical Biology*, **2**, 358–364.

17 Zhao, Z., Wu, H., Wang, L., Liu, Y., Knapp, S., Liu, Q., and Gray, N.S. (2014) Exploration of type II binding mode: a privileged approach for kinase inhibitor focused drug discovery? *ACS Chemical Biology*, **9**, 1230–1241.

18 Patel, R.Y. and Doerksen, R.J. (2010) Protein kinase-inhibitor database: structural variability of and inhibitor interactions with the protein kinase P-loop. *Journal of Protein Research*, **9**, 4433–4442.

19 Guimaraes, C.R.W., Rai, B.K., Munchhof, M.J., Liu, S., Wang, J., Bhattacharya, S.K., and Buckbinder, L. (2011) Understanding the impact of the P-loop conformation on kinase selectivity. *Journal of Chemical Information and Modeling*, **51**, 1199–1204.

20 Clark, J.D., Flanagan, M.E., and Telliez, J.-B. (2014) Discovery and development of Janus kinase (JAK) inhibitors for inflammatory diseases. *Journal of Medicinal Chemistry*, **57**, 5023–5038.

21 Ahn, Y.M., Clare, M., Ensinger, C.L., Hood, M.M., Lord, J.W., Lu, W.-P., Miller, D.F., Patt, W.C., Smith, B.D., Vogeti, L., Kaufman, M.D., Petillo, P.A., Wise, S.C., Abendroth, J., Chun, L., Clark, R., Feese, M., Kim, H., Stewart, L., and Flynn, D.L. (2010) Switch control pocket inhibitors of p38-MAP kinase: durable type II inhibitors that do not require binding into the canonical ATP hinge region. *Bioorganic & Medicinal Chemistry Letters*, **20**, 5793–5798.

22 Fraley, M.E., Steen, J.T., Brnardic, E.J., Arrington, K.L., Spencer, K.L., Hanney, B.A., Kim, Y., Hartman, G.D., Stirdivant, S.M., Drakas, B.A., Richert, K., Walsh, E.S., Hamilton, K., Buser, C.A., Hardwick, J., Tao, W., Beck, S.C., Mao, X., Lovell, R.B., Sepp-Lorenzino, L., Yan, Y., Ikuta, M., Munshi, S.K., Kuo, L.C., and Kreatsoulas, C. (2006) 3-(Indol-2-yl) indazoles as Chek1 kinase inhibitors: optimization of potency and selectivity via substitution at C6. *Bioorganic & Medicinal Chemistry Letters*, **16**, 6049–6053.

23 Michel, J., Tirado-Rives, J., and Jorgensen, W.L. (2009) Energetics of displacing water molecules from protein binding sites: consequences for ligand optimization. *Journal of the American Chemical Society*, **131**, 15403–15411.

24 Zak, M., Hurley, C.A., Ward, S.I., Bergeron, P., Barrett, K., Balazs, M., Blair, W.S., Bull, R, Chakravarty, P., Chang, C., Crackett, P., Deshmukh, G., DeVoss, J., Dragovich, P.S., Eigenbrot, C., Ellwood, C., Gaines, S., Ghilardi, N., Gibbons, P., Gradl, S., Gribling, P., Hamman, C., Harstad, E.,

Hewitt, P., Johnson, A., Johnson, T, Kenny, J.R., Koehler, M.F.T., Bir Kohli, P., Labadie, S., Lee, W.P., Liao, J., Liimatta, M., Mendonca, R., Narukulla, R., Pulk, R., Reeve, A., Savage, S., Shia, S., Steffek, M., Ubhayakar, S., van Abbema, A., Aliagas, I., Avitabile-Woo, B., Xiao, Y., Yang, J, and Kulagowski, J.J. (2013) Identification of C-2 hydroxyethyl imidazopyrrolopyridines as potent JAK1 inhibitors with favorable physicochemical properties and high selectivity over JAK2. *Journal of Medicinal Chemistry*, **56**, 4764–4785.

25 Fitzgerald, C.E., Patel, S.B., Becker, J.W., Cameron, P.M., Zaller, D., Pikounis, V.B., O'Keefe, S.J., and Scapin, G. (2003) Structural basis for p38α MAP kinase quinazolinone and pyridol-pyrimidine inhibitor specificity. *Nature Structural Biology*, **10**, 764–769.

26 Hansen, J.D., Grina, J., Newhouse, B., Welch, M., Topalov, G., Littman, N., Callejo, M., Gloor, S., Martinson, M., Laird, E., Brandhuber, B.J., Vigers, G., Morales, T., Woessner, R., Randolph, N., Lyssikatos, J., and Olivero, A. (2008) Potent and selective pyrazole-based inhibitors of B-Raf kinase. *Bioorganic & Medicinal Chemistry Letters*, **18**, 4692–4695.

27 Hoshino, R., Chatani, Y., Yamori, T., Tsuruo, T., Oka, H., Yoshida, O, and Shimada, Y., Ari-I, S., Wada, H., Fujimoto, J., Kohno, M. (1999) Constitutive activation of the 41-/43-kDa mitogen-activated protein kinase signaling pathway in human tumors. *Oncogene*, **18** (3), 813–822.

28 Davies, H., Bignell, G.R., Cox, C., Stephens, P., Edkins, S., Clegg, S., Teague, J., Woffendin, H., Garnett, M.J., Bottomley, W., Davis, N., Dicks, E., Ewing, R., Floyd, Y., Gray, K., Hall, S., Hawes, R., Hughes, J., Kosmidou, V., Menzies, A., Mould, C., Parker, A., Stevens, C., Watt, S., Hooper, S., Wilson, R., Jayatilake, H., Gusterson, B.A., Cooper, C., Shipley, J., Hargrave, D., Pritchard-Jones, K., Maitland, N., Chenevix-Trench, G., Riggins, G.J., Bigner, D.D., Palmieri, G., Cossu, A., Flanagan, A., Nicholson, A., Ho, J.W.C., Leung, S.Y., Yuen, S.T., Weber, B.L., Seigler, H.F., Darrow, T.L., Paterson, H., Marais, R., Marshall, C.J., Wooster, R., Stratton, M.R., and Futreal, P.A. (2002) Mutations of the BRAF gene in human cancer. *Nature*, **417**, 949–954.

29 Pollock, P.M., Harper, U.L., Hansen, K.S., Yudt, L.M., Stark, M., Robbins, C.M., Moses, T.Y., Hostetter, G., Wagner, U., Kakareka, J., Salem, G., Pohida, T., Heenan, P., Duray, P., Kallioniemi, O., Hayward, N.K., Trent, J.M., and Meltzer, P.S. (2003) High frequency of BRAF mutations in nevi. *Nature Genetics*, **33**, 19–20.

30 Wan, P.T.C., Garnett, M.J., Roe, S.M., Lee, S., Niculescu-Duvaz, D., Good, V.M., Jones, C.M., Marshall, C.J., Springer, C.J., Barford, D., and Marais, R. (2004) Mechanism of activation of the RAF-ERK signaling pathway by oncogenic mutations of B-RAF. *Cell*, **116**, 855–867.

31 Houben, R., Becker, J.C., Kappel, A., Terheyden, P., Broecker, E.-B., Goetz, R., and Rapp, U.R. (2004) Constitutive activation of the Ras-Raf signaling pathway in metastatic melanoma is associated with poor prognosis. *Journal of Carcinogenesis*, **3**, 6–18.

32 Bollag, G., Tsai, J., Zhang, J., Zhang, C., Ibrahim, P., Nolop, K., and Hirth, P (2012) Vemurafenib: the first drug approved for BRAF-mutant cancer. *Nature Reviews. Drug Discovery*, **11**, 873–886.

33 Rheault, T.R., Stellwagen, J.C., Adjabeng, G.M., Hornberger, K.R., Petrov, K.G., Waterson, A.G., Dickerson, S.H., Mook, R.A., Laquerre, S.G., King, A.J., Rossanese, O.W., Arnone, M.R., Smitheman, K.N., Kane-Carson, L.S., Han, C., Moorthy, G.S., Moss, K.G., and Uehling, D.E. (2013) Discovery of dabrafenib: a selective inhibitor of Raf kinases with antitumor activity against B-Raf-driven tumors. *Medicinal Chemistry Letters*, **4**, 358–362.

34 Wang, Z., Canagarajah, B.J., Boehm, J.C., Kassisa, S., Cobb, M.H., Young, P.R., Abdel-Meguid, S., Adams, J.L., and Goldsmith, E.J. (1998) Structural basis of inhibitor selectivity in MAP kinases. *Structure*, **6**, 1117–1128.

35 Kumar, S., Boehm, J, and Lee, J.C. (2003) p38 MAP kinases: key signalling molecules as therapeutic targets for inflammatory

diseases. *Nature Reviews. Drug Discovery*, **2**, 717–726.
36 Dambach, D.M. (2005) Potential adverse effects associated with inhibition of p38α/β MAP kinases. *Current Topics in Medicinal Chemistry*, **5**, 929–939.
37 Frantz, B., Klatt, T., Pang, M., Parsons, J., Rolando, A., Williams, H., Tocci, M.J., O'Keefe, S.J., and O'Neill, E.A. (1998) The activation state of p38 mitogen-activated protein kinase determines the efficiency of ATP competition for pyridinylimidazole inhibitor binding. *Biochemistry*, **37**, 13846–13853.
38 Knight, Z.A. and Shokat, K.M. (2005) Features of selective kinase inhibitors. *Chemistry & Biology*, **12**, 621–637.
39 Takle, A.K., Brown, M.J.B., Davies, S., Dean, D.K., Francis, G., Gaiba, A., Hird, A.W., King, F.D., Lovell, P.J., Naylor, A., Reith, A.D., Steadman, J.G., and Wilson, D.M. (2006) The identification of potent and selective imidazole-based inhibitors of B-Raf kinase. *Bioorganic & Medicinal Chemistry Letters*, **16**, 378–381.
40 Manning, G., Whyte, D.B., Martinez, R., Hunter, T., and Sudarsanam, S. (2002) The protein kinase complement of the human genome. *Science*, **6**, 1912–1934.
41 Newhouse, B.J., Hansen, J.D., Grina, J., Welch, M., Topalov, G., Littman, N., Callejo, M., Martinson, M., Galbraith, S., Laird, E.R., Brandhuber, B.J., Vigers, G., Morales, T., Woessner, R., Randolph, N., Lyssikatos, J., and Olivero, A. (2011) Non-oxime pyrazole based inhibitors of B-Raf kinase. *Bioorganic & Medicinal Chemistry Letters*, **21**, 3488–3492.
42 Namboodiri, H.V., Bukhtiyarova, M., Ramcharan, J., Karpusas, M., Lee, Y., and Springman, E.B. (2010) Analysis of imatinib and sorafenib binding to p38a compared with c-Abl and B-Raf provides structural insights for understanding the selectivity of inhibitors targeting the DFG-out form of protein kinases. *Biochemistry*, **49**, 3611–3618.
43 Bamborough, P., Drewry, D., Harper, G., Smith, G.K., and Schneider, K. (2008) Assessment of chemical coverage of kinome space and its implications for kinase drug discovery. *Journal of Medicinal Chemistry*, **51**, 7898–7914.
44 Huang, D., Zhou, T., Lafleur, K., Nevado, C., and Caflisch, A. (2010) Kinase selectivity potential for inhibitors targeting the ATP binding site: a network analysis. *Bioinformatics*, **26**, 198–204.
45 Koch, K. (2011) ARRY-380: a selective, oral HER2 inhibitor for the treatment of solid tumors. AACR 102nd Annual Meeting DDT01 New drugs on the Horizon.
46 Roskoski, R., Jr. (2014) The ErbB/HER family of protein-tyrosine kinases and cancer. *Pharmacological Research*, **79**, 34–74.
47 Harries, M. and Smith, I. (2002) The development and clinical use of trastuzumab (herceptin). *Endocrine-Related Cancer*, **9**, 75–85.
48 Wakeling, A.E. (2002) Epidermal growth factor receptor tyrosine kinase inhibitors. *Current Opinion in Pharmacology*, **2**, 382–387.
49 Johnston, J.B., Navaratnam, S., Pitz, M.W., Maniate, J.M., Wiechec, E., Baust, H., Gingerich, J., Skliris, G.P., Murphy, L.C., and Los, M. (2006) Targeting the EGFR pathway for cancer therapy. *Current Medicinal Chemistry*, **13**, 3483–3492.
50 Hynes, N.E. and Lane, H.A. (2005) ERBB receptors and cancer: the complexity of targeted inhibitors. *Nature Reviews. Cancer*, **5**, 341–354.
51 Burgess, A.W., Henis, Y.I., Hynes, N.E., Jovin, T., Levitzki, A., Pinkas-Kramarski, R, and Yarden, Y (2014) EGF receptor family: twisting targets for improved cancer therapies. *Growth Factors*, **32**, 74–81.
52 Huang, Y., Fu, P., and Fan, W. (2013) Novel targeted therapies to overcome trastuzumab resistance in HER2-overexpressing metastatic breast cancer. *Current Drug Targets*, **14**, 889–898.
53 Tse, C., Gauchez, A.-S., Jacot, W., and Lamy, P.-J. (2012) HER2 shedding and serum HER2 extracellular domain: biology and clinical utility in breast cancer. *Cancer Treatment Reviews*, **38**, 133–142.
54 Stamos, J., Sliwkowski, M.X., and Eigenbrot, C. (2002) Structure of the epidermal growth factor receptor kinase domain alone and in complex with a 4-anilinoquinazoline inhibitor. *The Journal*

of Biological Chemistry, **277**, 46265–46272.

55 Dunbrack, R.L., Jr. (1995) Conformational analysis of the backbone-dependence of protein sidechain rotamer preferences: applications to homology modeling and protein conformation. Book of Abstracts, 210th ACS National Meeting, Chicago, IL, August 20–24, COMP-006.

56 Aertgeerts, K., Skene, R., Yano, J., Sang, B.-C., Zou, H., Snell, G., Jennings, A., Iwamoto, K., Habuka, N., Hirokawa, A., Ishikawa, T., Tanaka, T., Miki, H., Ohta, Y., and Sogabe, S. (2011) Structural analysis of the mechanism of inhibition and allosteric activation of the kinase domain of HER2 protein. *The Journal of Biological Chemistry*, **286**, 18756–18765.

57 Wood, E.R., Truesdale, A.T., McDonald, O.B., Yuan, D., Hassell, A., Dickerson, S.H., Ellis, B., Pennisi, C., Horne, E., Lackey, K., Alligood, K.J., Rusnak, D.W., Gilmer, T.M., and Shewchuk, L. (2004) A unique structure of epidermal growth factor receptor bound to GW572016 (lapatinib): relationships among protein conformation, inhibitor off-rate, and receptor activity in tumor cells. *Cancer Research*, **64**, 6652–6659.

58 Blake, J.F., Xu, R., Bencsik, J.R., Xiao, D., Kallan, N.C., Schlachther, S., Mitchell, I.S., Spencer, K.L., Banka, A.L., Wallace, E.M., Gloor, S.L., Martinson, M., Woessner, R.D., Vigers, G.P.A., Brandhuber, B.J., Liang, J., Safina, B.S., Li, J., Zhang, B., Chabot, C., Do, S., Lee, L., Oeh, J., Sampath, D., Lee, B.B., Lin, K., Liederer, B.M., and Skelton, N.J. (2012) Discovery and preclinical pharmacology of a selective ATP-competitive Akt inhibitor (GDC-0068) for the treatment of human tumors. *Journal of Medicinal Chemistry*, **55**, 8110–8127.

59 Cheng, J.Q., Lindsley, C.W., Cheng, G.Z., Yang, H., and Nicosia, S.V. (2005) The Akt/PKB pathway: molecular target for cancer drug discovery. *Oncogene*, **24**, 7482–7492.

60 Altomare, D.A. and Testa, J.R. (2005) Perturbations of the AKT signaling pathway in human cancer. *Oncogene*, **24**, 7455–7464.

61 Degtyarev, M., De Mazière, A., Orr, C., Lin, J., Lee, B.B., Tien, J.Y., Prior, W.W., van Dijk, S., Wu, H., Gray, D.C., Davis, D.P., Stern, H.M., Murray, L.J., Hoeflich, K.P., Klumperman, J., Friedman, L.S., and Lin, K. (2008) Akt inhibition promotes autophagy and sensitizes PTEN-null tumors to lysosomotropic agents. *The Journal of Cell Biology*, **183**, 101–116.

62 Blake, J.F., Kallan, N.C., Xiao, D., Xu, R., Bencsik, J.R., Skelton, N.J., Spencer, K.L., Mitchell, I.S., Woessner, R.D., Gloor, S.L., Risom, T., Gross, S.D., Martinson, M., Morales, T.H., Vigers, G.P.A., and Brandhuber, B.J. (2010) Discovery of pyrrolopyrimidine inhibitors of Akt. *Bioorganic & Medicinal Chemistry Letters*, **20**, 5607–5612.

63 Reiken, S., Lacampagne, A., Zhou, H., Kherani, A., Lehnart, S.E., Ward, C., Huang, F., Gaburjakova, M., Gaburjakova, J., Rosemblit, N., Warren, M.S., He, K-l., Yi, G.-H., Wang, J., Burkhoff, D., Vassort, G., and Marks, A.R. (2003) PKA phosphorylation activates the calcium release channel (ryanodine receptor) in skeletal muscle: defective regulation in heart failure. *The Journal of Cell Biology*, **160**, 919–928.

64 Doe, C., Bentley, R., Behm, D.J., Lafferty, R., Stavenger, R., Jung, D., Bamford, M., Panchal, T., Grygielko, E., Wright, L.L., Smith, G.K., Chen, Z., Webb, C., Khandekar, S., Yi, T., Kirkpatrick, R., Dul, E., Jolivette, L., Marino, J.P., Jr., Willette, R., Lee, D., and Hu, E. (2007) Novel rho kinase inhibitors with anti-inflammatory and vasodilatory activities. *The Journal of Pharmacology and Experimental Therapeutics*, **320**, 89–98.

65 Gavrin, L.K. and Saiah, E. (2013) Approaches to discover non-ATP-site kinase inhibitors. *Medicinal Chemical Communications*, **4**, 41–51.

66 Fang, Z., Grüetter, C., and Rauh, D. (2013) Strategies for the selective regulation of kinases with allosteric modulators: exploiting exclusive structural features. *ACS Chemical Biology*, **8**, 58–70.

67 Liu, Q., Sabnis, Y., Zhao, Z., Zhang, T., Buhrlage, S.J., Jones, L.H., and Gray, N.S. (2013) Developing irreversible

inhibitors of the protein kinase cysteinome. *Chemistry and Biology*, **20**, 146–159.

68 Dar, A.C. and Shokat, K.M. (2011) The evolution of protein kinase inhibitors from antagonists to agonists of cellular signaling. *Annual Review of Biochemistry*, **80**, 769–795.

69 Knight, Z.A., Lin, H., and Shokat, K.M. (2010) Targeting the cancer kinome through polypharmacology. *Nature Reviews. Cancer*, **2010**, 130–137.

70 Morphy, R.S. (2010) Selectively nonselective kinase inhibition: striking the right balance. *Journal of Medicinal Chemistry*, **53**, 1413–1437.

Section 5
Examples of Clinical Translation

Antitargets and Drug Safety, First Edition. Edited by László Urbán, Vinod F. Patel, and Roy J. Vaz.

19
Torcetrapib and Dalcetrapib Safety: Relevance of Preclinical *In Vitro* and *In Vivo* Models

Eric J. Niesor, Andrea Greiter-Wilke, and Lutz Müller

19.1
Introduction

Early compounds that affected the activity of cholesteryl ester transfer protein (CETP) were CETP inhibitors (CETPi) [1–3] and these were shown to increase plasma high-density lipoprotein cholesterol (HDL-C) levels both in animal models and in clinical studies. Numerous epidemiological studies have demonstrated a correlation between high HDL-C levels and lower rates of cardiovascular disease (CVD) [4]; thus, CETP was considered recently as a therapeutic target to raise HDL-C [3] and to potentially decrease CVD risk [5]. Torcetrapib and dalcetrapib, compounds from two different chemical classes (Figure 19.1) [6], differing in lipophilicity and affecting CETP activity by two different mechanisms [1,2,7,8], entered large-scale outcome studies. The development of torcetrapib, the first CETP inhibitor (CETPi) to enter phase III outcome studies, was prematurely halted due to increased mortality in torcetrapib-treated patients during the phase III ILLUMINATE trial [9]. The dal-HEART phase III clinical trial program with dalcetrapib, the second compound entering phase III, was stopped more recently due to lack of efficacy, but no significant safety signal was observed in an outcome study of similar size to the one conducted for torcetrapib [10].

Here we focus on the effect of torcetrapib on blood pressure (BP) observed in both in *in vitro* and *in vivo* preclinical and clinical studies and briefly discuss the preclinical findings of dalcetrapib on lymph node macrophages and the molecular mechanisms supporting lack of relevance to the clinical setting.

19.2
Effect of Torcetrapib on Blood Pressure

Some modest increases in BP had been reported in phase II clinical studies with torcetrapib [11], but this was not considered a major risk based on the lack of a consistent treatment-related pattern over time; these findings suggested the

Antitargets and Drug Safety, First Edition. Edited by László Urbán, Vinod F. Patel, and Roy J. Vaz.

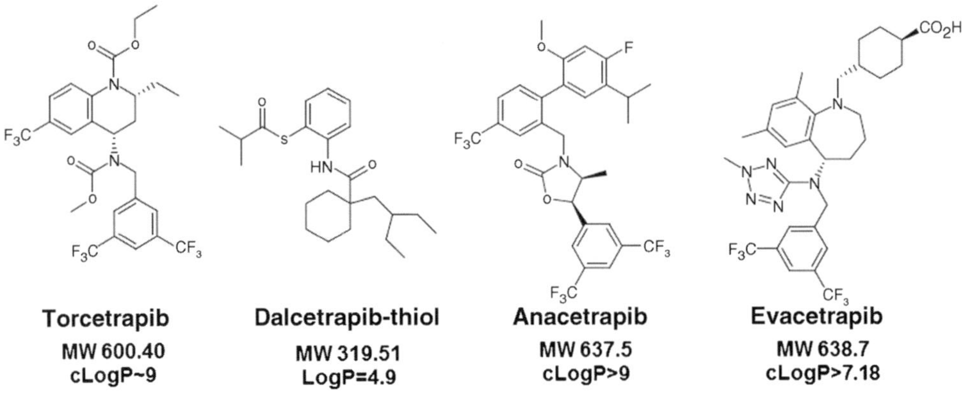

Figure 19.1 Torcetrapib, dalcetrapib, anacetrapib, and evacetrapib: differences in chemical structure and physicochemical properties.

effect to be of limited magnitude within the therapeutic dose range. It was also assumed that the effect on HDL-C would counteract any potential deleterious effects of higher BP. However, these assumptions could have been challenged upfront given that (a) some patients and animals displayed pathologic increases in BP with torcetrapib that were markedly greater than the mean; and (b) torcetrapib was the first CETPi to test the hypothesis that a higher HDL-C as a result of drug intervention may protect from CVD. HDL-C increase was not (and is not yet) recognized as a relevant biomarker of cardiovascular protection.

19.3 *In Vitro* Studies

At the time the phase III ILLUMINATE study of torcetrapib was stopped, changes in plasma aldosterone and electrolytes pointed strongly toward an adrenal effect, particularly in long-term clinical studies. The obvious step was to exclude or demonstrate a direct effect of torcetrapib on aldosterone synthesis and/or secretion by adrenal cells. A review of the literature for adrenocortical cells that could potentially be used for evaluating any action of torcetrapib on aldosterone production revealed that adrenal cell primary cultures were not suitable. The adrenal corticocarcinoma cell line H295R has, however, been rigorously studied for steroid hormone production [12] associated with the regulation of pathways culminating in aldosterone production [13]. Aldosterone offers the technical advantage that it is not stored, but is synthesized on demand through induction of expression of the messenger RNA (mRNA) coding for the Cyp11B2 gene, also known as aldosterone synthase (AS) [14]. Thus, the effect of torcetrapib, even on the molecular (transcription) level, could be investigated in such a cell line. This may also offer the possibility of screening for better drug candidates.

19.3.1 Direct Effect of Torcetrapib on Aldosterone Production *In Vitro* in Cultured H295R Adrenal Corticocarcinoma Cells

Unexpectedly, a dose–response study [14] demonstrated an immediate direct effect of torcetrapib on aldosterone production even at relatively low concentrations compared with those needed for CETP inhibition, (i.e., levels comparable to, or even lower than, plasma drug levels achieved in preclinical or clinical studies [15,16]). In this study, angiotensin II, the physiological inducer, was used as a positive control and torcetrapib was demonstrated to be the most potent "synthetic analogue" (IC50 17 nM) aldosterone-inducing compound tested. Interestingly, in the same assay, anacetrapib, a CETPi currently undergoing phase III studies, was also associated with an aldosterone release effect but required concentrations >3 μM to induce a weak increase in aldosterone production. As expected, dalcetrapib, which belongs to a fundamentally different chemical class than torcetrapib and anacetrapib, showed no induction of aldosterone up to 10 uM [14,17].

Further studies of structure–activity relationships showed evidence of aldosterone-inducing activity of torcetrapib and torcetrapib-like compounds, suggesting an as yet undiscovered antitarget activity of these compounds. As receptor chemistry most likely "drives" these interactions, it is not surprising that the fundamentally different chemical structure of dalcetrapib does not confer such antitarget activity.

Although practical and relevant, the H295R cell line has the disadvantage of producing several steroid hormones that are not as well regulated as Cyp11B2. For instance, parallel induction of Cyp11B1 (cortisol synthase) was seen for torcetrapib [17], although the clinical relevance of this observation is still not known.

19.3.2 Molecular Mechanism of Torcetrapib Induction of Aldosterone Secretion

Detailed molecular mechanistic studies by several investigators have demonstrated the direct effect of several derivatives of torcetrapib on aldosterone production through Cyp11B2 induction. Clerc *et al.* [14] showed that torcetrapib and angiotensin II elevated both Cyp11B2 mRNA and aldosterone production in H295R cells on 6 h incubation, while on days 1–5 torcetrapib was associated with a sustained increase of Cyp11B2 mRNA but not angiotensin II. Although torcetrapib and angiotensin II potentiated the effect of precursor 25-OH cholesterol and raised pregnenolone levels, torcetrapib increased neither cytosolic Ca nor extracellular signal-regulated kinase1/2 phosphorylation at 5 min, suggesting initially divergent pathways. Unlike angiotensin II, torcetrapib-induced steroidogenesis was not affected by angiotensin II receptor type 1 (AT1) receptor antagonism or voltage-gated T-type Ca channel antagonism, but was blocked by several L-type Ca channel antagonists. In unbiased genome-wide screening, torcetrapib and angiotensin II modulated an overlapping but distinct set of genes in H295R cells, but only torcetrapib upregulated mRNA levels of the L-type Ca channel known to be involved in smooth muscle cell contraction. Thus, a single mechanism may be involved in smooth muscle cell contraction and aldosterone secretion.

19.3.3 Development of Reproducible *In Vitro* Screening Models for Increase in Aldosterone and Cyp11B2 mRNA in a Human Adrenal Corticocarcinoma Cell Line

The human adrenal corticocarcinoma cell line H295R model provided consistent reproducible findings with torcetrapib and has thus been used as a research tool by many laboratories and pharmaceutical companies, including Lilly [18], Merck [19], Pfizer [20], and Roche [14], for example, to screen compounds for CETPi activity and evaluate potential to induce aldosterone secretion. The investigations performed for torcetrapib, as reviewed by Johns *et al.* [17], have allowed the development of *in vitro* and *in vivo* screening models to assess compounds in clinical development for potential torcetrapib-like side effects. Moreover, such screening has allowed the identification of novel compounds that lack the 1,2,3,4-tetrahydroquinoline scaffold present in torcetrapib and resulted in the identification of isonipecotic acid (PF-04445597) derivatives, which has improved oral pharmacokinetic properties and is devoid of aldosterone-inducing activity [21].

19.3.4 Application of *In Vitro* Models for the Successful Derisking of Dalcetrapib, Anacetrapib, and Evacetrapib

The dalcetrapib compound, which was from a chemical class unrelated to torcetrapib [6], was already in phase III clinical development when development of torcetrapib was stopped. Dalcetrapib, in contrast to torcetrapib, showed no aldosterone-inducing activity in H295R cells [14]. Anacetrapib also did not induce any increase in aldosterone production *in vitro* in primary cultures of rat adrenal cells [22] but displayed only weak Cyp11B2 and aldosterone-increasing activity in H295R cells [14].

Development of evacetrapib has, perhaps, benefited the most from research performed with the other CETPi since it has been elegantly designed to avoid any *in vitro* effect on aldosterone [18]. In addition, a potential weak point of anacetrapib and torcetrapib, that is, accumulation in adipose tissue in animal studies [23,24] due to high lipophilicity and slow metabolism of these agents, was avoided in designing a compound with a relatively short half-life and hence no accumulation in deep compartment [25].

In addition to the direct effect of CETPi on aldosterone secretion, studies should also consider their potential indirect effect via raised HDL-C level, a potential cholesterol provider to adrenal cells as precursor for aldosterone synthesis. This might be significant given that aldosterone production and Cyp11B2 expression in human adrenocortical cells can be stimulated by large mature HDL, also referred to as HDL_2 [26], a particle subtype generated following inhibition of CETP activity.

19.4 *In Vivo* Studies

19.4.1 Effect of Torcetrapib on Aldosterone and BP

At the time the torcetrapib ILLUMINATE trial was stopped, no preclinical data were published on its effects on BP. It was initially assumed, therefore, that the putative torcetrapib-induced BP increase was unique to humans. Indeed, if this was the case, research should have been directed toward identifying a human-specific and unique metabolite. Since torcetrapib is metabolized into more than 28 identified metabolites [27], this would have proved extremely difficult. Another hypothesis proposed to support a human-specific adverse effect was that torcetrapib affected a human-specific BP-regulating pathway. This was considered relatively unlikely since BP-, salt- and water-regulating pathways are known to be well conserved across species [28]. We reasoned, therefore, that torcetrapib may increase BP in species other than humans and re-evaluated this potential.

19.4.1.1 Immediate Increase (Transient) in BP in Normotensive Wistar Rats

We administered torcetrapib orally (10, 40, or 80 mg/kg per day for 5 consecutive days) to instrumented normotensive Wistar rats. These doses, which provided plasma drug concentrations generally comparable with clinical studies of torcetrapib [15], were associated with a modest and transient but clear increase in BP (+3.7 mmHg).

19.4.1.2 Sustained Increase in BP in Spontaneously Hypertensive and Zucker Diabetic Fatty Rats

The same experiment was performed in the spontaneously hypertensive rat (SHR), a more sensitive animal model to study both hypotensive and hypertensive compounds [16]. A sustained, dose-dependent increase in BP (+6.5 mmHg) was observed in SHR 1 day after oral dosing. This led to several conclusions:

1) Torcetrapib can increase BP in rats and may therefore use a pathway well conserved between rats and humans.
2) The torcetrapib effect does not involve CETP and HDL metabolism since rats do not express the CETP gene.
3) In normotensive animals (and possibly patients), the hypertensive effect of torcetrapib is minor and might have escaped early safety preclinical studies generally performed in healthy normotensive animals.

4) Its effect may be similarly increased in hypertensive patients if torcetrapib is more potent under hypertensive disease conditions.

19.4.1.3 Tissue mRNA Analysis Suggested Involvement of the Renin–Angiotensin–Aldosterone System (RAAS)

In order to investigate the potential pathways involved in the torcetrapib-induced increase in BP, we collected tissues from normotensive rats 5 days after oral administration of torcetrapib (i.e., when BP had returned to normal) [16]. In this context, the RAAS presents a prime pathway that may be inadvertently affected by drug candidates. Indeed, increased expression of RAAS-related genes (RNA transcript) was observed in the adrenal glands, that is, AT1, angiotensinogen, angiotensin-converting enzyme (ACE), endothelin-converting enzyme, and endothelin-1 (ET1, measured as preproET1). Torcetrapib also increased expression of RAAS-related genes in aortic samples, particularly ET1 and ACE. Since these changes occurred concomitantly with return of BP to normal values, torcetrapib may induce compensatory changes in genes involved in the RAAS to maintain normal BP. Notably, such compensatory changes in RAAS genes were not observed in the SHR model, in which a torcetrapib-mediated sustained increase in BP was observed.

Simic *et al.* [29] followed-up on our observations in SHR versus Wistar rats and confirmed that the off-target effects of torcetrapib are evident in SHR only and not in Wistar rats. In particular, sustained and marked impairment of endothelial function, decreased nitric oxide (NO) bioavailability, and increased production of reactive oxygen species, as well as activation of ET and aldosterone were reported. Cao *et al.* [18] investigated a number of rat strains and confirmed that the Zucker diabetic fatty rat (ZDFR) represented a sensitive model in which to examine the hypertensive potential of new compounds. In fact, in this model, torcetrapib produced a dose-dependent, sustained increase in BP after oral administration, supporting the concept of a higher sensitivity to torcetrapib in rats manifesting essential hypertension (SHR) or a metabolic profile characteristic of the metabolic syndrome (ZDFR). These findings may perhaps partly explain the increased mortality associated with torcetrapib treatment in patients with a higher burden of CV risk factors such as in the ILLUMINATE trial [9].

After studies in rodent models, dog models are often used in cardiovascular safety studies. Compared with the monkey, dog models offer the advantage of being deficient in the target, CETP, and thus permit study of the antitarget effects of torcetrapib undisturbed by its pharmacology. It was noted that during intravenous (i.v.) infusion to dogs, an acute effect of torcetrapib on BP was evident, implying a direct vascular effect of a hormone(s)-mediating vessel constriction [30]. The response of the adrenal gland in the acute increase in BP (i.e., within minutes following i.v. infusion of torcetrapib) and the fact that adrenalectomy abolished this effect in rats [22] revealed an intriguing role and link between the adrenal gland and torcetrapib-induced acute hypertension. In addition, despite a sustained BP response, it was also apparent that torcetrapib-induced secretion of aldosterone and corticosterone was blocked in rats treated with trilostane, an agent that inhibits the early step of adrenal steroidogenesis. These provocative data led Funder [30] to speculate that torcetrapib can raise BP by promoting adrenal release of a pressor agent(s) such as ouabain synthesized from cholesterol in the zona glomerulosa. Collectively, these findings suggest that torcetrapib does not act via any classical hormonal pathway.

19.4.1.4 Increase in BP and Aldosterone with Torcetrapib in All Species Tested

The observation that torcetrapib increased BP in different species led various pharmaceutical companies to develop "their preferred" animal models for the screening of CETPi for potential to raise BP, for example, the SHR (Roche) [16], ZDFR (Lilly) [18], monkey (Pfizer) [31], CETPtg mouse and rat (Merck) [22], and the rabbit (Johnson and Johnson) [32]. The effect of torcetrapib was, in fact, so robust that findings were generally comparable and consistent between laboratories. Interestingly, in general, compounds found to increase aldosterone production in H295R cells also increased BP in SHR [14], suggesting a unique link between these two phenomena or a common target linking both pathways.

In a series of investigations of torcetrapib and a close analogue CP-532,623, Blasi *et al.* showed that both compounds increased BP in cynomolgus monkeys and human subjects [33]. Moreover, administration of torcetrapib at 10 or 100 mg/kg daily for 2 weeks was associated with a dose-dependent increase in systolic BP, that is, up to 18 and 26 mmHg, respectively. Despite providing a similar maximal CETP inhibition to torcetrapib, single dose (420 mg/kg) CP-532,623 produced a significantly greater pressor effect, with increase in BP evident from 2 h; this peaked at 23 mmHg after 6–8 h and was sustained for up to 16 h [33]. In addition, while the highest dose of torcetrapib (100 mg/kg per day) was associated after 10 days with reduction in both aldosterone and renin, the dose of 10 mg/kg per day induced only a transient increase in aldosterone (on days 1–2) without any significant change in plasma renin. The transient nature of these hormonal changes suggests compensatory mechanisms exist and that increases in BP do not result directly from RAAS activation, but also possibly from direct effects on blood vessels. Thus, plasma aldosterone alone does not appear to be a suitable marker for a potential deleterious effect of torcetrapib-like compounds.

Ironically, the effect of torcetrapib on BP proved sufficiently reproducible in various animal species and across laboratories that Fryer *et al.* [34] proposed and integrated this effect into *in vivo* cardiovascular models. Two compounds, torcetrapib and a novel steroid hormone mimetic (SHM-1121X), both with off-target cardiovascular contraindications, with the potential to increase and decrease BP, respectively, were profiled in four distinct *in vivo* cardiovascular models (anesthetized rat, telemetry rat, anesthetized dog, and telemetry dog). Significant torcetrapib-induced changes in arterial BP were equally detectable in all four models independent of species tested, route of administration, and anesthesia used. Moreover, in all models tested, dose dependency was observed and equivalent changes in BP were demonstrated within a 1/2 log unit range of mean plasma concentrations. The predictive value of each model was validated with torcetrapib. When moving from dogs to the cynomolgus monkey, the nonrodent species proficient in CETP and hence also important in this context, torcetrapib treatment was associated with a clear increase in BP of 10–15 mmHg at 30 mg/kg (exposure 2700 ng/ml; Roche internal report). In the same study, aldosterone was mildly increased at 10 and 30 mg/kg. Cholesterol and HDL-C tended to be increased at 30 mg/kg, while low-density lipoprotein cholesterol (LDL-C) was generally decreased at the same dose.

Meyer *et al.* [35] even succeeded in detecting hemodynamic changes after administration of torcetrapib at 10 and 30 mg/kg to conscious dogs employing a noninvasive cuff methodology (high-definition oscillometry) to measure BP (increases of +9 and +16 mmHg in mean pressure). This was surprising, since handling *per se* increases pressure (similar to the "white coat" effect in humans) and could have readily masked the torcetrapib effect. Exposures at these dose levels were 918 and 1462 ng/ml, respectively, that is, 4.5–7-fold greater than the target human exposure of 210 ng/ml following a 60 mg dose [36].

This series of *in vivo* cardiovascular safety studies with torcetrapib in rats, dogs, and monkeys succinctly demonstrated the antitarget effects of the compound, that is, the independence of the effect of torcetrapib on BP from its desired pharmacology. A series of straightforward and mostly standard methods in safety pharmacology were suitable to reveal this serious antitarget effect, which materialized as an increase in side effects in humans in a large outcome study.

In the context of standard cardiovascular-related safety pharmacology studies, dalcetrapib has proved devoid of effects on BP in the CETP-proficient monkey (up to exposures in excess of 15 times the human C_{max} and AUC observed in the phase III clinical trial using a daily dose of 600 mg dalcetrapib). Due to effects on the autonomic nervous system at high doses, manifesting as diarrhea and soft stools, dalcetrapib-treated monkeys showed a distinct loss of BP "dipping" that is typically observed in normal humans and nonhuman primates with the onset of the night photoperiod (Figure 19.2). This resulted in a compromised decrease in systemic BP compared with individual time-matched vehicle controls, and although this occurred in most subjects who received dalcetrapib at 1000 mg/kg and in only few subjects who received 300 mg/kg, there was no clear dose relationship. In contrast, following treatment with torcetrapib, monkeys showed a dose-dependent increase in BP of 10–15 mmHg, again following a 30 mg/kg dose (Figure 19.3).

19.4.2
Molecular Mechanisms of Torcetrapib-Induced BP Increase

One of the most informative investigations of the pathway involved in the acute increase in BP produced by torcetrapib and CP-532,623 was performed by DePasquale *et al.* in male Sprague-Dawley rats [31]. Changes in BP were determined in conscious animals following both chronic oral and acute i.v. administration in conjunction with pharmacologic blockade of numerous pressor agents

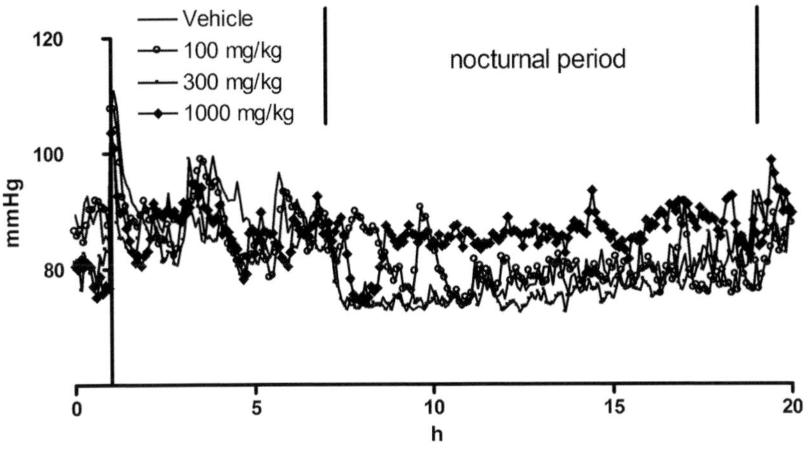

Figure 19.2 Effect of dalcetrapib (100, 300, 1000 mg/kg) on mean BP in conscious telemetered cynomolgus monkeys ($n = 6$). Dosing at 1 h; nocturnal period 7–19 h.

and pathways. Here, the torcetrapib-induced increase in BP was not attenuated by blockade of adrenergic, cholinergic, angiotensin, endothelin, NO synthase, Rho kinase, and thromboxane pathways. Only pretreatment with the Ca channel blocker nifedipine significantly attenuated the BP increase for CP-532,623.

We have demonstrated that the SHR is uniquely sensitive to the sustained hypertensive activity of torcetrapib, and this animal is characterized by relatively high-level expression of the voltage-gated Ca channel. Specifically, Clerc *et al.* showed that the Ca channel antagonist nifedipine completely attenuated the pressor effect of torcetrapib, supporting the hypothesis that the Ca messenger might be the primary trigger of torcetrapib action [14]. These findings are

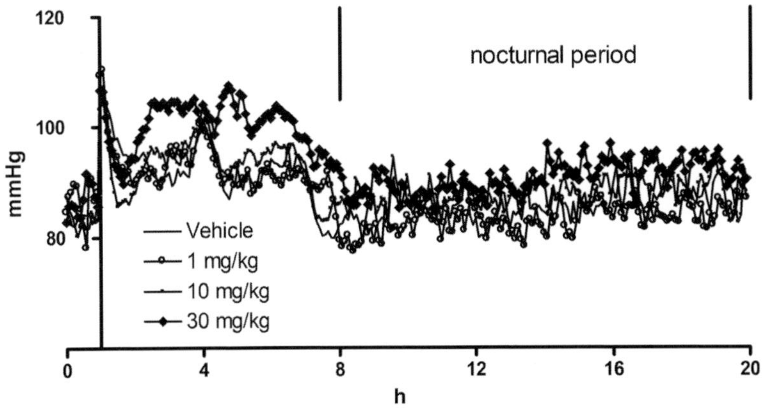

Figure 19.3 Effect of torcetrapib (1, 10, 30 mg/kg) on mean BP in conscious telemetered cynomolgus monkeys ($n = 6$). Dosing at 1 h; nocturnal period 8–20 h.

consistent with *post-hoc* analysis of the RADIANCE data [37] in which patients treated with torcetrapib/atorvastatin showed a decrease in BP when also treated with nifedipine or amlodipine. In contrast, patients administered a diuretic or other antihypertensive intervention showed no change, or even an increase, in BP.

19.4.2.1 Torcetrapib-Positive Inotropism and Increased Cardiac Work in a Dog Telemetry Study

The opening of L-type Ca channels appears to be a characteristic feature of torcetrapib and torcetrapib-like compounds, but not of dalcetrapib. Ca channel-opening compounds are generally known to act as positive inotropic compounds, that is, they increase contractility and cardiac output, which is most likely a mortality/morbidity risk factor [38]. This mechanistic link prompted further analysis of torcetrapib-related data from a dog telemetry study with specific focus on cardiac contractility. In the context of safety pharmacology studies, that is, when no routine echocardiography is performed, the first derivative of the left ventricular (LV) pressure signal (LV d*P*/d*t* max – delta pressure/delta time) is a well-established marker for cardiac contractility [39,40].

Administration of torcetrapib at 10 mg/kg to conscious Beagle dogs resulted not only in the expected increase in aortic pressure but also a clear increase in LV d*P*/d*t* max from 6 h post-dose onward (Figure 19.4). Changes in preload and afterload as potential confounding factors to the parameter LV d*P*/d*t* max have to be taken into account when interpreting LV pressure data. However, since no effects were noted either on LV end diastolic pressure or heart rate, this increase in LV d*P*/d*t* max can be regarded as an indicator for a true positive inotropic effect of torcetrapib.

Overall, it appears a reasonable hypothesis that increased cardiac work will represent a contributory factor for increased risk of cardiovascular adverse effects in a population already with increased cardiovascular risk at baseline.

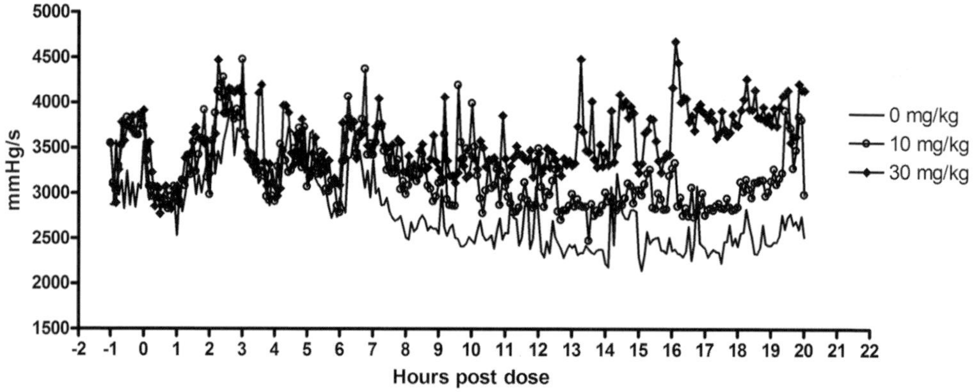

Figure 19.4 Effect of torcetrapib (10, 30 mg/kg) on positive LV d*P*/d*t* max in conscious telemetered dogs ($n = 6$). Dosing at 0 h.

There is, however, a lack of reliable clinical data on chronic use of positive inotropic compounds and their impact on cardiovascular risk outcomes.

19.4.2.2 A Common Molecular Mechanism for BP and Induction of Aldosterone Secretion?

The immediate effect of torcetrapib on the vessel wall and its direct *in vitro* effect on adrenal cells have proved difficult to explain, but suggest multiple molecular targets and tissue targets or a single target and/or pathway resulting in apparently different pharmacological toxicities. Due to the obvious link between aldosterone and BP regulation, we hypothesized that a potential unique target and pathway may exist. It has been shown previously that aldosterone synthesis and secretion is partly regulated by the slow Ca channel [41], in particular the T-type channel. Conversely, it is well established that Ca ion entry via the L-type Ca channel triggers vasoconstriction. The observation that the SHR, which displays an increase in L-type Ca channel, was markedly more sensitive to the hypertensive effect of torcetrapib supported this hypothesis [42].

The findings that the Ca channel subunit CACNAC1 is upregulated by torcetrapib but not angiotensin II and that downregulation of CACNAC1C and CACNAC1D decrease torcetrapib-induced steroidogenesis concur with the reported effect of nifedipine L-type Ca channel antagonist on torcetrapib-induced aldosterone production [14]. The demonstration that nifedipine has the unique property of diminishing the hypertensive effect of torcetrapib strongly suggests that the primary target of torcetrapib could be the direct or indirect activation of the L-type Ca channel as demonstrated in the positive inotropic effect in the dog telemetry study. Thus, the hypothesis of a common target or pathway associated with the two main off-target effects of torcetrapib and its analogue is plausible.

19.5 General Safety Risk with Increased Aldosterone and BP

19.5.1 Inappropriate Increase in Aldosterone Secretion May Increase CV Risks

The scientific delineation of the mode of action of torcetrapib goes beyond understanding the mechanism underlying a reported adverse effect. Aldosterone regulates several important physiological pathways related to BP regulation, but is also directly linked to cardiovascular mortality [43]. Indeed, patients suffering from an acute cardiovascular event can be protected for further morbidity and mortality if treated with an aldosterone receptor inhibitor such as ephlerenone [44]. This strongly supports a negative impact of aldosterone in human cardiovascular events [45]. It also seems obvious that an inappropriate aldosterone response (i.e., not triggered by a physiological need for sodium retention) may not only result in a positive inotropic response but also cause pathological changes in the RAAS and possible tissue and cell injuries. In fact, there is much literature to suggest such inotropic effects and also a direct toxic effect of aldosterone in promoting endothelial dysfunction and myocyte apoptosis in cardiomyocytes and skeletal muscle cells [40,46,47]. Nevertheless, it remains to be confirmed that drug-induced changes in aldosterone alone contribute to mortality risk and morbidity associated with CVD.

If some of the actions of torcetrapib were associated with positive inotropism, one could perhaps best compare the clinical risk situation as a sustained, non physiological chronic rise in adrenaline, not compatible with homeostasis. In a patient population with clearly increased cardiovascular risk factors, this could be associated with an effect on outcomes comparable to that leading to the discontinuation of the phase III clinical development program for torcetrapib.

In addition, Pratt [48] noted in a mouse model of aldosterone synthase overexpression ($AS^{hi/hi}$) that only a modest increase in aldosterone synthase/Cyp11B2 (such as that described by Makhanova *et al.* [49]) may participate in the development of hypertension and its complications. When maintained on a normal-salt diet, $AS^{hi/hi}$ mice relative to wild-type mice showed a 1.5-fold increase in adrenal Cyp11B2 mRNA, while BP and plasma aldosterone were unchanged. In this model, $AS^{hi/hi}$ mice had 10 mmHg higher BP on a high-salt diet compared with a low-salt diet and showed higher plasma aldosterone and lower plasma potassium levels on a high-salt diet, and maintained normal BP with less activation of the RAAS on a low-salt diet, compared with wild-type mice. Changes in dietary salt did not affect the BP of wild-type mice. Additionally, $AS^{hi/hi}$ mice were more susceptible than wild-type mice to infusion of angiotensin II, manifesting as higher BP, greater cardiac hypertrophy, and increased oxidative stress. Collectively, these observations suggest that a modest increase in AS expression renders BP maintenance increasingly sensitive to dietary salt, and that genetically increased AS expression in humans may contribute to hypertension and cardiovascular complications in societies with high-salt intake.

19.6
Relevance of BP and Aldosterone Preclinical Models to Clinical Observation with Dalcetrapib and Anacetrapib

As expected from preclinical studies, thorough investigation of both dalcetrapib and anacetrapib in clinical studies with regard to effect on plasma aldosterone level and BP showed no evidence of clinically relevant changes in either parameter. This was evident for dalcetrapib administered at a dose of 600 mg daily for up to 3 years [10] and in the case of anacetrapib, the DEFINE study [50] concluded an absence of increase in aldosterone in treated patients. Notably, however, the data did not account for the surprisingly very long half-life of anacetrapib of 2–3 days following multiple administration in human subjects [51], most likely due to accumulation in adipose tissue observed both in preclinical [52] and clinical [53] studies. Significantly, such accumulation could result in a sustained high plasma level and pharmacological activity after cessation of treatment. In addition, patients whose LDL-C levels fell below 25 mg/100 ml were excluded from the study and also from analysis of BP and aldosterone data [50]. One may argue that these patients were exposed the most or who responded the most to the lipid changes produced by anacetrapib. Interestingly, when these patients were included in the washout/reversal part of the DEFINE study, an increase in diastolic BP was measured, although this was interpreted by the investigators as a type one error [54].

It remains possible, however, that patients removed from the DEFINE study main protocol remained exposed during the putative washout/reversal period. Whether this is the case, and if this would have manifested as a sustained effect of anacetrapib, will be evaluated in the ongoing REVEAL (Randomized EValuation of the Effects of Anacetrapib through Lipid modification) morbidity and mortality phase III study. Here, patients are exposed to high concentrations of anacetrapib for a median of 4 years with no exclusion of cases of higher than anticipated exposure or responsiveness. Thus, confirmation of lack of any effect of anacetrapib on aldosterone and BP should await findings from this study. Long-term clinical safety data with evacetrapib are not yet available.

19.7 Similarities between Potent CETPi and Halogenated Hydrocarbons

The putative "potent" CETPi are mainly derived from a similar chemical class of highly fluorinated compounds (torcetrapib: 9, anacetrapib: 10, evacetrapib: 6/F per molecule) of high molecular weight (>600) and high lipophilicity ($\text{clog}\,P > 5$) (Figure 19.1). On reviewing available literature describing the use of the H295R cell line in screening for steroid hormone disruptive compounds, we were surprised to find that several chemicals [55], pharmaceuticals, and environmentally active compounds [56] also induce steroid production in these cells. For example, polychlorinated biphenyls (PCBs), a class of polyhalogenated compounds of considerable environmental impact and persistence, increase aldosterone [57,58], although to a much lesser extent than torcetrapib or some of its derivatives. Additionally, PCB118, PCB123, and PCB126 were found to induce aldosterone synthesis [58]. In this regard, detailed study of PCB126 has shown this compound to increase both basal and inducible aldosterone biosynthesis [57] via a mechanism involving increased expression of both Cyp11B2 and Cyp11B1 [59]. Interestingly, PCB126 was observed to have an adverse effect on the cardiovascular system in female rats, specifically causing increased cardiomyopathy and chronic active arteritis, manifesting lesions similar to those observed in humans [60,61]. As for polyfluorinated compounds, polychlorinated compounds share the property of being highly lipophilic and of accumulating in adipose tissue according to their degree of lipophilicity [62]. Coupled with high metabolic stability, these compounds demonstrate very long environmental persistence and in the human population, thus, even low exposure and low potency toward adverse effects can contribute to human risk.

Although no direct evidence exists, it is intriguing that increases in BP as well as cardiovascular mortality were observed in subjects exposed to environmental PCBs such as the dioxin-like PCB126 and PCB118, whether from employment in a PCB manufacturing environment [63] Goncharov or community exposure to PCBs [64] Everett. However, findings show some variability, with Akagi *et al.* reporting no association between PCB exposure for 9 years in 20 patients from the Yusho region [65], while Kreiss *et al.* observed a positive association between plasma PCB and BP, which was independent of sex, body mass index, and social class [66]. Generally comparable observations have been reported for aldosterone induction in H295R cells by flame-retardant polybrominated hydrocarbons [67,68], as well as for some metabolites.

19.7.1 The Macrophage Scavenger Receptor MARCO, a Possible Antitarget for Dalcetrapib, and Its Relevance to Humans

Treatment with dalcetrapib under conditions of repeated dose toxicity studies in rats, monkeys, mice, and hamsters produced macrophage changes in the small intestine and in the mesenteric lymph nodes. Macropathological effects (increased size and yellow discoloration of the mesenteric lymph nodes) were observed in mice and rats. Histologically, foamy macrophages were detected in the small intestine and the mesenteric lymph nodes and evidence shows that macrophages ingested dalcetrapib-adducted lipoproteins. In affected animals, the mesenteric lymph nodes were always the most affected organ with regard to lowest observable effect dose and severity. In monkeys, the macrophage changes slowly regressed over 6 months after cessation of 12 months' chronic treatment, but there was no evidence that the macrophage changes were associated with any degenerative organ or tissue toxicities. When comparing different species in studies of similar duration (4 weeks) and at comparable doses/exposure, macrophage changes were much more prominent in rats and mice than in monkeys and practically absent in hamsters. *In vitro* studies with macrophages from rats, mice, hamsters, and monkeys showed that dalcetrapib promoted the uptake of chylomicrons (CM). Uptake of dalcetrapib-treated CM was more prominent in rats and mice than in hamsters and monkeys. Hence, the results of *in vitro* studies resemble the order of sensitivity observed in nonclinical studies.

In vitro macrophages have been shown to take up dalcetrapib by a specific scavenger receptor, the macrophage receptor with collagenous structure (MARCO) [69]. This receptor shows extensive species- and tissue-specific differences in its expression and, therefore, differences in uptake between tissues and species have been recorded *in vitro* and *in vivo*. *In vivo* mesenteric lymph node enlargement based on this macrophage uptake has been found in mice and rats in a cumulative way. In monkeys, this enlargement has been less pronounced. However, the effect was of slow reversibility, consistent with the life span of the macrophages. In order to assist assessment of clinical relevance, imaging of lymph nodes in the gastrointestinal tract was performed in an extended phase II study with a duration of at least 6 months [70]. This imaging approach supported the nonclinical assessment of low relevance of the animal findings for the human situation. In the dalcetrapib phase III outcomes study, no safety issues potentially related to perturbation in lymph nodes and immunity were observed [10], confirming the lack of relevance of the preclinical finding to the clinical setting.

19.8 Conclusions

So far, with the exception of dalcetrapib, compounds that affect CETP have all been derived from similar chemical structures. Because the substrates of CETP are lipids (cholesteryl esters and triglycerides), with the exception of dalcetrapib ($\log P \sim 5$), compounds affecting this target are highly lipophilic, with clog$P$ greater than 7. Torcetrapib and most torcetrapib derivatives share the properties of directly increasing aldosterone secretion and BP in many animal species. Understanding the off-target activities of torcetrapib has allowed other candidates, such as dalcetrapib, anacetrapib, and evacetrapib, to be derisked and for development of this class to continue despite the torcetrapib results.

It should be noted that recently [71] the effects of torcetrapib, anacetrapib, and evacetrapib (not dalcetrapib) on two important regulators of LDL metabolism, namely, the LDL receptor and PCSK9 expression, were demonstrated to be off-target and unrelated to CETP inhibition, indicating a range of nontarget activities of highly lipophilic derivatives of torcetrapib.

References

1 Okamoto, H., Yonemori, F., Wakitani, K., Minowa, T., Maeda, K., and Shinkai, H. (2000) A cholesteryl ester transfer protein inhibitor attenuates atherosclerosis in rabbits. *Nature*, **406**, 203–207.

2 Clark, R.W., Ruggeri, R.B., Cunningham, D., and Bamberger, M.J. (2006) Description of the torcetrapib series of cholesteryl ester transfer protein inhibitors, including mechanism of action. *Journal of Lipid Research*, **47**, 537–552.

3 Barter, P.J., Brewer, H.B., Jr., Chapman, M.J., Hennekens, C.H., Rader, D.J., and Tall, A.R. (2003) Cholesteryl ester transfer protein: a novel target for raising HDL and inhibiting atherosclerosis. *Arteriosclerosis, Thrombosis, and Vascular Biology*, **23**, 160–167.

4 Gordon, T., Castelli, W.P., Hjortland, M.C., Kannel, W.B., and Dawber, T. R. (1977) High density lipoprotein as a protective factor against coronary heart disease: The Framingham Study. *The American Journal of Medicine*, **62**, 707–714.

5 Barter, P.J. and Kastelein, J.J. (2006) Targeting cholesteryl ester transfer protein for the prevention and management of cardiovascular disease. *Journal of the American College of Cardiology*, **47**, 492–499.

6 Shinkai, H. (2009) Cholesteryl ester transfer protein inhibitors as high-density lipoprotein raising agents. *Expert Opinion on Therapeutic Patents*, **19**, 1229–1237.

7 Niesor, E.J. (2011) Different effects of compounds decreasing cholesteryl ester transfer protein activity on lipoprotein metabolism. *Current Opinion in Lipidology*, **22**, 288–295.

8 Maugeais, C., Perez, A., von der Marker, E., Magg, C., Pflieger, P., and Niesor, E.J. (2013) Evidence for a role of CETP in HDL remodeling and cholesterol efflux: role of cysteine 13 of CETP. *Biochimica et Biophysica Acta*, **1831**, 1644–1650.

9 Barter, P.J., Caulfield, M., Eriksson, M., Grundy, S.M., Kastelein, J.J., Komajda, M., Lopez-Sendon, J., Mosca, L., Tardif, J.C., Waters, D.D., Shear, C.L., Revkin, J.H., Buhr, K.A., Fisher, M.R., Tall, A.R., and Brewer, B. (2007) Effects of torcetrapib in patients at high risk for coronary events. *The New England Journal of Medicine*, **357**, 2109–2122.

10 Schwartz, G.G., Olsson, A.G., Abt, M., Ballantyne, C.M., Barter, P.J., Brumm, J., Chaitman, B.R., Holme, I.M., Kallend, D., Leiter, L.A., Leitersdorf, E., McMurray, J.J., Mundl, H., Nicholls, S.J., Shah, P.K., Tardif, J.C., and Wright, R.S. (2012) Effects of dalcetrapib in patients with a recent acute coronary syndrome. *The New England Journal of Medicine*, **367**, 2089–2099.

11 Davidson, M.H., McKenney, J.M., Shear, C.L., and Revkin, J.H. (2006) Efficacy and safety of torcetrapib, a novel cholesteryl ester transfer protein inhibitor, in individuals with below-average high-density lipoprotein cholesterol levels. *Journal of the American College of Cardiology*, **48**, 1774–1781.

12 Lichtenauer, U.D., Shapiro, I., Osswald, A., Meurer, S., Kulle, A., Reincke, M., Riepe, F., and Beuschlein, F. (2013) Characterization of NCI-H295R cells as an *in vitro* model of hyperaldosteronism. *Hormone and Metabolic Research*, **45**, 124–129.

13 Romero, D.G., Plonczynski, M., Vergara, G.R., Gomez-Sanchez, E.P., and Gomez-Sanchez, C.E. (2004) Angiotensin II early regulated genes in H295R human adrenocortical cells. *Physiological Genomics*, **19**, 106–116.

14 Clerc, R.G., Stauffer, A., Weibel, F., Hainaut, E., Perez, A., Hoflack, J.C., Benardeau, A., Pflieger, P., Garriz, J.M., Funder, J.W., Capponi, A.M., and Niesor, E.J. (2010) Mechanisms underlying off-target effects of the cholesteryl ester transfer protein inhibitor torcetrapib involve L-type calcium channels. *Journal of Hypertension*, **28**, 1676–1686.

15 Clark, R.W., Sutfin, T.A., Ruggeri, R.B., Willauer, A.T., Sugarman, E.D., Magnus-Aryitey, G., Cosgrove, P.G., Sand, T.M., Wester, R.T., Williams, J.A., Perlman, M.E., and Bamberger, M.J. (2004) Raising high-density lipoprotein in humans through inhibition of cholesteryl ester transfer protein: an initial multidose study of torcetrapib. *Arteriosclerosis, Thrombosis, and Vascular Biology*, **24**, 490–497.

16 Stroes, E.S., Kastelein, J.J., Benardeau, A., Kuhlmann, O., Blum, D., Campos, L.A., Clerc, R.G., and Niesor, E.J. (2009) Dalcetrapib: no off-target toxicity on blood pressure or on genes related to the renin-angiotensin-aldosterone system in rats. *British Journal of Pharmacology*, **158**, 1763–1770.

17 Johns, D.G., Duffy, J., Fisher, T., Hubbard, B.K., and Forrest, M.J. (2012) On- and off-target pharmacology of torcetrapib: current understanding and implications for the structure activity relationships (SAR), discovery and development of cholesteryl ester-transfer protein (CETP) inhibitors. *Drugs*, **72**, 491–507.

18 Cao, G., Beyer, T.P., Zhang, Y., Schmidt, R.J., Chen, Y.Q., Cockerham, S.L., Zimmerman, K.M., Karathanasis, S.K., Cannady, E.A., Fields, T., and Mantlo, N.B. (2011) Evacetrapib is a novel, potent, and selective inhibitor of cholesteryl ester transfer protein that elevates HDL cholesterol without inducing aldosterone or increasing blood pressure. *Journal of Lipid Research*, **52**, 2169–2176.

19 Bird, I.M., Mathis, J.M., Mason, J.I., and Rainey, W.E. (1995) Ca(2+)-regulated expression of steroid hydroxylases in H295R human adrenocortical cells. *Endocrinology*, **136**, 5677–5684.

20 Hu, X., Dietz, J.D., Xia, C., Knight, D.R., Loging, W.T., Smith, A.H., Yuan, H., Perry, D.A., and Keiser, J. (2009) Torcetrapib induces aldosterone and cortisol production by an intracellular calcium-mediated mechanism independently of cholesteryl ester transfer protein inhibition. *Endocrinology*, **150**, 2211–2219.

21 Kalgutkar, A.S., Frederick, K.S., Hatch, H.L., Ambler, C.M., Perry, D.A., Garigipati, R.S., Chang, G.C., Lefker, B.A., Clark, R.W., Morehouse, L.A., Francone, O., and Hu, X. (2013) Identification of a novel, non-tetrahydroquinoline variant of the cholesteryl ester transfer protein (CETP) inhibitor torcetrapib, with improved aqueous solubility. *Xenobiotica*, **44**, 591–605.

22 Forrest, M.J., Bloomfield, D., Briscoe, R.J., Brown, P.N., Cumiskey, A.M., Ehrhart, J., Hershey, J.C., Keller, W.J., Ma, X., McPherson, H.E., Messina, E., Peterson, L.B., Sharif-Rodriguez, W., Siegl, P.K., Sinclair, P.J., Sparrow, C.P., Stevenson, A.S., Sun, S.Y., Tsai, C., Vargas, H., Walker, M., III, West, S.H., White, V., and Woltmann, R.F. (2008) Torcetrapib-induced blood pressure elevation is independent of CETP inhibition and is accompanied by increased circulating levels of aldosterone. *British Journal of Pharmacology*, **154**, 1465–1473.

23 Kumar, S., Tan, E.Y., Hartmann, G., Biddle, Z., Bergman, A.J., Dru, J., Ho, J.Z., Jones, A.N., Staskiewicz, S.J., Braun, M.P., Karanam, B., Dean, D.C., Gendrano, I.N., Graves, M.W., Wagner, J.A., and Krishna, R. (2010) Metabolism and excretion of anacetrapib, a novel inhibitor of the cholesteryl ester transfer protein, in humans. *Drug Metabolism and Disposition: The Biological Fate of Chemicals*, **38**, 474–483.

24 Dalvie, D., Chen, W., Zheng, C., Vaz, A.D., Smolarek, T.A., Cox, L.M., Lin, J., and Obach, R.S. (2008) Pharmacokinetics, metabolism, and excretion of torcetrapib, a cholesteryl ester transfer protein inhibitor, in humans. *Drug Metabolism and Disposition*, **36**, 2185–2198.

25 Nicholls, S.J., Brewer, H.B., Kastelein, J.J., Krueger, K.A., Wang, M.D., Shao, M., Hu, B., McErlean, E., and Nissen, S.E. (2011) Effects of the CETP inhibitor evacetrapib administered as monotherapy or in combination with statins on HDL and LDL cholesterol: a randomized controlled trial. *JAMA*, **306**, 2099–2109.

26 Xing, Y., Cohen, A., Rothblat, G., Sankaranarayanan, S., Weibel, G., Royer, L., Francone, O.L., and Rainey, W.E. (2011) Aldosterone production in human adrenocortical cells is stimulated by high-density lipoprotein 2 (HDL2) through increased expression of aldosterone synthase (CYP11B2). *Endocrinology*, **152**, 751–763.

27 Prakash, C., Chen, W., Rossulek, M., Johnson, K., Zhang, C., O'Connell, T., Potchoiba, M., and Dalvie, D. (2008) Metabolism, pharmacokinetics, and excretion of a cholesteryl ester transfer protein inhibitor, torcetrapib, in rats, monkeys, and mice: characterization of unusual and novel metabolites by high-resolution liquid chromatography–tandem mass spectrometry and 1*H* nuclear magnetic resonance. *Drug Metabolism and Disposition: The Biological Fate of Chemicals*, **36**, 2064–2079.

28 McCormick, S.D. and Bradshaw, D. (2006) Hormonal control of salt and water balance in vertebrates. *General and Comparative Endocrinology*, **147**, 3–8.

29 Simic, B., Hermann, M., Shaw, S.G., Bigler, L., Stalder, U., Dorries, C., Besler, C., Luscher, T.F., and Ruschitzka, F. (2012) Torcetrapib impairs endothelial function in hypertension. *European Heart Journal*, **33**, 1615–1624.

30 Funder, J. W. (2009) The off-target effects of torcetrapib. *Endocrinology*, **150**, 2024–2026.

31 DePasquale, M., Knight, D., Loging, W., Morehouse, L., Winter, S., Blasi, E., Perry, D., and Keiser, J. (2009) Mechanistic studies of hemodynamics with a series of cholesterol ester transfer protein inhibitors. *Drug Development Research*, **70**, 35–48.

32 Connelly, M.A., Parry, T.J., Giardino, E.C., Huang, Z., Cheung, W.M., Chen, C., Cools, F., van der Linde, H., Gallacher, D.J., Kuo, G.H., Sarich, T.C., Demarest, K.T., and Damiano, B.P. (2010) Torcetrapib

produces endothelial dysfunction independent of cholesteryl ester transfer protein inhibition. *Journal of Cardiovascular Pharmacology*, **55**, 459–468.

33 Blasi, E., Bamberger, M., Knight, D., Engwall, M., Wolk, R., Winter, S., Betts, A., John-Baptiste, A., and Keiser, J. (2009) Effects of CP-532,623 and torcetrapib, cholesteryl ester transfer protein inhibitors, on arterial blood pressure. *Journal of Cardiovascular Pharmacology*, **53**, 507–516.

34 Fryer, R.M., Harrison, P.C., Muthukumarana, A., Nodop Mazurek, S.G., Ng, K.J., Chen, R.R., Harrington, K.E., Dinallo, R.M., Chi, L., and Reinhart, G.A. (2012) Strategic integration of *in vivo* cardiovascular models during lead optimization: predictive value of 4 models independent of species, route of administration, and influence of anesthesia. *Journal of Cardiovascular Pharmacology*, **59**, 369–376.

35 Meyer, O., Jenni, R., Greiter-Wilke, A., Breidenbach, A., and Holzgrefe, H.H. (2010) Comparison of telemetry and high-definition oscillometry for blood pressure measurements in conscious dogs: effects of torcetrapib. *Journal of the American Association Laboratory Animal Science*, **49**, 464–471.

36 Polakowski, J.S., King, A.J., Campbell, T.J., Nelson, R.A., Preusser, L.C., Kempf-Grote, A.J., Marsh, K.C., Gintant, G.A., Cox, B.F., and Mittelstadt, S.W. (2009) Cardiovascular effects of torcetrapib in conscious and pentobarbital-anesthetized dogs. *Journal of Cardiovascular Pharmacology*, **54**, 543–551.

37 Vergeer, M., Bots, M.L., van Leuven, S.I., Basart, D.C., Sijbrands, E.J., Evans, G.W., Grobbee, D.E., Visseren, F.L., Stalenhoef, A.F., Stroes, E.S., and Kastelein, J.J. (2008) Cholesteryl ester transfer protein inhibitor torcetrapib and off-target toxicity: a pooled analysis of the rating atherosclerotic disease change by imaging with a new CETP inhibitor (RADIANCE) trials. *Circulation*, **118**, 2515–2522.

38 Muller, M., Junger, A., Brau, M., Kwapisz, M.M., Schindler, E., Akinturk, H., Benson, M., and Hempelmann, G. (2002) Incidence and risk calculation of inotropic support in patients undergoing cardiac surgery with cardiopulmonary bypass using an automated anaesthesia record-keeping system. *British Journal of Anaesthesia*, **89**, 398–404.

39 Markert, M., Klumpp, A., Trautmann, T., Mayer, K., Stubhan, M., and Guth, B. (2007) The value added by measuring myocardial contractility '*in vivo*' in safety pharmacological profiling of drug candidates. *Journal of Pharmacological and Toxicological Methods*, **56**, 203–211.

40 Cools, F., Dhuyvetter, D., Vanlommel, A., Janssens, S., Borghys, H., Geys, H., and Gallacher, D.J. (2014) A translational assessment of preclinical versus clinical tools for the measurement of cardiac contractility: comparison of LV dP/dt (max) with echocardiography in telemetry implanted beagle dogs. *Journal of Pharmacological and Toxicological Methods*, **69**, 17–23.

41 Rossier, M. F. (2006) T channels and steroid biosynthesis: in search of a link with mitochondria. *Cell Calcium*, **40**, 155–164.

42 Pratt, P.F., Bonnet, S., Ludwig, L.M., Bonnet, P., and Rusch, N.J. (2002) Upregulation of L-type Ca^{2+} channels in mesenteric and skeletal arteries of SHR. *Hypertension*, **40**, 214–219.

43 Milliez, P., Girerd, X., Plouin, P.F., Blacher, J., Safar, M.E., and Mourad, J.J. (2005) Evidence for an increased rate of cardiovascular events in patients with primary aldosteronism. *Journal of the American College of Cardiology*, **45**, 1243–1248.

44 Meier, D.J., Pitt, B., and Rajagopalan, S. (2004) Eplerenone: will it have a role in the treatment of acute coronary syndromes? *Current Cardiology Reports*, **6**, 259–263.

45 Palmer, B.R., Pilbrow, A.P., Frampton, C.M., Yandle, T.G., Skelton, L., Nicholls, M.G., and Richards, A. M. (2008) Plasma aldosterone levels during hospitalization are predictive of survival post-myocardial infarction. *European Heart Journal*, **29**, 2489–2496.

46 Burniston, J.G., Saini, A., Tan, L.B., and Goldspink, D.F. (2005) Aldosterone induces myocyte apoptosis in the heart and skeletal muscles of rats *in vivo*. *Journal of Molecular and Cellular Cardiology*, **39**, 395–399.

47 McGraw, A.P., Bagley, J., Chen, W.S., Galayda, C., Nickerson, H., Armani, A., Caprio, M., Carmeliet, P., and Jaffe, I.Z. (2013) Aldosterone increases early atherosclerosis and promotes plaque inflammation through a placental growth factor-dependent mechanism. *Journal of American Heart Association*, **2**, e000018.

48 Pratt, J. H. (2008) A not-so-modest proposal that a "modest" increase in aldosterone causes hypertension and more. *Hypertension*, **51**, 39–40.

49 Makhanova, N., Hagaman, J., Kim, H.S., and Smithies, O. (2008) Salt-sensitive blood pressure in mice with increased expression of aldosterone synthase. *Hypertension*, **51**, 134–140.

50 Cannon, C.P., Shah, S., Dansky, H.M., Davidson, M., Brinton, E.A., Gotto, A.M., Stepanavage, M., Liu, S.X., Gibbons, P., Ashraf, T.B., Zafarino, J., Mitchel, Y., and Barter, P. (2010) Safety of anacetrapib in patients with or at high risk for coronary heart disease. *The New England Journal of Medicine*, **363**, 2406–2415.

51 Krishna, R., Bergman, A.J., Jin, B., Fallon, M., Cote, J., Van Hoydonck, P., Laethem, T., Gendrano, I.N., III, Van Dyck, K., Hilliard, D., Laterza, O., Snyder, K., Chavez-Eng, C., Lutz, R., Chen, J., Bloomfield, D.M., De Smet, M., Van Bortel, L.M., Gutierrez, M., Al-Huniti, N., Dykstra, K., Gottesdiener, K.M., and Wagner, J.A. (2008) Multiple-dose pharmacodynamics and pharmacokinetics of anacetrapib, a potent cholesteryl ester transfer protein (CETP) inhibitor, in healthy subjects. *Clinical Pharmacology and Therapeutics*, **84**, 679–683.

52 Tan, E.Y., Hartmann, G., Chen, Q., Pereira, A., Bradley, S., Doss, G., Zhang, A.S., Ho, J.Z., Braun, M.P., Dean, D.C., Tang, W., and Kumar, S. (2010) Pharmacokinetics, metabolism, and excretion of anacetrapib, a novel inhibitor of the cholesteryl ester transfer protein, in rats and rhesus monkeys. *Drug Metabolism and Disposition: The Biological Fate of Chemicals*, **38**, 459–473.

53 Dansky, H.M., Bloomfield, D., Gibbons, P., Liu, S., Sisk, C.M., Tribble, D., McKenney, J.M., Littlejohn, T.W., III, and Mitchel, Y. (2011) Efficacy and safety after cessation of treatment with the cholesteryl ester transfer protein inhibitor anacetrapib (MK-0859) in patients with primary hypercholesterolemia or mixed hyperlipidemia. *American Heart Journal*, **162**, 708–716.

54 Gotto, A.M., Jr., Cannon, C.P., Li, X.S., Vaidya, S., Kher, U., Brinton, E.A., Davidson, M., Moon, J.E., Shah, S., Dansky, H.M., Mitchel, Y., and Barter, P. (2014) Evaluation of lipids, drug concentration, and safety parameters following cessation of treatment with the cholesteryl ester transfer protein inhibitor anacetrapib in patients with or at high risk for coronary heart disease. *The American Journal of Cardiology*, **113**, 76–83.

55 Hecker, M. and Giesy, J.P. (2008) Novel trends in endocrine disruptor testing: the H295R steroidogenesis assay for identification of inducers and inhibitors of hormone production. *Analytical and Bioanalytical Chemistry*, **390**, 287–291.

56 Gracia, T., Hilscherova, K., Jones, P.D., Newsted, J.L., Higley, E.B., Zhang, X., Hecker, M., Murphy, M.B., Yu, R.M., Lam, P.K., Wu, R.S., and Giesy, J.P. (2007) Modulation of steroidogenic gene expression and hormone production of H295R cells by pharmaceuticals and other environmentally active compounds. *Toxicology and Applied Pharmacology*, **225**, 142–153.

57 Li, L.A., Wang, P.W., and Chang, L.W. (2004) Polychlorinated biphenyl 126 stimulates basal and inducible aldosterone biosynthesis of human adrenocortical H295R cells. *Toxicology and Applied Pharmacology*, **195**, 92–102.

58 Kraugerud, M., Zimmer, K.E., Dahl, E., Berg, V., Olsaker, I., Farstad, W., Ropstad, E., and Verhaegen, S. (2010) Three structurally different polychlorinated biphenyl congeners (Pcb 118, 153, and 126) affect hormone production and gene expression in the human H295R *in vitro*

model. *Journal of Toxicology and Environmental Health A*, **73**, 1122–1132.

59 Lin, T.C., Chien, S.C., Hsu, P.C., and Li, L.A. (2006) Mechanistic study of polychlorinated biphenyl 126-induced CYP11B1 and CYP11B2 up-regulation. *Endocrinology*, **147**, 1536–1544.

60 Jokinen, M.P., Walker, N.J., Brix, A.E., Sells, D.M., Haseman, J.K., and Nyska, A. (2003) Increase in cardiovascular pathology in female Sprague-Dawley rats following chronic treatment with 2,3,7,8-tetrachlorodibenzo-*p*-dioxin and 3,3′,4,4′,5-pentachlorobiphenyl. *Cardiovascular Toxicology*, **3**, 299–310.

61 Yoshizawa, K., Heatherly, A., Malarkey, D.E., Walker, N.J., and Nyska, A. (2007) A critical comparison of murine pathology and epidemiological data of TCDD, PCB126, and PeCDF. *Toxicologic Pathology*, **35**, 865–879.

62 Bourez, S., van den Daelen, C., Le, L.S., Poupaert, J., Larondelle, Y., Thome, J.P., Schneider, Y.J., Dugail, I., and Debier, C. (2013) The dynamics of accumulation of PCBs in cultured adipocytes vary with the cell lipid content and the lipophilicity of the congener. *Toxicology Letters*, **216**, 40–46.

63 Goncharov, A., Pavuk, M., Foushee, H.R., Carpenter, D.O., and Anniston Environmental Health Reseach Consortium (2011) Blood pressure in relation to concentrations of PCB congeners and chlorinated pesticides. *Environmental Health Perspective*, **119** (3), 319–325.

64 Everett, C.J., Mainous, A.G., III, Frithsen, I.L., Player, M.S., and Matheson, E.M. (2008) Association of polychlorinated biphenyls with hypertension in the 1999–2002 National Health and Nutrition Examination Survey. *Environmental Research*, **108**, 94–97.

65 Akagi, K. and Okumura, M. (1985) Association of blood pressure and PCB level in yusho patients. *Environmental Health Perspectives*, **59**, 37–39.

66 Kreiss, K., Zack, M.M., Kimbrough, R.D., Needham, L.L., Smrek, A.L., and Jones, B.T. (1981) Cross-sectional study of a community with exceptional exposure to DDT. *JAMA*, **245**, 1926–1930.

67 Song, R., Duarte, T.L., Almeida, G.M., Farmer, P.B., Cooke, M.S., Zhang, W., Sheng, G., Fu, J., and Jones, G.D. (2009) Cytotoxicity and gene expression profiling of two hydroxylated polybrominated diphenyl ethers in human H295R adrenocortical carcinoma cells. *Toxicology Letters*, **185**, 23–31.

68 He, Y., Murphy, M.B., Yu, R.M., Lam, M.H., Hecker, M., Giesy, J.P., Wu, R.S., and Lam, P.K. (2008) Effects of 20 PBDE metabolites on steroidogenesis in the H295R cell line. *Toxicology Letters*, **176**, 230–238.

69 Perez, A., Wright, M.B., Maugeais, C., Braendli-Baiocco, A., Okamoto, H., Takahashi, A., Singer, T., Mueller, L., and Niesor, E.J. (2010) MARCO, a macrophage scavenger receptor highly expressed in rodents, mediates dalcetrapib-induced uptake of lipids by rat and mouse macrophages. *Toxicol In Vitro*, **24** (3), 745–750.

70 Stein, E.A., Roth, E.M., Rhyne, J.M., Burgess, T., Kallend, D., and Robinson, J.G. (2010) Safety and tolerability of dalcetrapib (RO4607381/JTT-705): results from a 48-week trial. *European Heart Journal*, **31**, 480–488.

71 Dong, B., Singh, A.B., Fung, C., Kan, K., and Liu, J. (2014) CETP inhibitors downregulate hepatic LDL receptor and PCSK9 expression *in vitro* and *in vivo* through a SREBP2 dependent mechanism. *Atherosclerosis*, **235**, 449–462.

20
Targets Associated with Drug-Related Suicidal Ideation and Behavior

Andreas Hartmann, Steven Whitebread, Jacques Hamon, Alexander Fekete, Christian Trendelenburg, Patrick Y. Müller, and László Urbán

20.1
Introduction

Some side effects of drug candidates are difficult to discover and study in the preclinical setting because of species differences in targets, pathways, and clinically relevant PK/PD correlations. A particularly difficult phenomenon is suicidality, including suicidal ideation, suicide attempts, and nonsuicidal self-injurious behavior. Suicide was the 10th leading cause of death in the United States in 2009; thus, addressing this matter when associated with drugs – even though this adverse drug reaction (ADR) is rare – has a high importance for patients, society, and healthcare authorities. Indeed, increased prevalence of suicidality may also occur as an ADR with a broad variety of drugs. For example, the US Food and Drug Administration (FDA) issued black box labeling of antidepressants based on clinical trial data with adolescents suffering from psychiatric disorders. This action was followed by several high-profile cases with nonpsychiatric drugs that were discovered to be responsible for increased incidence of suicidal behavior (isotretinoin, tretinoins, β-adrenergic blockers, reserpine, smoking cessation drugs, and drugs prescribed for weight loss).

Regarding the importance of suicidality assessment in psychiatric and nonpsychiatric drug trials, the FDA issued a Draft Guidance for the Industry on Prospective Assessment of Suicidality in clinical trials with revisions in August 2012 [1,2]. This guidance describes instruments and specific (nonbinding) clinical trial and indication recommendations for suicidality assessment. In addition to psychiatric and neurological indications, the FDA also recommends a prospective suicidality assessment for nonpsychiatric drugs that are pharmacologically similar to the above-mentioned class of drugs. The FDA guidance does not make a difference between healthy volunteer and patient studies and there is no recommendation for suicidality assessment of drugs that do not have central nervous system (CNS) effects. No similar guidance has been issued by the European Medicines Agency (EMA).

Antitargets and Drug Safety, First Edition. Edited by László Urbán, Vinod F. Patel, and Roy J. Vaz.

While the FDA guidance outlines clear requirements for prospective clinical assessment of suicidality, it leaves considerations open for preclinical evaluation. Since suicide is a complex behavior, it is impossible to fully reproduce it in animal models. To a limited extent, it is feasible to investigate traits that show strong cross-species parallels in addition to associations with suicide in humans. Traits linked with potential suicide in humans that can be modeled in rodents include aggression, impulsivity, irritability, and hopelessness/helplessness [3]. However, recently accumulating translational knowledge obtained in the clinic provides good foundation to create first-line screening of drug candidates at targets that have strong association with suicidal behavior. This is an inexpensive and scientifically well-justified approach in the absence of relevant animal experiments. Observations of increased incidence of suicidal behavior associated with drugs that have well-characterized effects at various CNS targets lead to the hypothesis that any drug candidate affecting these targets and crossing the blood–brain barrier (BBB) may be suspected to cause suicidal behavior. Here, we will discuss the evidence supporting this hypothesis and provide examples for practical use. In this chapter, the term target is used not only to denote the primary pharmacological target responsible for the intended pharmacological effect, but also for targets at which the drug was not intentionally designed to be active [4].

20.2 Targets Associated with Increased Suicidal Intent and Behavior

Determining the effect of drug candidates and drugs on suicidal behavior is a daunting task, particularly in the case when the patient population has already an increased prevalence. This includes consideration of age, gender, and the characteristics of the disease. The combination of all three is demonstrated with the treatment of difficult-to-manage acne in teenagers [5]. While increase of suicidal intent by a drug is not necessarily a roadblock for development, it would generate hurdles toward clinical registration and would require a box warning in case of positive findings when the drug is marketed. Furthermore, the cost implications would be significant because psychiatric support would be necessary for the clinical management of patients. Table 20.1 provides a complete list of targets addressed in this chapter.

20.2.1 G-Protein-Coupled Receptors

20.2.1.1 Dopamine D_1 and D_2 Receptors (DRD1 and DRD2)

Dopamine is a major neurotransmitter with a critical role in the regulation of locomotor, neuroendocrine, cognitive, and emotional functions. Dysfunctions of the dopaminergic system may result in neurological disorders such as Parkinson's disease (PD), schizophrenia, and Tourette's syndrome and in the

Table 20.1 Targets associated with suicidality (clinical evidence is used for annotation).

Target (OMIM)	Associated CNS effects (MoA; agonism/antagonism)	Clinical evidence
HTR1A	Some evidence exists for suicidal behavior in patients with $5\text{-}HT_{1A}$ hypoactivity	Aripiprazole (Abilify) is a *partial dopamine agonist* with additional effects at 5-HT receptors. It is also an agonist of the D2L and D_4 receptors. It is a third-generation atypical antipsychotic used for the treatment of schizophrenia, bipolar disorder, and clinical depression. It carries a *box warning for suicidal behavior.*
HTR2A	Some evidence exists for suicidal behavior in patients with $5\text{-}HT_{2A}$ hyperexcitability	
SLC6A4	5-HTT inhibitors are associated with suicidal ideation in children, insomnia, anxiety, nausea and vomiting, and sexual dysfunction	All SSRIs carry *label for suicidal ideation* in adolescent population.
CACNA1B	CaN channel blockers are associated with somnolence, ataxia, weakness, and may cause suicidal ideation	Ziconotide (Prialt) is an N-type ($Ca_v2.2$) calcium channel *blocker.* The most severe, but rare side effects are hallucinations, thoughts of suicide, new or worsening depression, meningitis, and seizures. Gabapentin and pregabalin block subunits of $Ca_v2.1$ and $Ca_v2.2$ channels after chronic administration. They carry *warning for suicidal ideation.*
CNR1	CB1 antagonism or inverse agonism is associated with emesis, weight loss, depression, and suicidal tendencies	Rimonabant is an *inverse agonist* of the CB1 receptor. *Withdrawn* from clinical use.
DRD1; DRD5	Tremor, sedation, depression, anxiety, and suicidal ideation were observed with D_1 and D_5 antagonists	Ecopipam, a $D_{1,5}$ receptor *antagonist,* was tested in clinical trials for weight management. *Phase III studies were discontinued* because of psychiatric adverse events, including *suicidal ideation.*
SLC6A2	NET inhibition is associated with depression and suicidal ideation	Atomoxetine (Strattera), a NET inhibitor for ADHD, carries a *box warning for suicidal intent.*
CHRNA4	Nicotinic $\alpha4\beta2$ receptor agonists may increase suicidal ideation, aggressiveness, hostility, and depression	Varenicline (Chantix) is a nicotinic $\alpha4\beta2$ *partial agonist* for smoking cessation. It stimulates dopamine release, leading to the pleasurable

(continued)

Table 20.1 (*Continued*)

Target (OMIM)	Associated CNS effects (MoA; agonism/antagonism)	Clinical evidence
		effects of smoking. It attenuates the craving and withdrawal symptoms that occur with abstinence from nicotine. Clinical evidence suggests *suicidal tendencies* and other psychiatric adverse reactions leading to *box warning* by FDA.
SLC18A2	Chronic inhibition of VMAT2 may induce parkinsonism, tremor, suicidal ideation, and depression	Tetrabenazine (Nitoman, Xenazina, and Xenazine) is a VMAT2 inhibitor for the treatment of tardive dyskinesia, Huntington's disease, Tourette's disease, and extrapyramidal disorders. The compound carries a *black box warning of the increased risk of depression and suicidal tendencies.* Reserpine, a crystalline alkaloid of *Rauwolfia*, is an irreversible VMAT2 inhibitor that has been used for the treatment of hypertension. Its label carries a warning for *depression and suicide.*

development of pituitary tumors. The actions of dopamine are mediated by five distinct receptor subtypes that belong to the G-protein-coupled receptor (GPCR) superfamily and are divided into two major subgroups, D_1-like and D_2-like, on the basis of their structure and pharmacology [6]. The D_1-like subfamily consists of the D_1 and D_5 subtypes, both of which transduce their signals by increasing intracellular cAMP levels, and the D_2-like family consists of D_2, D_3, and D_4 receptor subtypes that inhibit cAMP levels [7].

By a mechanism of alternative splicing, the D_2 receptor gene encodes two molecularly distinct isoforms, D2S (short) and D2L (long), which display similar pharmacological characteristics but serve different functions *in vivo* [8]. Signaling through dopamine D_2 receptors governs physiological functions related to locomotion, hormone production, and drug abuse.

Agonists of D_1 and D_2 receptors may induce dyskinesia [9,10], extreme arousal, flushing, locomotor activation, vasodilation, bradycardia, hypotension (renal effect), and diminished pituitary hormone secretions (e.g., prolactin). D_2 agonists may cause drowsiness, dizziness, and nausea/vomiting especially with the first dose and some psychosis may occur after long-term treatment. D_1 antagonist/inhibitor activity manifests in tremor. Sedation, depression, anxiety, and suicidal ideation were observed with D_1 and D_5 antagonists. Furthermore, D_2 antagonism is associated with tardive dyskinesia (impairment of voluntary movement), akathisia (an inability to sit still or remain motionless) and other extrapyramidal effects

(Parkinson-like syndrome), gastrointestinal prokinetic properties, and hyperprolactinemia.

Clinical Relevance

Levodopa, which is used for the treatment of symptoms associated with Parkinson's disease, is nearly always effective, but has a high incidence of adverse effects with long-term use, including response fluctuations (on/off phenomena) and dyskinesias (after several years of treatment).

Ecopipam, a dopamine $D_{1,5}$ receptor antagonist, was tested in clinical trials for weight management. Phase III studies were discontinued because of unexpected psychiatric adverse events (ecopipam 31% versus placebo 15%), including depression, anxiety, and suicidal ideation [11].

Nonselective dopamine D_2-like agonists such as the ergoline derivatives (bromocriptine, cabergoline, pergolide, and lisuride) or the nonergoline derivatives (pramipexole) are useful in the treatment of PD or for the treatment of hyperprolactinemia. The main side effects include drowsiness, dizziness, and nausea especially with the first dose and some psychosis may occur after long-term treatment. Problematic compulsive behaviors (e.g., obsessive gambling) also occur during treatment with dopamine receptor agonists [12].

All clinically effective antipsychotic drugs selectively bind to and block the D_2 receptor family at concentrations that correlate well with clinically effective antipsychotic doses (clozapine (D_2–5-HT_2 antagonist) is a good example). Interestingly, clozapine treatment of chronic schizophrenic patients has been shown to reduce the rate of suicide by 80–85% possibly due to a reduction in impulsive aggressive behavior [13,14]. Aripiprazole (Abilify, Aripiprex) is a unique partial dopamine agonist (D2L, D_4) with additional effects at 5-hydroxytryptamine (5-HT) receptors (5-HT_{1A} partial agonist; 5-HT_{2A} antagonist; 5-HT_{2C} partial agonist; 5-HT_6 and 5-HT_7 antagonist). It represents the third generation of atypical antipsychotics used for the treatment of schizophrenia, bipolar disorder, and clinical depression. Aripiprazole also has antidepressant effects; however, it carries a boxed warning for suicidal behavior.

Based on the above clinical observations, it is anticipated that D_1 (D_5) antagonism (based on the clinical observation with ecopipam) and possibly D_2 activation might be responsible for increased incidence for suicidal intent and behavior. There is supportive evidence for the involvement of the D_2 dopaminergic receptor in suicidal behavior [15,16] and this is further supported by the higher incidence of suicidality in patients taking Abilify. Bowden *et al.* [17] found increased numbers and decreased affinity of D_2 receptors in the brain of antidepressant-treated suicide victims. On the other hand, there is no confirmation on D_4 receptor association with suicidal behavior [18].

So far, there is no clear consensus on the primary dopaminergic target or combination of targets for suicidal behavior [19]. Indeed, atypical antipsychotic drugs are highly promiscuous as demonstrated by aripiprazole and further contribution of 5-HT, muscarinic, and adrenergic receptors and transporters could generate a combined effect in brain function that will manifest in psychosis,

	Preclinical Data view all 1362	Clinical Data view all 6743	Post-Marketing Reports (AERS) view all 19568
⊟ Psychiatric disorders	56	832	5265
⊞ Adjustment disorders (incl subtypes)	no data	1	3
⊞ Anxiety disorders and symptoms	no data	135	985
⊞ Changes in physical activity	55	55	607
⊞ Cognitive and attention disorders and disturbances	1	2	11
⊞ Communication disorders and disturbances	no data	2	79
⊞ Deliria (incl confusion)	no data	38	330
⊞ Depressed mood disorders and disturbances	no data	49	334
⊞ Developmental disorders NEC	no data	no data	3
⊞ Dissociative disorders	no data	7	26
⊞ Disturbances in thinking and perception	no data	61	867
⊞ Eating disorders and disturbances	no data	no data	39
⊞ Impulse control disorders NEC	no data	5	73
⊞ Manic and bipolar mood disorders and disturbances	no data	66	424
⊞ Mood disorders and disturbances NEC	no data	52	362
⊞ Personality disorders and disturbances in behaviour	no data	70	477
⊞ Psychiatric and behavioural symptoms NEC	no data	3	298
⊞ Psychiatric disorders NEC	no data	7	187
⊞ Schizophrenia and other psychotic disorders	no data	36	955
⊞ Sexual dysfunctions, disturbances and gender identity disorders	no data	41	99
⊞ Sleep disorders and disturbances	no data	85	971
⊞ Somatoform and factitious disorders	no data	no data	16
⊞ Suicidal and self-injurious behaviours NEC	no data	111	701

Figure 20.1 Postmarketing psychiatric side effect profile of aripiprazole obtained from the FDA Adverse Event Reporting System (FAERS) accessed via PharmaPendium.

dyskinesia, and personality disorders. Figure 20.1 demonstrates the associated psychiatric ADR profile of aripiprazole.

20.2.1.2 **Cannabinoid CB1 Receptor (CNR1)**

CB1 and CB2 cannabinoid receptors have been described as two prime sites of action for endocannabinoids. Both the localization and pharmacology of these two GPCRs are well described, and numerous selective ligands have been characterized [20]. The physiological effects of *Cannabis sativa* (cannabis) and a thorough study of the endocannabinoid system have enabled several pathophysiological conditions to be determined, including obesity, dyslipidemia, addictions, inflammation, and allergies, in which blocking the cannabinoid receptors might be beneficial.

CB1 receptors are widely expressed in the brain, predominantly presynaptically. They are expressed to a lesser degree in the periphery, where they are found on cells of the immune system, vascular endothelium, liver, small intestine, reproductive organs, and peripheral presynaptic sites [21]. The activation of presynaptic CB1 receptors by synthetic agonists or low concentration of anandamide results in inhibition of transmitter release from nociceptive primary sensory neurons [22]. In general, cannabinoids participate in the control of neuronal hyperexcitability by inhibiting glutamatergic transmission in the brain [23]. The endocannabinoid system is associated with the control of emotional behavior and mood by functional coupling with the monoaminergic system [24].

Known agonists of the CB1 receptor include δ-9-tetrahydrocannabinol (THC, dronabinol, schedule II), which is the main psychoactive substance found in the cannabis plant, and a group of endocannabinoid neurotransmitters including anandamide [25]. Activation of the CB1 receptor is involved in alteration of cognition and memory, sleep disturbance, drowsiness, sedation, locomotor dysfunction, bronchodilation, cardiovascular regulation (hypotension and bradycardia), increased appetite, and mild to moderate antihyperalgesic effect. Euphoric mood and enhancement of sensory perception of THC and other cannabinoids are well documented but somewhat controversially interpreted [26,27]. Antagonists induce emesis, weight loss, depression, and increased suicidal tendencies [28].

Clinical Aspects

Rimonabant is the first selective blocker (an inverse agonist) of the cannabinoid CB1 receptors primarily for the treatment of obesity [29]. Therapy with rimonabant is also associated with favorable changes in serum lipids and in glycemic control in type 2 diabetes [30]. Rimonabant was well positioned with its novel mechanism of action to be useful in the treatment of obesity and metabolic syndrome [31]. It was generally well tolerated, with mild side effects such as nausea and diarrhea, but incidence of anxiety and depression became a major concern for regulatory authorities. At a dose of 20 mg per day, rimonabant increased the risk of psychiatric adverse events, although depression and anxiety were exclusion criteria in clinical trials [32]. Postmarketing observations identified increased risk of suicide during treatment with rimonabant (Figure 20.2), which resulted in withdrawal by the manufacturer due to a recommendation by EMA. Merck also discontinued the development of taranabant in phase III trials due to

⊟ **Psychiatric disorders**	179
⊞ **Anxiety disorders and symptoms**	34
⊞ **Changes in physical activity**	2
⊞ **Depressed mood disorders and disturbances**	48
⊞ **Disturbances in thinking and perception**	14
⊞ **Eating disorders and disturbances**	no data
⊞ **Mood disorders and disturbances NEC**	19
⊞ **Personality disorders and disturbances in behaviour**	17
⊞ **Psychiatric disorders NEC**	2
⊞ **Schizophrenia and other psychotic disorders**	2
⊞ **Sleep disorders and disturbances**	25
⊞ **Suicidal and self-injurious behaviours NEC**	15

Figure 20.2 FAERS data segment representing psychiatric disorders of rimonabant treatment prior to voluntary withdrawal from the market. A significant number of cases describing anxiety disorders, depression, and suicidal ideation or behavior were reported. Total number of FAERS reports is 457.

similar adverse drug reactions [33]. The clean off-target profile of rimonabant suggests that the inhibition of the intended therapeutic target, CB1, was responsible for suicidal behavior.

20.2.1.3 Serotonin (5-HT$_{1A}$) Receptor (HTR1A)

Serotonin (5-HT) produces its effects through a variety of membrane-bound receptors. Serotonin and its receptors are found both in the central and peripheral nervous system (CNS/PNS) and in a number of non-neuronal tissues including the GI tract, cardiovascular system, and blood cells. The serotonergic system has been implicated in many psychiatric disease states such as depression, anxiety, schizophrenia, and migraine. The 5-HT receptors, except for the 5-HT$_3$ subtype, a ligand-gated ion channel, belong to the GPCR superfamily. It represents one of the most complex families of neurotransmitter receptors and is divided, according to the NC-IUPHAR Committee, into seven distinct classes (5-HT$_1$ to 5-HT$_7$) with at least 14 different members [34,35].

The 5-HT$_{1A}$ receptors are coupled with G$_i$/G$_0$ subunits. The 5-HT$_{1A}$ receptor-mediated autoregulation of 5-HT neuronal activity is well known [36] and the involvement of 5-HT$_{1A}$ receptors in a number of physiological and behavioral effects has been established, including psychosis, anxiety, depression, sleep, locomotor activity, alcohol consumption, feeding behavior, water intake, drug addiction, cognition, pain perception, temperature regulation, and sexual activity [36,37].

Central activation of 5-HT$_{1A}$ receptors decreases arterial blood pressure in experimental hypertensive rat models via systemic vasodilation. Low doses of serotonin cause tachycardia, while high doses can induce hypotension in anaesthetized rats. Central activation of 5-HT$_{1A}$ receptors decreases arterial blood pressure in experimental hypertensive models via systemic vasodilation. Cardiovascular effects of serotonin and its receptors are discussed in a review by Villalón and Centurión [38].

The most frequent ADRs associated with 5-HT$_{1A}$ agonists are headache, lightheadedness, miosis, nervousness or agitation, nausea, and diarrhea. Most agonists may induce hypothermia, decrease blood pressure and heart rate (flesinoxan was initially developed as an antihypertensive agent [39]), or induce a behavioral syndrome characterized by flat body posture and head weaving in rats.

There are no clear side effects recorded with 5-HT$_{1A}$ receptor antagonists. However, there is accumulating evidence for increased incidence for suicidal behavior in patients with 5-HT$_{1A}$ hypoactivity [40]. 5-HT$_{1A}$ receptor gene expression dysregulation is implicated in the mechanisms of mental disorders. The human 5-HT$_{1A}$ gene transcription is modulated by a common C(−1019)G single nucleotide polymorphism in its promoter regulatory region. C(−1019)G polymorphism in the 5-HT$_{1A}$ receptor gene was associated with major depression and suicide. The homozygous G(−1019) allele was found about twofold more frequently in depressed patients and fourfold more frequently in suicide victims. The G(−1019) allele might depress 5-HT$_{1A}$ receptor expression and consequently reduces 5-HT neurotransmission that will result in depression and suicide [40]. While more observations support the involvement of 5-HT_{1A} receptors in suicidal behavior, there are still a reasonable number of conflicting publications [41,42]. It is intriguing that chronic treatment with selective serotonin reuptake inhibitors (SSRIs) reduces the number and signaling of 5-HT_{1A} autoreceptors, which enhances 5-HT release [43] and may correlate with the increased incidence of SSRI-associated suicidal behavior.

Clinical Aspects

The most frequent, mild to moderate ADRs of buspirone (5-HT_{1A} receptor partial agonist) are headaches, nervousness, agitation, lightheadedness, and nausea [44]. No suicidal behavior was reported in a randomized, double-blind, placebo-controlled trial [44]. Flesinoxan (7 and 14 μg/kg), another 5-HT_{1A} receptor agonist, administered intravenously in 11 healthy volunteers, elicited a dose-related decrease in body temperature and increases in growth hormone, adrenocorticotropic hormone (ACTH), cortisol, and prolactin plasma levels [45]. Clinical trials with flesinoxan also support the role of 5-HT_{1A} receptor in suicidal behavior [46].

Side effects of lecozotan, another 5-HT_{1A} antagonist, were mild or moderate, but did not include suicidal ideation [47]. These clinical data, although not conclusive in the absence of large well-controlled trials, suggest that 5-HT_1 receptor antagonists are safe in the management of psychiatric disorders and further data are required to establish a firm association of 5-HT_{1A} receptor inhibition, mimicking receptor hypoactivity, with suicidal behavior.

20.2.1.4 **5-HT_{2A} (HTR2A)**

The 5-HT_2 receptor subfamily consists of the 5-HT_{2A}, 5-HT_{2B}, and 5-HT_{2C} receptors. These three receptors exhibit considerable homology: 46–50% in their overall amino acid sequence and more than 70% within the transmembrane domains. They all couple to the G_q family of G-proteins and activate phospholipase C, leading to increases in intracellular levels of Ca^{2+} and phosphoinositol hydrolysis. 5-HT_2 receptors exhibit distinct expression profiles [48] with distribution in the cortex, basal ganglia, hippocampus, platelets, and vascular smooth muscle. They mediate contractile responses in various smooth muscle preparations, including vascular, bronchial, uterine, and urinary smooth muscle. Centrally, 5-HT_{2A} receptor activation stimulates hormone secretion, for example, ACTH, corticosterone, oxytocin, renin, and prolactin. It mediates certain behavioral syndromes *in vivo*: head twitching in mice and wet-dog shakes and back muscle contractions in rats.

The 5-HT_{2A} receptor mediates the effects of the "classical" hallucinogens such as LSD, psilocin, and mescaline, which act as full or partial agonists at this receptor [35]. Agonist effects at the 5-HT_{2A} receptor may be associated with suicidal ideation, based on genetic fingerprints obtained from suicide victims. Smooth muscle contraction (resulting in increased blood pressure), tachycardia, and a serotonin syndrome [49] were also observed. The serotonin syndrome is a drug-induced condition resulting from coadministration of SSRIs and monoamine oxidase inhibitors (MAOIs) that increase the level of intrasynaptic serotonin acting at the 5-HT_{2A} receptors. Depending on the degree to which intrasynaptic serotonin is elevated, symptoms can range from mild serotonin-induced side effects (agitation, tremor, hyperreflexia, mydriasis, fever, and tachycardia) to life-threatening toxicity [50]. There is a correlation between diminished 5-HT_{2A} receptor binding in platelets, tryptophan/amino acid ratio in plasma, and suicidal ideation, lethality of suicide attempts [51]. Shoval *et al.* [52] found strong association between LSD, (±)-3,4-methylenedioxymethamphetamine (MDMA), and suicidality in the high-risk population of adolescent psychotic inpatients.

5-HT_{2A} antagonism is one component explaining the antipsychotic activity of drugs such as clozapine and olanzapine. There is an effort to capitalize on the synergistic actions of 5-HT_{2A} antagonists (risperidone, olanzapine, and mianserin) and SSRIs in neuropsychiatric disorders [53]. Inhibition of the 5-HT_{2A} receptor may also cause hemorrhage [54] and decrease in blood pressure in hypertensive rats (effect of ketanserin).

Clinical Aspects

Clozapine, the first atypical antipsychotic, was introduced to the market in 1971. It blocks the D_2 and 5-HT_{2A} receptors, which makes it void of movement-related side effects. The primary indications for clozapine are treatment-resistant schizophrenia and patients with schizophrenia who are at high risk for suicide [55]. However, safety considerations such as idiosyncratic agranulocytosis are responsible for the restriction of wider use of clozapine. Recently, clozapine has been found in epidemiological studies to have the lowest mortality of any antipsychotic drug, which is considered mainly due to its effect to reduce the risk for suicide most probably due to inhibition of the 5-HT_{2A} receptor [56]. Preliminary reports indicate improvements in suicidality in schizophrenia patients treated with other atypical antipsychotics, for example, risperidone and olanzapine; however, these data remain anecdotal in comparison with the clinical reports of clozapine. The effect of clozapine is supported by findings that 5-HT_{2A} receptor expression is enhanced in the brain of teenage suicide victims [57].

Taken together, a hyperactive 5-HT_{2A} receptor population might be at least partly responsible for suicidal behavior; therefore, activating the receptor in this patient population might enhance the incidence of suicidal intent and behavior.

20.2.2 Transporters

20.2.2.1 Serotonin Transporter (SLC6A4)

The serotonin transporter (SERT, 5-HTT), an integral membrane protein that recycles serotonin in a sodium-dependent manner back into the presynaptic terminals from the synaptic space, belongs to the solute carrier 6 gene family, encoded by the SLC6A4 gene. 5-HTT is an important target of psychomotor stimulants, such as amphetamine, cocaine, and MDMA (ecstasy). A repeat length polymorphism in the promoter of the 5-HTT gene has been shown to affect the rate of serotonin uptake and may play a role in sudden infant death syndrome, aggressive behavior in Alzheimer's disease patients, post-traumatic stress disorder, and depression susceptibility in people experiencing emotional trauma. Serotonin transporter polymorphism has also been linked to vascular smooth muscle proliferation in patients with primary pulmonary hypertension [58].

Drugs that target this transporter protein can be divided into two basic classes: reuptake inhibitors and substrate-type releasers. SSRIs, which inhibit the 5-HTT, act by binding to the transporter and blocking the reuptake of serotonin, resulting in decreased intracellular concentrations. At the same time, however, the extracellular level of serotonin is increased, which is available to bind in excess to postsynaptic 5-HT receptors. The increased 5-HT receptor activation caused by increased levels of serotonin is thought to be the main mechanism by which the side effects of SSRIs are mediated [59]. Side effects of SSRIs include suicidal ideation in adolescents, insomnia, anxiety, nausea and vomiting, sexual dysfunction, GI cramps/diarrhea, headache, and primary pulmonary hypertension in newborns due to treatment during pregnancy.

Substrate-type releasers (e.g., fenfluramine [60]) not only bind to transporter proteins, but also are subsequently transported into the nerve terminals. They elevate intersynaptic concentration by promoting transmitter efflux via transporter-mediated exchange and increase cytoplasmic levels of 5-HT by disrupting storage in synaptic vesicles [61].

Clinical Aspects

SSRIs, which act through the serotonin transporter, are among the most frequently prescribed therapeutic agents for depression, obsessive–compulsive disorder, panic disorder, bulimia, and prevention of premature ejaculation. All SSRIs carry label warnings for suicidal ideation in teenagers: citalopram (Celexa, Cipramil, Emocal, and Sepram), escitalopram oxalate (Lexapro and Cipralex), fluoxetine (Prozac, Fontex, Seromex, Seronil, Sarafem, and Fluctin), fluvoxamine maleate (Luvox and Faverin), paroxetine (Paxil, Seroxat, Aropax, Deroxat, and Paroxat), and sertraline (Zoloft, Lustral, and Serlain). Based on a meta-analysis of clinical trials and postmarketing reports, Healy and Aldred [62] found that there is clear association between SSRIs and the rise to a relative risk of suicide over placebo. There is particular precaution with SSRIs in pediatric indications [63,64].

The precise mode of action of SSRIs in conjunction with suicidal ideation and behavior is not completely understood as all of the SSRIs affect other targets than 5-HTT, such as 5-HT, dopaminergic histamine and muscarinic receptors, and other transporters. However, 5-HTT, the common primary target for this class of drugs, defines suicide as a shared ADR. A comprehensive analysis on the role of the serotonergic system in suicidal behavior is available in a review [65].

20.2.2.2 Norepinephrine Transporter (SLC6A2)

The norepinephrine transporter (NET) is encoded by the solute carrier family 6 member 2 (SLC6A2) gene. NET is responsible for the sodium chloride (Na^+/Cl^-)-dependent reuptake of extracellular norepinephrine and dopamine. Many antidepressants and recreational drugs bind to NET or are a substrate of it.

NET blockade is primarily associated with cardiovascular side effects, and NET deficiency/inhibition is linked to tachycardia in familial orthostatic intolerance [66,67] and in normal subjects [68]. NET inhibition selectively reduces baroreflex control of sympathetic vasomotor tone and attenuates the responsiveness to sympathetic stimuli. The reduction in baroreflex buffering increases the sensitivity to vasoactive medications [69]. Concerning stimulation or upregulation of NET, no safety related clinical information exists. Antagonists may be useful for the treatment of ADHD (atomoxetine) and depression. There is clinical evidence that NET inhibition could be associated with suicidal ideation.

Clinical Relevance

Atomoxetine (Strattera), an ADHD medicine, carries a box warning for suicidal intent in adolescent population. It is also associated with onset of a motor tic [70] and hypertension [71]. Interestingly, methylphenidate does not increase the incidence of suicidal intent, which might be due to the different transmitter transporter profile of the two drugs (IC_{50} values for methylphenidate: 0.08 μM at DAT,0.8 μM at NET, and no effect at 5-HTT; IC_{50} values for atomoxetine: 4.4 μM at DAT, 0.01 μM at NET, and 0.02 μM at 5-HTT).

Sibutramine, a 5-HT reuptake inhibitor used for the indication of obesity, also causes hypertension as a common side effect [72,73]. It is no longer available in the United States because of increased risk of cardiovascular events such as heart attack and stroke. There is evidence for increased incidence of suicidal intent in adolescents associated with sibutramine treatment as well [74].

20.2.2.3 Vesicular Monoamine Transporter, VMAT2 (SLC18A2)

The vesicular monoamine transporter VMAT2 is a member of the solute carrier family and encoded by the SLC18A2 gene. It helps to maintain intravesicular concentrations of monoamines such as dopamine, serotonin, and epinephrine [75] and actively transports such molecules against a gradient from the cytoplasm of the presynaptic nerve terminal to storage vesicles for subsequent release into the synaptic cleft. A blocker of VMAT2 causes the intravesicular monoamine concentrations to fall. Thus, neurotransmitters not stored in the vesicle are unprotected from metabolism by enzymes such as monoamine oxidase.

Reduction of vesicular dopamine levels can lead to Parkinson's disease. A 95% partial VMAT2 knockout mouse (complete deletion is lethal) is used as an adequate animal model [76]. A recent positron emission tomography (PET) study demonstrated a significantly lower level of striatal VMAT2 in

Parkinson's patients and the PET ligand used is considered to be a good biomarker [77].

Cocaine, in addition to binding to DAT, NET, and 5-HTT, depletes the VMAT2 protein, which might damage striatal dopamine fibers. These neuronal changes could play a role in causing disordered mood and motivational processes in more severely dependent patients [78]. Human pancreatic beta cells are also highly enriched in VMAT2 transporters and the PET ligand used as a Parkinson's biomarker is also a good biomarker for beta cell mass [79].

Amphetamines (e.g., MDMA) are substrates of VMAT2. When amphetamines are taken up by VMAT2, the vesicle releases dopamine molecules into the cytosol in exchange. The redistributed dopamine can interact with DAT to promote reverse transport [80,81]. Chronic inhibition of VMAT2 may induce parkinsonism, tremor, suicidal ideation, depression, and hypoglycemia.

Clinical Aspects

Tetrabenazine (Xenazine) is a VMAT2 inhibitor that was approved in 2008 for the treatment of tardive dyskinesia, Huntington's disease, Tourette's disease, and extrapyramidal disorders. The compound carries a box label warning of the increased risk of depression and suicidal tendencies.

Reserpine is a pure crystalline alkaloid of *Rauwolfia serpentina* (Indian snakeroot), used as an antihypertensive. It acts by irreversibly blocking VMAT2. In most countries, it is no longer used as a single-ingredient preparation. The reserpine label also carries a warning for depression and suicide.

The appetite suppressant fenfluramine is a substrate for the vesicular monoamine transporter. By disrupting compartmentalization of serotonin into vesicles, fenfluramine increases the pool of cytoplasmic transmitter available for release [75]. This may contribute to the cardiac valvulopathy effects of this drug acting as an agonist of the 5-HT_{2B} receptor [82].

For more details on the mechanism of action of addictive drugs and their common effects, consult a recent review by Sulzer [83]. Figure 20.3 demonstrates the assembly of the various transmitter transporters in the synaptic junction.

20.2.3 Ion Channels

20.2.3.1 Neuronal Nicotinic α4β2 Channel (CHRNA4)

Neuronal nicotinic receptors (nAChRs) form a large, heterogeneous family of ligand-gated ion channels that are differently expressed in various regions of the CNS and the peripheral nervous system. All nAChRs are pentameric, thus composed of five membrane-spanning subunits arranged around a central pore that serves as the cation channel. These channels are comprised of homomeric or heteromeric combinations of 13 known different subunits [84–86]. The α-subunits (α2, α4, and α6) carry the principal component of the acetylcholine-binding site [86].

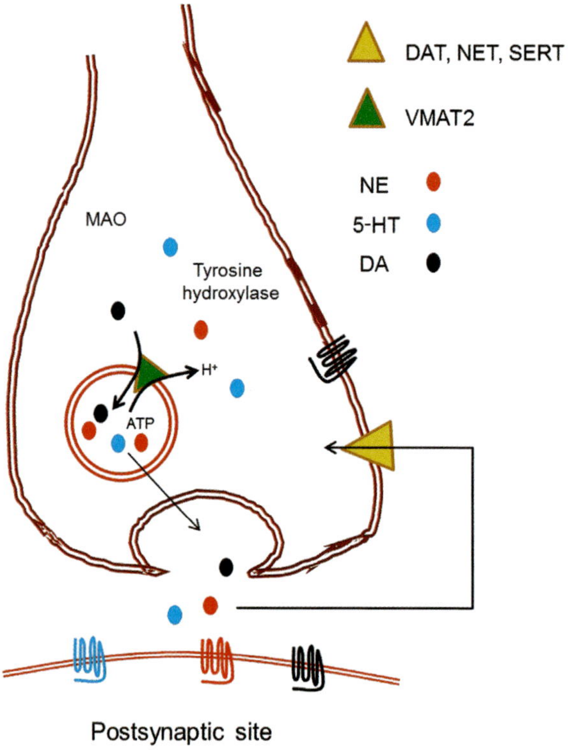

Figure 20.3 Schematic representation of the assembly of various transmitter transporters in the synaptic junction. DAT: dopamine transporter; NET: norepinephrine transporter; SERT: serotonin transporter; NE: norepinephrine; 5-HT: serotonin; DA: dopamine; MAO: monoamine oxidase.

By responding to the endogenous neurotransmitter acetylcholine, nAChRs contribute to a wide range of brain activities and influence a number of physiological functions. The perturbation of the cholinergic nicotinic neurotransmission leads to various diseases, including Alzheimer's disease, Parkinson' disease, anxiety disorders, ADHD, schizophrenia, and chronic pain conditions [87]. The predominant nAChRs in the human brain are $\alpha4\beta2$, a bungarotoxin-insensitive channel, followed by the $\alpha7$ pentamer, which, on the other hand, is bungarotoxin sensitive.

Agonists/activators of nicotinic acetylcholine receptors may play a role in the modulation of a number of neurotransmitters (e.g., dopaminergic, serotonergic, and glutamatergic) with effects on cognitive and motor functions. They exhibit analgesic activity (epibatidine) and may stimulate autonomic cardiovascular, respiratory, and gastrointestinal functions (palpitation/nausea). Nicotinic receptor agonists may increase depression, aggressiveness, hostility, and suicidal ideation. A number of neurotoxins (e.g., bungarotoxin and conotoxins) also display antagonist action on different nicotinic acetylcholine receptor subtypes [88].

The development of nicotinic agents for the enhancement of alertness, reduction of anxiety, muscle relaxation, and analgesia has been hampered by serious central and peripheral side effects, fast desensitization, and the abuse potential of nicotine. Only recent generations of selective agonists or positive modulators can be considered for broader clinical use [87,89]. In Alzheimer's disease and dementia with Lewy bodies, cortical loss of epibatidine binding was associated with reductions in both α and β subunits. In Parkinson's disease, striatal deficits in $\alpha6$ and $\beta3$ subunits tend to be greater than those for $\alpha4$ and $\beta2$ [90].

Clinical Aspects

There are two major groups of medications intended for smoking cessation: partial agonists and antagonists of the nicotinic $\alpha4\beta2$ receptors. Varenicline (Chantix), a nicotinic $\alpha4\beta2$ partial agonist, causes dopamine release, leading to the pleasurable effects of smoking. As an nAChR partial agonist, varenicline attenuates the craving and withdrawal symptoms that occur with abstinence from nicotine and reduces the rewarding effects of nicotine obtained from smoking in patients who lapse. Clinical studies suggest that varenicline is unlikely to induce a potential for abuse [91]; however, clinical evidence of suicidal tendencies emerged and other psychiatric adverse reactions such as depression, hostility, and aggression were reported [92], leading to a boxed warning by the FDA [93].

Antagonists offer an alternative approach in smoking cessation by blocking the nAChR subtypes that mediate neurotransmitter release associated with the reward of tobacco use. $\alpha4\beta2$ subtype-selective antagonists inhibit mesolimbic dopamine release and norepinephrine release induced by nicotine. This approach is more likely to prevent relapses [94]. Bupropion, an antidepressant (DAT and NET inhibitor) with an inhibitory effect at the nicotinic $\alpha4\beta2$ and $\alpha3\beta2$ (ganglionic) subtypes, has been successfully introduced for smoking cessation. However, the FDA issued warnings on increased incidence of suicidal behavior in the same communication for both varenicline and bupropion (Zyban). Thus, agonists, partial agonists, and antagonists of the nAChR subtypes are not devoid of suicidal adverse reactions. A review on drugs intended for smoking cessation is available [95].

20.2.3.2 Neural-Type Voltage-Gated Calcium Channel, $Ca_v2.2$ (CACNA1B)

Voltage-gated calcium channels are broadly distributed, found in excitable cells such as cardiomyocytes and neurons. They selectively permeate calcium ions, with a closed state at resting membrane potential. When the membrane potential is depolarized, voltage-gated calcium channels open and allow calcium ions to enter into the cell. The increased intracellular calcium concentration depending on the cell type triggers muscular contraction in muscle cells or secretion of transmitters or hormones in neurons and endocrine cells. There are several kinds of voltage-gated calcium channels with diverse electrophysiological characteristics [96].

N-type ("N" for neural) calcium channels ($Ca_v2.2$) are found primarily at presynaptic terminals and are involved in neurotransmitter release [97].

Depolarization by an action potential causes these channels to open and allow influx of Ca^{2+}, initiating vesicle fusion and neurotransmitter release. The CACNA1B gene encodes the pore-forming subunit of the N-type calcium channel that forms a complex with α2, β, and δ subunits to form the high-voltage activated channel. The channel is sensitive to both Ω-conotoxin-GVIA and Ω-agatoxin-IIIA, but insensitive to dihydropyridines [98].

Inhibitors of the N-type calcium channel may be an anticonvulsant, analgesic [99] and may cause somnolence, ataxia, weakness, and suicidal ideation.

Clinical Aspects

Ziconotide (Prialt) is a strong analgesic devoid of opioid, NSAID, or conventional local anesthetic effects. It is used for the amelioration of severe chronic pain by intrathecal infusion [100]. Derived from the cone snail *Conus magus*, it is the synthetic form of the cone snail peptide ω-conotoxin M-VII-A, an N-type calcium channel blocker [101]. The most common side effects of ziconotide are dizziness, nausea, confusion, and headache. Other side effects may include weakness, hypertonia, ataxia, abnormal vision, anorexia, somnolence, unsteadiness on feet, and memory problems. The most severe, but rare side effects are hallucinations, suicidal ideation, new or worsening depression, seizures, and meningitis. Prialt carries a label for severe side effects and contraindications: "Prialt is contraindicated in patients with a preexisting history of psychosis. Severe psychiatric symptoms and neurological impairment may occur during treatment with Prialt. Monitor all patients frequently for evidence of cognitive impairment, hallucinations, or changes in mood or consciousness." Cases with suicidal intent and behavior have been reported [102]. Based on increased alertness for suicidal behavior, all N-type Ca channel blockers are required to undergo prospective suicidality assessment by the FDA.

The analgesic and antiepileptic drug gabapentin has been shown to bind to and block the trafficking of the α2/δ1 (CACNA2D1) and α2/δ2 (CACNA2D2) subunits of $Ca_v2.1$ and $Ca_v2.2$ channels [103]. It blocks calcium currents only after chronic administration [104]. Gabapentin carries a warning for suicidal behavior and ideation. Pregabalin (Lyrica) has a similar mechanism of action and carries the same warning. Although FDA recommends prospective suicidality for all antiepileptics, there are significant differences between their relation with suicidal intent and behavior. While incidence of suicidal ideation and behavior is significantly higher in epileptic patients, other antiepileptic drugs such as carbamazepine, oxcarbazepine, valproate, and lamotrigine with different mode of action rather decrease the incidence of suicide in this patient population [105].

20.3 Conclusions

This chapter aimed at providing a comprehensive summary of known central nervous system targets associated with suicidal behavior with the understanding that the strength of clinical evidence may vary and literature often provides conflicting information on these targets. It is also important to consider that a majority of antipsychotic drugs are highly promiscuous with variable clinical phenotypes. The association of these targets with suicidal behavior is further complicated by psychiatric patients often having increased incidence of suicidal behavior with significant baseline variations. Nevertheless, our approach was to provide an overview of the present knowledge about targets involved in suicidality and support drug discovery projects with relevant information for assessing and mitigating this important drug-related side effect whenever possible.

References

1 Center for Drug Evaluation and Research (CDER) (2010) FDA Draft Guidance for Industry. Suicidality: Prospective Assessment of Occurrence in Clinical Trials. CDER, FDA.

2 Center for Drug Evaluation and Research (CDER) (2012) FDA Draft Guidance for Industry. Suicidal Ideation and Behavior: Prospective Assessment of Occurrence in Clinical Trials. Revision 1, CDER, FDA.

3 Malkesman, O., Pine, D.S., Tragon, T., and Austin, D.R. (2009) Animal models of suicide-trait-related behaviors. *Trends in Pharmacological Sciences*, **30**, 165–173.

4 Bowes, J., Brown, A.J., Hamon, J. *et al.* (2012) Reducing safety-related drug attrition: the use of *in vitro* pharmacological profiling. *Nature Reviews. Drug Discovery*, **11**, 909–922.

5 Halvorsen, J.A., Stern, R.S., Dalgard, F. *et al.* (2011) Suicidal ideation, mental health problems, and social impairment are increased in adolescents with acne: a population-based study. *The Journal of Investigative Dermatology*, **131**, 363–370.

6 Beaulieu, J.M. and Gainetdinov, R.R. (2011) The physiology, signaling, and pharmacology of dopamine receptors. *Pharmacological Reviews*, **63**, 182–217.

7 Emilien, G., Maloteaux, J.-M., Geurts, M. *et al.* (1999) Dopamine receptors–physiological understanding to therapeutic intervention potential. *Pharmacology & Therapeutics*, **84**, 133–156.

8 Usiello, A., Baik, J.-H., Rougé-Pont, F., Picetti, R., Dierich, A., LeMeur, M., Pier Piazza, V., and Borrelli, E. (2000) Distinct functions of the two isoforms of dopamine D_2 receptors. *Nature*, **408**, 199–203.

9 Peacock, L. and Gerlach, J. (2001) Aberrant behavioral effects of a dopamine D_1 receptor antagonist and agonist in monkeys: evidence of uncharted dopamine D_1 receptor actions. *Biological Psychiatry*, **50**, 501–509.

10 Rascol, O., Nutt, J.G., Blin, O., Goetz, C.G., Trugman, J.M., Soubrouillard, C., Carter, J.H., Currie, L.J., Fabre, N., Thalamas, C., Giardina, W.W., and Wright, S. (2001) Induction by dopamine D1 receptor agonist ABT-431 of dyskinesia similar to levodopa in patients with Parkinson disease. *Archives of Neurology*, **58**, 249–254.

11 Astrup, A., Greenway, F.L., Ling, W., Pedicone, L., Lachowicz, J., Strader, C.D., and Kwan, R. (2007) Randomized controlled trials of the D_1/D_5 antagonist ecopipam for weight loss in obese subjects. *Obesity*, **15**, 1717–1731.

12 Kolla, B.P., Mansukhani, M.P., Barraza, R., and Bostwick, J.M. (2010) Impact of dopamine agonists on compulsive behaviors: a case series of pramipexole-induced pathological gambling. *Psychosomatics*, **51**, 271–273.

13 Fakra, E. and Azorin, J.M. (2012) Clozapine for the treatment of schizophrenia. *Expert Opinion on Pharmacotherapy*, **13**, 1923–1935.

14 Spivak, B., Shabash, E., Sheitman, B., Weizman, A., and Mester, R. (2003) The effects of clozapine versus haloperidol on

measures of impulsive aggression and suicidality in chronic schizophrenia patients: an open, nonrandomized, 6-month study. *Journal of Clinical Psychiatry*, **64**, 755–760.
15 Suda, A., Kawanishi, C., Kishida, I., Sato, R., Yamada, T., Nakagawa, M., Hasegawa, H., Kato, D., Furuno, T., and Hirayasu, Y. (2009) Dopamine D_2 receptor gene polymorphisms are associated with suicide attempt in the Japanese population. *Neuropsychobiology*, **59**, 130–134.
16 Allard, P. and Norlén, M. (2001) Caudate nucleus dopamine D_2 receptors in depressed suicide victims. *Neuropsychobiology*, **44**, 70–73.
17 Bowden, C., Theodorou, A.E., Cheetham, S.C., Lowther, S., Katona, C.L., Crompton, M.R., and Horton, R.W. (1997) Dopamine D_1 and D_2 receptor binding sites in brain samples from depressed suicides and controls. *Brain Research*, **752**, 227–233.
18 Persson, M.L., Geijer, T., Wasserman, D., Rockah, R., Frisch, A., Michaelovsky, E., Jönsson, E.G., Apter, A., and Weizman, A. (1999) Lack of association between suicide attempt and a polymorphism at the dopamine receptor D_4 locus. *Psychiatric Genetics*, **9**, 97–100.
19 Bennett, R.R. (2011) The prefrontal–limbic network in depression: modulation by hypothalamus, basal ganglia and midbrain. *Progress in Neurobiology*, **93**, 468–487.
20 Pacher, P., Bátkai, S., and Kunos, G. (2006) The endocannabinoid system as an emerging target of pharmacotherapy. *Pharmacological Reviews*, **58**, 389–462.
21 Croxford, J.L. (2003) Therapeutic potential of cannabinoids in CNS disease. *CNS Drugs*, **17**, 179–202.
22 Morisset, V., Ahluwalia, J., Nagy, I., and Urban, L. (2001) Possible mechanisms of cannabinoid-induced antinociception in the spinal cord. *European Journal of Pharmacology*, **429**, 93–100.
23 Shen, M., Piser, T.M., Seybold, V.S., and Thayer, S.A. (1996) Cannabinoid receptor agonists inhibit glutamatergic transmission in rat hippocampal cultures. *Journal of Neuroscience*, **16**, 4322–4334.
24 Esteban, S. and García-Sevilla, J.A. (2012) Effects induced by cannabinoids on monoaminergic systems in the brain and their implications for psychiatric disorders. *Progress in Neuro-Psychopharmacology and Biological Psychiatry*, **38**, 78–87.
25 McPartland, J.M., Glass, M., and Pertwee, R.G. (2007) Meta-analysis of cannabinoid ligand binding affinity and receptor distribution: interspecies differences. *British Journal of Pharmacology*, **152**, 583–593.
26 Ameri, A. (1999) The effects of cannabinoids on the brain. *Progress in Neurobiology*, **58**, 315–348.
27 Robson, P. (2011) Abuse potential and psychoactive effects of δ-9-tetrahydrocannabinol and cannabidiol oromucosal spray (Sativex), a new cannabinoid medicine. *Expert Opinion on Drug Safety*, **10**, 675–685.
28 Nathan, P.J., O'Neill, B.V., Napolitano, A., and Bullmore, E.T. (2011) Neuropsychiatric adverse effects of centrally acting antiobesity drugs. *CNS Neuroscience & Therapeutics*, **17**, 490–505.
29 Boyd, S.T. and Fremming, B.A. (2005) Rimonabant – a selective CB1 antagonist. *Annals of Pharmacotherapy*, **39**, 684–690.
30 Lafontan, M., Piazza, P.V., and Girard, J. (2007) Effects of CB1 antagonist on the control of metabolic functions in obese type 2 diabetic patients. *Diabetes and Metabolism*, **33**, 85–95.
31 Gelfand, E.V. and Cannon, C.P. (2006) Rimonabant: a selective blocker of the cannabinoid CB1 receptors for the management of obesity, smoking cessation and cardiometabolic risk factors. *Expert Opinion on Investigational Drugs*, **15**, 307–315.
32 Christensen, R., Kristensen, P.K., Bartels, E.M., Bliddal, H., and Astrup, A. (2007) Efficacy and safety of the weight-loss drug rimonabant: a meta-analysis of randomised trials. *The Lancet*, **370**, 1706–1713.
33 Trainor, K. (2007) Panel advises against rimonabant approval. *American Journal*

of Health-System Pharmacy, **15**, 1460–1461.

34 Barnes, N.M. and Sharp, T. (1999) A review of central 5-HT receptors and their function. *Neuropharmacology*, **38**, 1083–1152.

35 Hoyer, D., Hannona, J.P., and Martin, G.R. (2002) Molecular, pharmacological and functional diversity of 5-HT receptors. *Pharmacology Biochemistry and Behavior*, **71**, 533–554.

36 Popova, N.K. and Naumenko, V.S. (2013) 5-HT_{1A} receptor as a key player in the brain 5-HT system. *Reviews in the Neurosciences*, **24**, 191–204.

37 Lacivita, E., Leopoldo, M., Berardi, F., and Perrone, R. (2008) 5-HT_{1A} receptor, an old target for new therapeutic agents. *Current Topics in Medicinal Chemistry*, **8**, 1024–1034.

38 Villalón, C. and Centurión, D. (2007) Cardiovascular responses produced by 5-hydroxytriptamine: a pharmacological update on the receptors/mechanisms involved and therapeutic implications. *Naunyn-Schmiedeberg's Archives of Pharmacology*, **376**, 45–63.

39 van Zwieten, P.A., Blauw, G.J., and van Brummelen, P. (1992) Serotonergic receptors and drugs in hypertension. *Pharmacology & Toxicology*, **70**, S17–S22.

40 Lemonde, S., Turecki, G., Bakish, D., Du, L., Hrdina, P.D., Bown, C.D., Sequeira, A., Kushwaha, N., Morris, S.J., Basak, A. *et al.* (2003) Impaired repression at a 5-HT_{1A} receptor gene polymorphism associated with major depression and suicide. *Journal of Neuroscience*, **23**, 8788–8799.

41 Underwood, M.D., Kassir, S.A., Bakalian, M.J., Galfalvy, H., Mann, J.J., and Arango, V. (2012) Neuron density and serotonin receptor binding in prefrontal cortex in suicide. *International Journal of Neuropsychopharmacology*, **15**, 435–447.

42 Angles, M.R., Ocaña, D.B., Medellín, B.C., and Tovilla-Zárate, C. (2012) No association between the HTR1A gene and suicidal behavior: a meta-analysis. *Revista Brasileira de Psiquiatrica*, **34**, 38–42.

43 Albert, P.R. and Lemonde, S. (2004) 5-HT_{1A} receptors, gene repression, and depression: guilt by association. *Neuroscientist*, **10**, 575–593.

44 Ghaleiha, A., Noorbala, A.A., Farnaghi, F., Hajiazim, M., and Akhondzadeh, S. (2010) A double-blind, randomized, and placebo-controlled trial of buspirone added to risperidone in patients with chronic schizophrenia. *Journal of Clinical Psychopharmacology*, **30**, 678–682.

45 Seletti, B., Benkelfat, C., Blier, P. *et al.* (1995) Serotonin 1A receptor activation by flesinoxan in humans. Body temperature and neuroendocrine responses. *Neuropsychopharmacology*, **13**, 93–104.

46 Hansenne, M., Pitchot, W., Pinto, E., Reggers, J., Scantamburlo, G., Fuchs, S., Pirard, S., and Ansseau, M. (2002) 5-HT_{1A} dysfunction in borderline personality disorder. *Psychological Medicine*, **32**, 935–941.

47 Patat, A., Parks, V., Raje, S., Plotka, A., Chassard, D., and Le Coz, F. (2009) Safety, tolerability, pharmacokinetics and pharmacodynamics of ascending single and multiple doses of lecozotan in healthy young and elderly subjects. *British Journal of Clinical Pharmacology*, **67**, 299–308.

48 Landolt, H.P. and Wehrle, R. (2009) Antagonism of serotonergic 5-$HT_{2A/2C}$ receptors: mutual improvement of sleep, cognition and mood? *European Journal of Neuroscience*, **29**, 1795–1809.

49 González-Maeso, J., Ang, R.L., Yuen, T. *et al.* (2008) Identification of a serotonin/glutamate receptor complex implicated in psychosis. *Nature*, **452**, 93–97.

50 Sun-Edelstein, C., Tepper, S.J., and Shapiro, R.E. (2008) Drug-induced serotonin syndrome: a review. *Expert Opinion on Drug Safety*, **7**, 587–596.

51 Lauterbach, E., Brunner, J., Hawellek, B., Lewitzka, U., Ising, M., Bondy, B., Rao, M.L., Frahnert, C., Rujescu, D., Müller-Oerlinghausen, B., Schley, J., Heuser, I., Maier, W., Hohagen, F., Felber, W., and Bronisch, T. (2006) Platelet 5-HT_{2A} receptor binding and tryptophan availability in depression are not associated with recent history of suicide attempts but with personality traits

characteristic for suicidal behavior. *Journal of Affective Disorders*, **91**, 57–62.
52 Shoval, G., Sever, J., Sher, L., Diller, R., Apter, A., Weizman, A., and Zalsman, G. (2006) Substance use, suicidality, and adolescent-onset schizophrenia: an Israeli 10-year retrospective study. *Journal of Child and Adolescent Psychopharmacology*, **16**, 767–775.
53 Marek, G.J., Carpenter, L.L., McDougle, C.J., and Price, L.H. (2003) Synergistic action of 5-HT_{2A} antagonists and selective serotonin reuptake inhibitors in neuropsychiatric disorders. *Neuropsychopharmacology*, **28**, 402–412.
54 Adams, J.W., Ramirez, J., Ortuno, D., Shi, Y., Thomsen, W., Richman, J.G., Morgan, M., Dosa, P., Teegarden, B.R., Al-Shamma, H., Behan, D.P., and Connolly, D.T. (2008) Anti-thrombotic and vascular effects of AR246686, a novel 5-HT_{2A} receptor antagonist. *European Journal of Pharmacology*, **586**, 234–243.
55 Kerwin, R.W. and Bolonna, A.A. (2004) Is clozapine antisuicidal? *Expert Review of Neurotherapeutics*, **4**, 187–190.
56 Meltzer, H.Y. (2012) Clozapine: balancing safety with superior antipsychotic efficacy. *Clinical Schizophrenia & Related Psychoses*, **6**, 134–144.
57 Pandey, G.N., Dwivedi, Y., Rizavi, H.S., Ren, X., Pandey, S.C., Pesold, C., Roberts, R.C., Conley, R.R., and Tamminga, C.A. (2002) Higher expression of serotonin 5-HT_{2A} receptors in the postmortem brains of teenage suicide victims. *American Journal of Psychiatry*, **159**, 419–429.
58 Rabinovitch, M. (2001) Linking a serotonin transporter polymorphism to vascular smooth muscle proliferation in patients with primary pulmonary hypertension. *Journal of Clinical Investigation*, **108**, 1109–1111.
59 Stahl, S.M. (1998) Mechanism of action of serotonin selective reuptake inhibitors: serotonin receptors and pathways mediate therapeutic effects and side effects. *Journal of Affective Disorders*, **51**, 215–235.
60 Rothman, R.B. and Baumann, M.H. (2002) Therapeutic and adverse actions of serotonin transporter substrates. *Pharmacology & Therapeutics*, **95**, 73–88.
61 Rudnick, G. (1997) Mechanisms of biogenic amine transporters, in *Neurotransmitter Transporters: Structure, Function and Regulation* (ed. M.E.A. Reith), Humana Press, Ottawa, pp. 73–100.
62 Healy, D. and Aldred, G. (2005) Antidepressant drug use and the risk of suicide. *International Review of Psychiatry*, **17**, 163–172.
63 Adegbite-Adeniyi, C., Gron, B., Rowles, B.M., Demeter, C.A., and Findling, R.L. (2012) An update on antidepressant use and suicidality in pediatric depression. *Expert Opinion on Pharmacotherapy*, **13**, 2119–2130.
64 Cooper, W.O., Callahan, S.T., Shintani, A., Fuchs, D.C., Shelton, R.C., Dudley, J.A., Graves, A.J., and Ray, W.A. (2014) Antidepressants and suicide attempts in children. *Pediatrics*, **133**, 204–210.
65 Sadkowski, M., Dennis, B., Clayden, R.C., Elsheikh, W., Rangarajan, S., Dejesus, J., and Samaan, Z. (2013) The role of the serotonergic system in suicidal behavior. *Neuropsychiatric Disease and Treatment*, **9**, 1699–1716.
66 Keller, N.R., Diedrich, A., Appalsamy, M., Tuntrakool, S., Lonce, S., Finney, C., Caron, M.G., and Robertson, D. (2004) Norepinephrine transporter-deficient mice exhibit excessive tachycardia and elevated blood pressure with wakefulness and activity. *Circulation*, **110**, 1191–1196.
67 Mayer, A.F., Schroeder, C., Heusser, K., Tank, J., Diedrich, A., Schmieder, R.E., Luft, F.C., and Jordan, J. (2006) Influences of norepinephrine transporter function on the distribution of sympathetic activity in humans. *Hypertension*, **48**, 120–126.
68 Strempel, S., Schroeder, C., Hemmersbach, R., Boese, A., Tank, J., Diedrich, A., Heer, M., Luft, F.C., and Jordan, J. (2008) Norepinephrine transporter inhibition alters the hemodynamic response to hypergravitation. *Journal of Applied Physiology*, **104**, 756–760.
69 Tank, J., Schroeder, C., Diedrich, A., Szczech, E., Haertter, S., Sharma, A.M., Luft, F.C., and Jordan, J. (2003) Selective impairment in sympathetic vasomotor control with norepinephrine transporter inhibition. *Circulation*, **107**, 2949–2954.

70 Ledbetter, M. (2005) Atomoxetine use associated with onset of a motor tic. *Journal of Child and Adolescent Psychopharmacology*, **15**, 331–333.

71 Shibao, C., Raj, S.R., Gamboa, A., Diedrich, A., Choi, L., Black, B.K., Robertson, D., and Biaggioni, I. (2007) Norepinephrine transporter blockade with atomoxetine induces hypertension in patients with impaired autonomic function. *Hypertension*, **50**, 47–53.

72 Sramek, J.J., Leibowitz, M.T., Weinstein, S.P., Rowe, E.D., Mendel, C.M., Levy, B., McMahon, F.G., Mullican, W.S., Toth, P.D., and Cutler, N.R. (2002) Efficacy and safety of sibutramine for weight loss in obese patients with hypertension well controlled by beta-adrenergic blocking agents: a placebo-controlled, double-blind, randomised trial. *Journal of Human Hypertension*, **16**, 13–19.

73 Scholze, J., Grimm, E., Herrmann, D., Unger, T., and Kintscher, U. (2007) Optimal treatment of obesity-related hypertension – the hypertension–obesity–sibutramine (HOS) study. *Circulation*, **115**, 1991–1998.

74 Rihmer, Z., Pureb, G., Faludi, G., and Halmy, L. (2008) Association of obesity and depression. *Neuropsychopharmacologia Hungarica*, **10**, 183–189.

75 Partilla, J.S., Dempsey, A.G., Nagpal, A.S., Blough, B.E., Baumann, M.H., and Rothman, R.B. (2006) Interaction of amphetamines and related compounds at the vesicular monoamine transporter. *The Journal of Pharmacology and Experimental Therapeutics*, **319**, 237–246.

76 Colebrooke, R.E., Humby, T., Lynch, P.J., McGowan, D.P., Xia, J., and Emson, P.C. (2006) Age-related decline in striatal dopamine content and motor performance occurs in the absence of nigral cell loss in a genetic mouse model of Parkinson's disease. *European Journal of Neuroscience*, **24**, 2622–2630.

77 Bohnen, N.I., Albin, R.L., Koeppe, R.A., Wernette, K.A., Kilbourn, M.R., Minoshima, S., and Frey, K.A. (2006) Positron emission tomography of monoaminergic vesicular binding in aging and Parkinson disease. *Journal of Cerebral Blood Flow and Metabolism*, **26**, 1198–1212.

78 Little, K.Y., Krolewski, D.M., Zhang, L., and Cassin, B.J. (2003) Loss of striatal vesicular monoamine transporter protein (VMAT2) in human cocaine users. *American Journal of Psychiatry*, **160**, 47–55.

79 Freeby, F., Goland, R., Ichise, M., Maffei, A., Leibel, R., and Harris, P. (2008) VMAT2 quantitation by PET as a biomarker for β-cell mass in health and disease. *Diabetes, Obesity and Metabolism*, **10**, 98–108.

80 Sulzer, D., Chen, T.K., Lau, Y.Y., Kristensen, H., Rayport, S., and Ewing, A. (1995) Amphetamine redistributes dopamine from synaptic vesicles to the cytosol and promotes reverse transport. *Journal of Neuroscience*, **15**, 4102–4108.

81 Riddle, E.L., Fleckenstein, A.E., and Hanson, G.R. (2006) Mechanisms of methamphetamine-induced dopaminergic neurotoxicity. *AAPS Journal*, **8**, E413–E418.

82 Rothman, R.B. and Baumann, M.H. (2002) Therapeutic and adverse actions of serotonin transporter substrates. *Pharmacology & Therapeutics*, **95**, 73–88.

83 Sulzer, D. (2011) How addictive drugs disrupt presynaptic dopamine neurotransmission. *Neuron*, **69**, 628–649.

84 Kormelink, P.J.G. and Luyten, W.H.M.L. (1997) Cloning and sequence of full-length cDNAs encoding the human neuronal nicotinic acetylcholine receptor (nAChR) subunits β3 and β4 and expression of seven nAChR subunits in the human neuroblastoma cell line SH-SY5Y and/or IMR-32. *FEBS Letters*, **400**, 309–314.

85 Paterson, D. and Nordberg, A. (2000) Neuronal nicotinic receptors in the human brain. *Progress in Neurobiology*, **61**, 75–111.

86 Greenbaum, L. and Lerer, B. (2009) Differential contribution of genetic variation in multiple brain nicotinic cholinergic receptors to nicotine dependence: recent progress and emerging open questions. *Molecular Psychiatry*, **14**, 912–945.

87 Arneric, S.P., Holladay, M., and Williams, M. (2007) Neuronal nicotinic receptors: a perspective on two decades of drug

discovery research. *Biochemical Pharmacology*, **74**, 1092–1101.

88 Tsetlin, V., Utkin, Y., and Kasheverov, I. (2009) Polypeptide and peptide toxins, magnifying lenses for binding sites in nicotinic acetylcholine receptors. *Biochemical Pharmacology*, **78**, 720–731.

89 Buccafusco, J.J. (2004) Neuronal nicotinic receptor subtypes: defining therapeutic targets. *Molecular Interventions*, **4**, 285–295.

90 Gotti, C., Moretti, M., Bohr, I. *et al.* (2006) Selective nicotinic acetylcholine receptor subunit deficits identified in Alzheimer's disease, Parkinson's disease and dementia with Lewy bodies by immunoprecipitation. *Neurobiology of Disease*, **23**, 481–489.

91 McColl, S.L., Burstein, A.H., Reeves, K.R. *et al.* (2008) Human abuse liability of the smoking cessation drug varenicline in smokers and nonsmokers. *Clinical Pharmacology and Therapeutics*, **83**, 607–614.

92 Ohmura, Y., Tsutsui-Kimura, I., and Yoshioka, M. (2012) Impulsive behavior and nicotinic acetylcholine receptors. *Journal of Pharmacological Sciences*, **118**, 413–422.

93 Anonymous (2009) The Smoking Cessation Aids Varenicline (Marketed as Chantix) and Bupropion (Marketed as Zyban and Generics): Suicidal Ideation and Behavior. *FDA Postmarket Reviews*, vol. 2, no. 1. Available at http://www.fda.gov/Drugs/DrugSafety/DrugSafetyNewsletter/ucm110235.htm (accessed September 15, 2014).

94 Dwoskin, L.P., Rauhut, A.S., King-Pospisil, K.A., and Bardo, M.T. (2006) Review of the pharmacology and clinical profile of bupropion, an antidepressant and tobacco use cessation agent. *CNS Drug Reviews*, **12**, 178–207.

95 Dwoskin, L.P., Smith, A.M., Wooters, T.E., Zhang, Z., Crooks, P.A., and Bardo, M.T. (2009) Nicotinic receptor-based therapeutics and candidates for smoking cessation. *Biochemical Pharmacology*, **78**, 732–743.

96 Kaczorowski, G.J. and Garcia, M.L. (1999) Pharmacology of voltage-gated and calcium-activated potassium channels. *Current Opinion in Chemical Biology*, **3**, 448–458.

97 Reid, C.A., Bekkers, J.M., and Clements, J.D. (2003) Presynaptic Ca^{2+} channels: a functional patchwork. *Trends in Neurosciences*, **26**, 683–687.

98 Williams, M.E., Brust, P.F., Feldman, D.H., Patthi, S., Simerson, S., Maroufi, A., McCue, A.F., Veliçelebi, G., Ellis, S.B., and Harpold, M.M. (1992) Structure and functional expression of an omega-conotoxin-sensitive human N-type calcium channel. *Science*, **257**, 389–395.

99 Schroeder, C.I., Doering, C.J., Zamponi, G.W., and Lewis, R.J. (2006) N-type calcium channel blockers: novel therapeutics for the treatment of pain. *Medicinal Chemistry*, **2**, 535–543.

100 Miljanich, G.P. (2004) Ziconotide: neuronal calcium channel blocker for treating severe chronic pain. *Current Medicinal Chemistry*, **11**, 3029–3040.

101 Dubel, S.J., Starr, T.V., Hell, J., Ahlijanian, M.K., Enyeart, J.J., Catterall, W.A., and Snutch, T.P. (1992) Molecular cloning of the alpha-1 subunit of an omega-conotoxin-sensitive calcium channel. *Proceedings of the National Academy of Sciences of the United States of America*, **89**, 5058–5062.

102 Maier, C., Gockel, H.H., Gruhn, K., Krumova, E.K., and Edel, M.A. (2011) Increased risk of suicide under intrathecal ziconotide treatment? A warning. *Pain*, **152**, 235–237.

103 Taylor, C.P. (2009) Mechanisms of analgesia by gabapentin and pregabalin – calcium channel alpha2-delta [$Ca_v\alpha2$-δ] ligands. *Pain*, **142**, 13–16.

104 Hendrich, J., Tran Van Minh, A., Heblich, F., Nieto-Rostro, M., Watschinger, K., Striessnig, J., Wratten, J., Davies, A., and Dolphin, A.C. (2008) Pharmacological disruption of calcium channel trafficking by the $\alpha2\delta$ ligand gabapentin. *Proceedings of the National Academy of Sciences of the United States of America*, **105**, 3628–3633.

105 Kalinin, V.V. (2007) Suicidality and antiepileptic drugs: is there a link? *Drug Safety*, **30**, 123–142.

Index

Antitargets and Drug Safety, First Edition. Edited by László Urbán, Vinod F. Patel, and Roy J. Vaz.

e

f

g

i